Atlas of Artifacts in Clinical Neurophysiology

Atlas of Artifacts in Clinical Neurophysiology

Editor

William O. Tatum, IV, DO
Professor of Neurology
Mayo Clinic College of Medicine
Director, Comprehensive Epilepsy Center
Mayo Clinic
Jacksonville, Florida

demosMEDICAL
An Imprint of Springer Publishing

Visit our website at www.springerpub.com

ISBN: 9780826169341
ebook ISBN: 9780826169358

Acquisitions Editor: Beth Barry
Compositor: diacriTech, Chennai

Medicine is an ever-changing science. Research and clinical experience are continually expanding our knowledge, in particular our understanding of proper treatment and drug therapy. The authors, editors, and publisher have made every effort to ensure that all information in this book is in accordance with the state of knowledge at the time of production of the book. Nevertheless, the authors, editors, and publisher are not responsible for errors or omissions or for any consequences from application of the information in this book and make no warranty, expressed or implied, with respect to the contents of the publication. Every reader should examine carefully the package inserts accompanying each drug and should carefully check whether the dosage schedules mentioned therein or the contraindications stated by the manufacturer differ from the statements made in this book. Such examination is particularly important with drugs that are either rarely used or have been newly released on the market.

Library of Congress Cataloging-in-Publication Data
Names: Tatum, William O., IV, editor.
Title: Atlas of artifacts of clinical neurophysiology / editor, William O. Tatum, IV.
Description: New York : Demos, 2018. | Includes bibliographical references and index.
Identifiers: LCCN 2018028988| ISBN 9780826169341 (alk. paper) | ISBN 9780826169358 (ebook)
Subjects: | MESH: Nervous System Diseases—diagnosis | Electrodiagnosis | Diagnostic Techniques, Neurological | Nervous System Physiological Phenomena
Classification: LCC RC387.5 | NLM WL 141 | DDC 616.8/0475—dc23 LC record available at https://lccn.loc.gov/2018028988

Publisher's Note: New and used products purchased from third-party sellers are not guaranteed for quality, authenticity, or access to any included digital components.

Printed in the United States of America.
18 19 20 21 22 / 5 4 3 2 1

The chapters in this atlas are dedicated to our patients who are the "innocent bystanders" when artifact serves to challenge us and interfere in providing the best care humanly possible.
The book is dedicated to my amazing family and the memory of my mother who continue to serve as my constant source of strength in life.

DKWILY

Contents

Contributors

Michel AlHilani, MD
Research Fellow
Laboratory of Children's Brain Dynamics, Division of Newborn Medicine
Boston Children's Hospital
Boston, Massachusetts

Erika Takle Axeen, MD
Assistant Professor of Neurology
University of Virginia
Charlottesville, Virginia

William P. Cheshire, Jr., MD
Professor of Neurology
Mayo Clinic College of Medicine
Mayo Clinic
Jacksonville, Florida

David Freeman, MD
Professor of Neurology, Neurosurgery, and Critical Care
Medical Director, Neurocritical Care Unit
Mayo Clinic College of Medicine
Mayo Clinic
Jacksonville, Florida

Gloria Galloway, MD, MBA
Professor of Neurology
Wexner Medical Center
The Ohio State University
Columbus, Ohio

Madeleine Grigg-Damberger, MD
Professor of Neurology
Medical Director of Pediatric Sleep Services, Associate Medical Director, Neurodiagnostic Laboratory
University of New Mexico School of Medicine
Albuquerque, New Mexico

Jonathan J. Halford, MD
Professor of Neurology
Director, Neurophysiology Laboratory
Medical University of South Carolina
Ralph H. Johnson Veterans Affairs Medical Center
Charleston, South Carolina

Tasneem F. Hasan, MD, MPH, CPH
Resident Physician
Department of Neurology
Louisiana State University Health Sciences Center
Shreveport, Louisiana

Lawrence J. Hirsch, MD
Professor of Neurology
Chief, Division of Epilepsy and EEG
Co-Director, Comprehensive Epilepsy Center
Co-Director, Critical Care EEG Program
Yale University School of Medicine
New Haven, Connecticut

Aatif M. Husain, MD
Professor of Neurology
Director, Neurodiagnostic Department
Duke University Health System
Veterans Affairs Medical Center
Durham, North Carolina

Emily B. Kale, BS, R. EP T, CNIM
Manager of Neuromonitoring Service
Neurodiagnostics Department
Duke University Health System
Durham, North Carolina

Ruple S. Laughlin, MD
Assistant Professor of Neurology
Mayo Clinic College of Medicine
Mayo Clinic
Rochester, Minnesota

Alan D. Legatt, MD, PhD
Professor of Neurology
Albert Einstein College of Medicine
Montefiore Medical Center
Bronx, New York

Carolina B. Maciel, MD
Assistant Professor of Neurology
University of Florida
Gainesville, Florida

Edward C. Mader, Jr., MD
Associate Professor of Neurology
Louisiana State University Health Sciences Center
New Orleans, Louisiana

Daniella Miller, MD, MPH
Assistant Professor of Neurology
Louisiana State University Health Sciences Center
New Orleans, Louisiana

Piotr W. Olejniczak, MD, PhD
Professor of Neurology
Louisiana State University Health Sciences Center
New Orleans, Louisiana

Christos Papadelis, PhD
Assistant Professor of Neurology
Director, Laboratory of Children's Brain Dynamics
Harvard Medical School
Boston Children's Hospital
Boston, Massachusetts

Phillip L. Pearl, MD
Professor of Neurology
Harvard Medical School
William G. Lennox Chair
Director of Epilepsy and Clinical Neurophysiology
Boston Children's Hospital
Boston, Massachusetts

Nishi Rampal, MD
Assistant Professor of Neurology
Assistant Director, Critical Care EEG Program
Yale University School of Medicine
New Haven, Connecticut

Devon I. Rubin, MD
Professor of Neurology
Mayo Clinic College of Medicine
Mayo Clinic
Jacksonville, Florida

Stephanie L. Schwartz, BS, CNIM
Neuromonitorist
Neurodiagnostics Department
Duke University Health System
Durham, North Carolina

Jason Siegel, MD
Assistant Professor of Neurology
Mayo Clinic College of Medicine
Mayo Clinic
Jacksonville, Florida

William O. Tatum, IV, DO
Professor of Neurology
Mayo Clinic College of Medicine
Director, Comprehensive Epilepsy Center
Mayo Clinic
Jacksonville, Florida

Thoru Yamada, MD
Emeritus Professor of Neurology
University of Iowa
Iowa City, Iowa

Preface

The unique ability to enlighten a diagnostic question of neural function, clarify a disease process, or characterize the course of a disease state over time is one unmatched benefit of procedures involving clinical neurophysiology (CNP). Since the inception of CNP, artifact has been recognized in essentially every study utilized to evaluate signals generated by the nervous system. Many important procedures in CNP covered in this atlas add essential information to assessing neurological function. The importance of artifact cannot be overstated due to its ubiquitous nature in each recording involving a CNP procedure. The type of artifact is related to the technique, recording site, and specificity of the signals produced by biological tissue. The prevalence is relative to the duration of the procedure and the ability for a technologist to intervene and identify, localize, and eliminate the artifact in question. The presence of "noise" in a study involving a CNP procedure produced by artifact may interfere with the results of a CNP study; worse yet, it may potentially lead to misinterpretation of the results that could lead to CNP-based management of the patient. In the *Atlas of Artifacts in Clinical Neurophysiology*, a series of informative chapters highlight the traps and pitfalls associated with artifact when interpreting studies involving CNP. Various forms of neurophysiological procedures are performed routinely at local CNP laboratories throughout the world. They are interpreted by neurologists and neurophysiologists including studies involving electroencephalography (EEG), electromyography (EMG), nerve conductions studies (NCS), sleep, autonomic neurophysiology, evoked potentials (EP), and magnetoencephalography (MEG). Prolonged studies in the operating room (OR), intensive care unit (ICU), and epilepsy monitoring unit (EMU) may increasingly be "contaminated" by artifact, the longer the procedure is continued. This atlas is designed to illustrate common and rare types of artifacts that may be encountered by the clinical practitioner during the course of performing CNP studies.

The goal of the *Atlas* is to provide an explanatory text with samples of artifact that emphasize essential principles existing within individual fields of CNP. The book is developed in atlas form to facilitate easy interpretation for the busy clinician practitioner. Each chapter addresses a common topic in CNP, and is written by an expert in that area of subspecialty. Illustrative examples of artifact were chosen to support information contained in each chapter. In the initial chapter, Dr. Mader and colleagues nicely summarize the basis for artifact in CNP studies. The technical aspects are subsequently addressed by Dr. Halford to translate the basis of electrophysiology into resultant artifacts. In Chapter 3 provided by Drs. Galloway and Yamada, they illustrate the impact of artifact in pediatric studies involving the peripheral nervous system in and out of the OR. An excellent chapter involving children includes Drs. Axeen and Pearl's experience with artifact and pediatric EEG. In a unique chapter involving CNP in special care units, Drs. Seigel and Freeman discuss artifacts in neuromonitoring used in combination with additional CNP techniques employed for critically ill hospitalized patients. Focusing on an important area of CNP used by neurologists and clinical neurophysiologists, Dr. Rampal and colleagues address continuous EEG monitoring in ICU patients to illustrate the importance in recognition, and the potential of artifact to mimic abnormal waveforms. In Chapter 7, artifacts in the adult EEG are discussed by Dr. Tatum with a large collection of samples to illustrate various forms. Artifacts seen with MEG are discussed by Drs. Papadelis and Pearl to highlight the presence of artifact in specialty studies and the influence they have in medical decision making. Drs. Rubin and Laughlin provide an outstanding chapter to review the difficulties encountered with artifact involved when performing EMG and NCS.

Electrophysiologic metrics of the autonomic nervous system has artifactual pitfalls that may lead to misinterpretation. This is well outlined by Dr. Cheshire in a dedicated chapter examining multiple studies necessary to comprise an evaluation. Sleep studies combining DC channel non-CNP sensors with standard CNP monitoring are covered in an excellent chapter by Dr. Grigg-Damberger discussing the impact of artifact in polysomnography. Artifact in EP studies is well represented with robust samples supplied by Dr. Legatt. Neurological intraoperative monitoring (NIOM) overlaps with EP studies and is increasingly utilized in complex cases, which is presented by Dr. Husain and colleagues. In the end, artifact reduction is an essential part after recognition and identification of the source and is covered by Dr. Hasan and Tatum in the final chapter.

These dedicated chapters are written by experts with relevant examples and descriptive interpretations of each study performed for a clinical complaint raised during the course of routine patient management. This atlas will be useful for learners who are best taught by pattern recognition. The significant integration of CNP into diagnostic neurology and potential impact on clinical management has significantly advanced our need to remain knowledgeable about artifact. By providing examples in atlas form, samples of CNP artifact may help trigger recall of a similar waveform or series of waveforms when faced with similar features encountered during clinical practice. The need for practitioners to keep up with the spectrum of artifactual features in a CNP procedure has been compounded by transformation of the field toward longer recording times. Because of the potential limitations imposed by artifact, the clinical need for an atlas of CNP is self-evident. We seek to provide a practical text to serve as a useful reference for a wide range of procedures performed by neurologists and neurophysiologists, from beginners to advanced practitioners. With artifact present in virtually every CNP procedure, it is time for an atlas to help guide accurate diagnosis and management of patients with neurological disorders.

William O. Tatum, IV, DO

Acknowledgment

I am grateful to the authors who volunteered their precious time to share their expertise and thank them very much for their contribution to this book. In addition to the notable experts involved in the chapters within it, we wish to acknowledge the many additional experts involved in the various fields in CNP who have contributed to our understanding of the presence and impact of artifact in the care of our patients.

CHAPTER 1

Clinical Neurophysiology: An Overview

Edward C. Mader, Jr., Daniella Miller, and Piotr W. Olejniczak

CLINICAL NEUROPHYSIOLOGIC TESTING

Clinical neurophysiology (CNP) is a time-honored medical specialty that continues to make great strides, bolstered by rapid advances in neuroscience, biomedical engineering, and computer technology. It encompasses a wide range of methods and techniques for recording, presenting, and analyzing neurophysiologic signals in order to diagnose sensory, motor, autonomic, and central nervous system disorders. Testing performed in CNP or procedures used in current neurological practice include a variety of modality-specific and mixed-modality tests (**Table 1.1**).

Modality-specific CNP tests are performed to assess *specific functional modalities* using biomedical instruments that measure changes in neurophysiologic signals that occur spontaneously or with activation. Spontaneous fluctuations in electrical and magnetic fields during brain cortical activity are detected with EEG and *magnetoencephalography* (MEG) (1,2). Changes in electrical potentials with nerve and muscle activity are measured with *electromyography* (EMG) and *nerve conduction studies* (NCSs) (3). Subtle changes in the function of signaling pathways can be detected with *evoked potentials* (EPs), of which the most clinically useful are somatosensory (SSEPs), brainstem auditory (BAEPs), visual (VEPs), and motor (MEPs) evoked potentials (4). SSEPs are elicited by electrical stimulation of the median nerve (M-SSEP), the tibial nerve (T-SSEP), and rarely from other peripheral nerves. MEPs are activated by means of transcranial electrical stimulation (TES-MEP) or transcranial magnetic stimulation (TMS-MEP). The brain's ability to anticipate or respond to cognitive events is examined using *event-related potentials* (ERPs), such as the Bereitschaftspotential (BSP), contingent negative variation (CNV), P300 (P3), and mismatch negativity (MN) (5). CNP *autonomic function testing* includes measurement of heart rate variability with deep breathing (HR-DB), recording of blood pressure (BP) and heart rate (HR), response to head-up tilt (HUT) and Valsalva (VAL) maneuver, and sudomotor function by means of the quantitative sudomotor axon reflex test (QSART) and the thermoregulatory sweat test (TST) (6).

Mixed-modality (aka multi-modality) CNP tests utilize two or more test modalities to assess complex states (e.g., sleep, coma), to track multiple physiologic parameters, or to obtain more accurate results. During *sleep studies*, scalp EEG, chin EMG, and EOG (electrooculogram) allow tracking of sleep–wake stages; additional physiologic processes, such as nasal airflow, ventilatory effort, snoring, blood oxygen saturation, ECG, and anterior tibialis EMG, are recorded during polysomnography (PSG) (7). As a rule, *neurophysiologic intraoperative monitoring* (NIOM) is unimodal with the test modality chosen based on the structures at risk during the procedure, but multimodal NIOM may be superior for selected surgical procedures, such as combining SSEP and MEP monitoring during surgery on the spine (8). In *multimodal neuromonitoring* (MNM), cerebral blood flow, brain tissue oxygenation, and brain tissue metabolism are monitored, in addition to intracranial pressure (ICP) and EEG, to improve outcome in acute brain injury (9). The multimodal approach, known as *coregistration*, involves superimposing the data of two or more test modalities to achieve a level of accuracy that is not attainable if each modality is analyzed separately (10). Examples of coregistration techniques are electric source imaging (ESI), magnetic source imaging (MSI), and combined electric-magnetic source imaging (EMSI).

Specific test methods or protocols are selected based on test objectives, patient characteristics, clinical setting, and other factors (11–14). While the routine approach is sufficient in most cases, some clinical problems and

TABLE 1.1: Clinical Neurophysiologic Tests in Current neurological Practice

EEG Routine scalp EEG (adult/pediatric/neonatal) Ambulatory scalp EEG monitoring Electrocorticography Stereo-electroencephalography Epilepsy monitoring unit EEG ICU-EEG monitoring Intraoperative EEG monitoring	Cortical electrical potential (EEG) EEG recorded on the scalp EEG recorded with subdural electrodes EEG recorded with depth electrodes EEG recorded on the scalp or intracranially Same as scalp EEG Same as scalp EEG
MEG Spontaneous MEG Evoked MEG	Cortical magnetic flux density (MEG) Cortical magnetic flux density (MEG)
EMG Needle EMG Single-fiber EMG Surface EMG	Motor unit action potential Single-muscle-fiber action potential Myogenic electrical potential (surface EMG)
NCS Sensory nerve conduction studies Motor nerve conduction studies Including repetitive stimulation and F-wave studies Sensory-motor reflex studies including H reflex, blink reflex, and LLR studies Intraoperative CMAP monitoring	Sensory nerve action potential CMAP: M wave CMAP: M wave, F wave CMAP: H wave CMAP: R1 and R2 responses, LLR response Same as M-NCS
EP studies Pattern-shift VEPs Flash VEPs FVEPs BAEPs SSEP via median/tibial nerve stimulation MEP via transcranial electric/magnetic stimulation Intraoperative MEP monitoring Intraoperative SSEP monitoring Intraoperative BAEP monitoring Intraoperative FVEP monitoring	Cortical electrical potential (P100, N100) Electrical potentials I, II, III, IV, V, VI Auditory nerve (I), brainstem (II–V) potential Peripheral nerve (N9/N8), cord (N13/N22), subcortical (P14, N18/P31, N34), cortical (N20/P37) Direct wave, indirect waves, and CMAP: M wave Same as MEP Same as M-SSEP/T-SSEP Same as BAEP Same as FVEP

(*continued*)

TABLE 1.1: Clinical Neurophysiologic Tests in Current Neurological Practice(*continued*)

Event-related potential studies Readiness or BSP CNV Oddball paradigm MN	 Cortical electrical potential (BSP or premotor potential) Cortical electrical potential (CNV) Cortical electrical potential (P300 or P3) Cortical electrical potential (MN)
Autonomic function tests HR variability with deep breathing Head-up tilt or tilt table test Valsalva maneuver Quantitative sudomotor axon reflex test Thermoregulatory sweat test	 Cardiac electric potential (ECG) BP, HR BP, HR Sweat volume Sweat distribution
Polygraphic sleep studies PSG Multiple sleep latency test Maintenance of wakefulness test	Sleep stage: scalp EEG, chin EMG, and EOG Other parameters (PSG): respiratory airflow and effort, blood oxygenation, ECG, tibialis anterior EMG, etc.
Multimodal neuromonitoring Multimodal intensive care neuromonitoring Multimodal intraoperative neuromonitoring	Intracranial pressure, brain perfusion, oxygenation, etc. Two or more types of signal or test parameters
Multimodal coregistration Electric source imaging Magnetic source imaging Electric and magnetic source imaging	 EEG coregistered with brain neuroimage MEG coregistered with brain neuroimage EEG and MEG coregistered with brain neuroimage

Note: The first seven categories comprise *modality-specific tests*, and the last three categories consist of *mixed-modality tests* (see text for explanation). Listed under each test category are test methods or protocols aimed at specific clinical settings and test objectives. The right column shows the signal of interest or physiologic parameter(s) recorded during neurophysiologic testing.

BAEP, brainstem auditory evoked potential; BP, blood pressure; BSP, Bereitschaftspotential; CMAP, compound motor action potential; CNV, contingent negative variation; EMG, electromyography; EOG, electrooculogram; EP, evoked potential; FVEP, flash visual evoked potential; HR, heart rate; LLR, long-latency reflex; MEG, magnetoencephalography; MEP, motor evoked potential; MN, mismatch negativity; M-NCS, motor nerve conduction study; M-SSEP, median nerve somatosensory evoked potentials; NCS, nerve conduction study; PSG, polysomnography; SSEP, somatosensory evoked potentials; T-SSEP, tibial nerve somatosensory evoked potentials; VEP, visual evoked potentials.

situations require modifications or refinements in the routine method. For example, the following EEG methods and protocols are aimed at *different clinical scenarios*: routine scalp EEG, extended EEG recording, ambulatory EEG, neonatal EEG, brain death study, ICU-EEG monitoring, IOM-EEG monitoring, long-term monitoring (LTM) of video and EEG in the epilepsy monitoring unit (EMU), electrocorticography (ECoG), stereo-EEG, and coregistration techniques, such as ESI and EMSI. It may be prudent to combine different test modalities to obtain more accurate results, such as simultaneous EEG and EMG recording to better define the seizure type and EEG recording during HUT to distinguish postsyncopal convulsions from epileptic seizures and psychogenic events.

CNP tests measure *specific biosignals or physiological parameters* (**Table 1.1**) allowing clinicians to probe and assess selected facets of the patient's *functional anatomy* (**Table 1.2**). The biosignals or physiological parameters recorded reflect the function of *specific anatomical structures* (**Table 1.3**). Based on recorded *signal characteristics* (**Figures 1.2** and **1.3**), the clinical neurophysiologist can tell if anatomical structures, circuits, or pathways are functioning normally or are affected by pathological processes (**Tables 1.4** and **1.5**).

Brain function is reflected in the EEG, MEG, ERP, and EP cortical and subcortical components (1,2,6,8). Even when EEG and MEG signals arise from the same cellular processes in the *cerebral cortex*, there are differences in the way EEG and MEG data are recorded and interpreted (15). A *reference* is required to record EEG, but not MEG. Because the skull and scalp do not distort magnetic fields as much as electrical fields, the spatial resolution of MEG is superior to EEG (1,2). EEG can detect activity in *"more"* brain areas by recording radial dipoles, but MEG is more sensitive to tangential dipolar activity in the superficial cortical sulci, making it superior for *source localization*; for example, MEG is used for MSI and more precise localization of the epileptogenic focus (2). While EEG is widely used in clinical practice, MEG is available only in far fewer centers. The constant interaction between cortical and subcortical structures implies that *diencephalic-brainstem disturbances* will also affect the EEG/MEG. Assessment of *modality-specific brain structures* is performed with VEP, BAEP, SSEP, LLR, ERP, and other CNP tests (see later) (3–6). Brain function assessment is the goal of IOM-EEG, sleep studies, and MNM of cerebral perfusion, oxygenation, and metabolism (1,7–9).

Muscle, peripheral nerve, and lower motor neuron function is routinely tested with needle EMG and NCS (3,16). During needle EMG, motor unit action potential (MUAP) number and firing rate increase with the force of muscle contraction. Each MUAP represents activation of a *motor unit* (i.e., one motor neuron, its nerve fiber, and all muscle fibers innervated by branches of the same nerve fiber). NCS is performed to assess signal conduction along *fast-conducting large-diameter nerve fibers*: S-NCS for sensory and M-NCS for motor nerve fibers. *Neuromuscular junction transmission* is evaluated by repetitive nerve stimulation and single-fiber EMG (3,16). F-wave recording extends the utility of M-NCS for evaluating *lower motor neurons*, *motor nerve roots*, and *proximal motor nerves*. These motor structures, along with the *sensory nerve roots* and *central components* of reflex pathways, can be evaluated with the H reflex, long-latency reflex, or blink reflex (3,17).

Modality-specific neural pathway or circuit activity is reflected in the EP or ERP signals that are generated when components of the pathway or circuit are activated (4,5,8). The *dorsal column pathway* is evaluated with M-SSEP and T-SSEP (18), the *visual pathway* with pattern-shift or flash VEP (19), the *auditory pathway* with BAEP (20), and the *central motor pathway* with TES-MEP or TMS-MEP (21). IOM-SSEP and IOM-MEP can be combined if both dorsal and ventral territories of the spinal cord are surgically at risk (22). The *neurophysiological substrates of ERP* have not yet been identified with certainty. BSP and CNV correlate with movement preparation and motor processing in the frontal lobe, P300 with selective attention and stimulus discrimination in the parietal lobe, and MN with sound feature discrimination, sensory learning, and perceptual accuracy (5,23).

Autonomic regulation of somatic and visceral function by the parasympathetic and sympathetic nervous system is mediated via *slow-conducting small-fiber autonomic nerves* that innervate most organs and tissues (6,24). Some autonomic function tests are organ specific, such as pupillometry, lacrimation tests, tests of saliva production, gastric motility tests, and urodynamic studies. In CNP, autonomic testing is performed to evaluate *parasympathetic cardiovagal reflexes* (HR-DB and VAL), *sympathetic vasomotor reflexes* (VAL and HUT), and *sympathetic sudomotor function* (QSART and TST). QSART evaluates the *sympathetic axon reflex* and TST evaluates the integrity of the *sympathetic thermoregulatory pathway* from the hypothalamus to eccrine sweat glands (6,24).

The *sensitivity of CNP tests* is remarkable and most tests will show abnormal results before the onset of clinical signs and symptoms. Unfortunately, CNP tests are also sensitive to technical factors and to noise. Exceptional care should therefore be exercised always to avoid overinterpreting neurophysiologic data. The *specificity of CNP tests* is limited to the identification of physiological disturbances or disorders in functional anatomy. To reach an etiologic diagnosis, neurophysiological data should always be interpreted in the context of the clinical history, physical examination, and other laboratory test results.

TABLE 1.2: Classification of Clinical Neurophysiologic Tests Based on Functional Anatomy or Neural Pathway Tested

Tests of global/focal cortical, diencephalic, and/or brainstem function

EEG–spontaneous, scalp-based cortical activity, including influence of diencephalic and brainstem structures
ECoG–focal/regional brain activity, including influence of diencephalic and brainstem structures
Stereo-EEG–focal limbic or deep-brain activity influenced by other cortical and noncortical structures
Epilepsy monitoring unit EEG–same as EEG, ECoG, or stereo-EEG
ICU-EEG–same as EEG
IOM-EEG–same as EEG
MEG–same as EEG, but superior for detecting localized cortical activity
MNM–global cerebral perfusion, oxygenation, metabolism, neocortical activity (see EEG)
Sleep studies–same as EEG, with emphasis on the function of the brain's sleep and wake centers

Tests of muscle, peripheral nerve, motor neuron, and/or reflex function

Needle EMG–motor units activated by volition, spontaneous activity of muscle fibers/motor units
Single-fiber EMG–neuromuscular junction and muscle fiber activity
Surface EMG–multiple motor units activated spontaneously or volitionally
S-NCS–large-fiber sensory peripheral nerve fibers
M-NCS–large-fiber motor peripheral nerve fibers, neuromuscular junction, and muscle fibers
Repetitive stimulation–same as motor NCS, with emphasis on neuromuscular junction transmission
F-wave study–large-fiber motor peripheral nerve fibers, muscle fibers, multiple motor units
IOM-CMAP–same as motor NCS
H reflex–large-fiber peripheral sensory nerve fibers and multiple motor units (H wave)
Long-latency reflex–large-fiber sensory pathway, somatomotor cortex, corticospinal tract, multiple motor units
Blink reflex–trigeminal nerve V_1 branch, nuclei and tracts in pons and medulla, facial nerve, orbicularis oculi fibers

Tests of central sensory/motor pathway and/or focal cortical function

VEP–QSART, quantitative sudomotor axon reflex testion, visual cortex
BAEP–auditory pathway: ear, auditory nerve, cochlear nucleus, lateral lemniscus, inferior colliculus
M-SSEP–somatosensory pathway: median nerve, dorsal column, medial lemniscus, thalamus, somatosensory cortex
T-SSEP–somatosensory pathway: tibial nerve, dorsal column, medial lemniscus, thalamus, somatosensory cortex
TES-MEP–motor pathway: motor cortex, corticospinal tract, multiple motor units
TMS-MEP–motor pathway: motor cortex, corticospinal tract, multiple motor units
IOM-SSEP–same as M-SSEP/T-SSEP
IOM-MEP–same as TES-MEP/TMS-MEP
BSP–frontal lobe premotor cortex circuits involved with movement preparation and execution
CNV–frontal lobe premotor cortex circuits involved with movement preparation
P300–parietal lobe circuits for selective attention and stimulus discrimination
MN–temporal lobe auditory cortex circuits for sound feature discrimination
ESI, MSI, or EMSI–focal area of cerebral cortex generating signal of interest (e.g., epileptiform discharges)

(*continued*)

TABLE 1.2: Classification of Clinical Neurophysiologic Tests Based on Functional Anatomy or Neural Pathway Tested (*continued*)

Tests of autonomic function
HR-DB–parasympathetic cardiovagal reflexes
HR-VAL–parasympathetic cardiovagal pathways
BP-VAL–sympathetic baroreflex afferent and efferent pathways
BP-HUT–sympathetic baroreflex afferent and efferent pathways
QSART–sympathetic postganglionic sudomotor axon reflex
TST–sympathetic central, preganglionic, postganglionic pathways and eccrine sweat glands

Note: Modality-specific tests assess the function of specific structures or neural circuits and mixed-modality tests assess multiple functional modalities or complex states (see **Table 1.1**). Physiological function is assessed by measuring signals generated by specific anatomical structures during a brief time interval (routine method) or by tracking how signals change over time (continuous monitoring).

BAEP, brainstem auditory evoked potential; BSP, Bereitschaftspotential; BP-HUT, blood pressure head-up tilt; BP-VAL, blood pressure Valsalva; CMAP, compound motor action potential; CNV, contingent negative variation; ECoG, electrocorticography; EMG, electromyography; EMSI, Electric and magnetic source imaging; ESI, electric source imaging; HR-DB, heart rate variability with deep breathing; HR-VAL, heart rate Valsalva; IOM, intraoperative monitoring; MEP, motor evoked potential; M-NCS, motor nerve conduction studies; NCS, nerve conduction study; MEG, magnetoencephalography; MN, mismatch negativity; MNM, multimodal neuromonitoring; M-SSEP, median nerve somatosensory evoked potential; MSI, magnetic source imaging; QSART, quantitative sudomotor axon reflex test; S-NCS, sensory nerve conduction study; T-SSEP, tibial nerve somatosensory evoked potential; TES-MEP, transcranial electrical stimulation MEP; TMS-MEP, transcranial magnetic stimulation motor evoked potential; TST, thermoregulatory sweat test; VEP, visual evoked potential.

TABLE 1.3: Generators and Sources of Signal and Test Parameters Measured in Clinical Neurophysiology

EEG/MEG		
EEG, ECoG	Cortical electrical potential[a]	Cortical pyramidal cell synaptic potential
MEG	Cortical magnetic flux density[b]	Cortical pyramidal cell electric currents
EMG/NCS		
Needle EMG	Motor unit action potential	MFAP
Single-fiber EMG	MFAP	MFAP
Surface EMG	Myogenic electric potential	MFAP
Sensory NCS	Sensory nerve action potential	Nerve fiber action potential
Motor NCS	CMAP[c]	MFAP
F waves	CMAP: F waves[b]	MFAP
H reflex	CMAP: H response[b]	MFAP
Long-latency reflex	CMAP: LL responses[b]	MFAP
Blink reflex	CMAP: R1 and R2 responses	MFAP

(*continued*)

TABLE 1.3: Generators and Sources of Signal and Test Parameters Measured in Clinical Neurophysiology (*continued*)

EP/ERP		
VEP	Cortical potential (P100, N100)	Cortical pyramidal cell synaptic potential
FVEP BAEP	Electrical potentials I, II, III, IV, V, VI[c] Auditory nerve action potential (I) Brainstem farfield potential (II[c], III, IV, V)	Nerve fiber and synaptic potentials Nerve fiber action potential Brainstem electric potential
M-SSEP	Peripheral nerve potential (N9) Cervical cord dorsal horn potential (N13) Subcortical potential (P14, N18)[c] Somatosensory cortical potential (N20)	Nerve fiber action potential Dorsal horn cell synaptic potential Synaptic/action potential Cortical pyramidal cell synaptic potential
T-SSEP	Peripheral nerve potential (N8) Thoracic cord dorsal horn potential (N22) Subcortical potential (P31, N34)[c] Somatosensory cortical potential (P37)	Nerve fiber action potential Dorsal horn cell synaptic potential Synaptic/action potential Cortical pyramidal cell synaptic potential
MEP	Pyramidal tract potential (D wave, I waves) Compound motor action potential (CMAP)	Nerve fiber action potential MFAP
ERP	Cortical potential	Cortical pyramidal cell synaptic potential
Autonomic tests HR-DB HUT/VAL QSART/TST	Electrocardiographic potential (ECG) Arterial BP (mmHg), heart rate (/min) Eccrine gland output (sweat)	Cardiac MFAP Not applicable Not applicable

(*continued*)

TABLE 1.3: Generators and Sources of Signal and Test Parameters Measured in Clinical Neurophysiology (*continued*)

Sleep studies		
EEG (scalp) EMG (chin) EOG (near eye)	Cortical electric potential[a] Myogenic electric potential Oculoelectric dipole	Cortical pyramidal cell synaptic potential[a] MFAP Corneal–retinal potential
Other parameters[d]	Respiratory airflow Respiratory effort Blood oxygenation Cardioelectric potential (ECG) Tibialis anterior muscle potential	Not applicable Not applicable Not applicable Cardiac MFAP MFAP
Neuromonitoring Unimodal NIOM Multimodal NIOM MNM	Same as EEG, CMAP, MEP, SSEP, etc. ≥2 modalities, e.g., IOM-SSEP and MEP ICP, brain perfusion, brain tissue oxygenation, cellular metabolism, etc.	Same as modality-specific test Same as modality-specific test Not applicable Not applicable
Coregistration ESI MSI EMSI	Same as EEG + electromagnetic Same as MEG + electromagnetic Same as EEG and MEG + electromagnetic	See EEG above See MEG above See EEG and MEG above

Note: This table shows (a) CNP test or test modality (left column); (b) the macroscopic generator and signal or physiologic parameter measured by the test (middle column); and, whenever applicable, (c) the microscopic SGU and the microscopic signal or "building block" of the macroscopic signal (right column).

BAEP, brainstem auditory evoked potential; BP, blood pressure; CMAP, compound motor action potential; ECoG, electrocorticography; EMG, electromyography; EMSI, electric-magnetic source imaging; EOG, electrooculogram; EP, evoked potential; ERP, event-related potentials; ESI, electric source imaging; FVEP, flash visual evoked potentials; HR, heart rate; HR-DB, heart rate variability with deep breathing; HUT, head-up tilt; ICP, intracranial pressure; IOM-SSEP, intraoperative somatosensory evoked potentials monitoring; MEG, magnetoencephalography; MEP, motor evoked potential; MFAP, muscle fiber action potential; MNM, multimodal neuromonitoring; MSI, magnetic source imaging; M-SSEP, median nerve somatosensory evoked potentials; NCS, nerve conduction study; NIOM, neurophysiologic intraoperative monitoring; QSART, quantitative sudomotor axon reflex test; SGU, signal-generating unit; SSEP, somatosensory evoked potentials; TST, thermoregulatory sweat test; T-SSEP, tibial nerve somatosensory evoked potentials; VAL, Valsalva; VEP, visual evoked potentials.

[a]Nonsynaptic and nonneuronal mechanisms may also play a role in EEG/MEG generation.

[b]Late responses are CMAPs that occur after the classic CMAP known as M wave.

[c]Generator(s) of FVEP waves I–VI, BAEP wave II, and SSEP subcortical components remain controversial.

[d]Physiologic parameters recorded during PSG in addition to EEG, EOG, and chin EMG (list is incomplete).

Translating *bioelectric and biomagnetic signals* into physiological information requires *a priori* knowledge of where and how signals are generated (discussed earlier) and how signals spread from the generator to the recording site. Once generated, *bioelectric and biomagnetic fields* propagate from the generator to other parts of the body. This mechanism of signal propagation, known as *volume conduction*, must be distinguished from another mechanism of signal propagation, known as *neural transmission*. These two mechanisms of signal propagation in biological tissue are quite distinct and result in waveforms with different spatiotemporal characteristics (**Figure 1.4**).

TABLE 1.4: Spatiotemporal Characteristics of Bioelectric Signals Measured in Clinical Neurophysiology

EEG	Cortical electric potential[a]	Stationary nearfield
MEG	Cortical magnetic flux density[a]	Stationary nearfield
Needle EMG Single-fiber EMG	Motor unit action potential MFAP[b]	Traveling nearfield Traveling nearfield
Sensory NCS Motor NCS Reflexes: H, LL, and blink	Sensory nerve action potential CMAP[c] CMAP[c]	Traveling nearfield Traveling nearfield Traveling nearfield
Pattern-shift VEP	Cortical potential (P100, N100)	Stationary nearfield
BAEP	Auditory nerve action potential (I) Brainstem farfield potential (II[c], III, IV, V)	Traveling nearfield Stationary farfield
M-SSEP/T-SSEP	Peripheral nerve action potential (N9/N8) Cervical cord dorsal horn potential (N13/N22) Subcortical potential (P14, N18/P31, N34)[d] Somatosensory cortical potential (N20/P37)	Traveling nearfield Stationary nearfield Stationary farfield Stationary nearfield
TES-MEP/TMS-MEP	Corticospinal tract action potential (D wave, I waves) CMAP	Traveling nearfield Traveling nearfield
ERP	Cortical electric potential	Stationary nearfield
ECG[e]	Cardiac electric potential	Stationary farfield[d]

[a]Nonsynaptic and non-neuronal mechanisms may play a role in the generation of EEG, MEG, ERPs, and cortical EPs

[b]The micro/macro stereotype is not applicable since the microscopic signal (MFAP) is also the signal that is recorded.

[c]Late responses (F waves, H reflex, LL response, R1/R2 responses) are CMAPs that occur after the classic CMAP or M wave.

[d]No definite consensus on the generator(s) of BAEP wave II and SSEP subcortical components and of FVEP waves I-VI

[e]ECG is a traveling nearfield signal near its generator but behaves as a farfield stationary signal when recorded in CNP.

Note: For each CNP test or test modality (left column), the macroscopic signal recorded (middle column) and the spatiotemporal characteristics of the recorded signal (right column) are shown.

BAEP, brainstem auditory evoked potential; CMAP, compound motor action potential; EMG, electromyography; ERP, event-related potentials; MEG, magnetoencephalography; MFAP, muscle fiber action potential; M-SSEP, median nerve somatosensory evoked potentials; NCS, nerve conduction study; TES-MEP, transcranial electrical stimulation motor evoked potential; TMS-MEP, transcranial magnetic stimulation motor evoked potential; T-SSEP, tibial nerve somatosensory evoked potentials; VEP, visual evoked potentials.

TABLE 1.5: Classification of Electrophysiologic Abnormalities[a]

Signal amplitude
Abnormally low amplitude Loss of SGUs–e.g., low SNAP with loss of nerve fibers, EEG attenuation with loss of pyramidal cells Decrease in number of SGUs activated–e.g., low CMAP amplitude with loss of nerve fibers SGU asynchrony–e.g., low CMAP amplitude due to temporal dispersion of signals in motor nerve fibers Changes in volume conductor–e.g., edema increasing distance between generator and electrode *Abnormally high amplitude* Increase in number of SGUs activated–e.g., giant MUAP with muscle reinnervation of fibers Pathologic hypersynchrony of SGUs–e.g., high-amplitude epileptiform waves, giant N20 or P100 Decrease in impedance of conducting medium–e.g., accentuation of fast EEG waveforms with skull defects
Signal conduction time
Abnormally long latency Conduction slowing in peripheral nerve–e.g., prolonged SNAP, CMAP, SSEP, or P100 absolute latency Conduction slowing in central tract–e.g., increase in BAEP III-V and SSEP N13-N20 interpeak latencies, temporal dispersion and asynchronous activation of SGUs–usually only mild prolongation in latency *Abnormally short latency* Not easy to account for with pathology; a technical reason must be excluded–e.g., electrode placement or artifact
Wave morphology or configuration
Abnormal wave morphology Combination of abnormalities–e.g., wave amplitude, duration, contour, number of phases/turns *Increase in wave duration* and *number of phases* SGU desynchrony–e.g., long CMAP duration due to temporal dispersion of signals in motor nerve fibers *Short wave duration and sharp contour* SGU hypersynchrony–e.g., EEG and MEG epileptiform discharges, spikes, and sharp waves

(continued)

TABLE 1.5: Classification of Electrophysiologic Aabnormalities[a] (*continued*)

Wave activation, modulation, and repetition
Abnormal activation or recruitment Reduced SGU activation–e.g., decreased MUAP recruitment with motor neuron or nerve fiber pathology Increased SGU activation–e.g., increased MUAP recruitment due to muscle fiber pathology Reduced and increased SGU activation–e.g., release of latent slow rhythms with loss of pyramidal cell input *Abnormal spontaneous activity* Hyperexcitability of SGUs–e.g., fibrillation potentials, positive sharp waves, complex repetitive discharge Hyperexcitability of non-SGU circuit components–e.g., fasciculation potentials, myokymia Hyperexcitability of circuit–e.g., EEG or MEG epileptiform activity *Abnormal repetition rate* Perturbation in network dynamics–e.g., disorganization of EEG or MEG rhythms with encephalopathy
Spatial characteristics
Abnormal spatial distribution Often due to the same factors affecting the time-domain characteristics of waves *Apparent displacement of signal generator* Technical factors–e.g., improper electrode placement State change–e.g., drowsiness can manifest as "anterior displacement" of EEG alpha rhythm.
Clinical and physiological context
Physiological state Often due to the same factors affecting the time-domain characteristics of waves *Age or developmental period* Maturational–e.g., dysmature features in the neonatal EEG

[a]When the above framework is used to classify abnormalities in the "raw" MEG record, one must be aware of its limits; for example, magnetic signals are not sensitive to changes in volume conductor properties. The above framework is not suitable for signals that are the product of complex transduction events between the biological source and the signal-sensing probe.

Note: Graphical features, clinical context, and pathophysiology are all taken into consideration in this classification scheme. Macroscopic abnormalities appear in the record as aberrations in amplitude, latency, or configuration of otherwise physiological waves, as a change in activation, modulation, or repetition pattern of physiologically recurring waves, as distortion of the spatial characteristics of waves, or as normally appearing but out-of-context waves in terms of physiologic state or age. Each of these abnormalities occurs because of impairment in SGU or non-SGU circuit components or because of changes in the properties of the volume conductor.

BAEP, brainstem auditory evoked potential; CMAP, compound motor action potential; MEG, magnetoencephalography; MUAP, motor unit action potential; SGU, signal-generating unit; SNAP, sensory nerve action potential; SSEP, somatosensory evoked potentials.

SIGNAL RECORDING AND GRAPHICAL DISPLAY

The *signal* that must be recorded and analyzed, or the "signal of interest," is often simply called "signal." Any other signal contaminating and potentially distorting the signal of interest is considered "noise." *Noise* entering the recording system may appear on the record as *artifact*. Because signal and noise are physically similar (both are electromagnetic signals), neurophysiologic instruments are intricately engineered to maximize the *signal-to-noise ratio* during signal recording and processing (25). Moreover, CNP technologists and specialists are trained to distinguish signal from artifact by visual inspection and, if necessary, digital reformation of the record. Chapter 2 is dedicated to *instrumentation and signal processing*. In this chapter, it is sufficient to mention that neurophysiological recording involves four processes: analog signal acquisition, analog signal conditioning, analog-to-digital conversion, and digital signal processing (**Figure 1.1**).

Signal analysis and interpretation is performed by professionals trained in CNP. Neurophysiologic data are usually presented and analyzed in the *time domain* (**Figure 1.2**). Recorded signals are displayed as *waveforms* on a computer or oscilloscopic screen (paper recording is nearly obsolete and is omitted from our discussion). *CNP records* contain one or more lines of tracing, called channels. Each *channel* is a graph of signal amplitude versus time, with waves rising above and falling below the baseline, indicating fluctuations in signal amplitude with time. When *differential amplification* is employed in biopotential recording, the wave amplitude at any given time is proportional to the voltage difference between the amplifier inputs, G1 and G2, multiplied by the amplification factor or *gain* (see Chapter 2) (25).

Quantitative analysis of "raw" data can extract additional information that can complement or supplement basic time-domain data. The *fast Fourier transform* (FFT) converts data in the time domain to an alternative representation of the same data in the *frequency domain* (26). Decomposing EEG into its frequency components and using *compressed spectral array* (CSA) to track the changes in amplitude/power of EEG frequency bands is a useful *quantitative EEG* (qEEG) technique for detecting cerebral ischemia and seizures during ICU-EEG monitoring (11). EEG trending in neonates is commonly performed using *amplitude-integrated EEG* (aEEG), a qEEG technique that involves filtering, rectification, smoothing, and compression of time-domain data. Quantitative analysis of MUAP, compound motor action potential (CMAP), HR-DB, and other data can also be performed. Although *waveform analysis in the time domain* is still the bread and butter of the clinical neurophysiologist, rapidly advancing computer technology and machine learning, and the increasing availability of automated algorithms, will inevitably transform the future practice of CNP.

Spontaneously generated signals represent oscillating physiologic processes, appear graphically as sinusoidal waves, and are referred to as *rhythmic activity* or *rhythms* (**Figure 1.2A**) (27). In EEG/MEG, sustained rhythmic activity is considered "background." Background activity, not individual waves, serves as the framework for time-domain analysis. Additional waves and rhythms may appear spontaneously or with activation and are mixed with, or replace, the background. Both background activity and emergent waves are signals of interest that are analyzed collectively. The most important graphical descriptor of rhythmic activity is *frequency*, the number of wave repeats per second, which is reported as Hertz (Hz) or cycles per second (cps or c/s). Frequency is described in precise terms (e.g., 60 Hz) or in terms of *frequency bands*, including EEG/MEG: less than 4 Hz is delta, 4 to less than 8 Hz is theta, 8 to 13 Hz

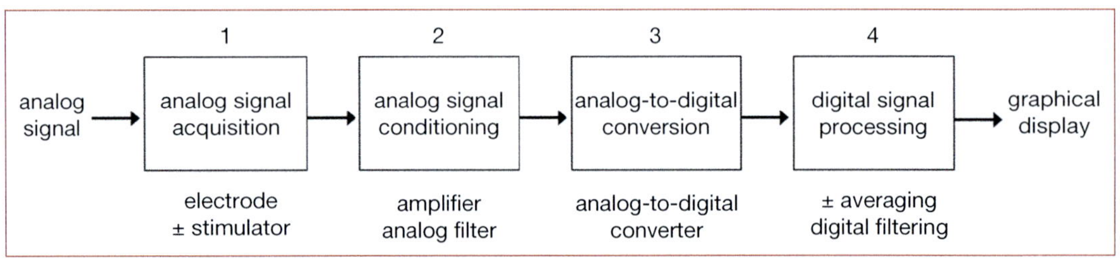

FIGURE 1.1: Signal recording in clinical neurophysiology. The analog signal recorded includes the signal of interest and noise. Signal recording involves four general processes: (1) analog signal acquisition, (2) analog signal conditioning, (3) analog-to-digital conversion, and (4) digital signal processing. The end product of the recording process is a graphical representation or record of the signals (see **Figure 1.2**).

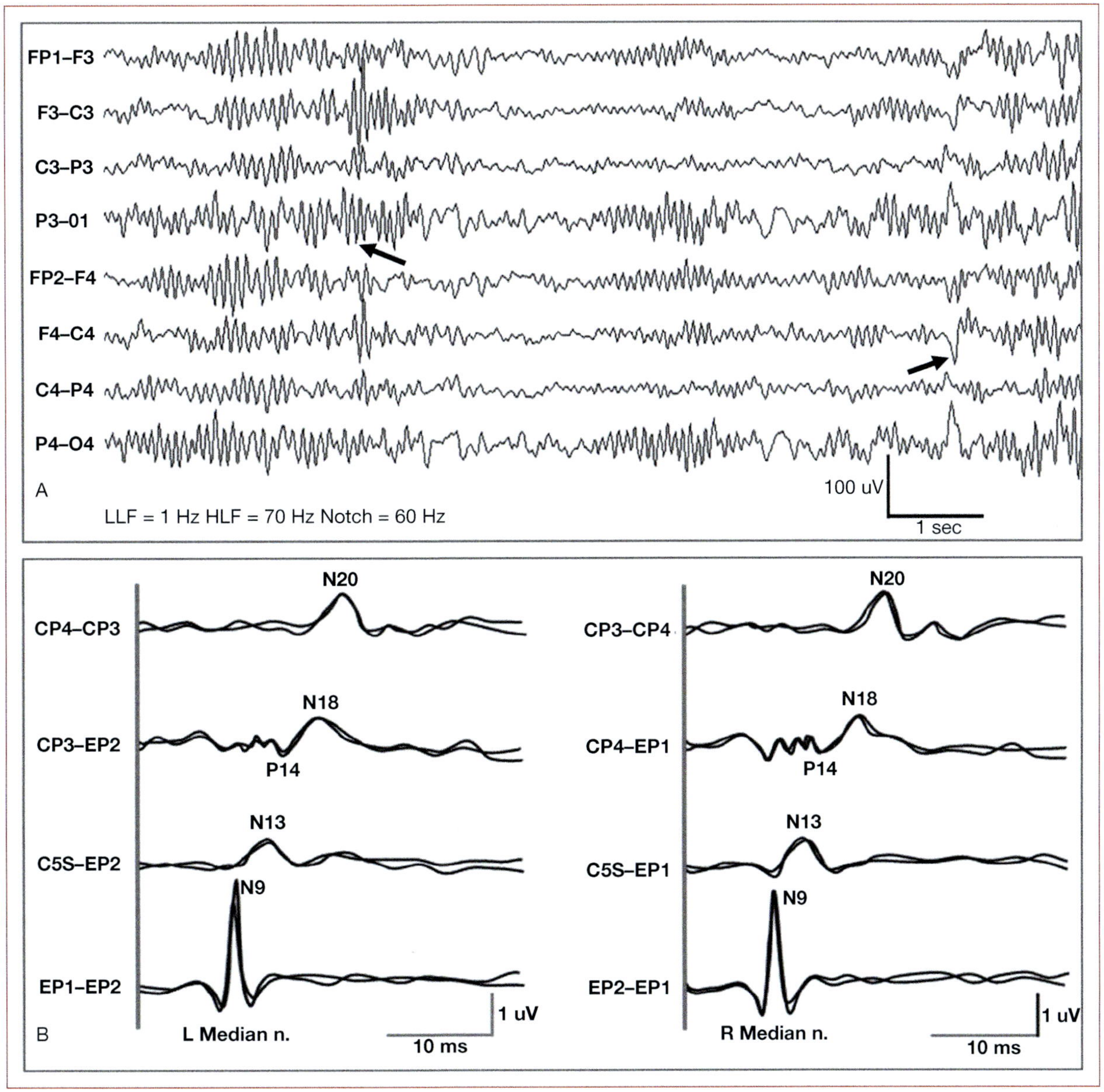

FIGURE 1.2: Graphical display of neurophysiologic signals. Recorded signals are usually displayed as a graph of signal amplitude (y-axis) versus time (x-axis) with each line of tracing (channel) showing how amplitude varies with time. A: Spontaneously generated signals (e.g., scalp EEG) are displayed as continuous tracings. The EEG sample shown is an 8-channel, 10-second epoch extracted from a 30-minute recording using the 10–20 system of electrode placement [11]. Background rhythm (left arrow) and emergent waves (right arrow) on the left (upper four channels) and right (lower four channels) sides of the head are analyzed collectively. The most important descriptor of rhythmic activity is *frequency*, the number of wave repeats per second, reported as Hertz (Hz). B: *Stimulus-evoked signals* (e.g., M-SSEP) are displayed as short-interval tracings, called *sweeps*. In the figure, each line of tracing is the average of 200 sweeps obtained by stimulating the median nerve, one side at a time, and recording from standard sites [11]. Two tracings are overlapped to prove *replicability*. Five SSEP peaks, N9, N13, P14, N18, and N20, are identified based on morphology and time of occurrence. The absolute and interpeak latencies and the degree of left-right asymmetry in SSEP latencies are analyzed using laboratory-specific normative values.

M-SSEP, median nerve somatosensory evoked potential.

is alpha, and greater than 13 Hz is beta (28). By interpreting a wave as a basic unit of a rhythm, an *isolated waveform* can be assigned a frequency that is equal to the reciprocal of its *duration*.

Stimulus-evoked signals, representing neurophysiological *events* that occur in response to specific stimuli, are typically displayed as waveform tracings *one sweep at a time* (**Figure 1.2B**) (27). The *evoked waves* or *wave complexes* are stereotypical—they are activated only by appropriate stimulus, they are time-locked to the stimulus, and they have a distinctive graphical appearance (29). While a *single acquisition sweep* is unlikely to capture very low amplitude signals that are buried in noise, *averaging many sweeps* can increase the signal-to-noise ratio and reveal these tiny signals. *Latency* is the time between two events. It is called *absolute latency* if the first event is a stimulus presentation and the second event is wave onset (*onset latency*) or wave peak or trough (*peak latency*), or *interpeak latency* if both events are wave peaks or troughs. *Duration* is the time from the onset to the termination of a wave or wave complex. *Phase* is the portion of the wave between two baseline crossings. *Turns* or *serrations* are reversals in the direction a waveform "flows" relative to the baseline. The amplitude, duration, and number of phases and turns of a wavelet or waveform complex determine its *configuration* or *morphology*.

CNP test result interpretation is the artful integration of clinical, technical, and graphical information. Most CNP records are simple two-dimensional graphs of signal amplitude versus time (**Figure 1.2**). The *optimal display configuration*, including number of channels, montage, sensitivity, time base, and filter settings, is different for each CNP test modality or procedure (**Figure 1.3**) (1–15). *Interpreting CNP records* requires skills and abilities in pattern recognition, spatial localization, contextual analysis, visual approximation, and computer-assisted measurements. The following is an overview of the common *graphical display and analysis methods* employed in CNP practice.

EEG/MEG signals are simultaneously recorded from multiple cranial sites and displayed as a multichannel record (**Figure 1.3**: top). Each line of tracing in the EEG record represents the difference in voltage between a pair of electrodes (30). Since MEG is reference free, each line of tracing in the MEG record corresponds to the fluctuation of magnetic flux density detected by a superconducting quantum interference device (SQUID) detector. The "raw" time-domain EEG/MEG record is displayed and read *one page (epoch) at a time*. In the process, EEG/MEG waves are characterized based on spatial distribution and time-domain characteristics, including amplitude, frequency, polarity, and morphology. Spontaneous and sustained rhythmic activity is considered *background activity*. Waveforms appearing spontaneously or with activation are analyzed in the context of the background and other waveforms. MEG signals are often processed, coregistered with a neuroimage (e.g., MRI), and displayed as an *MSI image* (not shown in **Figure 1.3**) (31).

EMG/NCS signals are acquired with needle or surface electrodes and displayed as a tracing with the option to superimpose or stack several tracings on the screen (**Figure 1.3**: second row). In *needle EMG*, a *fully relaxed muscle* is "silent" if the electrode is not picking up endplate noise (**Figure 1.3**: EMG relaxed). With slight *muscle contraction*, an MUAP appears with a low firing rate and, as effort increases, firing rate increases and more MUAPs are recruited (**Figure 1.3**: EMG activated). Abnormal spontaneous and exertional activity is identified by visualizing the waveforms and listening to the sounds emitted by a synthesizer (32). In *M-NCS/S-NCS*, electrical stimulation of a motor/sensory peripheral nerve triggers a CMAP/sensory nerve action potential (SNAP), which is displayed on the screen *one sweep at a time* (**Figure 1.3**: CMAP, SNAP). Latency and amplitude are measured and conduction velocity is calculated (16).

EP/ERP responses are obtained using standardized activation-recording protocols and displayed as waves that are time-locked to the stimulus (**Figure 1.3**: third row). Peripheral nerve, spinal cord, subcortical, and cortical *SSEPs* are evoked with median/tibial nerve stimulation (**Figure 1.3**: SSEP), cortical *VEPs* with monocular pattern-shift stimulation (**Figure 1.3**: VEP), *BAEPs* with monoaural stimulation (**Figure 1.3**: BAEP), pyramidal tract and myogenic *MEPs* with transcranial electric/magnetic stimulation (**Figure 1.3**: MEP), and cortical *ERPs* with cognitive processes or tasks (not shown in **Figure 1.3**). EP/ERP requires *signal averaging* and juxtaposition of two or more averages to demonstrate *replicability*. Although the most reliable indicator of pathology in routine EP studies is *latency prolongation*, the most sensitive indicator of impending injury during EP monitoring is *decreasing amplitude* of response (33).

Autonomic function test results are commonly displayed as graphs in the time domain (**Figure 1.3**: bottom) (34). In *HR-DB*, a graph of ECG R-R interval shows how HR changes with respiration (**Figure 1.3**). The BP and HR are plotted as a function of expiratory pressure in *VAL* (**Figure 1.3**) and as a function of the time of tilt in *HUT* (**Figure 1.3**). The *QSART* record is a graph of sweat output or rate of sweating in response to iontophoresis of acetylcholine through the skin (**Figure 1.3**). In *TST*, a body surface map of sweat density is constructed based on the change in color of an indicator as it reacts with sweat (not shown).

Mixed-modality tests display the results of different test modalities in one record or in separate records (not shown in **Figure 1.3**). In *PSG*, cross-modal correlation is facilitated by displaying EEG, chin EMG, EOG, respiratory airflow and effort, oxygen saturation, snoring, ECG, and tibialis anterior EMG in the same record. *MNM* employs a variety of techniques for monitoring ICP, cerebral hemodynamics, brain tissue oxygenation, brain biochemistry and metabolic markers, EEG, and other parameters. With the advent of multiparameter probes and other advances in biomedical engineering, we can look forward to more integrated and less invasive approaches to MNM (35).

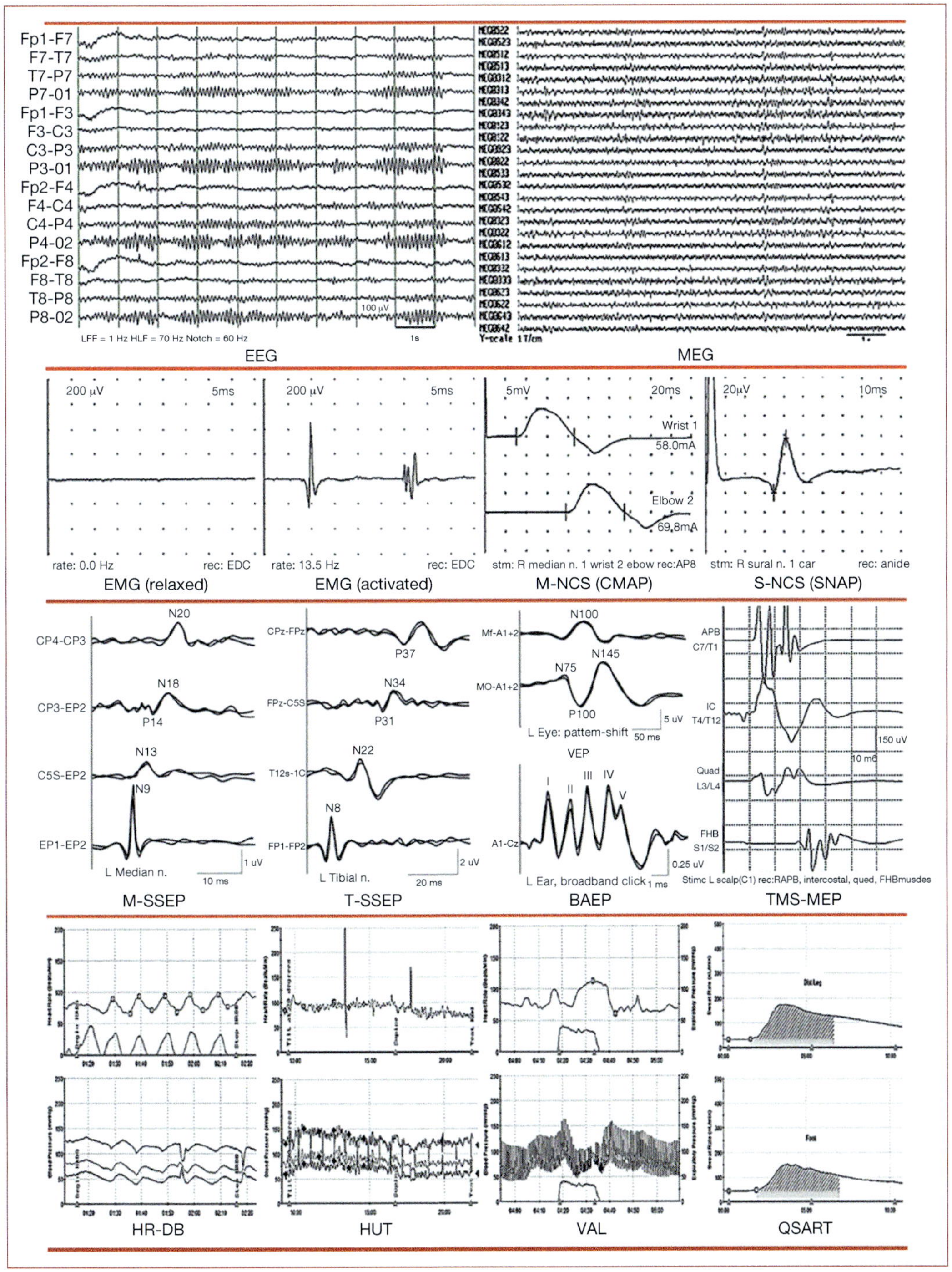

FIGURE 1.3: Clinical neurophysiologic records. Sample records showing how test results are typically displayed in EEG/MEG (top), EMG/NCS (second row), EP studies (third row), and autonomic function tests (bottom). All records are time-domain graphs of signal amplitude (y-axis) versus time (x-axis). Also shown are the amplitude/time scale and, when necessary, the parameter measured, recording site, and channel derivation. Although both sides are tested in routine EMG, NCS, and EP studies, only one side is shown. Image credits: MEG-Dr. Michael M. Quach*; EMG/NCS-Dr. John D. England** and Dr. Christopher O. Edwards**; MEP-Dr. Leo T. Happel** and Kelly M. Clement, CNIM, R.EEG-T***; Autonomic testing: HR-DB, HUT, VAL, and QSART-Dr. Paul A. Lelorier**; the rest are from the teaching files of the authors**. Institutions: *Baylor College of Medicine, **Louisiana State University Health Sciences Center, ***Children's Hospital of New Orleans.

BAEP, brainstem auditory evoked potentials; EMG, electromyography; EP, evoked potential; HR-DB, heart rate variability with deep breathing; HUT, head-up tilt; MEG, magnetoencephalography; NCS, nerve conduction study; M-NCS, motor nerve conduction study; M-SSEP, median nerve somatosensory evoked potential; QSART, quantitative sudomotor axon reflex test; S-NCS, sensory nerve conduction study; TMS-MEP, transcranial magnetic stimulation motor evoked potential; T-SSEP, tibial nerve somatosensory evoked potential; VAL, Valsalva.

NORMAL SIGNAL GENERATION AND PROPAGATION

In CNP, the word *generator* without a qualifier means *signal generator*, not rhythm generator. The signal generator is the biological structure directly generating the signal that is recorded by the instrument (36). It can be a gross structure, a circuit or network, a tissue or cell type, or a cell substructure (**Table 1.3**). The generator paradigm works well if the recorded *macroscopic signal* represents the linear superposition of many elementary *microscopic signals*. This is the case with bioelectric and biomagnetic signals in which the macroscopic signal is the sum of many microscopic signals, each of which is contributed by a *signal-generating unit* (SGU). The notion of a generator is not suitable if the recorded signal is a product of complex transduction events occurring between the biological source and the signal-sensing probe.

Bioelectric and biomagnetic signals can be traced to a *change in the membrane potential* of cells as ion currents flow across the cell membrane in response to a change in the conductance of ion channels (37). A change in membrane potential (depolarization or hyperpolarization) occurs at a focal site of the membrane (e.g., postsynaptic site) and spreads passively and locally (electrotonic conduction). Spatiotemporal summation of local *synaptic potentials* can lead to suprathreshold depolarization and trigger an actively propagating potential, known as *action potential*.

The *SGU and elementary signal is firmly established* for some CNP signals (**Table 1.3**). In needle EMG, the *MUAP* is a compound muscle action potential, the sum of the action potentials of muscle fibers belonging to the same motor unit. The *muscle fiber* is the SGU and the *muscle fiber action potential* (MFAP) is the elementary signal producing the MUAP. The signals recorded in NCS are also compound action potentials. Like the MUAP, the *CMAP*, the *F waves*, and the *H response* are the sum of MFAPs. In contrast, the *SNAP* is the sum of the action potentials of fast-conducting sensory nerve fibers. The *nerve fiber* is the SGU and the *nerve fiber action potential* (NFAP) is the elementary signal producing the SNAP. Like the SNAP, the BAEP *wave I*, the M-SSEP *N9*, and the T-SSEP *N8* are compound nerve action potentials. The direct waves (*D waves*) and indirect waves (*I waves*) in MEP are compound nerve action potentials arising from corticospinal or pyramidal tract fibers. The *CMAP* in MEP is analogous to the CMAP in NCS. The M-SSEP *N13* and the T-SSEP *N22* are the sum of *dorsal horn cell synaptic potentials* and are not generated from the dorsal column (33).

Even if the *principal SGU and elementary signal is known*, the contribution of other SGUs in shaping the macroscopic signal may not be fully understood (**Table 1.3**). For example, the main SGU of the *EEG* is the *cortical pyramidal cell* and the elementary signal is the postsynaptic potential. There is, however, evidence that *glial cells* and *nonsynaptic neural events*, such as action potentials, calcium spikes, voltage-dependent intrinsic oscillations, intrinsic spikes after hyperpolarization, and ephaptic effects, have some role in shaping the EEG (38). The same argument applies to other signals generated in the *cerebral cortex*, including *MEG*, *ERPs*, the VEP *P100*, the M-SSEP *N20*, and the T-SSEP *P37*. There is consensus on the brainstem generators of BAEP *waves III*, *IV*, and *V*, but the *generator and SGU remain controversial* for BAEP *wave II* and for the subcortical SSEPs *P14*, *N18*, *N34*, and *P31*. Despite decades of experience with *BSP*, *CNV*, *P300*, and *MN* recording, the neural generators of cognitive ERPs are still not fully understood.

The *generator concept is not suitable* for some CNP signals and physiological parameters, such as the HR, BP, and sweat output measured during autonomic testing; the nasal airflow, ventilation, and oxygen saturation detected with PSG; and the ICP, ultrasonic flow and near-infrared signals, and chemical compounds monitored during MNM. The mechanisms by which biophysical parameters (e.g., temperature, pressure, flow, volume, stretch) are transduced to electronic current, processed in the circuitry of the apparatus, and transformed into a readable graph are outside the scope of this chapter (39).

Volume conduction is the propagation of an electrical or magnetic field inside a *volume conductor*. It can be represented by a simple model, such as a point source generating a field that spreads in a homogeneous infinite volume conductor. More realistic models take into account the complexities of the source (e.g., charge distribution) and the volume conductor (e.g., varying tissue resistance) (40). Biological tissue responds to a propagating field by inducing an *electrical current*, the magnitude of which is inversely related to tissue *resistance*. Because the *speed of volume conduction* is only slightly less than the speed of light in a vacuum, as soon as a field is generated, it will propagate to the rest of the body almost *instantaneously*. In the case of an electrical field, the *potential* recorded depends on the distance of the recording site from the generator and on the properties of the generator (e.g., field strength, charge distribution) and the volume conductor (e.g., tissue resistance). The *spatial rate of change of electrical potential* reflects the shifting properties of tissues that the field encounters as it spreads inside the body. A *nearfield signal* is characterized by rapid potential drop and substantial loss in signal amplitude even when it is recorded at locations that are not too far from the generator. By contrast, a *farfield signal* is characterized by a slow potential drop and relative preservation in amplitude when recorded far from the generator (41). The extent of volume conduction (nearfield vs. farfield) and the electrode positions (E1 and E2) determine how much of the electrical potential is recorded (**Figure 1.4**).

Neural transmission is a physiological process involving excitation of the cell membrane of nerve, muscle, or other excitable cells. Unlike volume

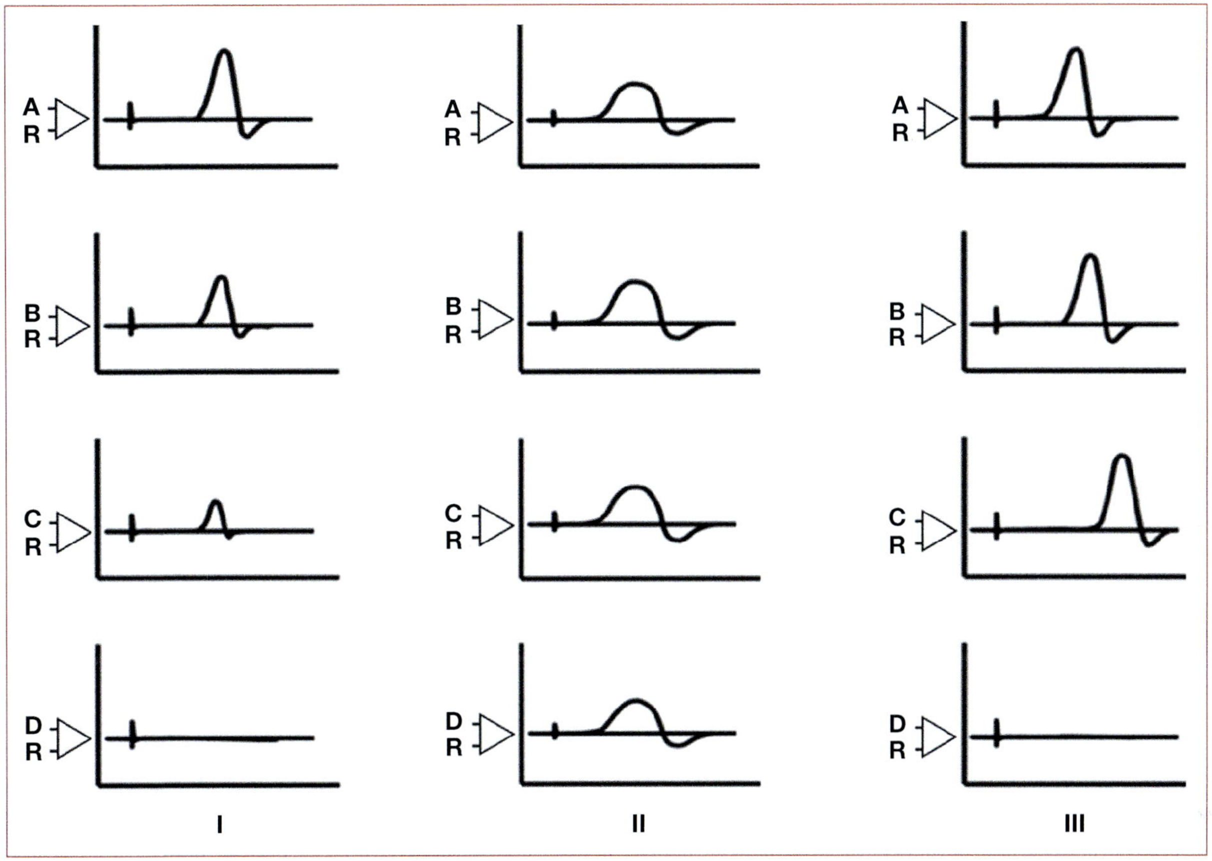

FIGURE 1.4: Spatiotemporal characteristics of signals. Recording the signal close to its generator may be enough to discern its *time-domain characteristics* but, to appreciate its *spatial characteristics*, the signal must be recorded from multiple sites (A, B, C, D in the diagram; R = reference) and the tracings displayed to show the location of signal recording relative to the location of signal generation (top to bottom in diagram). A *stationary nearfield signal* (I) will exhibit decreasing peak amplitude with increasing distance from the generator (A–C) and disappear when no longer detectable (D). A *stationary farfield signal* (II) will have no change or a slight change in peak amplitude with increasing distance from the generator (A–D). A *signal transmitted via neural mechanisms* (III), namely a propagated potential or traveling wave, will show increasing peak latency with increasing distance from the signal generator (A–C) and will not be detected at a site that is located far from the propagating signal (D).

conduction, neural transmission is the result of active signal generation and regeneration along the cell membrane. Because neural transmission involves active processes, its speed is many orders of magnitude lower than the speed of volume conduction (42). A signal spreading by neural transmission is called a *propagating potential* or a *traveling wave*, terms that are both misleading. The electrical potential (potential energy per unit charge) is measured at a point in the field, and its value is always relative to another point (a point at infinity is often used as reference). Although the value of the potential changes from one point to another, it is the electrical field that *physically propagates in space*. The trace or waveform displayed on each channel represents fluctuations of electrophysiologic potential in time, not in space. Unlike in physics, a *traveling wave* in CNP is not a wave propagating in a medium but a series of waves that are actively generated each time a different part of the cell membrane is activated (**Figure 1.4C**).

The *spatiotemporal characteristics of a signal* can be appreciated if the signal is recorded from a few strategic locations and the tracings are displayed "topographically" (**Figure 1.4**). The location of the generator is approximated by the site of maximum signal amplitude. A *stationary nearfield signal* has a peak amplitude that decreases with increasing distance from the generator (**Figure 1.4A**). The abrupt amplitude drop-off with distance of a nearfield signal may render the signal undetectable a few centimeters from the generator (site D). On the other hand, a *stationary farfield signal* will show no change or only very slight change in amplitude with increasing distance from the generator (**Figure 1.4B**). During neural transmission, a *"traveling" nearfield signal* (usually called "propagating potential" or "traveling wave") will show increasing peak latency as the signal "travels" from the initial generation site onward to a series of recording sites (**Figure 1.4C**). The signal is undetectable when recorded far from the path of signal transmission (site D). Clinical neurophysiologic testing methods and protocols differ in terms of *test parameters*, *range of normality*, and *criteria for abnormality* (1–14).

ABNORMAL TEST RESULTS AND CLINICAL IMPLICATIONS

Electrophysiologic signal abnormalities may appear as (a) waves with abnormal amplitude, latency, duration, or morphology; (b) waves recurring with abnormal repetition rate or pattern; (c) waves that emerge de novo due to pathological processes, or (d) wave patterns that are incompatible with the mode of activation or the patient's physiologic state or age (**Table 1.5**). Each of these macroscopic signal abnormalities can be traced to a disturbance in the activity of microscopic SGUs or to an alteration in the properties of the *volume conductor* (43).

Signal amplitude depends on the number of SGUs activated in synchrony and on the fidelity of signal propagation from the generator to the recording electrode. An *abnormally low amplitude* indicates loss of SGUs (e.g., low SNAP amplitude with nerve fiber loss, EEG attenuation with pyramidal cell loss), a decrease in the number of activated SGUs (e.g., low CMAP amplitude with nerve fiber loss or conduction block), desynchrony in SGU activity (e.g., low CMAP amplitude due to temporal dispersion of MFAPs), or changes in the conducting medium increasing the impedance or distance between the generator and electrode (e.g., edema, blood). An *abnormally high amplitude* indicates an increase in the number of SGUs activated (e.g., giant MUAP with muscle reinnervation), abnormal hypersynchrony of SGUs (e.g., epileptiform EEG/MEG waves), or the presence of a low-impedance path of signal propagation from the generator to the recording electrode (e.g., breach rhythm due to skull defect) (43).

Signal conduction time, the time between initial and subsequent signal generation via nonsynaptic and synaptic mechanisms, is quantified as *absolute latency* or *interpeak latency* in the tracing (43). An *abnormally long latency* indicates conduction slowing. For example, an increase in SNAP, CMAP, or SSEP wave latency is seen with peripheral nerve demyelination; an increase in VEP P100 latency with optic nerve demyelination; and an increase in BAEP III-V and SSEP N13-N20 interpeak latencies with central tract demyelination. Mild prolongation in latency may occur with temporal dispersion and asynchronous activation of SGUs. Since an *abnormally short latency* cannot easily be attributed to a pathologic process, a technical explanation should be sought to explain this finding (43).

Wave morphology or configuration is influenced by the duration or frequency, the number of phases or turns, and the contour of waveform components. A normal CNP waveform has a characteristic configuration. For example, SNAPs and VEP P100 waves are typically triphasic, whereas CMAPs and EEG vertex waves are usually biphasic. Because most waveforms have a wide range of acceptable configurations, spatial distribution and other wave characteristics must always be considered in deciding if a wave is normal. An *increase in wave duration and number of phases* imply asynchronous SGU activation (e.g., temporal dispersion from demyelination). Conversely, *shorter wave duration and apiculate contour* indicate SGU hypersynchrony (e.g., EEG/MEG epileptiform sharp waves).

Wave activation, modulation, and repetition pattern reflect recurrent SGU activity resulting from the intrinsic oscillatory behavior of SGUs and the extrinsic influences of other circuit components (44). The pattern of *abnormal activation and recruitment* may be simple (e.g., MUAP recruitment is reduced with motor neuron or nerve pathology and increased with muscle pathology) or complex (e.g., loss of pyramidal cell afferent input suppresses some and releases other activation patterns, such as slow wave rhythms). So-called *abnormal spontaneous activity* indicates hyperexcitability of SGUs (e.g., fibrillation potentials due to muscle denervation hypersensitivity), of non-SGU circuit components (e.g., fasciculation potentials from nerve irritability), or of the entire functional circuit including SGUs (e.g., epileptiform activity). Perturbations in network dynamics may appear as rhythmic/periodic waves with *abnormal repetition rate* (e.g., slower rhythms are seen in the EEG/MEG tracings with encephalopathy).

Spatial distribution is demonstrated by recording the signal from multiple body locations. Pathologic processes that disturb the time-domain characteristics of a signal can also affect the signal's spatial characteristics. It is always prudent to exclude technical factors (e.g., improper electrode placement) and normal physiologic changes (e.g., anterior displacement of the EEG alpha rhythm in drowsiness) before attributing spatial abnormalities to pathological processes. Lastly, signals with time-domain and spatial characteristics that appear "normal" are considered abnormal if their characteristics do not conform to the *age* and *physiologic state* of the patient (**Table 1.5**).

Modality-specific CNP tests are performed to assess the *functional integrity of signaling pathways*. Most of these tests can also assess *specific parts of the pathway* to determine which structures are involved in the pathologic process. A general scheme for classifying electrophysiologic test abnormalities was described earlier (**Table 1.5**). We will now describe the salient abnormalities encountered in each test category and their *clinical implications* (**Table 1.6**).

EEG and MEG are sensitive to pathologic processes that implicate the *cerebral cortex*, either directly or indirectly through its connections with the *diencephalon/brainstem*. By and large, abnormal EEG and MEG waveforms have the same clinical implications. However, differences in the physics of electrical and magnetic fields prevent us from extrapolating all EEG "interpretation rules" to MEG. Abnormal EEG/MEG waves are either epileptiform or nonepileptiform. *Epileptiform activity* indicates ongoing epileptic disturbances of the brain, either interictal (spikes or sharp waves) or ictal (seizures) (45). *Nonepileptiform abnormalities* include changes in background rhythm, abnormal slow waves, abnormal response to activation, and asymmetries in amplitude or other parameters (46). As a rule, focal nonepileptiform abnormalities indicate localized cerebral dysfunction if intermittent and structural lesions if persistent while diffuse bihemispheric changes imply encephalopathy, encephalitis, or neurodegeneration. *Periodic discharges* are either epileptiform or nonepileptiform (47) and, if epileptiform, they are either ictal, interictal, or due to an epileptic disturbance that lie somewhere along the *ictal–interictal continuum* (48).

EMG and NCS have been, and are still, the best tools for assessing *peripheral nerve and muscle* physiology. Needle EMG findings, particularly abnormalities in *MUAP morphology and recruitment pattern*, can distinguish a myopathy from a neuropathy or motor neuronopathy. *Abnormal spontaneous activity* implies nerve fiber irritability if motor units are involved and denervation hypersensitivity if individual muscle fibers are affected. *Increased jitter* in single-fiber EMG is diagnostic of a neuromuscular junction disorder. The pattern of *CMAP/SNAP amplitude and the latency abnormalities in NCS* will clarify if a neuropathy is focal, multifocal, or diffuse; if it is sensory, motor, or mixed; and if it is primarily due to demyelination or axonal loss. *CMAP amplitude increment/decrement* with repetitive nerve stimulation can differentiate a presynaptic from a postsynaptic neuromuscular junction disorder. If the routine NCS is normal, the finding of *abnormal F waves* implies more proximal involvement of the motor pathway (e.g., a radiculopathy or motor neuronopathy). *Abnormal H, blink*, or *long-latency reflexes* indicate peripheral nerve pathology or a lesion in the intra-axial segment of the reflex pathway.

EP and ERP can detect a disease in its early stages if it involves structures in the signaling pathway. Conduction slowing *increases absolute latency* if present between the sensory receptor and EP generator (e.g., peripheral nerve demyelination) and *increases interpeak latency* if present between two EP generators (e.g., central tract demyelination). A *loss of amplitude* is particularly significant if it represents a left–right asymmetry or a relative change from baseline, such as during intraoperative monitoring (IOM). *Giant SSEP or VEP cortical potentials* indicate cortical hyperexcitability (46). Impairment in attentional or cognitive processing from neurodegeneration or psychopathology may *increase P300 latency* or *decrease P300 amplitude*, or it may result in *abnormal MN morphology* (47). Brain disorders that cause psychomotor retardation often manifest as an early *decrease in BSP or CNV amplitude*.

Autonomic function tests evaluate cardiovagal, adrenergic, and sudomotor autonomic functions. In *HR-DB*, disorders that impair the cardiovagal reflex manifest as *reduced or absent HR* with deep breathing. Certain *abnormal BP and HR patterns* during HUT or VAL are valuable for diagnosing sympathetic dysfunction or generalized dysautonomias due to diabetes mellitus, amyloidosis, and other diseases (6,34). In QSART, *low sweat output* indicates sympathetic sudomotor failure, as in distal small-fiber neuropathy and idiopathic anhidrosis, and *high sweat output* indicates sweat gland hypersensitivity, as in reflex sympathetic dystrophy. The *pattern of anhidrosis and hyperhidrosis* in TST allows the differential diagnosis to be narrowed down to a few dysautonomias (6,34).

Sleep studies involve multimodal tracking of sleep stage to detect *abnormalities in sleep* latency, efficiency, and architecture (7). In PSG, *other physiologic disturbances* can also be detected, such as apneas, increased airway resistance, blood oxygen desaturation, cardiac arrhythmias, abnormal movements, and parasomnias. During *MNM*, changes in ICP, cerebral blood flow, brain tissue oxygenation, and/or biochemical markers of brain metabolism indicate impending brain injury or exacerbation of previous injury (9,35).

TABLE 1.6: Abnormal Neurophysiologic Test Results and Their Clinical Implications

EEG/MEG
Epileptiform activity–epileptic brain disturbance with or without structural brain lesion or encephalopathy
Periodic discharges–epileptic brain disturbance often with structural brain lesion or encephalopathy
Altered background rhythm–usually encephalopathy if generalized and structural brain lesion if focal
Abnormal slow-wave activity–usually encephalopathy if generalized and structural brain lesion if focal
Abnormal response to activation–usually encephalopathy if generalized and structural brain lesion if focal
Amplitude and other asymmetries–structural brain lesion if persistent and physiologic disturbance if transient
Needle EMG
Abnormal insertional activity–increased with muscle fiber irritability and decreased with muscle fiber loss
Abnormal spontaneous activity–muscle fiber denervation hypersensitivity or motor neuron or nerve irritability
High-amplitude, short-duration MUAPs–neuropathic MUAPs with collateral reinnervation of muscle fibers
Low-amplitude, long-duration MUAPs–myopathic MUAPs with loss of muscle fibers
Decreased recruitment of MUAPs–motor neuron or nerve fiber pathology preventing motor unit activation
Increased recruitment of MUAPs–loss of muscle fibers with compensatory early motor unit recruitment
Increased jitter with single-fiber EMG–neuromuscular junction disorder
NCS
Decreased CMAP amplitude–motor neuron or axonal loss, motor conduction block or temporal dispersion
Decreased SNAP amplitude–sensory axonal loss, sensory conduction block or temporal dispersion
Increased CMAP latency–motor conduction slowing with demyelination of large motor nerve fibers
Increased SNAP latency–sensory conduction slowing with demyelination of large sensory nerve fibers
Increased F wave latency–motor conduction slowing with demyelination of distal or proximal motor nerve fibers
Absent F waves–conduction failure due to motor nerve or axon pathology or to motor conduction block
Absent H reflex–conduction failure due to a lesion in the sensory, central, or motor part of the stretch reflex circuit
Abnormal repetitive stimulation–presynaptic or postsynaptic disorder of neuromuscular junction transmission
EP
Increased absolute latency–delayed signal conduction from peripheral stimulation site to EP generator
Increased interpeak latency–delayed signal conduction between two EP generators due to a central tract disorder
Decreased EP amplitude–conduction failure in central tract fibers (e.g., compression or ischemia) or loss of SGUs
Increased EP amplitude–hypersynchrony (e.g., giant SSEPs or VEPs with cortical hyperexcitability)
Absent EP response–generator dysfunction or disconnection from signaling pathway
Abnormal wave configuration–most of the above processes will also affect wave morphology and duration

(continued)

TABLE 1.6: Abnormal Neurophysiologic Test Results and Their Clinical Implications (*continued*)

ERP
Increased P300 latency–cognitive dysfunction due to dementia or psychiatric disorder
Decreased P300 amplitude–cognitive dysfunction due to dementia or psychiatric disorder
Altered MN morphology–attentional perceptual processing deficit due to dementia or psychiatric disorder
Decreased amplitude of BSP early components–psychomotor retardation due to psychiatric or movement disorder
Decreased amplitude of CNV late component–psychomotor retardation due to psychiatric or movement disorder
Autonomic testing
Reduced or absent HR-DB–impairment of cardiovagal reflex
Abnormal HR response to VAL–impairment of vagal component of baroreflex
Abnormal BP response to HUT/VAL–sympathetic adrenergic dysfunction (e.g., generalized dysautonomias)
Reduced sweat secretion rate in QSART–sympathetic sudomotor dysfunction (e.g., distal small-fiber neuropathy)
Increased sweat secretion rate in QSART–sympathetic sudomotor hyperactivity (e.g., reflex sympathetic dystrophy)
Abnormal sweat patterns in TST–anhidrosis or hyperhidrosis (e.g., generalized dysautonomias)
Sleep studies
Abnormal sleep continuity or pattern–impairment in chronophasic, homeostatic, and/or afferent sleep-wake drives
Decreased or absent respiratory airflow and/or effort–increased upper airway resistance, obstructive/central apnea
Blood oxygenation desaturation–hypoxia from obstructive/central apnea, cardiac insufficiency, etc.
ECG changes–tachyarrhythmia or bradyarrhythmia from sleep apnea, cardiac disease, etc.
Anterior tibialis EMG–periodic limb disorder of sleep, other movement disorders
Neuromonitoring
Elevation of ICP–cerebral edema, space-occupying lesion, impaired autoregulation, abnormal CSF flow dynamics
Abnormal cerebral blood flow–increased ICP, vasospasm, impaired autoregulation, reperfusion
Abnormal brain oxygenation–ischemia/hyperemia, abnormal oxygen extraction, flow-metabolism decoupling
Abnormal biochemistry–impaired energy-substrate metabolism, cell injury, cell membrane breakdown

Note: Listed for each test modality are the most commonly encountered test result abnormalities and associated pathological processes, not specific diseases.

BSP, Bereitschaftspotential; CMAP, compound motor action potential; CNV, contingent negative variation; CSF, cerebral spinal fluid; EMG, electromyography; EP, evoked potential; ERP, event-related potentials; HR, heart rate; HR-DB, heart rate variability with deep breathing; HUT, head-up tilt; ICP, intracranial pressure; MEG, magnetoencephalography; MN, mismatch negativity; MUAP, motor unit action potential; NCS, nerve conduction study; QSART, quantitative sudomotor axon reflex test; SGU, signal-generating unit; SNAP, sensory nerve action potential; SSEP, somatosensory evoked potentials; TST, thermoregulatory sweat test; VAL, Valsalva; VEP, visual evoked potentials.

ARTIFACT RECOGNITION AND OTHER TECHNICAL CHALLENGES

Although the terms "artifact" and "noise" are used interchangeably, an *artifact* is, strictly speaking, the graphical depiction of *noise* entering the system and mixing with the desired signal (**Table 1.7**). Simply put, *noise* is the undesired analog signal and *artifact* is the undesired digital trace or waves. *Separating noise from desired signal* is achieved with modern technology and proper technique (25,26,49,50). The use of finely engineered signal transducers and recording equipment, the optimal placement of electrodes and sensors, proper grounding, and the ability to recognize and avoid potential sources of noise are crucial for maximizing the signal-to-noise ratio during neurophysiologic testing (**Figure 1.1**).

Despite the best technology and technique, some amount of noise will still enter the recording system and appear in the record as an artifact. *Separating artifact from "useful waves"* is accomplished by direct inspection of the record and, if necessary, by additional digital signal processing (26). Visual analysis involves artifact recognition based on the spatiotemporal characteristics of waves. Depending on the test, postacquisition digital signal processing, such as averaging, artifact rejection, digital filtering, and quantitative analysis, may be performed to eliminate or reduce artifact (see Chapter 2).

Artifact classification is based on the physical properties and source of noise causing the artifact and on the mechanism by which noise gains access to the recording system (**Table 1.7**) (25,27,49). Any part of the recording system is a potential *portal for noise* but the most vulnerable sites are the movable wires outside the chassis of the recording apparatus and the interface between machine and body where transduction of biological signals to electronic current takes place. The *electrode–tissue interface* is usually the site of biological to electronic signal transduction during CNP testing (50).

Environmental and instrument noise originates from sources outside the patient's body (49). In the hospital, the most significant source of *environmental noise* is alternating current (AC) from wires and equipment in the building (27,49). *AC noise* entering the recording system, via its inductive effects on electrode wires or via poorly applied electrodes, result in *60-Hz artifact* (50 Hz in Europe) (27). Electric-powered equipment in the room or building, such as radiological scanners and surgical devices, may contribute to environmental noise (27,49). *Instrument noise*, such as thermal noise and amplifier noise, originates from the electronics of the recording apparatus. Good engineering design keeps instrument noise to a minimum but it can be an issue if the equipment is old, malfunctioning, or poorly maintained (49).

Noise generated at the signal transduction site, usually the electrode–tissue interface, is a common source of artifacts in CNP (49,50). *Slight movement* of electrodes and other instabilities in the electrode–tissue interface, such as electrode polarization or impedance mismatch, may affect charge distribution and currents at the electrode–tissue interface and lead to *signal distortion* or *electrode artifact* (50). Gross movements of multiple electrodes, wires, or cable connections may appear as a *movement artifact* in the record. An electrode with high impedance can be "replaced" by the ground electrode, resulting in *ground lead artifact*.

Medical devices that deliver current to the patient can be the source of artifacts (25,49). In some neurophysiologic studies (e.g., NCS, EP), the *stimulus artifact* indicates the time of stimulation, but excessive stimulus artifacts can interfere with and distort the signal (3,16). *Implanted medical devices*, such as pacemakers and stimulators, produce characteristic artifacts. During CNP testing, some *normal physiological processes* in the patient's body may be captured in the record as *physiological artifacts* (27). Note that a waveform can represent desired signal in one test or in one channel and the same waveform can be a physiological artifact in another test or in a different channel in the same record.

Other technical issues encountered in CNP include (a) *improper placement of recording electrodes* causing artifactual changes in signal or signal distortion; (b) *improper stimulus delivery* leading to insufficient activation, cross-activation of other structures, or contamination by stimulus artifact; and (c) *failure to recognize the cause of signal distortion*, such as temperature, humidity, and other physical factors, the presence of a low-impedance path or an intervening substance between the generator and recording electrode, or technical factors, such as poor equipment maintenance and calibration (**Table 1.7**). This book and atlas will provide students and professionals of CNP a deep understanding of artifacts and technical issues that are encountered during each of the CNP tests introduced in this chapter.

TABLE 1.7: Sources of Aartifacts in Clinical Neurophysiologic Testing

Sources of Artifacts
Environmental sources–electric, magnetic, or electromagnetic field from wires and equipment in the building AC noise–AC artifact: 60-cycle artifact in the United States, 50-cycle artifact in Europe Scanners and other equipment–AC artifact, high-frequency artifact Fluorescent light–if light intensity is strong it can contribute to AC artifact Strobe light–artifact is time-locked to the flash and reflects the photic frequency of the source Television and video monitors–usually high-frequency artifacts (e.g., 300 Hz) Diathermy or cautery device–usually high-frequency artifacts (e.g., 120 Hz) Dripping fluid–inductive effects on electrode wires result in artifact (e.g., intravenous fluid drip artifact) Radiofrequency noise–audible and can often be identified (e.g., paging system, phone ringing)
Recording instrument–electronic circuitry and components of the recording apparatus Thermal noise–random motion of charges in any part of the apparatus may result in high-frequency artifact Shot noise–charges crossing a junction (e.g., n-p junctions in a transistor, may result in artifact) Equipment wiring noise–AC noise from wires in apparatus; produces 60-Hz artifact (50 Hz in Europe) Amplifier noise–intrinsic noise of an operational amplifier Filter noise–ringing artifacts that appear as spurious signals near sharp transitions Quantization noise–arises from digitization; often negligible with respect to other sources of noise Switching artifact–opening and closing of control switches on equipment
Signal transduction site–electrochemical change at the interface between the probe and the patient's tissue Increased impedance–loss of signal, electrode artifacts, AC artifact, and other artifacts Poor electrode contact–electrode can be "replaced" by ground electrode resulting in ground lead artifact Impedance mismatch–reduced cancellation of common-mode noise resulting in AC and other artifacts Salt bridge or short circuit–increased cancellation resulting in reduced signal amplitude or signal loss Electrode polarization–altered charge distribution and current at the interface resulting in signal distortion Junctional potential–altered charge distribution and current at the interface resulting in signal distortion Slight electrode movement–altered charge distribution resulting in signal distortion or electrode artifact Gross movement–multiple electrodes, wires, or cable box connections affected resulting in movement artifact Mechanical vibrations–motion artifact from ventilator, compressors, and other hospital equipment
Current delivering devices–external or implanted medical device injecting current to the patient's body Neurodiagnostic stimulator–excessive stimulus artifact can interfere with the signal (e.g., SNAP or CMAP) Implanted cardiac device–distinctive artifact frequency and morphology (e.g., pacemaker/defibrillator artifact) Implanted nerve stimulator–distinctive artifact frequency and morphology (e.g., vagus nerve stimulator) Transcutaneous stimulator–distinctive artifact frequency; transcutaneous electrical nerve stimulation

(*continued*)

TABLE 1.7: Sources of Artifacts in Clinical Neurophysiologic Testing (*continued*)

Normal physiological processes–normal activity of biological structures in the patient's body Eye movement–eye blink, slow lateral eye movements, eye flutter, and other optokinetic artifacts Oropharyngeal activity–glossokinetic, talking, biting, chewing, teeth-grinding, snoring, and other artifacts Skeletal muscle activity–EMG artifact, tremor artifact, photomyogenic artifact, motor artifact in SNAP Cardiovascular activity–ECG artifact, pulse artifact, cardioballistic artifact Sudomotor activity–sweat artifact, galvanic skin response or electrodermal artifact Movement of body parts–movement artifacts (see Signal transduction site section)
Other technical factors–not considered noise but can result in artifactual signal distortion Improperly placed electrodes–artifactual change in signal amplitude, latency, and other characteristics Suboptimal stimulus delivery–insufficient activation, cross-activation of other structures, stimulus artifact Altered volume conduction–fluid or substance between generator and electrode, low impedance path Temperature effects–artifactual change in amplitude and latency if not recognized and remedied Humidity and other physical factors–e.g., QSART is sensitive to humidity Poor equipment maintenance–uncalibrated apparatus, old corroded sensors

Noise entering the recording system may appear as an artifact in the record. Potential sources of noise during clinical neurophysiological testing include (a) electrical, magnetic, or electromagnetic fields from wires and equipment in the building (environmental noise); (b) circuit components of the recording apparatus (instrument noise); (c) electrochemical change in the interface between the recording apparatus and the patient (transduction site noise); (d) current delivered to the patient from diagnostic and therapeutic devices (e.g., pacemaker and stimulator); and (e) normal activity of biological structures in the patient's body (physiological source of artifact). To these five groups, we can add (f) technical factors that are not considered noise but can degrade test results.

AC, alternating current; CMAP, compound motor action potential; EMG, electromyography; QSART, quantitative sudomotor axon reflex test; SNAP, sensory nerve action potential.

REFERENCES

1. Ebersole JS, Husain AM, Nordli DR, eds. *Current Practice of Clinical Electroencephalography*. 4th ed. Philadelphia, PA: Wolters Kluwer Health; 2014.
2. Papanicolaou AC, ed. *Clinical Magnetoencephalography and Magnetic Source Imaging*. Cambridge, UK: Cambridge University Press; 2009.
3. Kimura J. *Electrodiagnosis in Diseases of Nerve and Muscle: Principles and Practice*. 4th ed. New York, NY: Oxford University Press; 2013.
4. Husain AM. Evoked potentials overview. In: Ebersole JS, Husain AM, Nordli DR, eds. *Current Practice of Clinical Electroencephalography*. 4th ed. Philadelphia, PA: Wolters Kluwer Health; 2014:442-487.
5. Luck SJ. *An Introduction to the Event-Related Potential Technique*. 2nd ed. Cambridge, MA: MIT Press; 2014.
6. Benarroch EE, ed. *Autonomic Neurology*. New York, NY: Oxford University Press; 2014.
7. Chokroverty S, Radtke R, Mullington J. Polysomnography: technical and clinical aspects. In: Schomer DL, Lopes da Silva FH, eds. *Niedermeyer's Electroencephalography: Basic Principles, Clinical Applications, and Related Fields*. 6th ed. Philadelphia, PA: Lippincott Williams & Wilkins; 2011:817-864.
8. Husain AM, ed. *A Practical Approach to Neurophysiologic Intraoperative Monitoring*. New York, NY: Demos Medical Publishing; 2008.

9. Le Roux PD, Levine JM, Kofke WA. *Monitoring in Neurocritical Care*. Philadelphia, PA: Elsevier; 2013.

10. He B, Liu Z. Multimodal functional neuroimaging: integrating functional MRI and EEG/MEG. *IEEE Rev Biomed Eng*. 2008;1:23-40. doi:10.1109/RBME.2008.2008233.

11. American Clinical Neurophysiology Society (ACNS) Guidelines and Consensus Statements. American Clinical Neurophysiology Society website. https://www.acns.org/practice/guidelines. Updated: August 11, 2016.

12. Deuschl, G, Eisen A, eds. Recommendations for the practice of clinical neurophysiology: guidelines of the International Federation of Clinical Neurophysiology. *Electroencephalogr Clin Neurophysiol Suppl*. 1999;52:1-304.

13. American Association of Neuromuscular & Electrodiagnostic Medicine (AANEM) Practice Guidelines and Quality. American Association of Neuromuscular & Electrodiagnostic Medicine (AANEM) website. http://www.aanem.org/Practice/Guidelines-and-Performance-Measures. .

14. American Academy of Neurology. Assessment: clinical autonomic testing report of the Therapeutics and Technology Assessment Subcommittee of the American Academy of Neurology. *Neurology*. 1996;46(3):873-880.

15. Malmivuo J. Comparison of the properties of EEG and MEG in detecting the electric activity of the brain. *Brain Topogr*. 2012;25(1):1-19. doi:10.1007/s10548-011-0202-1.

16. Preston DC, Shapiro BE, eds. *Electromyography and Neuromuscular Disorders: Clinical-Electrophysiological Correlations*. 3rd ed. London, UK: Elsevier Saunders; 2013.

17. Hallett M. Electrophysiologic evaluation of movement disorders. In: Aminoff MJ, ed. *Aminoff's Electrodiagnosis in Clinical Neurology*. 6th ed. Amsterdam, the Netherlands: Elsevier Saunders; 2012:437-454.

18. Emerson RG. Somatosensory evoked potentials. In: Levins KH, Luders HO, eds. *Comprehensive Clinical Neurophysiology*. Philadelphia, PA: W.B. Saunders Company; 2000:543-564.

19. Epstein CM. Visual evoked potentials. In: Levins KH, Luders HO, eds. *Comprehensive Clinical Neurophysiology*. Philadelphia, PA: W.B. Saunders Company; 2000:507-524.

20. Luders HO, Terada K. Auditory evoked potentials. In: Levins KH, Luders HO, eds. *Comprehensive Clinical Neurophysiology*. Philadelphia, PA: W.B. Saunders Company; 2000:525-541.

21. Galloway GM, Nuwer MR, Lopez JR, et al., eds. *Intraoperative Neurophysiologic Monitoring*. Cambridge, UK: Cambridge University Press; 2010.

22. Nuwer MR, Emerson RG, Galloway G, et al. Evidence-based guideline update: intraoperative spinal monitoring with somatosensory and transcranial electrical motor evoked potentials. *J Clin Neurophysiol*. 2012;29(1):101-108.doi:10.1212/WNL.0b013e318247fa0e.

23. Lopez da Silva FH. Event-related potentials: general aspects of methodology and quantification. In: Schomer DL, Lopes da Silva FH, eds. *Niedermeyer's Electroencephalography: Basic Principles, Clinical Applications, and Related Fields*. 6th ed. Philadelphia, PA: Lippincott Williams & Wilkins; 2011:923-934.

24. Buijs RM, Swaab DF, eds. *Autonomic Nervous System*. Amsterdam, the Netherlands: Elsevier BV; 2013. *Handbook of Clinical Neurology*; vol 117 (3rd series).

25. Mainardi LT, Bianchi AM, Cerutti S. Digital biomedical signal acquisition and processing. In: Liang H, Bronzino JD, Peterson DR, eds. *Biosignal Processing Principles and Practices*. Boca Raton, FL: CRC Press; 2013:1.1-1.23.

26. Lagerlund TD. Digital signal processing. In: Daube JR, Rubin DI, eds. *Clinical Neurophysiology*. 3rd ed. New York, NY: Oxford University Press; 2009:53-68.

27. Daube JR. Waveforms and artifacts, In: Daube JR, Rubin DI, eds. *Clinical Neurophysiology*. 3rd ed. New York, NY: Oxford University Press; 2009:103-114.

28. Fisch BJ. *Fisch and Spehlmann's EEG Primer: Basic Principles of Digital and Analog EEG*. 3rd ed. Amsterdam, the Netherlands: Elsevier; 1999.

29. Chiappa KH. Principles of evoked potentials. In: Chiappa KH, ed. *Evoked Potentials in Clinical Medicine*. 3rd ed. Philadelphia, PA: Lippincott-Raven; 1997:1-30.

30. Tatum WO. *Handbook of EEG Interpretation*. 2nd ed. New York, NY: Demos Medical Publishing; 2014.

31. Bagić AI, Bowyer SM, Kirsch HE, et al. American Clinical MEG Society (ACMEGS) position statement #2: the value of magnetoencephalography (MEG)/magnetic source imaging (MSI) in noninvasive presurgical mapping of eloquent cortices of patients preparing for surgical interventions. *J Clin Neurophysiol*. 2017;34(3):189-195. doi:10.1097/WNP.0000000000000366.

32. Rubin DI. Needle electromyography: basic concepts and patterns of abnormalities. *Neurol Clin*. 2012;30(2):429-456. doi:10.1016/j.ncl.2011.12.009.

33. Yamada T, Meng E, Seaba P. Principles of evoked potentials. In: Yamada T, Meng E, eds. *Practical Guide for Clinical Neurophysiologic Testing: EP, LTM, IOM, PSG and NCS*. Philadelphia, PA: Lippincott Williams & Wilkins; 2011.

34. Low PA, Tomalia VA, Park K. Autonomic function tests: some clinical applications. *J Clin Neurol*. 2013;9(1):1-8. doi:10.3988/jcn.2013.9.1.1.

35. Kirkman MA, Smith M. Multimodal intracranial monitoring: implications for clinical practice. *Anesthesiol Clin*. 2012;30(2):269-287. doi:10.1016/j.anclin.2012.05.007.

36. Lagerlund TD. Electrophysiological generators in clinical neurophysiology. In: Daube JR, Rubin DI, eds. *Clinical Neurophysiology*. 3rd ed. New York, NY: Oxford University Press; 2009:97-101.

37. Daube JR, Stead SM. Basic neurophysiology. In: Daube JR, Rubin DI, eds. *Clinical Neurophysiology*. 3rd ed. New York, NY: Oxford University Press; 2009:69-95.

38. Buzsáki G, Anastassiou CA, Koch C. The origin of extracellular fields and currents—EEG, ECoG, LFP and spikes. *Nat Rev Neurosci*. 2012;13(6):407-420.

39. Hansman RJ Jr. Characteristics of instrumentation. In: Webster JG, Eren H, eds. *Measurement, Instrumentation, and Sensors Handbook: Spatial, Mechanical, Thermal, and Radiation Measurement*. 2nd ed. Boca Raton, FL: CRC Press/Taylor & Francis Group; 2014:2:1-9.

40. Lagerlund TD, Rubin DI, Daube JR. Volume conduction. In: Daube JR, Rubin DI, eds. *Clinical Neurophysiology*. 3rd ed. New York, NY: Oxford University Press; 2009:33-51.

41. Rutkove SB. Introduction to volume conduction. In: Blum AS, Rutkove SB, eds. *The Clinical Neurophysiology Primer*. Totowa, NJ: Humana Press Inc.; 2007:43-53.

42. Stegeman DF, Dumitru D, King JC, et al. Near- and far-fields: source characteristics and the conducting medium in neurophysiology. *J Clin Neurophysiol*. 1997;14(5):429-442. doi:10.1097/00004691.

43. Quian Quiroga R, Panzeri S. *Principles of Neural Coding*. Boca Raton, FL: CRC Press; 2013.

44. Ashwin P, Coombes S, Nicks RJ. Mathematical frameworks for oscillatory network dynamics in neuroscience. *J Math Neurosci*. 2016;6(1):2. doi:10.1186/s13408-015-0033-6.

45. Mader EC Jr., Olejniczak PW. Epilepsy syndromes. In: Fisch BJ, ed. *Epilepsy and Intensive Care Monitoring: Principles and Practice*. New York, NY: Demos Medical Publishing; 2010:119-150.

46. Benbadis SR. Abnormal nonepileptiform EEG. In: Tatum WO, ed. *Handbook of EEG Interpretation*. 2nd ed. New York, NY: Demos Medical Publishing; 2014:57-78.

47. Hirsch LJ, LaRoche SM, Gaspard N, et al. American clinical neurophysiology society's standardized critical care EEG terminology: 2012 version. *J Clin Neurophysiol*. 2013;30(1):1-27. doi:10.1097/WNP.0b013e3182784729.

48. Rodríguez V, Rodden MF, LaRoche SM. Ictal-interictal continuum: a proposed treatment algorithm. *Clin Neurophysiol*. 2016;127(4):2056-2064. doi:10.1016/j.clinph.2016.02.003.

49. Semmlow J. Signals and systems: Noise and variability. In: Ratner BD, Hoffman AS, Schoen FJ, et al., eds. *Biomedical Engineering Desk Reference*. Oxford, UK: Academic Press; 2009:73-76.

50. Button V. *Principles of Measurement and Transduction of Biomedical Variables*. Oxford, UK: Elsevier; 2015.

CHAPTER 2

Equipment and Instrumentation

Jonathan J. Halford

INTRODUCTION

The recognition of noncerebral signals in clinical neurophysiology (CNP) requires both the ability to recognize artifactual patterns and an understanding of the physics and engineering principles that are involved. Although most clinical neurophysiologists are adept at recognizing patterns, few have formal engineering or physics training. This should not discourage practitioners in the field of CNP, because most of the concepts relevant to clinical practice which underlie the technical aspect of their instruments can be supported using simple equations. The challenge is that the number of important concepts required to understand how the equipment works increases every year. Over the last several decades, the major driver of this evolution has been the digitization of recording. We all live in an *analog* world in which measured electrophysiologic values can take an infinite number of positive or negative values. Neurophysiological recordings began as a completely analog enterprise with equipment that channeled electrical currents which could take on an infinite set of values. Obviously, several decades ago this abruptly changed. Now all of the neurophysiology equipment on the market has a substantial *digital* component, meaning that the equipment operates using one or more internal computers that measures a limited number of possible discrete quantities.

As every year passes, we see more analog components of neurophysiology-recording equipment replaced by digital components. An example of this is the spread of digital equipment beyond the amplifier, storage, and visualization stages of the recording to the electrodes themselves in recent research using EEG recording systems. Another example is the change in how signals are filtered. Previously, this required only an understanding of analog electronics. Now, signal filtering is performed by both analog and digital equipment. The reason for this *"digital spread"* is that, although digital systems force the recorded signal to become discrete (potentially leading to a loss of relevant information), they are faster than analog systems, offer lower power consumption, allow greater control on signal information flow, and are less susceptible to noise.

Despite this digital spread, most artifacts in neurophysiology recordings have their source in the initial stages of the recording process, which are analog and will probably remain analog for a long time or indefinitely. For this reason, this chapter focuses on an explanation of analog recording concepts but also provides explanation of important digital recording concepts. Additionally, certain mathematical concepts in information theory will be presented when they are relevant to artifacts due to digital signal postprocessing and display.

ANALOG RECORDING

Basic Electrical Principles

The movement of electrical charge in currents within the nervous system leads to the electromyography (EMG), EEG, and magnetoencephalography (MEG) signal. Electric charges exist in two forms (with either positive or negative polarity) and are found in packages or "quanta" of a particular unit size—the negative charge of one electron or the positive charge of one proton. Protons are usually fixed within atoms and cannot move, but some electrons from each atom, especially in certain elements, are free to move between atoms. Their movement creates electrical current flow. Charges also create electrical fields which cause them to act at a distance upon other charges, with like charges repelling each other and opposite charges attracting. Electrical current flows best through materials called *conductors*, which are composed primarily of metals or solutions. When electric current flows through a conductor, it also creates a magnetic field around it. The measurement unit for charge (Q) is the *coulomb*, which carries the charge of 6.24×10^{18} electrons. Flow of electrical current (I) is measured in *amperes*, also called "amps," and is equal to the flow of one coulomb of charge per second.

$$I = \frac{dQ}{dt} \qquad \text{(}dQ\text{ is the change in }Q\text{; }dt\text{ is the change in time)}$$

Electrical current does not flow very fast, only approximately 0.25 mm/second, but the field of distribution spreads out within the conductor at the speed of light. This is similar to what happens in a pipe filled with water in which, when a small quantity of water is forced into one end of the pipe, the pressure increase within the water spreads very rapidly and a small quantity of water is immediately forced out of the other end of the pipe, despite the water itself in the pipe not having travelled far. Any changes to a magnetic field created by changes in the movement of electrical charge also spreads out from the conductor at the speed of light.

Electrical devices work by causing current to flow around in a circle, called a *circuit*. The *voltage* (V) is the amount of potential energy between two points in that circuit. The unit measure of V is the *volt*, which is the energy that is measured in *joules* which will be delivered per coulomb of charge when that charge passes between two points in the circuit. A common analogy to understand electric current flow is water flow to and from a water tank. The volume of water is equivalent to Q, the rate of flow is equivalent to I, and V is equivalent to the difference in the pressure of water between two points in the flow system (such as between the top of the water tank and the pipe in your home). Like an electrical circuit, water delivery in a city runs in a circle, with water flowing down from the tank to various destinations from which it is eventually recollected and pumped back into the tank. But unlike water, which usually flows only one way through pipes, electronic circuits are often designed to create current flow which alternates in direction very rapidly. A direct current (DC) is current that flows only in one direction. Alternating current (AC) rapidly switches direction of flow.

The electrical *resistance* (R) is a measure of the difficulty of passing an electrical current through a conductor. Generally, the amount of current (I) is linearly proportional to V and inversely linearly proportional to R:

$$I = \frac{V}{R} \qquad \text{(This can also be represented as } V = I \times R\text{)}$$

The unit of measure for R is ohm (Ω), which equals 1 volt per ampere of current. A *resistor* is an electrical circuit element added to create an impediment to current flow, like a sponge or filter placed in a pipe to slow the flow of water. A material with a high R, such as rubber, is called an *insulator*. Conductance (G) is defined as the opposite of resistance such that $G = 1/R$. The human body predominantly consists of salt water, which acts as a passive *volume conductor*, a relatively low-R medium for electric current through which an electric field can spread easily throughout. This is the reason why signals generated in one area of the body (such as the heart) can be measured in completely different areas of the body (such as on the head or foot).

Two circuit elements serve to store electric charge, capacitors, and inductors. *Capacitors* are devices used to store charge, consisting of one or more pairs of conductors (usually metal plates) separated by a thin insulator (**Figure 2.1**).

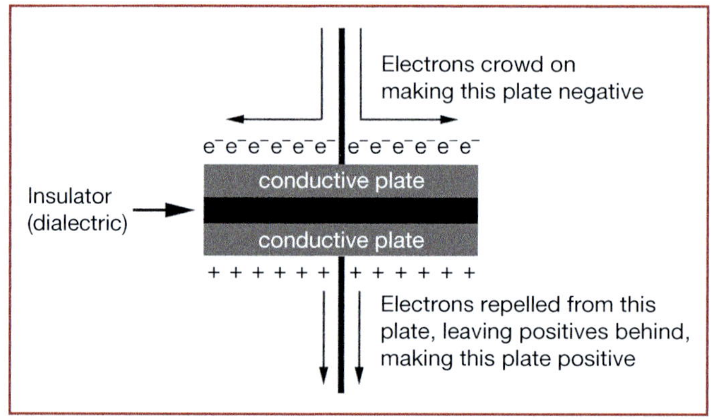

FIGURE 2.1: Diagram of a capacitor.

A voltage source, such as a battery, pushes electrons (negative charge) onto one of the conductive plates, creating an electrical field that pushes electrons off the opposite plate, leaving positive charges behind. How much charge a capacitor can store, or its *capacitance* (C), is linearly proportional to the amount of charge stored in the capacitor (Q) and inversely linearly proportional to the voltage difference (V) between the two metal plate conductors.

$$C = \frac{Q}{V}$$

The unit of measurement of capacitance is the farad (F), which equals the capacitance in which one coulomb of charge causes a potential difference across the capacitor of one volt. A capacitor will resist the flow of DC but will allow AC to "flow" through, although this AC flow is more of an illusion since it is caused by electric charge accumulating or leaving the two plates of the capacitor. This apparent "flow" of current across a capacitor is termed *capacitive coupling*.

Inductors are electrical components that store energy in a magnetic field when electrical current is flowing through it. Typically they consist of a coil of wire wrapped around a magnet. When electrical current flows through an inductor, a magnetic field is created around it (**Figure 2.2**).

If the electrical current flowing through the inductor decreases or stops, the magnetic field quickly collapses and induces a current in the coil which resists that decrease in current flow. In this way, an inductor resists *changes* in the current, therefore resisting AC but permitting DC. The strength of an inductor to perform this function is termed *inductance* (L) and its unit of measurement is in henrys. In a circuit in which the current is decreasing at a constant rate of one ampere per second, an inductance of one henry results in the generation of one volt of potential difference across the inductor. This induced voltage, called the *electromotive force*, is directly proportional to L and is also directly proportional to the inverse of the change in current ($-dI$).

$$V = L\frac{-dI}{dt}$$ (dI is the change in current; dt is the change in time)

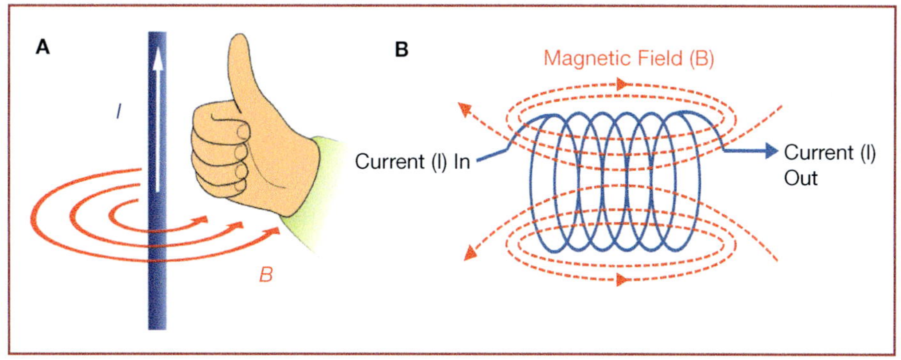

FIGURE 2.2: (A) The right-hand rule illustrates the direction of the magnetic field if the electrical current is flowing upwards. (B) The magnetic field generated by electrical current flow through a coiled conductor.

Often there are multiple circuit elements that store charge in an electrical circuit and these sum in different ways, depending on whether they are in series or in parallel, as described in **Table 2.1**.

TABLE 2.1: Rules for Combining Resistors, Inductors, and Capacitors in Electronic Circuits

	Resistors and Inductors	Capacitors
In Series 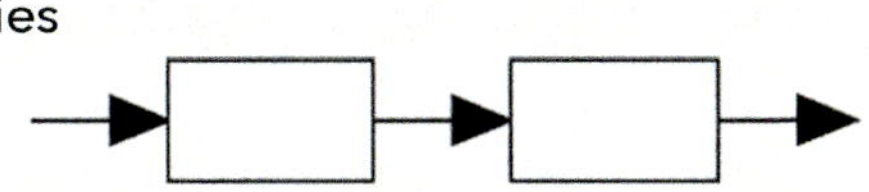	$R = R_1 + R_2 + R_3$ $L = L_1 + L_2 + L_3$	$\frac{1}{C} = \frac{1}{C_1} + \frac{1}{C_1} + \frac{1}{C_1}$
In Parallel 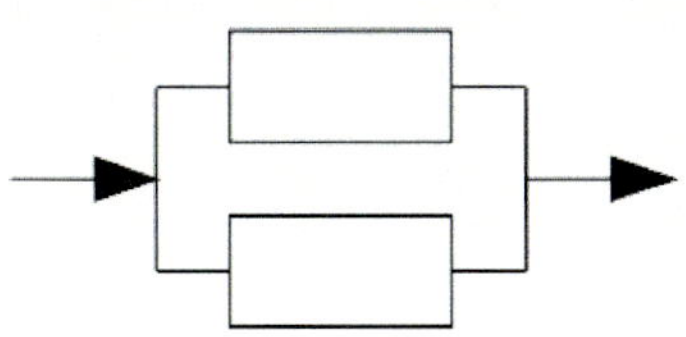	$\frac{1}{R} = \frac{1}{R_1} + \frac{1}{R_2} + \frac{1}{R_3}$ $\frac{1}{L} = \frac{1}{L_1} + \frac{1}{L_2} + \frac{1}{L_3}$	$C = C_1 + C_2 + C_3$

The fundamental circuit for understanding the analogue components of neurophysiology recording is the resistor–capacitor (RC) circuit (**Figure 2.3**). The current flow in this circuit varies over time when a voltage change occurs.

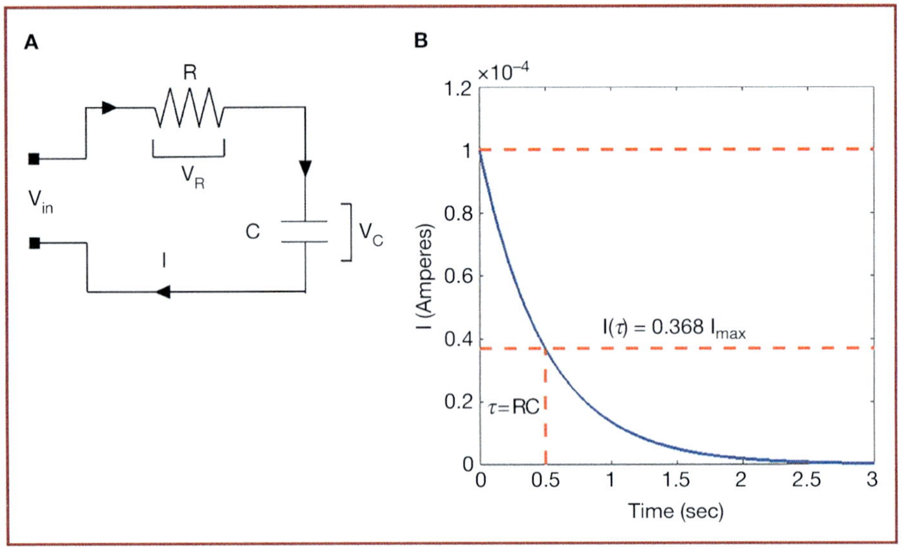

FIGURE 2.3: (A) A series RC circuit is shown with three circuit elements: the resistor (*R*), capacitor (*C*), and a power source (V_{in}). Three voltage potential changes are labeled: the voltage potential increase from a power source (V_{in}), the voltage potential decrease across a resistor (V_R), and the voltage potential decrease across a capacitor (V_C). The current (*I*) flows clockwise around the circuit (1). (B) The current flow as a capacitor charges. Since the time constant for the RC circuit (τ) is 0.5 seconds, current drops to the 1/e (0.368) fraction of the starting current by that time point.

Analog Amplifiers

The changes in the current in an AC electrical signal are sinusoidal, meaning they follow the shape of a sine wave. Many biological signals have a sinusoidal pattern as well, and any time-varying signal can be broken down into a combination of sinusoidal waves of different frequencies and times of occurrence. One of the primary functions of neurophysiology instruments is to *amplify* a biological signal, which means to increase the power of the voltage and/or current of the time-varying biological signals. Neurophysiology amplifiers are predominantly voltage amplifiers and therefore the output of the amplifier is measured in volts. The *gain* of an amplifier (*G*) is the factor by which the amplifier increases the amplitude of the input signal. A voltage amplifier with a *G* of 2, for example, outputs a signal with double the voltage of the input signal.

Because amplifiers are constructed with resistors, capacitors, and inductors, they provide resistance to the flow of electrical current, which is dependent on *frequency* of the waves in the biological signal. (Frequency is a measurement of the number of sinusoidal waves passing per unit time and is measured in hertz, which is the number of cycles or waves per second.) The *impedance* of an amplifier is a measure of the overall resistance of the amplifier to current flow. It is quite complicated to calculate impedance because it involves multiple factors including the resistance of the resistors, capacitors, and inductors in the amplifier system, as well as the frequency of the waveforms that the amplifier is acting on. The impedance of an amplifier is important because, ideally, a recording device should not disturb the electrical current flow that it is trying to measure. If an amplifier has a high impedance, it will not allow much current to flow into it, and therefore not disturb the current it is trying to measure. This leads to a more accurate measurement of the voltage of the source. The following equation and subsequent **Figure 2.4** depict the relationship of the impedance of the biological source and the measurement device (which includes an amplifier).

$$V_{meas} = V_s \times \frac{Z_{in}}{(Z_{in} + Z_{out})}$$

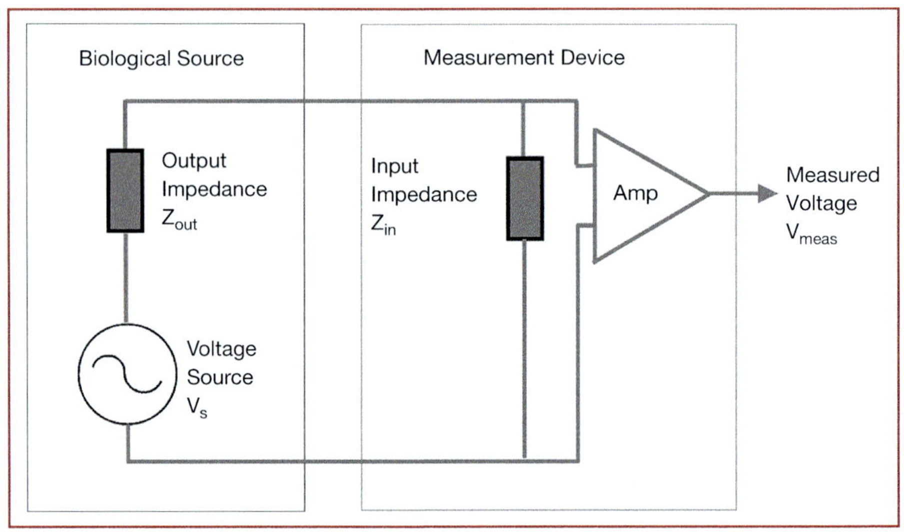

FIGURE 2.4: Schematic of impedances and biological voltage source for a measurement device, which includes an amplifier.

Note that if the Z_{in} is much higher than the Z_{out}, the impedance component of the equation is driven toward a value of one, causing the measured voltage to closely approximate the source voltage. If the value of Z_{in} is near to the value of Z_{out}, substantial current is shunted through the measurement device, disturbing the current flow through the biological source and decreasing the measured voltage.

As shown in Figure 2.4, an amplifier (also called an "amp") has two input lines, which are usually wires, and it amplifies the voltage potential difference between these two lines to produce one output signal, which is called a *channel*. Each line is connected to an electrode placed on or in biological tissue. Usually one line is connected to a signal electrode, which is placed in a region of interest in the biological tissue, and one line is connected to a reference electrode, which is placed in a location with relatively low voltage. Biosignal recording equipment contains multiple amplifiers which permits recording from multiple signal electrodes. The reference electrode is connected to the second input of all of the amplifiers. This arrangement is called a *referential recording*. A ground electrode is also usually placed on the forehead in EEG recording. The location of the reference electrode in a referential EEG recording is usually chosen to be at the top of the head, at a distance remote from eye movement artifacts near the front of the head, muscle artifacts in the temporal regions, and the posterior dominant background rhythm in the posterior head region. Figure 2.5 contains a diagram of the wiring of an amplifier system in a referential recording setup with two signal electrodes, one referential electrode, and two amplifier output channels. This figure also shows the setup for *bipolar recording*, in which three electrodes are connected in a chain in which the middle electrode is connected to both amplifiers.

Because there is so much ambient noise in the environment during neurophysiologic recordings, a special type of amplifier, called a *differential amplifier*, is used in neurophysiology-recording equipment to minimize noise. This type of amplifier is essentially a combination of three amplifiers wired together. In the first stage of a differential amplifier, two amplifiers working in parallel amplify the potential difference between (a) the signal electrode and the patient ground electrode and (b) the reference electrode and the patient ground electrode. In the second stage, a third amplifier amplifies the difference between the outputs of the two first-stage amplifiers. A differential amplifier can be used for both a referential and a bipolar recording. Figure 2.6 depicts only the referential recording.

Environment noise usually causes a voltage potential difference between the recording electrodes and the ground electrode, which is called the *common mode signal*, and this is of relatively similar magnitude among the recording channels. The *differential signals* are the voltage potential differences between each signal electrode and the reference electrode, which are the signals of interest. Differential amplifiers work to cancel out much of the common mode signal, a process called *common mode rejection*. The degree to which a differential amplifier rejects the common mode signal is called the *common mode rejection ratio* (CMRR). This is calculated using the amplification of the common mode signal, called the *common mode gain* (G_{cm}) versus the amplification of the referential signal, called the *referential gain* (G_d). The CMMR is usually expressed in the unit of decibels (dB), which expresses the ratio of two numbers (usually signal magnitude) on a logarithmic scale multiplied by a factor of 20.

$$\text{CMMR} = 20\log_{10}\left(\frac{G_d}{G_{cm}}\right)$$

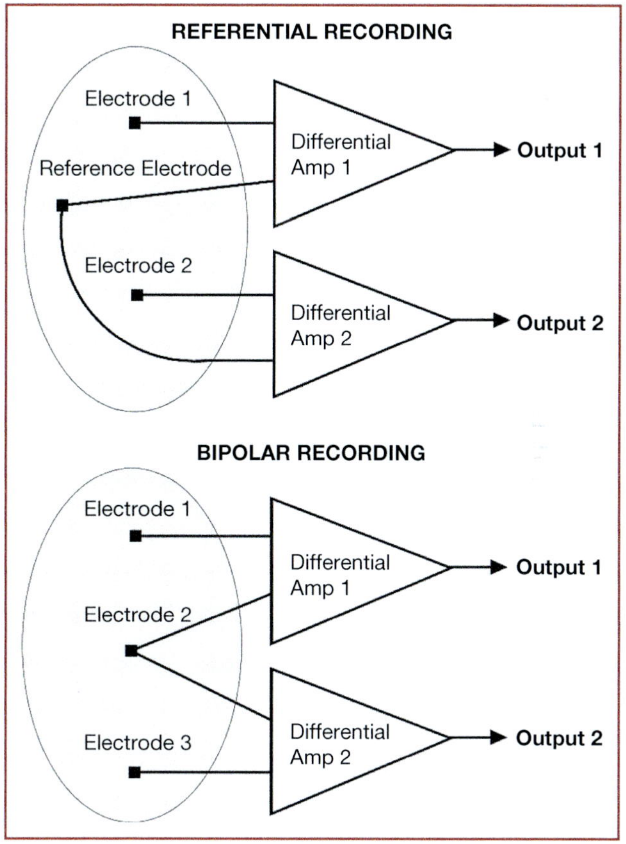

FIGURE 2.5: Schematic depicting referential and bipolar recordings.

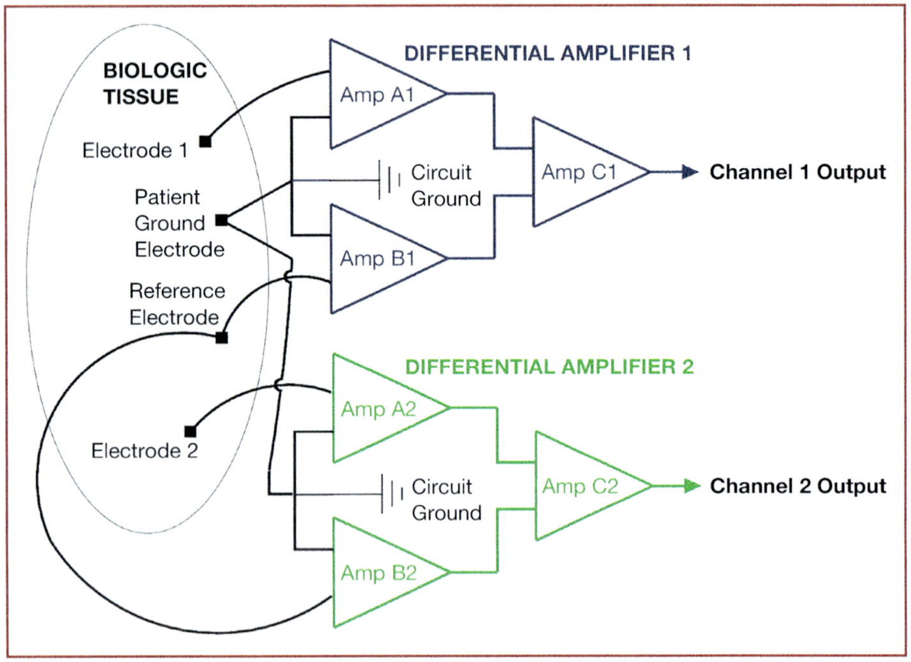

FIGURE 2.6: Diagram of a differential amplifier showing two recording electrodes arranged in a referential montage.

An amplifier that reduces the common mode signal by a factor of 10,000 (10^4) relative to the differential signals has a CMRR of 80 dB. Most modern biosignal amplifiers have a CMRR of over 100 dB. The entire amplifier (consisting of multiple channels) has a total input impedance (I_{in}) as described earlier. The I_{in} is designed to be as high as possible, in order to improve the performance of the amplifier. Most modern amplifiers have an I_{in} of 100 MΩ or more. But a high I_{in} is not sufficient to assure a high-quality recording. Each electrode has an impedance value as well, which is primarily due to skin resistance and electrode capacitive and resistive impedance. If there is a difference between the impedance of the electrodes, this can cause leakage of common mode signal into the output of the differential amplifiers. For this reason, it is important to keep the impedance of each electrode as low as possible, and keep the impedance of each electrode within a similar range (such that a few electrodes do not have significantly higher impedance than the other electrodes).

Electrodes

Recording electrodes provide an interface point between biological tissues and the metal wires which are usually connected to amplifiers. Within biological tissues, electrical current flows in a low-resistance salt water solution by the movement of positively and negatively changed ions. The metal of electrodes and the wires that connect them to amplifiers also provide a low-resistance media in which current can flow. But the boundary between these two media is difficult to bridge electrically because of multiple sources of impedance to current flow which must be overcome. An electrolyte solution or gel is placed between the skin and the electrode to help improve conduction. The first source of impedance is the outer layer of the skin, the epidermis, which contains keratin and is covered in natural oils, both of which are good insulators. Skin preparation by gentle abrasion removes some of this keratin by removing dead skin cells and the natural oils that cover the epidermis. At the boundary between the electrolyte solution and the metal electrode, current can pass back and forth either through the movement of electrons due to chemical reactions between the metal and the electrolyte (called *redox reactions*) or through capacitive coupling. Movement of charge through capacitive coupling is preferred, because redox reactions at the electrolyte solution/electrode boundary can produce toxic chemicals which can damage tissues. Capacitive coupling can occur because a charge imbalance develops between the electrolyte solution and the metal electrode, either from redox chemical reactions or the exchange of electrons between ions in solution and the metal. This charge imbalance, which acts as a capacitor, is called the *half-cell potential*.

An ideal electrode develops only a small half-cell potential because if this potential is too large, it leads to problems due to the intrinsic properties of capacitors and due to the instability of this capacitance. This half-cell potential can break down abruptly for uncertain reasons, leading to discharges of current, which causes "electrode pop" artifacts or can be altered unpredictably by the influx of sweat into the electrolyte. Because capacitance acts to impede the flow of DC current, the half-cell potential also decreases the transmission of low-frequency signals. Silver–silver chloride electrodes, which have silver salt intermixed with the silver metal within the electrode, produce the lowest half-cell potentials and make the best scalp EEG electrodes, particularly if DC potentials need to be recorded. Because electrical charges flow directly between the silver–silver chloride electrode and the electrolyte gel, not much of a charge imbalance develops between the electrode and the biological media and there is no polarization of charge between the electrode and the conductive media (therefore less capacitance develops). For this reason, silver–silver chloride electrodes are termed *nonpolarizing electrodes*. Nonpolarizing electrodes are good for recording both high frequencies and *DC potentials* (very low frequencies).

Gold and platinum electrodes are low-resistance conductors and do not cause chemical reactions with the electrolyte. Electrical charges do not move between these metals and the electrolyte media because these metals are inert. Electrical current flows between the metals and biologic media through capacitive coupling due to the large half-cell potential, which develops between the electrode and the biologic media. This charge imbalance produces capacitance and therefore capacitive impedance, which impedes the transmission of low-frequency signals. Gold, platinum, and stainless steel electrodes are termed polarizing electrodes. The larger half-cell potentials of polarizing electrodes make them more susceptible to electrode pop and movement artifacts, due to rapid unpredictable release of charge from the electrode. Gold electrodes (which are actually gold plated over silver) are considered acceptable for recordings, although their recording properties are not as good as silver–silver chloride electrodes, because they are cheaper to fabricate. Needle electrodes for EEG and EMG recording are usually made of stainless steel to control cost (these electrodes are disposable) and because the electrode must be thin but strong, although the relatively high capacitive impedance of stainless steel decreases its ability to record lower frequencies. The high impedance of stainless steel electrodes is less of a problem due to the higher impedance of modern amplifiers. Polarizing electrodes are used for intracranial recordings because they do not cause chemical redox reactions which could damage tissues. Stainless steel is not commonly used for intracranial electrodes because it is not completely inert like gold and platinum, and can therefore be involved in chemical reactions, particularly during stimulation (2). Also, stainless steel electrodes are more ferromagnetic, leading to greater MRI artifact.

MEG Sensors

MEG measures the magnetic fields generated by the electrical currents produced by the brain. The detectors of these magnetic field changes are called *superconducting quantum interference devices* (SQUIDs). Loops of superconducting material are immersed within a container of liquid helium (called a dewar) and kept at a temperature near absolute zero kelvin. The SQUIDS transduce magnetic flux into alternating electrical current, which can be amplified and visualized like typical bioelectric signals. Because the SQUIDs have to be kept so cold, they must be thermally insulated from the head and therefore kept at a distance of around 2 cm from the scalp. The magnetic flux produced by the brain is very small in comparison to the ambient magnetic noise in the environment and the magnetic signal from the heart. The magnetic flux recorded by a MEG system is in the range of 10^{-12} to 10^{-13} T. Movement of large metal objects near a MEG system (sometimes even hundreds of feet away) as well as magnetic thermal noise generated by nonneuronal electrical currents in the human subject and SQUID sensor usually generate noise in the 1 to 3 µT range (3), which is many orders of magnitude higher than the magnetic signal from the brain. For this reason, the MEG system must be housed in a magnetically shielded room. Even small movements of metal in the room, such as the movement of metal buttons on clothing or manipulation of metal switches in the environment of the MEG system, can cause MEG signal artifact.

Analog Filters

An analog signal filter is a device that removes some unwanted components in an electrical signal, usually certain frequencies. Analog filters are built using a combination of resistors and capacitors. The design of a simple analog filter is based on the concept of the *voltage divider* (**Figure 2.7A**), which is a circuit consisting of two resistors that produces an output voltage (V_{out}) which is a fraction of its input voltage (V_{in}).

$$V_{out} = V_{in}\left(\frac{R_1}{R_1 + R_2}\right)$$

A *high-pass filter*, which allows high frequencies to pass on through (and blocks lower frequencies), is a circuit with a combination of a capacitor and resistor similar to a voltage divider, as illustrated in **Figure 2.7B**. In this design, all current flow must pass through the capacitor, which will only pass current through capacitive coupling, and therefore preferentially passes AC current of higher frequencies better than that of lower frequencies. Additionally, the resistor, which does not impede lower frequencies,

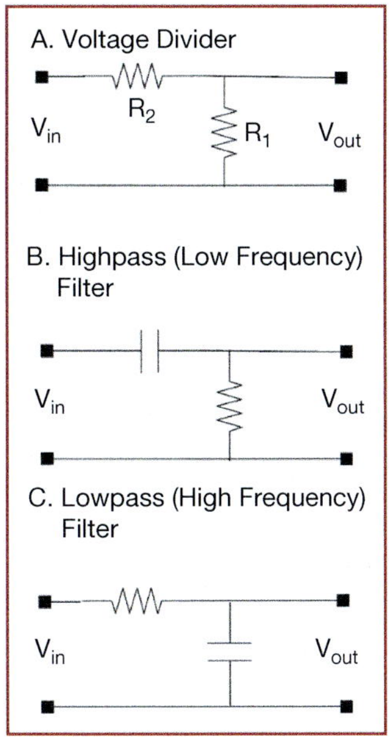

FIGURE 2.7: Voltage divider and simple high-pass and low-pass analog filters.

lets a certain amount of the lower frequency content of the signal leak through and therefore it does not get passed on to the output of the circuit. A *low-pass filter* is designed with the resistor and capacitor in opposite positions in the circuit (**Figure 2.7C**). For signals containing lower frequencies, since the resistor does not alter the transmission of current based on its frequency content, lower frequencies are allowed to pass through without much attenuation. But for higher frequencies, some or all of the current leaks through the capacitor (which preferentially passes higher frequencies) and the higher frequency components of the signal do not appear as much in the output of the circuit.

Filters are defined mainly by three design characteristics—filter type, cutoff frequency (or frequencies), and filter order. There are four main filter types, as illustrated by **Figure 2.8**. The first two filter types (high-pass and low-pass) have already been discussed. **Figure 2.8** illustrates the frequency response of the four types of filters. Both high-pass and low-pass filters have one cutoff frequency, which is defined as the frequency at which the voltage output of the filter is −3 dB (or 0.707) of the voltage of the input signal. The cutoff frequency can be calculated from the time constant of the filter (τ). As described earlier in the discussion of RC circuits, $\tau = \text{RC}$.

$$f_{\text{cutoff}} = \frac{1}{2\pi \text{RC}} = \frac{1}{2\pi\tau}$$

A *band-pass* filter, as depicted in **Figure 2.8C**, is a combination of a low-pass and a high-pass filter, which has two cutoff frequencies, and frequencies between the two cutoffs are allowed to pass. A *band-stop* (or notch) filter is designed to block frequencies in a very narrow range and is usually used to remove 60-Hz power line noise.

The order of a filter describes how rapidly the output amplitude of various frequencies drops off beyond the cutoff frequency. The order of a filter also approximately equals the number of resistors and capacitors that would be needed to build the analog filter circuit. **Figure 2.9** depicts the frequency response of different 100-Hz low-pass filters with three different orders (1st, 3rd, and 5th). Note how the frequency response decreases more rapidly as the filter order increases. The filter order is also called the *roll-off* of the filter such that filters of higher order have a "steeper" roll-off (4). Filters can also change the timing of when certain features appear in an input signal. This is called the *phase-response* of a filter. Generally, all analog filters change the appearance of the signal so as to make waveforms in the input signal appear to occur slightly earlier or slightly later than in the original signal, and this is termed *phase advance* and *phase delay*, respectively. Whether a filter causes phase advance or delay depends on the frequency of the waves in the signal and on whether the filter is a low-pass or high-pass filter. Generally, this has become less of a problem in modern equipment because, unlike for analog filters, most modern digital filters do not induce much change in the phase of the signal for signal frequency components which are within the band-pass of the filters.

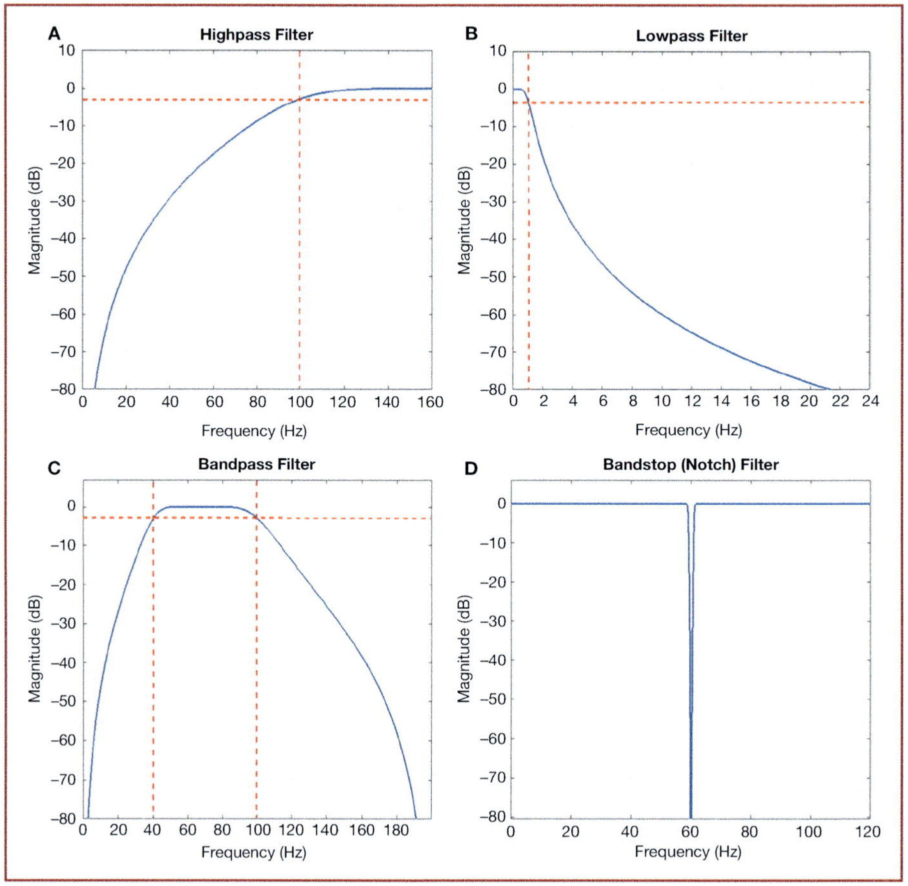

FIGURE 2.8: (A) High-pass filter with cutoff frequency of 100 Hz. (B) Low-pass filter with cutoff frequency 1 Hz. (C) Band-pass filter with cutoff frequencies of 40 and 100 Hz (high-pass and low-pass, respectively). (D) 60-Hz band-stop (notch) filter. All filters are Butterworth 3rd order except for the band-stop filter, which is 10th order.

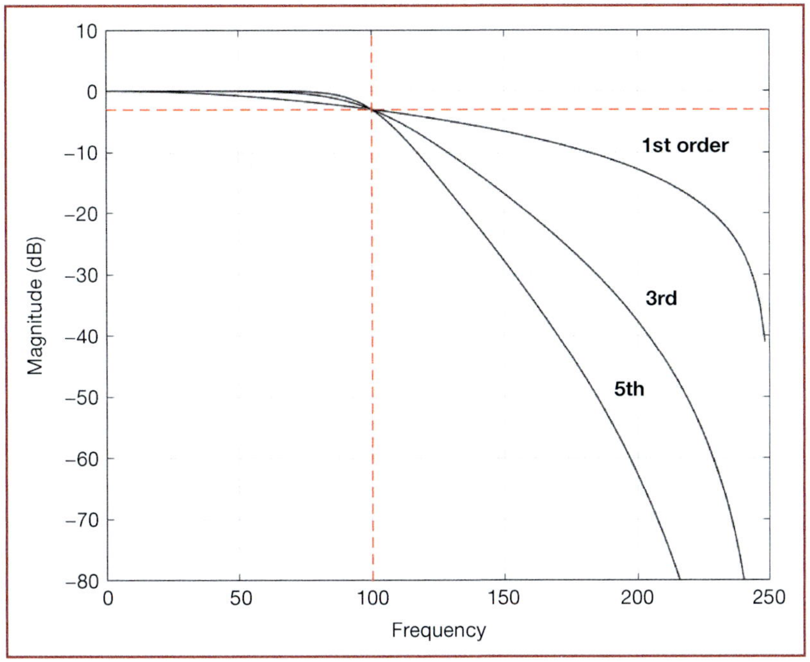

FIGURE 2.9: Frequency response of three 100-Hz cutoff low-pass Butterworth filters of three different orders: 1st, 3rd, and 5th. The higher the order of the filter, the greater the roll-off.

Grounding

In electrical engineering, the *ground* is the reference point in an electrical circuit from which voltages are measured and is a common path for electrical current. Connecting a circuit to *earth ground* means physically connecting to the earth through conductors. Patients connected to a modern biosignal amplifier system are usually not connected to earth ground but connected to the *amplifier common ground*. Amplification is performed in two stages. The first stage involves differential amplification within the preamplifier, which is connected to the amplifier common ground. The second stage of amplification is performed by a more powerful amplifier, which is connected to earth ground. This second amplifier includes an *isolator* that transmits the signal through a nonelectrical mode of signal transmission, such as light waves. This isolates the patient from the more powerful second amplifier and earth ground. This protects the patient from exposure to accidental electrical currents in the environment, which are not from the neurophysiologic recording equipment (and want to flow to earth ground) and isolates the delicate preamplifier stage from connection to the more powerful isolation amplifier equipment, decreasing noise. Figure 2.10 is a diagram of a typical connection between one channel of a biosignal amplifier and the two types of ground.

Because the body of the recording subject, power lines, lines connecting the electrodes to amplifiers, and ground lines all contain electrical charge, capacitive coupling can develop between them all, even if there is not a physical connection through which electrical charge can flow. This creates multiple potential circuit loops through which current can flow due to magnetic induction generated by any magnetic field in the environment. These circuit loops are called *ground loops*. Note in Figure 2.10 how many potential loops there are just for one biosignal recording channel. The magnetic flux noise in the environment, which creates the current in these ground loops, is usually caused by other electrical equipment nearby.

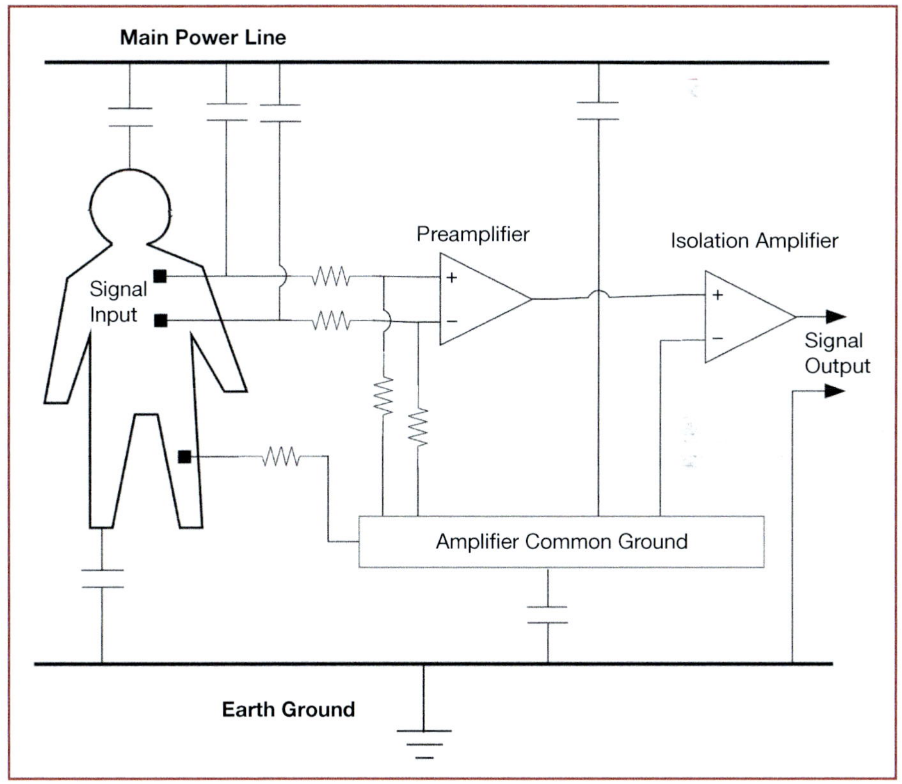

FIGURE 2.10: Connection between the main power line, the patient, amplifiers, and two types of ground.

Source: From Metting van Rijn A, Peper A, Grimbergen C. High-quality recording of bioelectric events. *Med Biol Eng Comput*. 1990;28(5):389-397. doi:10.1007/BF02441961.

DIGITAL RECORDING

Basic Digital Recording Principles

Digital electronic systems represent the amplitude of time-based signals (such as EEG, EMG, or MEG) in discrete bands, as opposed to the continuous ranges used in analog electronics. As depicted in Figure 2.11, the time-based signal is sampled at discrete points, which are arranged to occur at regular intervals in time. Additionally, the amplitude of the signal (usually in volts) is discretized at certain specified levels within a minimum and maximum range.

The frequency at which the system measures the amplitude of the input signal is called the *sampling rate*, which is expressed as the number of measurements per second in hertz. EEG is typically recorded with a sampling rate between 256 and 2,048 Hz (2 kHz). Since digital computers work using the base two number system, technical specifications for the features in digital systems, such as sampling rate, are often numbers of base two such as $2^8 = 256$ or $2^{11} = 2{,}048$. The Nyquist theorem states that in order to adequately reproduce a signal, it should be periodically sampled at a rate that is at least two times the highest frequency you wish to record. In practice, the sampling rate must be at least three to five times the highest frequency of interest for faithful *analog to digital* (A–D) conversion of the signal.

The minimum number of points at which the signal amplitude is discretized is termed the *bit depth*. Figure 2.12 depicts two approximately 1-Hz sine waves that have been sampled with two different bit depths. One sine wave has been sampled at a bit depth of 2^{10} (1,024 discrete levels of amplitude) and the other sine wave has been sampled at a bit depth of 2^5 (32 discrete levels of amplitude). For the sine wave sampled at a bit depth of 5, it is clear that the bit depth is not sufficient to fully render the shape of the wave, and the wave appears "jagged" with abrupt transitions from discrete levels of amplitude clearly visible. A bit depth of 10 is sufficient to represent the biosignals of most EEG recordings. Most modern EEG amplifiers have a bit depth that exceeds 20. A much higher bit depth than 10 is helpful because biosignal amplifiers must record more than just signals from the nervous system—noise and artifactual signals commonly have a much higher amplitude than signals from the brain.

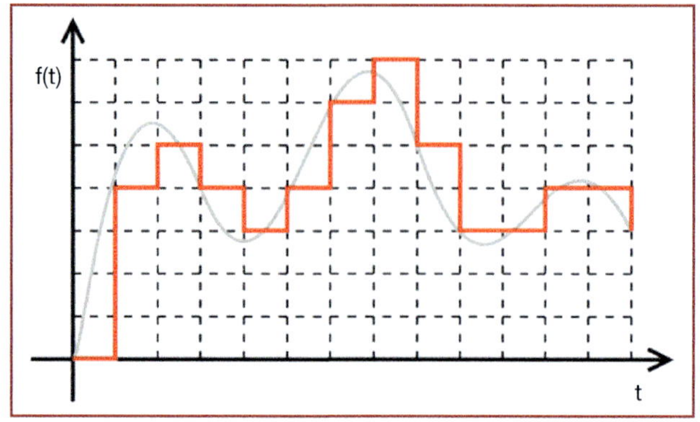

FIGURE 2.11: An analog signal (in red) and a discrete digital representation of that signal. The horizontal axis is time (*t*) and the vertical axis is the quantity of the signal, *f*(*t*).

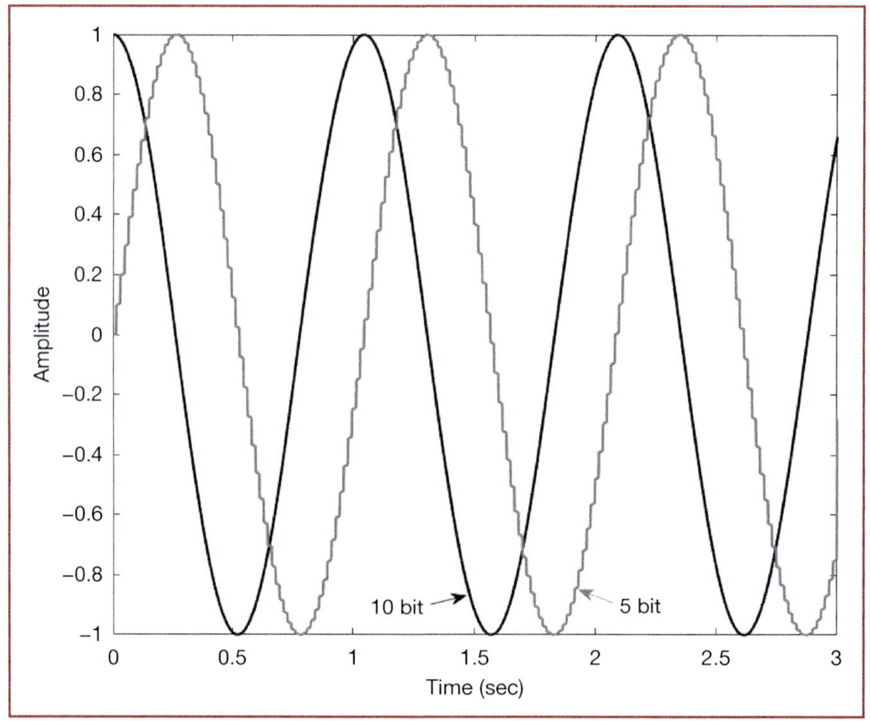

FIGURE 2.12: Sine waves of approximately 1 Hz frequency rendered with two sampling rates. The black sine wave is rendered at a bit depth of 10 and the gray sine at bit depth of 5.

Signal Digitization

The basic stages of biosignal recording are depicted in Figure 2.13. The signal from the electrodes is initially amplified to a small degree by the preamplifier, using a combination of amplifiers in the differential amplification process as described earlier (6). The purpose of this preamplifier stage is to (a) use a very high amplifier impedance (so as to accurately measure the signal),

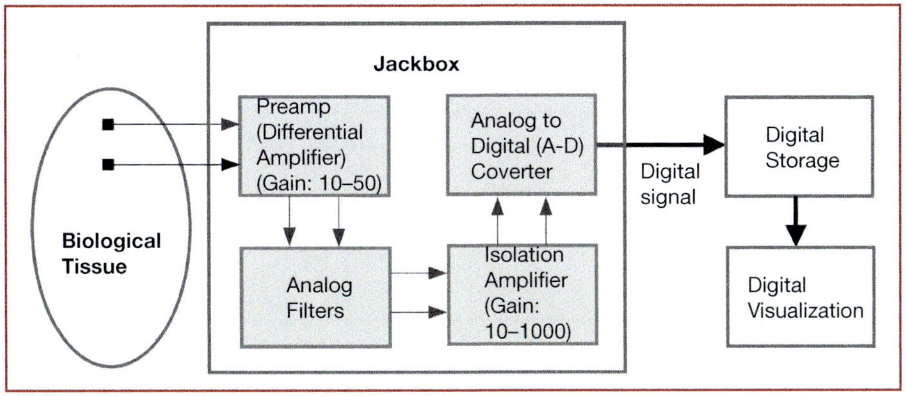

FIGURE 2.13: The basic components of a digital biosignal amplifier in a recording jack box (for one recording channel).

(b) remove the common mode signal, and (c) boost the amplitude of the signal to provide sufficient input amplitude to the next amplifier stage. Next (either before or after the next amplification stage, depending on the system), analog filters are applied. A high-pass analog filter with a low cutoff frequency is used to remove the very low-frequency upward or downward voltage drift of each channel (called the "DC shift"). A low-pass analog filter with a high cutoff near the Nyquist frequency is used to remove noise and to improve the accuracy of A–D conversion. The second amplifier stage brings the signal voltage up to the level needed by the A–D converter (usually in the −5 to +5 V range) and uses built-in signal *isolation*. Within this amplifier is a complete (isolation) barrier to electrical current flow across which the signal is carried by light (optical isolation) or using a transformer to transmit the signal using changing magnetic flux (transformer isolation). The output of the isolation amplifier is directed to the A–D converter where the analog electrical signal is discretized at a specified sampling rate and at a set of amplitudes and then transmitted out as digital information. The digital information is stored in computer memory or hard drive. From there, the digital signal information is visualized using computer software and displayed on a monitor.

Digital Filtering

Once a digital signal is stored, it can be processed mathematically by a computer. Digital filtering is the process of using mathematical algorithms to apply filters to remove certain frequency components. This process acts in a similar way to analog filtering but unlike analog filters, which can process incoming signals quickly in real time, digital filters are only applied to the signal after the recording is completed. Digital filters have some advantages over analog filters. First, a well-designed digital filter has a very "flat" response in the band-pass of the filter, meaning that digital filters do not affect some frequency components more than others (as much as analog filters) in the range of frequencies that are intended to be passed through the filter without attenuation. Second, digital filters can be designed to avoid any effect on the phase of the signals in the frequency ranges of the passband (low phase distortion). Analog filters, on the other hand, often cause slight phase delay or phase advance in the signal, even for those signal frequency components that are intended to pass through filters without modification. Third, digital filters can adapt their characteristics to match characteristics of the input signal, whereas analog filters are not as flexible.

Digital Display

EEG is displayed using modern neurophysiology equipment on computer monitors, which depict information as individual points of light, called *pixels*. Characteristics of computer monitors include *luminance* (brightness), *aspect ratio* (ratio of the height to width of the viewable screen), and display *resolution* (measured based on the number of pixels along the height axis versus the number of pixels on the width axis). Equipment manufacturers agree to standard display specifications, which are listed in Table 2.2. Note that the total number of pixels on a screen (and therefore the amount of memory required to store the information in the video) is increasing exponentially as video specification formats are advancing.

In a digital review system, the reviewer sets the height at which a unit of voltage is rendered on the screen, called the *vertical scaling* or *digital display gain*. A standard setting for the digital display gain would be 7 microvolts per mm of computer monitor screen. Additionally, the reviewer can set the *time base* for review, which is the number of seconds of neurophysiology signal that is viewed on the monitor, which defines the horizontal time scaling. A sufficient screen resolution is necessary to render a neurophysiology waveform clearly, as illustrated in Figure 2.14. Inadequate screen resolution can limit rendering of neurophysiology waveforms if the time base and/or gain are set insufficiently low by the reviewer. Note in Figure 2.14 that the screen resolution is insufficient to clearly render these waveforms, particularly for the higher frequency waves on the right.

Aliasing

During the process of A–D conversion, and also during the process of signal display on a computer monitor, a time-based signal is forced to take

TABLE 2.2: Computer Monitor Screen Resolutions, Aspect Ratios, and Total Number of Pixels Per Frame

Video Standard	Width	Height	Aspect Ratio	Pixels
8K UHD (4320p)	7,680	4,320	16:9	33,177,600
4K HD (2160p)	3,840	2,160	16:9	8,294,400
FHD+(WQHD) (1440p)	2,560	1,440	16:9	3,686,400
FHD (FullHD) (1080i, 1080p),	1,920	1,080	16:9	2,073,600
HDV (1080i)	1,440	1,080	4:3	1,555,200
WXGA-H (720p)	1,280	720	16:9	921,600
"High" VGA	640	480	4:3	307,200
QVGA	320	240	4:3	76,800
QQVGA	160	120	4:3	19,200

certain discrete values, as explained earlier in the process of discretization. Aliasing can occur when the sampling rate for this discretization is insufficient to represent the frequencies of the analog signal or digital signal being converted or displayed, respectively. The Nyquist theorem states that the highest frequency that can be represented in a digital time-based signal is half of the sampling rate. Of course, sampling at twice the frequency of the original analog waveform is not nearly enough to guarantee an accurate representation of the waveform (as illustrated in the right side of Figure 2.14), and usually a minimum of five sampling points per cycle of a waveform is suggested. So, for example, the minimum adequate sampling frequency to record a 10-Hz signal would be approximately 30 to 50 Hz (Figure 2.15).

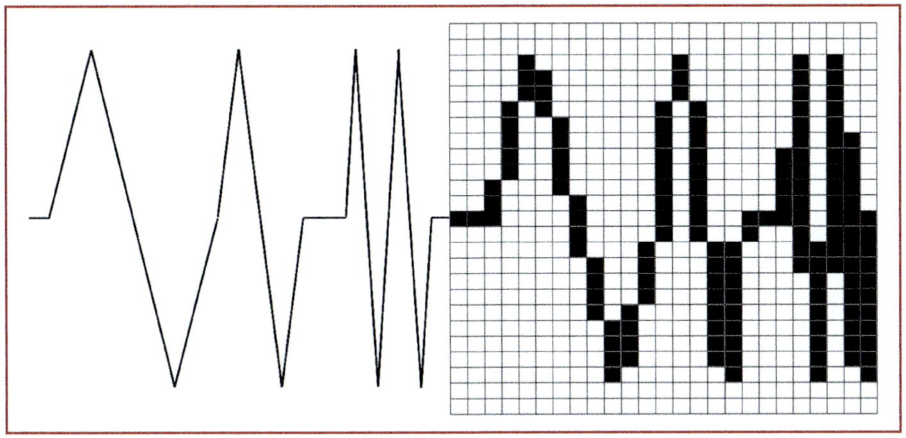

FIGURE 2.14: Inadequate rending of waveforms in pixels because of inadequate screen resolution.

Signals of frequency close to or higher than the Nyquist frequency that are present in the signal before digitization can appear in the signal after digitization at lower frequencies, and this is called *aliasing*. This artifactual aliased signal (f_a) appears at a frequency lower than the Nyquist frequency (f_N) based on the magnitude of the original signal frequency, (f_o) as described in the following equation.

$$f_a = |f_o - f_N|$$

The problem of aliasing in A–D conversion can be minimized by applying an analog low-pass filter with a cutoff near the Nyquist frequency before the signal undergoes digitization, as portrayed in Figure 2.13. This decreases the amplitude of the frequencies, which are most likely to be aliased before the A–D conversion process.

Aliasing of a digital signal can also occur during the process of display on a computer monitor. The resolution of the computer monitor used to display a time-based signal imposes a sampling frequency on the signal to be displayed. This sampling frequency is best understood as the maximum frequency that a monitor can display. This maximum display frequency (f_d) can be calculated from the number of horizontal pixels dedicated to the display (h) and the number of seconds (s) of time-based signal displayed:

$$f_d = \frac{1}{2}(h / s)$$

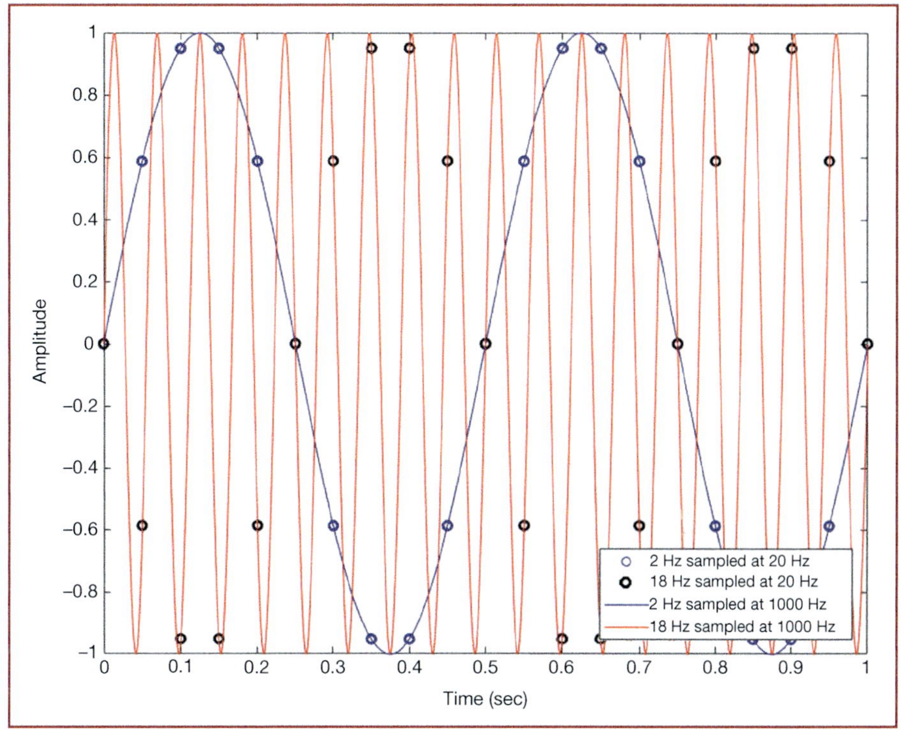

FIGURE 2.15: Aliasing of an 18-Hz signal that is acquired at a 20-Hz sampling rate reduces the true waveform to a frequency of 2 Hz. The red sinusoidal wave is the 18-Hz signal sampled at 1,000 Hz. The blue signal is the 2-Hz signal sampled at 20 Hz as well as 1,000 Hz. The black circles represent the 2-Hz sinusoidal wave created by aliasing of the 18-Hz sinusoidal wave because it is sampled at 20 Hz, a frequency below the Nyquist frequency.

Signals of frequency near this maximum display frequency are not rendered well on the computer monitor in many cases and aliasing can occur. This aliasing is prevented by a digital antialiasing filter which is built into the neurophysiology review software. This digital filter can be quite complex and in some systems performs a type of "intelligent down-sampling," such that when the frequency of the signal to be rendered exceeds the maximum display frequency, the system uses an algorithm to render the waveform such that certain frequencies that are above the maximum display frequency are rendered at precisely the maximum display frequency. The use of modern high-resolution widescreen monitors can minimize the problems caused by a suboptimal monitor maximum display frequency. Monitors with Full HD Plus (FHD+ or WQHD) resolution at 2,560 × 1,440 or higher resolutions offer many more pixels than traditional monitors and are now inexpensive enough for most labs.

CONCLUSIONS

Digitization has created new stages in the clinical review process in which problems can occur because of how easy it is to store and manipulate digital signals once they are recorded. In the field of EEG, new stages in the interpretation process include interpreter specification of the review montage and filtering, the calculation of mathematical transforms for the creation of trends, and automated artifact suppression. Although each of these new stages has been designed to help the EEG interpreter review data more efficiently and to identify artifact, these stages themselves can create new artifacts. For example, an automated artifact reduction algorithm can remove components of an EEG signal that are artifactual and improve a reviewer's ability to observe the underlying electroencephalographic signal of interest. But what if the artifact reduction algorithm also removes part of the EEG signal? How would a reviewer know this had happened? How could this affect the biosignal to measured?

Additionally, as digital equipment becomes more complex, equipment in the clinical recording environment can create artifactual signals that are quite complex and easy to mistake for biological signals. Ultimately, a clinical neurophysiologist's ability to recognize artifacts is bolstered by a firm understanding of the technical background of neurophysiology data acquisition. But since new technologies and artifacts are constantly emerging, the ability to recognize the difference between a biological signal and a signal generated by a machine is also important. In probability theory, a *stochastic* (or random) process is a collection of random variables used to represent the evolution of a value over time. It is not possible to predict how a stochastic process will evolve over time if you do not know the starting conditions. A *deterministic* process is a process in which, given the starting point, you can know with certainty how the process will evolve over time. Biological signals have a strong stochastic component, which is due partially to noise but also due to complexity of the system generating the signal. Artifactual signals generated by equipment in the environment often have the appearance of deterministic signals, which appear in a mathematically predictable pattern. Understanding this basic difference in types of signals is key to identifying many types of artifacts.

REFERENCES

1. Inductiveload. RC series filter (with V&I labels).svg [Image file]. Available at: https://commons.wikimedia.org/w/index.php?curid=5801614. Accessed August 1, 2018.
2. White RL, Gross TJ. An evaluation of the resistance to electrolysis of metals for use in biostimulation microprobes. *IEEE Trans Biomed Eng*. 1974;21(6): 487-490. doi:10.1109/TBME.1974.324339.
3. Taula S, Simola J, Nenonen J, Parkkonen L. Novel noise reduction methods. In: Supek S, Aine CJ, eds. *Magnetoencephalography: From Signals to Dynamic Cortical Networks*. Berlin, Heidelberg: Springer-Verlag; 2014:35-71.
4. Maus D, Litt B. Engineering principles. In: Ebersole JS, Husain AM, Nordli DR, eds. *Current Practice of Clinical Electroencephalography*. Philadelphia, PA: Lippincott Williams & Wilkins; 2014:45-77.
5. Van Rijn AM, Peper A, Grimbergen CA. High-quality recording of bioelectric events. *Med Biol Eng Comput*. 1990;28(5):389-397.
6. Epstein CM. Analog signal recording principles. In: Schomer DL, Da Silva FL, eds. *Niedermeyer's Electroencephalography: Basic Principles, Clinical Applications, and Related Fields*. Philadelphia, PA: Lippincott Williams & Wilkins; 2011:111-118.

CHAPTER 3

Pediatric Clinical Neurophysiology

Gloria Galloway and Thoru Yamada

INTRODUCTION

Artifacts in the pediatric population are often similar in many ways to those encountered in adults. However, some artifacts are more commonly seen in the pediatric population. One reason for this is the short distance used between stimulation and recording electrodes in the very young patient with a small body size. Therefore, this chapter attempts to describe a number of age-specific artifacts that can cause significant difficulties in interpretation of clinical neurophysiologic studies involving both electromyogram (EMG) recordings and intraoperative monitoring.

ELECTROMYOGRAPHY

Obtaining an EMG in a child or young adult patient can be challenging due to the discomfort involved and the need to avoid inadvertent movement. The presence of artifacts during an EMG procedure increases the challenge involved and likely increases the amount of time needed for the procedure to eliminate these artifacts (1). Artifacts can often be difficult to eliminate completely and may cause misinterpretation of the data. This can be particularly problematic in pediatric cases and especially in the very young patient where cooperation cannot always be depended upon during the procedure or over the length of time it takes to accomplish adequate real-time artifact reduction. In young children, certain artifacts (e.g., movement) may be seen more commonly than in adults. These may be unintentional despite attempting to exert volitional control. In this chapter, several case examples are provided in which the presence of an artifact led to confusion in the interpretation of the EMG evaluation. It is important first to recognize when an EMG finding is due to the presence of an artifact, and then to determine what measures need to be taken to eliminate or reduce the frequency or intensity of that artifact, optimizing interpretation of the EMG evaluation.

Several clues help guide the examiner to suspect that certain features in an EMG are physiologic or due to the presence of an artifact. The first clue a waveform is artifactual involves having a finding which is unexpected from the clinical scenario. It is important to remember that the EMG is an extension of the physical, neurological, and neuromuscular examinations (2). Therefore, the EMG should be interpreted with the clinical context in mind. It is unusual that after a thoughtful history and neuromuscular examination, the EMG finding is contrary to or inappropriate for the clinical situation. The second clue that the EMG features are due to the presence of an artifact stems from observation of the patient. This involves observing whether the patient is participating in movement that may cause the corresponding artifact either voluntarily or involuntarily. The third clue is recognized by observing the patient surroundings. In observing the patient surroundings, it is important to observe what equipment is attached to the patient, as well as what electrophysiologically active sources may be in the surrounding environment that could introduce artifacts in the EMG signal. These sources may include other machinery, devices, or people. The strongest clue involves a successful attempt to minimize a suspected artifact that correlates to reduction or elimination of the artifact, such as unplugging an electrical device or moving equipment away from the patient in order to eliminate interference. Artifacts therefore can be divided into intrinsic sources involving the patient and external sources that are not patient induced.

ARTIFACTS IN THE ELECTROMYOGRAM

Intrinsic Sources

Intrinsic sources of artifacts involve electrophysiological activity generated by the patient that interferes with the recording. Common sources of artifacts in the EMG are summarized in Table 3.1 and include the following:

Voluntary Muscular Contraction

Muscular contraction can be attributed to voluntary or involuntary muscle activity. One example of a patient-induced myogenic artifact shown in Figure 3.1 is due to voluntary muscle contraction. This may initially go unnoticed as it can involve small muscles and be unintentional. In some cases, particularly in a young patient, muscle contraction can be a response to pain or in anticipation of pain despite the absence of pain itself. During voluntary muscle contraction, the EMG response is sustained for a variable period of time but can be eliminated by relaxation of the muscle. This can often be accomplished by speaking calmly to the patient if an older child or by distracting a younger patient. Elimination of the muscle contraction through relaxation is critical to interpretation (3). This is critical not only because muscle contraction makes it difficult to recognize abnormal spontaneous electrical activity, but excessive involuntary muscle contractions can be seen in several neuromuscular disorders as well and therefore may confuse rendering an appropriate interpretation. In disorders involving hypocalcemia, hypomagnesemia, and hyperkalemia, cramps induce electrical discharges in the EMG during the needle examination. These are briefly sustained involuntary muscular contractions lasting seconds to minutes in duration. Because they are involuntary, eliminating the contraction through distraction or relaxation can help differentiate these from voluntary muscle contractions. Myoclonus may introduce another type of movement artifact that may be confused with involuntary muscle contraction. Myoclonus is a sudden brief and often intense involuntary muscle contraction which can be peripheral, cortical, or spinal in origin. In addition, in the congenital form of Stiff person syndrome, sustained muscle contractions are seen. Therefore, recognizing this finding as a voluntary muscle contraction as opposed to an artifact by making unsuccessful attempts to eliminate it will allow appropriate interpretation of the EMG (4).

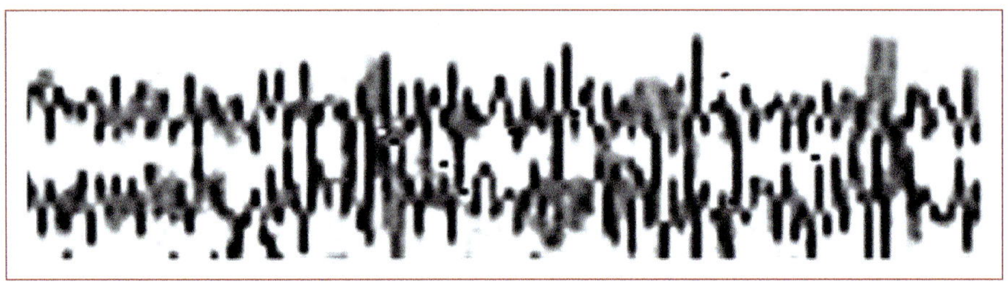

FIGURE 3.1: This is an example of an artifact caused by voluntary muscle contraction sustained for a variable period of time but eliminated by relaxation of the muscle.

Startle Response

Another example of an intrinsic source of artifact is produced by a startle response, as shown in Figure 3.2. Startle occurs most commonly in infants without an inciting factor. When it is associated with anxiety disorders, an increased auditory startle response, along with increased sweat response and enhancement of other autonomic responses, may be seen in young adults (5). In general, a startle response can be differentiated from an abnormal neuromuscular or myogenic response in that it is transient, becomes habituated, and usually is associated with a sudden movement involving the upper body of the patient. It generally does not recur. If not recognized it may be misinterpreted as a polyphasic motor unit in the EMG suggesting the presence of chronic change or reinnervation in that muscle. Since some polyphasic motor unit activity is expected at percentages that vary depending on the sampled muscle, when they occur infrequently, this could lead to a misdiagnosis (6).

Chewing/Sucking Movements

Chewing and sucking movements can be subtle and missed clinically as young patients may make chewing movement with their tongues without much mouth movement being noticed (7,8). If obtaining an EMG recording near the mouth or along upper shoulder girdle muscles, one may notice artifact appearing in bursts of motor unit activity that varies in amplitude and duration (see Figure 3.3). Complex repetitive discharges in the EMG in contrast have a polyphasic pattern of discharge that is uniform from one waveform to another with a constant firing rate starting and stopping abruptly. These complex repetitive discharges can be seen in the chronic neuropathies including various polyneuropathies, motor neuron disease (including spinal muscular atrophy and muscular dystrophy), as well as chronic radiculopathies (9,10).

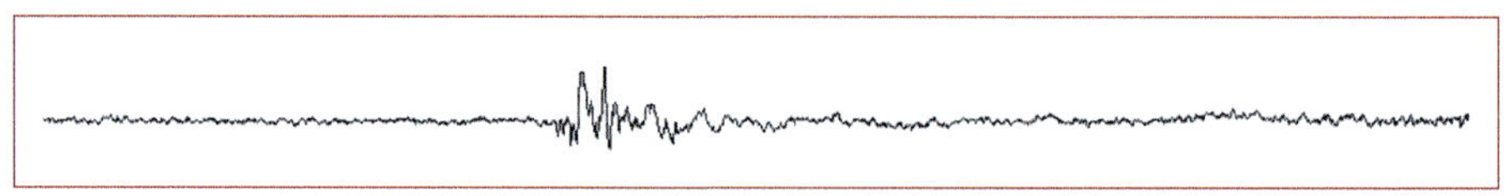

FIGURE 3.2: Startle responses during needle examination can be differentiated from an abnormal neuromuscular or myogenic response in that it is transient, becomes habituated, and usually is associated with a sudden movement.

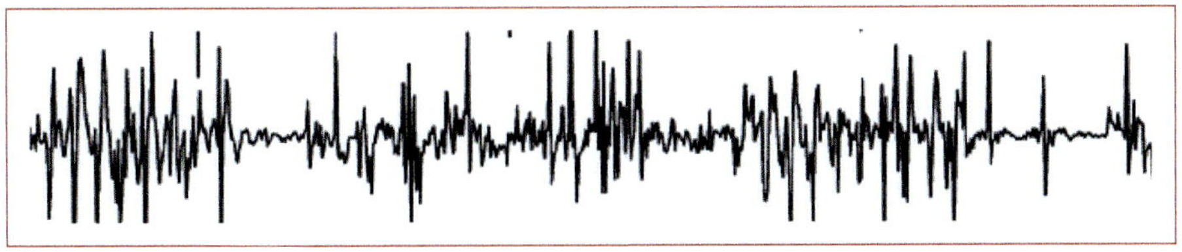

FIGURE 3.3: Chewing and sucking artifact in an infant during electromyogram can be associated with movement of their tongues without much mouth movement being noticed.

Chewing or sucking movements may be misinterpreted as complex repetitive discharges if the configuration of the EMG pattern is not closely analyzed, or if the patient is not observed to have apparent mouth or tongue movements (9).

Extrinsic Sources

The next group of artifacts is one caused by objects or electrical activity in the environment or around the patient that interferes with the recording. Common causes of artifact in the EMG include the following extrinsic sources:

Cardiac Monitors

Cardiac monitors attached to the patient may produce a regular cardiac rhythm superimposed upon the EMG signal, as shown in Figure 3.4. These can be recognized by the regular periodic pattern that is synchronous with the patient's heart rate. Furthermore, it is able to be eliminated by temporarily removing the cardiac leads or by moving the cardiac monitoring equipment further away from the surface electrode or EMG needle recording electrode. If not recognized, these could be misinterpreted as fibrillation potentials, suggesting the presence of denervation and leading to inaccurate diagnosis. Fibrillation potentials may be seen in a wide variety of neuromuscular disorders and usually indicate active, ongoing denervation. These may occur in acute radiculopathies, inflammatory myopathies, axonal degeneration in peripheral neuropathies, and motor neuron disease (11).

60 Hz Artifact

A common source of EMG artifact is due to electrical equipment near the patient. Interference from nearby equipment may include mechanical ventilators, blood warming machines, and infusion pumps. A common type of artifact in EMG is 60-Hz artifact. This artifact occurs at a frequency of 60 cycles per second or a multiple of 60 Hz as seen in Figure 3.5. Similar to artifacts produced by cardiac monitors, these artifacts are recognized by their regular

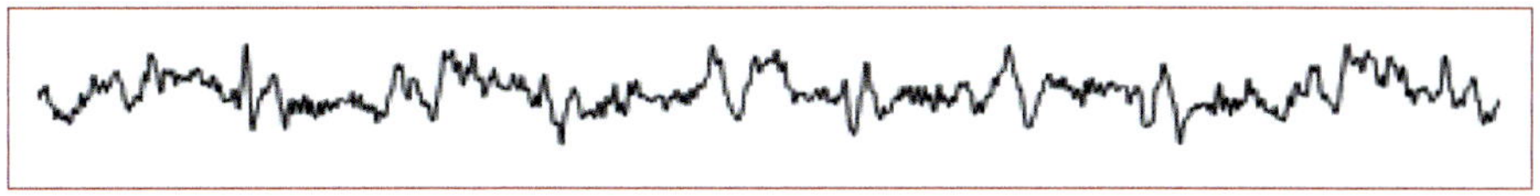

FIGURE 3.4: Cardiac monitor producing extrinsic artifact in the needle recording of the electromyogram, recognized by the regular periodic pattern that is synchronous with the patient's heart rate.

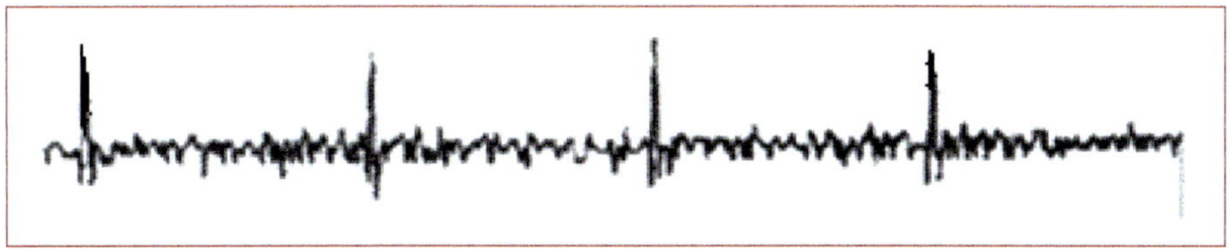

FIGURE 3.5: Artifact in the electromyogram produced by a nearby motorized device, which in this case was due to an intravenous infusion pump.

rate and successful elimination if the offending equipment is removed or moved further away from the patient (12). If not recognized during the EMG procedure, these superimposed discharges may be misinterpreted as positive sharp discharges or fibrillations suggesting the presence of denervation, leading to inaccurate diagnosis. Positive, sharp wave discharges and fibrillations can be seen in a number of neuromuscular disorders including axonal degeneration and motor neuron diseases, acute and subacute neuropathies, and inflammatory myopathic disorders.

Artifacts in Neurophysiologic Intraoperative Monitoring

In the operating room (OR), multiple devices such as infusion pumps and cardiac monitors may produce electrical noise. These artifacts are similar to what may be encountered during the performance of EMG. These extraneous signals can act as interference-producing artifacts in monitoring electrophysiological potentials during neurophysiologic intraoperative monitoring (NIOM), including the EEG, and during evoked potential (EP) monitoring. These artifacts can be confused with abnormal biological potentials suggesting nerve injury and therefore can cause misinterpretation if they remain unrecognized. In the OR, the surgical field may produce a local artifact during electrophysiological recording due to movement induced by fluid during irrigation or from electrocautery equipment. Electrocautery during routine use of a Bovie has the potential to cause amplifier overload and the signals may be added to the signal averages erroneously. Therefore, NIOM is usually stopped during its use (13).

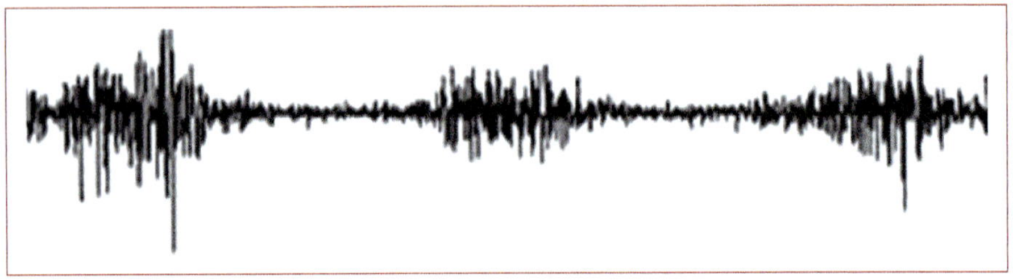

FIGURE 3.6: Galvanic artifact or "cross-talk" in a free-running electromyogram recording obtained during NIOM. Galvanic artifact occurs when metal instruments are rubbed together or a metal electrode records an artifact during irrigation or in the presence of blood or body fluid in the surgical field.

NIOM, neurophysiologic intraoperative monitoring.

In addition, artifact can occur during the use of free-running EMG in the intraoperative setting when metal instruments are rubbed together or a metal electrode records an artifact during irrigation or in the presence of blood or body fluid in the surgical field. This type of artifact in Figure 3.6 has been referred to as galvanic coupling or "cross talk." It is of significance in that it can mimic a polyphasic motor potential and lead to misinterpretation of the waveforms. If the contact is brief, the artifact may look like an electrode "pop" similar to what is seen on an EEG when an electrode loses contact with the scalp.

Artifacts During EP Monitoring

Artifacts encountered during NIOM are very different from those seen with outpatient clinical neurophysiology (CNP) recording. In outpatient EEG recordings, artifacts are due generally to physiological factors that measure eye movements (electrooculogram), tongue movements (movement monitor), and muscle movements (electromyography) which are not problematic during NIOM where the patient is anesthetized. However, NIOM recordings are obtained in an electrically "hostile" environment where many different electrical devices are present that are either attached to, or functioning around, the patient. Therefore, it is not surprising that most NIOM artifacts are due to electrical interference from external sources. These common artifacts can be differentiated by the underlying cause as noted here.

Stimulus Artifact

A common artifact present during EP monitoring is due to an electrical stimulus. It is therefore referred to as a stimulus artifact (Figure 3.7). This can be exacerbated with short interelectrode distances as in very young patients. Somatosensory evoked potential (SEP) studies require electrical stimulation applied to the skin overlying a peripheral nerve (e.g., median, posterior tibial nerve). The electrical current can spread over the cutaneous surface causing a large stimulus artifact at the recording electrodes. This may occur even when the recording electrodes are distant from the stimulus electrodes. Although the presence of stimulus artifacts assures the delivery of stimulus, large stimulus artifacts may shift the baseline and obscure the early components of an evoked response. Fortunately, most of the stimulus artifact is cancelled out if both electrodes (inputs 1 and 2) have low impedances and are balanced. To minimize the presence of stimulus artifacts, the electrode impedance (14) should be less than 10 kΩ and be balanced between two electrodes (15). If stimulus artifact is seen in all recording channels, the impedance of the ground electrode should be checked to ensure proper function.

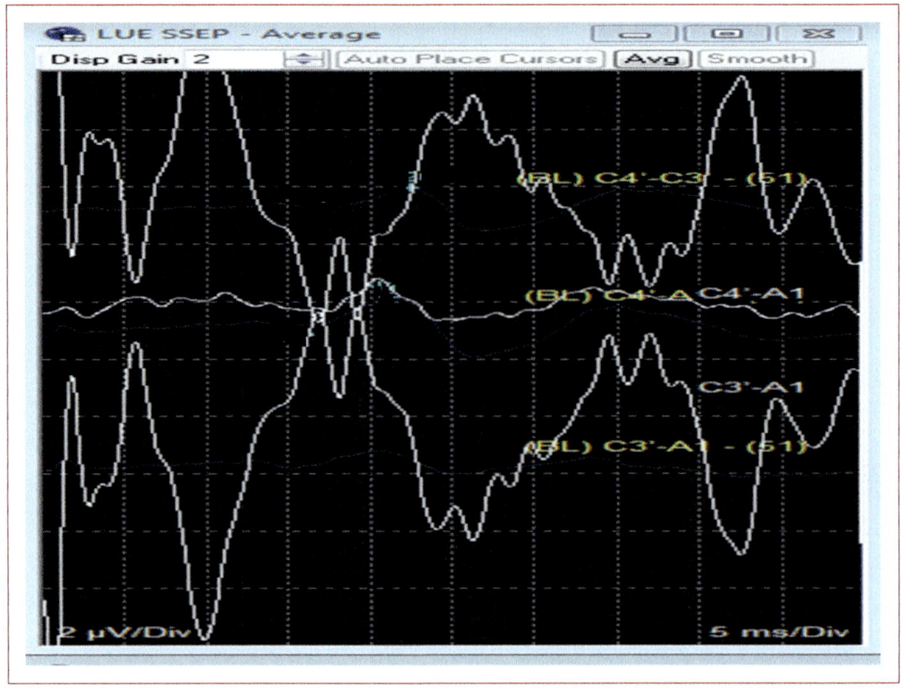

FIGURE 3.7: SEP I after left ulnar nerve stimulation. Channels 1 and 3 show high-amplitude slow waves (three waves in 50-ms sweep) corresponding to 60 Hz. This is due to high electrode impedance at C3 which are common to both channels 1 and 3. The channel 2 tracing from C4-A1 derivation shows a normal N18 waveform.

SEP, somatosensory evoked potential.

In addition, physically separating the input and stimulus cables can reduce the presence of stimulus-induced artifact. If stimulus artifact cannot be minimized using standard methods to limit interference with the early waveforms of the EP, the final solution may be switching the stimulus electrodes of cathode and anode. This may be successful when half of the averaging is done with the cathode proximal to the anode, and then reversing the polarity of stimulus electrodes is performed for the second half of the averaging. The same can be accomplished by adding the two final tracings obtained using standard and subsequent reversal of the anode and cathode stimulus locations.

1. 60-Hz artifact
   Another common artifact is "60-cycle" or 60-Hz artifact. It is impossible to eliminate this artifact completely from the NIOM environment because of the presence of an alternating current (AC) power supply that is ubiquitous in the OR. Similar to stimulus artifact, most of 60-Hz interference activity is canceled out as long as the impedance of the two input electrodes is low and balanced. This scenario does not differ in pediatric cases from those in adulthood. Figure 3.8 shows a large degree of 60-Hz artifact due to high electrode impedance at the C3 recording electrode. In order to avoid synchronization with 60 Hz, the stimulus rate is usually set at a rate that is not a harmonic of 60 Hz. For example, a rate of 2.1 Hz or 3.1 Hz may be utilized instead of a whole number such as 2 Hz or 3 Hz, so it is not entrained as a similar frequency. If a 60-Hz artifact increases during the averaging process, changing the stimulus rates and increasing the number of averages could help to reduce this artifact. Physically separating cables that conduct AC, including input cables and power mains and outlets, can help minimize the 60-Hz artifact. Although the use of a 60-Hz notch filter is not recommended for most EP recordings, in some cases they may be necessary when all efforts and measures fail to eliminate the artifact. In this case, we may encounter "60-Hz ringing," which consists of rhythmic 60-Hz waveforms that rapidly decline in amplitude following the stimulus artifact (Figure 3.8) (16). The artifact encountered by ringing tends to be greater with higher stimulus rates. Unfortunately, the presence of 60-Hz ringing may obscure the identification of the early components in the EPs.
2. Cautery artifacts
   Cautery artifacts are another type of artifact encountered in the NIOM setting. Its presence does not differ in the pediatric patient compared to adults. Cautery artifacts produce an intermittent artifact. As expected, the use of cautery introduces a high-amplitude, fast frequency artifact. Practically, all trials obtained will be rejected from averaging EPs during the time cautery is used. It is not possible to collect measurable tracings when cautery is taking place. Fortunately, the use of cautery occurs most often during the early stages of surgery and therefore not typically during periods of surgical manipulation or intervention when SEP and motor evoked potential (MEP) monitoring is required. Using an auto-rejection program, it may be possible to obtain measurable responses, but it takes a considerable amount of time to record one response when the majority of trials are rejected from averaging due to artifact (17). Figure 3.9 shows

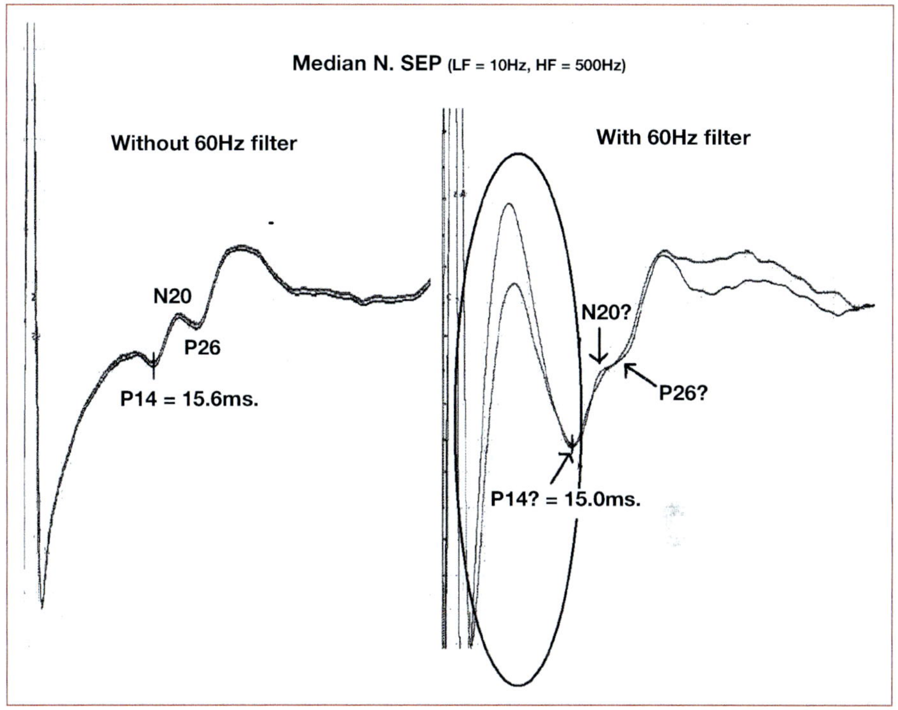

FIGURE 3.8: Median nerve SEP recording. The left tracing was recorded without a 60-Hz notch filter. The right tracing was simultaneously recorded from the same electrodes with the use of a 60-Hz notch filter. This tracing shows high-amplitude sinusoidal waves immediately after the stimulus artifact, obscuring the identification of P14, N20, and P26 potentials. The high-amplitude sinusoidal wave is an initial wave in a series of 60-Hz sine waves ("ringing"), which sequentially decreases over time.

Source: From Yamada T, Meng E. Basic EEG technology. In: Yamada T, Meng E, eds. *Practical Guide for Clinical Neurophysiologic Testing: EEG*. Vol. 1. Philadelphia, PA: Wolters Kluwer, Lippincott Williams & Wilkins; 2010:5-39, with permission.

SEP, somatosensory evoked potential.

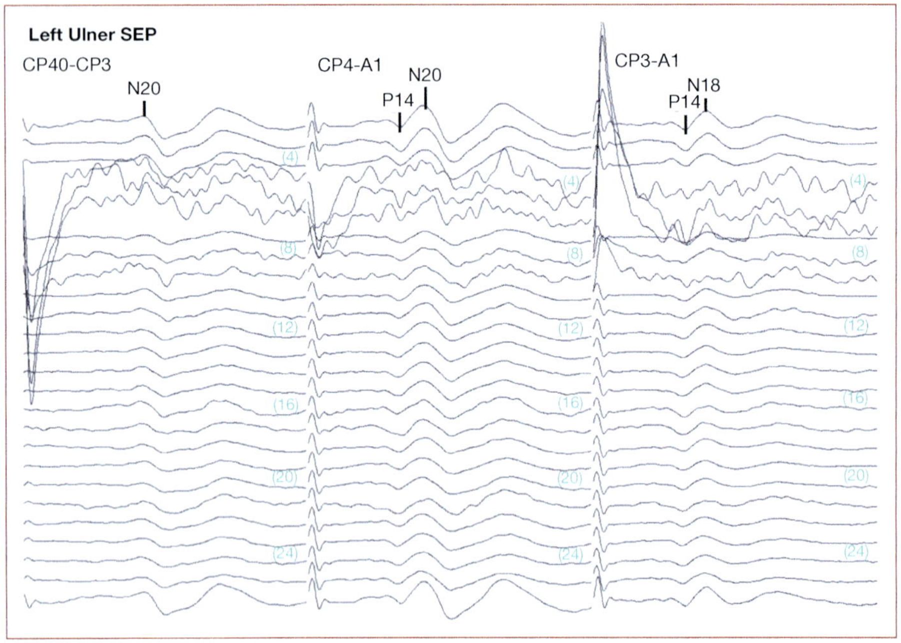

FIGURE 3.9: Serial ulnar SEP tracings during surgery. The tracings 4 to 6 (from the top) were recorded without the use of autorejection mode during cautery. Therefore, the responses were totally obscured by cautery artifact.

SEP, somatosensory evoked potential.

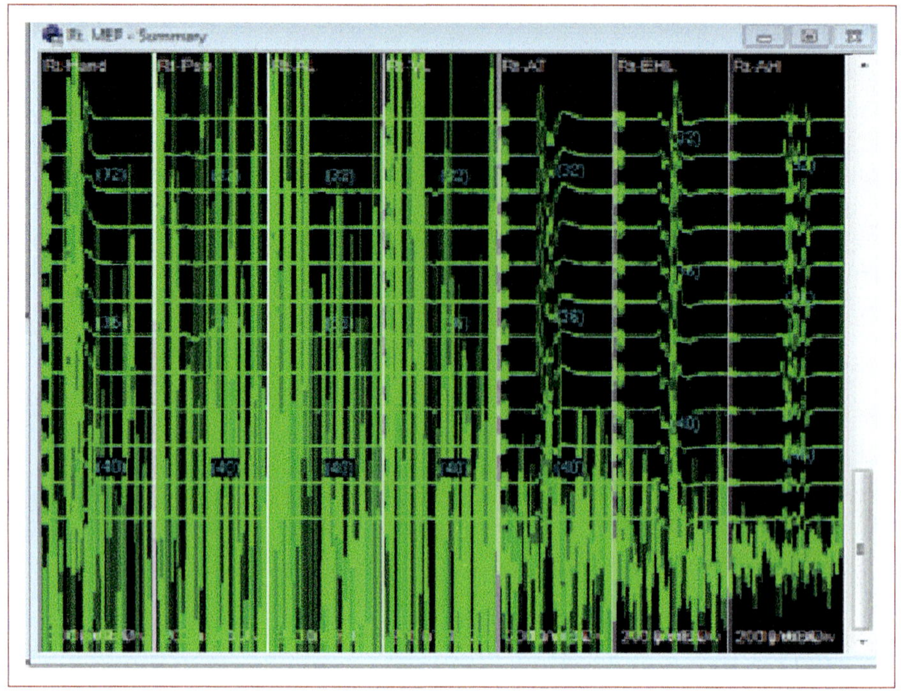

FIGURE 3.10: Serial tracings of MEPs from extremity muscles on the left recorded after transcranial stimulation. The bottom tracing was captured by inadvertent stimulation during the use of cautery. Extremely high-amplitude fast frequency activity was registered in all the muscles recorded.

MEP, motor evoked potential.

three tracings that were recorded without the use of autorejection mode during cautery. The responses that resulted are unreliable. In this case, when an artifact is introduced and is not rejected, one commonly used phrase to reflect this situation is "garbage in-garbage out." Figure 3.9 shows an example of cautery artifact that was obtained accidentally during the delivery of transcranial electrical stimulation for MEP monitoring.

Other Intraoperative Monitoring Equipment

It is crucial to be aware of the number of machines, variety of equipment in the OR, and their proximity to the patient and other intraoperative monitoring equipment (18). Electrical interference from any number of other instruments can occur and interfere with reliable collection of NIOM data.

Some medical devices may send high-amplitude signals that interfere with identification of the target waveforms, even when the device is a distance away from recording instruments and from the patient. The frequencies vary depending on the particular medical device. Figure 3.10 shows a rhythmic 80-Hz artifact that did not disappear even after 1,000 averages. The artifact was eliminated only after the AC power to the cardiac echo machine was turned off. In this scenario, an increase in the number of averages and altering the stimulus rate may attenuate but not eliminate the artifact. External interference artifacts usually affect all channels but the degree of artifact may vary depending on the electrode impedance and impedance balance between two electrodes (note 80-Hz artifacts are most prominent in Fz and Cz channels as compared to others in Figure 3.11).

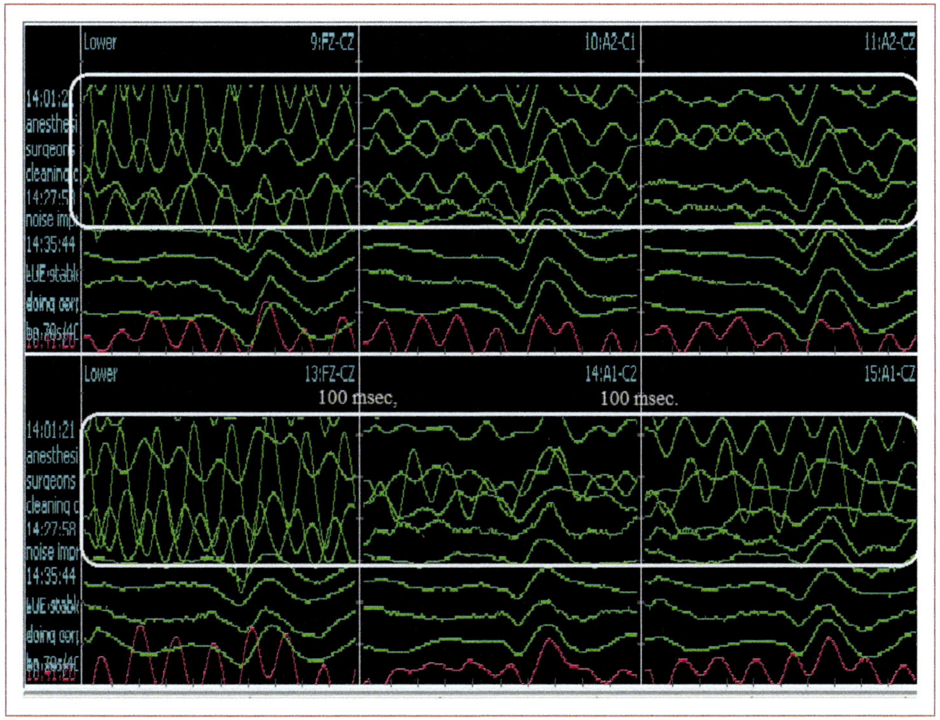

FIGURE 3.11: This figure demonstrates tibial nerve SEP monitoring. The first 4 to 5 tracings were contaminated by rhythmic 80-Hz (eight waves in 100-msec window) artifacts (highlighted by rectangular boxes). This interference pattern was created by the echocardiographic machine placed nearby the EPs instrument. Note that the wave forms and wave phases vary depending on the trial and are reflected by the time difference between stimulus and interference pattern for each trial.

EP, evoked potential; SEP, somatosensory evoked potential.

TABLE 3.1: Summary of Artifacts Encountered During EMG Recording and the Resultant Potential for Misinterpretation of the Findings

Artifact	Etiology	Misinterpretation
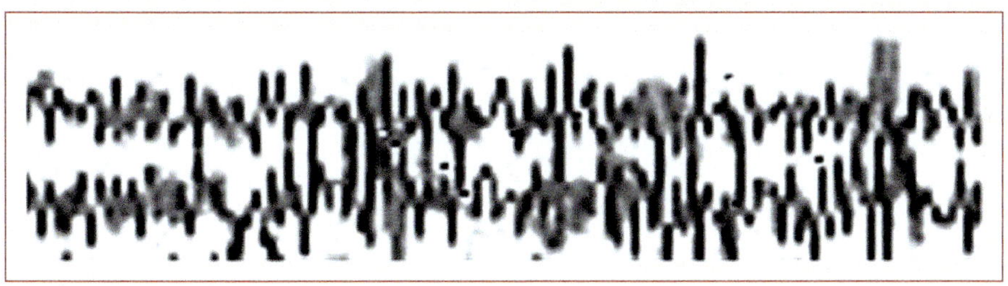	Voluntary muscle contraction	Cramp potential Pathologic–contracture

(*continued*)

TABLE 3.1: Summary of artifacts encountered during EMG recording and the resultant potential for misinterpretation of the findings. (*continued*)

Artifact	Etiology	Misinterpretation
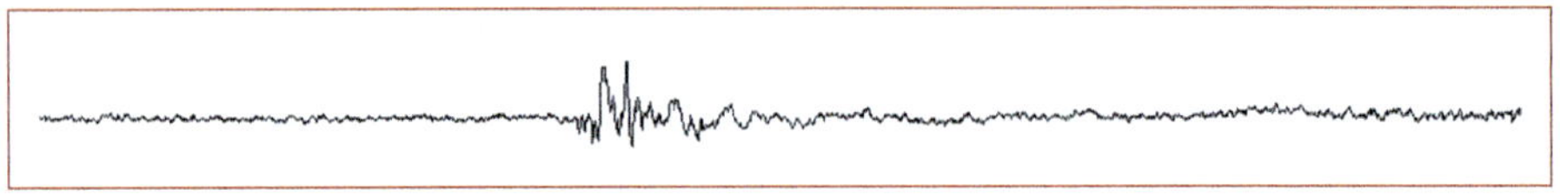	Startle	Polyphasic motor potential
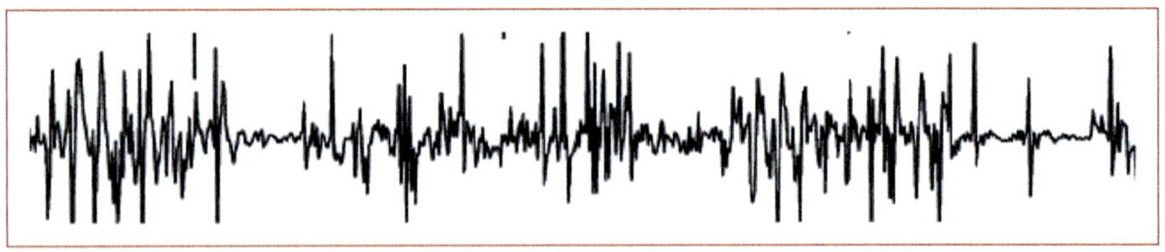	Chewing Sucking	Complex repetitive discharge
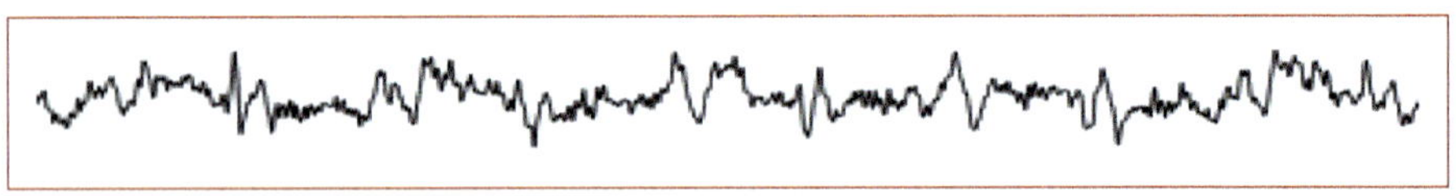	Cardiac monitor	Fibrillations
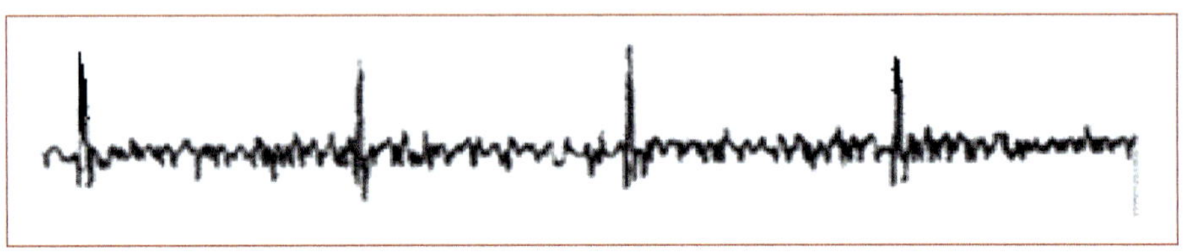	Intravenous infusion pumps, mechanical ventilators, blood warmers	Positive sharp discharges Fibrillations
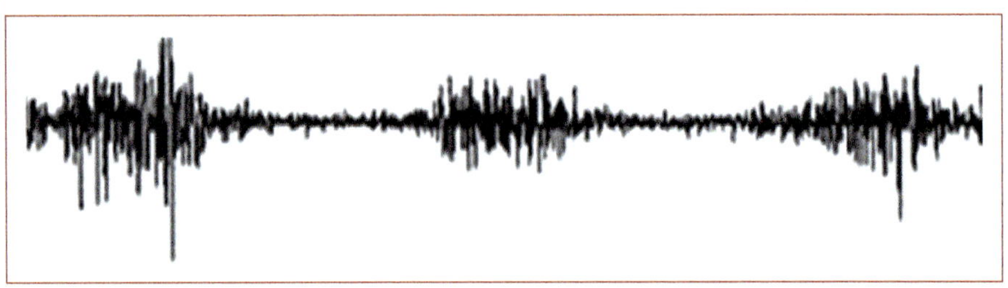	Metal electrodes Irrigation fluid Body fluids	Polyphasic activity

CONCLUSION

In the pediatric population, some artifacts may be seen more commonly than in adults due to shorter interelectrode distances, the presence of startle reflexes, and the need for multiple unique types of monitoring devices. The key to interpretation is first to recognize that the data being evaluated have artifact present. Subsequent efforts involve determining the likely cause in order to eliminate or reduce the source of an artifact. Awareness of the surrounding environment and observation of the patient should be the first step in the search for reducing artifact in pediatric clinical neurophysiological procedures.

REFERENCES

1. Pitt MC. Nerve conduction studies and needle EMG in very small children. *Eur J Paediatr Neurol*. 2017;16:285-291. doi:10.1016/j.ejpn.2011.07.014.
2. Kimura J. *Electrodiagnosis in Diseases of Nerve and Muscle: Principles and Practice*. 4th ed. New York, NY: Oxford University Press; 2013.
3. Galloway GM. EMG considerations in the pediatric patient. In: Galloway GM, ed. *Clinical Neurophysiology in Pediatrics: A Practical Approach to Neurodiagnostic Testing and Management*. New York, NY: Demos Medical; 2015:147-152.
4. McDonald CM. Electrodiagnosis in pediatrics. In: Alexander MA, Matthews DJ, Murphy KP, eds. *Pediatric Rehabilitation: Principles and Practice*. 5th ed. New York, NY: Demos Medical; 2015:113-152.
5. Bakker MJ, Tijssen MA, van der Meer JN, et al. Increased whole-body auditory startle reflex and autonomic reactivity in children with anxiety disorders. *J Psychiatry Neurosci*. 2009;34:314-322.
6. McEvoy K, Hasenstab K, Senturk D, et al. Physiologic artifacts in resting state oscillations in young children: methodological considerations for noisy data. *Brain Imaging Behav*. 2015;9:104-114. doi:10.1007/s11682-014-9343-7.
7. Hellmann M, von Kleist-Retzow J-C, Haupt WF, et al. Diagnostic value of electromyography in children and adolescents. *J Clin Neurophysiol*. 2005;22:43-48. doi:10.1097/01.WNP.0000151146.91147.A1.
8. Rubin DI, Daube JR. *Clinical Neurophysiology*. 4th ed. New York, NY: Oxford University Press; 2016.
9. King, PB. Pediatric nerve conduction studies and EMG. In: Blum AS, Rutkove SB, eds. *The Clinical Neurophysiology Primer*. New York, NY: Humana Press; 2007:369-389.
10. Komur M, Okuyaz C, Makharoblidze K. Consistency between referral diagnosis and post-ENMG diagnosis in children. *J Pak Med Assoc*. 2014; 64:179-183.
11. Ghosh PS, Sorenson EJ. Use of clinical and electrical myotonia to differentiate childhood myopathies. *J Child Neurol*. 2015;30:1300-1306. doi:10.1177/0883073814559646.
12. Galloway G. Electromyography. In: Husain A, ed. *A Practical Approach to Neurophysiologic Intraoperative Monitoring*. 2nd ed. New York, NY: Demos Medical; 2015:66-75.
13. Pearlman RC, Isley MR, Ganley JC. Electrical artifact during intraoperative EMG monitoring. *Am J Electroneurodiagnotic Tech*. 2008;48:107-118.
14. Seaba P. Basic electronics and electrical safety. In: Yamada T, Meng E, eds. *Practical Guide for Clinical Neurophysiologic Testing: EEG*. Philadelphia, PA: Wolters Kluwer, Lippincott Williams & Wilkins; 2010:40-53.
15. Sinha SR, Sullivan L, Sabau D, et al. American Clinical Neurophysiology Society Guideline 1: minimum technical requirements for performing clinical electroencephalography. *J Clin Neurophysiol*. 2016;33:303-307. doi:10.1097/WNP.0000000000000308.
16. Yamada T, Meng E. Basic EEG technology. In: Yamada T, Meng E, eds. *Practical Guide for Clinical Neurophysiologic Testing: EEG*. Philadelphia, PA: Wolters Kluwer, Lippincott Williams & Wilkins; 2010:5-39.
17. Yamada T, Meng E, Seaba P. Principle of evoked potentials. In: Yamada T, Meng E, eds. *Practical Guide for Clinical Neurophysiologic Testing: EP, LTM, IOM, PSG and NCS*. Philadelphia, PA: Wolters Kluwer, Lippincott Williams & Wilkins; 2011:1-12.
18. Kale EB. Introduction to the operating room. In: Hussain AM, ed. *Practical Approach to Neurophysiologic Intraoperative Monitoring*. 2nd ed. New York, NY: Demos Medical; 2015:3-17.

CHAPTER 4

Artifacts of Neuromonitoring

Jason Siegel and David Freeman

INTRODUCTION

The neurocritical care unit (NCCU) houses patients with the ability for rapid neurological decompensation, often requiring continuous monitoring with clinical and neurophysiologic monitoring technology. In addition to standard patient monitors such as continuous invasive blood pressure, central venous pressures, cardiac output, and ventilator management, the NCCU employs highly specialized neurological monitors. These monitors collect information on intracranial pressure (ICP), cerebral blood flow (CBF), cerebral spinal fluid (CSF) analysis, brain tissue oxygen monitoring, and electrophysiology. As with any type of biological monitoring, interpretation relies not only on knowledge of normal and pathological signals but also on the presence of artifacts. Deviation in measurements obtained by technological support supplied by a monitor may represent neither normal neurophysiology nor pathology. This chapter will discuss several types of invasive and noninvasive techniques for NCCU neurophysiologic monitoring, with relevant examples of common and rare artifacts.

INTRACRANIAL PRESSURE

ICP monitoring is pertinent for a variety of diseases, including malignant edema in large territorial ischemic strokes, mass effect from hemorrhagic strokes and tumors, and global cerebral edema from hypoxic brain injury, severe hepatic encephalopathy, and traumatic brain injury.

According to the Monro–Kellie doctrine, there is a fixed volume of intracranial space that is occupied by the brain, CSF, and blood. When a new component enters this space, one of these must be sacrificed (usually CSF first, then brain or blood) (1). Because cerebral perfusion pressure (CPP) is the difference between mean arterial pressure (MAP) and ICP, as the ICP increases, the CPP decreases, further limiting blood flow to the brain and subsequently causing secondary ischemia and edema, which in turn further increases ICP.

Depending on the underlying disease, availability, comorbidities, and goals of monitoring, there are many choices for ICP monitoring.

Invasive ICP Monitoring

There are several options available for invasive ICP monitoring. These are placed by neurosurgeons, or experienced neurocritical care physicians (Figure 4.1).

External Ventricular Drainage

The external ventricular drain (EVD) is the gold standard for ICP monitoring. An added benefit to ICP monitoring is the ability to drain CSF to therapeutically relieve ICP. A catheter is typically placed into the right lateral ventricle in the brain, and is connected to sterile tubing that meets a three-way stopcock on the collection apparatus. The stopcock allows the system to either be opened to the collection bag or opened to the electronic transducer, which reports the ICP and waveform via continuous electronic display. The ICP and waveforms generated can also be deduced by the features of the CSF that are present in the tubing between the stopcock and the collection bag.

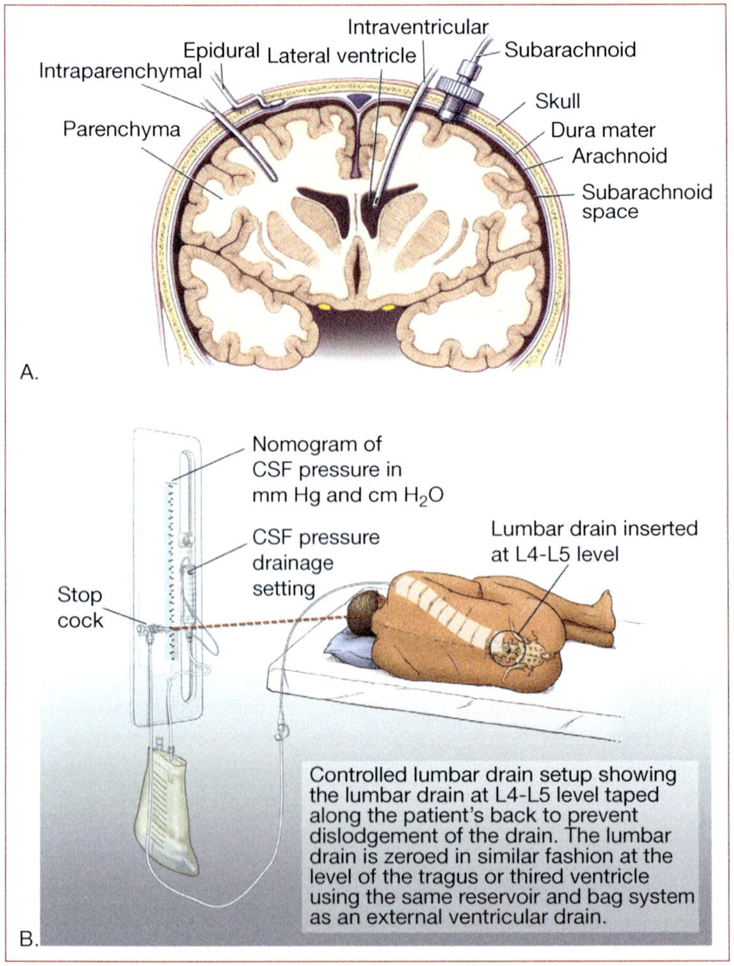

FIGURE 4.1: (A) Types and placement of invasive ICP monitors. These include intraparenchymal, subarachnoid, intraventricular, and epidural. EVD is considered the gold standard. (B) Typical setup and positioning of a patient with an EVD (note the patient does not need to remain in the lateral decubitus position after insertion, as along as the stopcock is leveled at the tragus).

CSF, cerebral spinal fluid; EVD, external ventricular drain; ICP, intracranial pressure.

Before the tubing drains into the bag, it runs vertically along a graduated scale for measurement. The level where the CSF equilibrates along the scale represents the tidal ICP. One can also appreciate the rhythmic variations in CSF level, which correspond to the waveform.

Normal CSF waveforms have three peaks (**Figure 4.2**). The percussion wave (P1) represents the arterial pulsation transmitting through the choroid plexus into the ventricle. The tidal wave (P2) reflects the venous compartment, translating into the compliance of the ventricular system. The P2 wave should be 80% of the height of P1. Finally, the dicrotic wave (P3) represents the aortic valve closure.

Normally, the P1 is the highest point, followed by P2 and P3 (2). Peaked P2 waves could be a sign of poor ventricular compliance due to increased ICP. Alternatively, this pattern can be seen in jugular venous compression (which can occur during central line placement or incorrect head or neck positioning), the Valsalva maneuver (in an incompletely sedated patient who is agitated, or in a constipated patient who is straining to have a bowel movement), or in an underventilated patient with carbon dioxide

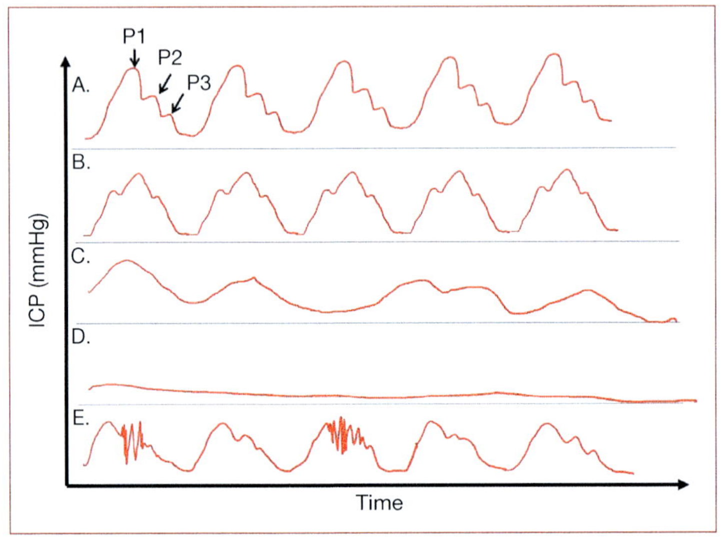

FIGURE 4.2: (A) Normal wave forms with P1 (arterial pulsation), P2 (venous compartment), and P3 (aortic valve closure) waves. (B) Peaked P2 waves, which can symbolize jugular compression artifact or Valsalva physiology. (C) Broad-based, low-amplitude waves, which suggest drainage occlusion artifact. (D) A flat line represents a severe occlusion artifact, or that the 3-way stopcock is closed to the transducer and is draining CSF. (E) Fast, sharp waveforms which do not correlate with respiration or heart rate suggest movement of the patient or transducer system.

CSF, cerebral spinal fluid; ICP, intracranial pressure.

accumulation. Broad-based, low-amplitude waveforms with indistinct P waves should raise the concern of drainage occlusion either from cellular debris, blood clots, tissue fragments, or as an artifact from kinking of the catheter (3). However, a flat line may mean severe pathology such as the absence of CBF and brain death. The EVD only transduces a wave form if it is not draining into a collection bag. Therefore, if a flat line is seen on the monitor, check to make sure the EVD is draining properly. If it is not draining, stop drainage and reassess the monitor. Finally, sharp, rapid wave forms that are asynchronous with heart rate imply a movement artifact of the EVD system or the monitor (Figure 4.2A–E).

Transduced and tidal ICPs that are inconsistent with the patient's clinical situation (normal or low ICP in a patient with hydrocephalus, or high ICPs in a patient who is awake, neurologically intact, and without headache) should raise the question of incorrect transducer positioning. The transducer should be leveled at the tragus of the ear, which represents the foramen of Monroe. If the transducer is too high, the ICPs will be falsely low, and vice versa.

Noninvasive Monitoring

Optic Nerve Sheath Diameter

The pia and arachnoid meningeal layers surround the optic nerve (ON). When the ICP increases, we can noninvasively observe the effects on the ON (4). The ON is typically 3 mm in diameter, and is surrounded by 0.1 to 0.2 mm of subarachnoid space, and a 0.3-mm-thick optic nerve sheath (ONS) (5,6). An ONS diameter of less than 5 mm is considered normal, but the sensitivity, specificity, and reproducibility are variable (6–9).

Measurements of the ONS diameter are obtained 3 mm posterior to the back wall of the globe, in the axial plane of the ON (5,10). The anatomical structures of the ON complex should be clearly identified, including retina; lamina cribrosa (hyperechoic); the ON fibers (hypoechoic); the subarachnoid space (hyperechoic); the ONS (hypoechoic); and the central retinal artery, which can be identified (Figure 4.3) using Doppler ultrasonography (11). The lamina cribrosa is a dense fiber layer that is hyperechoic and can cast a shadow artifact, mimicking the hypoechoic ON (Figure 4.4). The central retinal artery runs through the center of the ON and will show the true direction of the ON despite lamina cribrosa artifact.

Time may be a further source of artifact as it has been suggested that there is a delayed reversal of nerve sheath distension, especially in patients with rapidly fluctuating ICP (commonly seen in patients with poor compliance) (12).

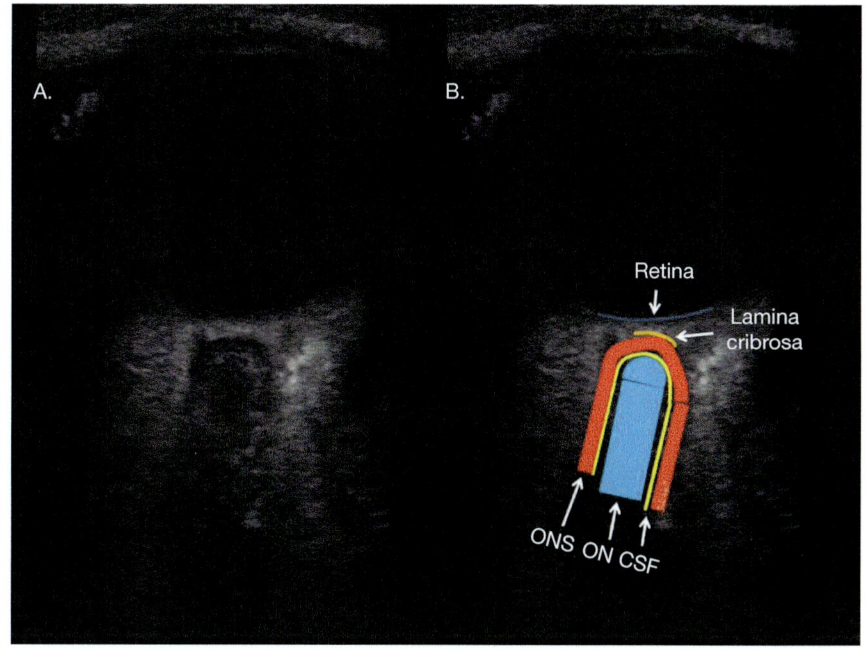

FIGURE 4.3: (A) Normal ON anatomy. (B) Labeled figure with retina, lamina cribrosa, ONS, ON, and subarachnoid space (CSF).

CSF, cerebral spinal fluid; ON, optic nerve; ONS, optic nerve sheath.

Transcranial Doppler Ultrasound

Transcranial Doppler ultrasound (TCD) uses low-frequency Doppler over four thin acoustic windows: transtemporal, suboccipital, transorbital, and submandibular (13). TCDs can be useful in identifying increased ICP, in addition to cerebral artery vasospasm (VSP), a condition that commonly occurs after aneurysmal subarachnoid hemorrhage (aSAH). When the intracranial vessels are isonated through these bone windows, the peak systolic velocity (PSV) and end diastolic velocity (EDV) can be directly measured (Figure 4.5). From these measurements, a variety of other indices can be calculated, including mean flow velocity (MFV), the Gosling pulsatility index (PI), the Pourcelot resistivity index (RI), and the Lindegaard ratio (LR) (13–16).

The most common source of artifact is poor bone windows, which occur in 10% to 15% of patients (6) and are due to thickness of the cancellous component of the temporal bone (17). The thickness prevents efficient transduction of ultrasound waves, decreasing the clarity of the cerebral vasculature

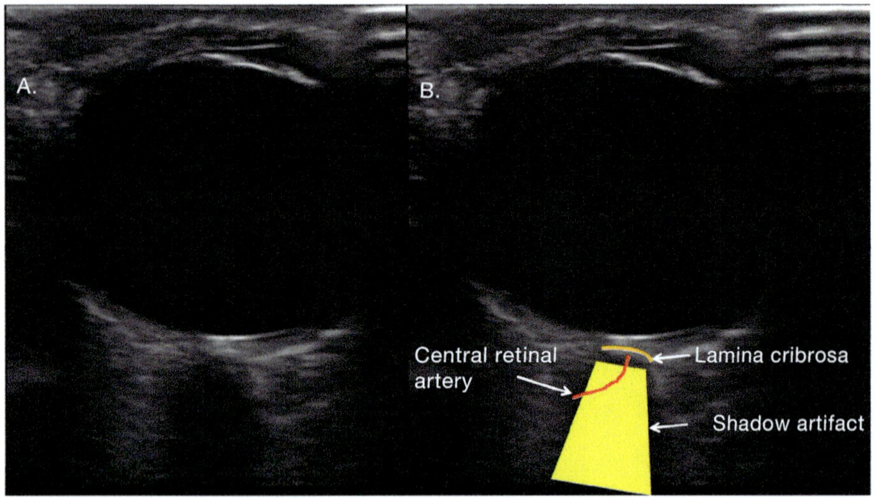

FIGURE 4.4: (A) The hypoechoic streak behind the globe appears to be the ON. (B) The central retinal artery tracks medially, revealing the true route of the ON and that the hypoechoic streak is a shadow artifact from the lamina cribrosa.

ON, optic nerve.

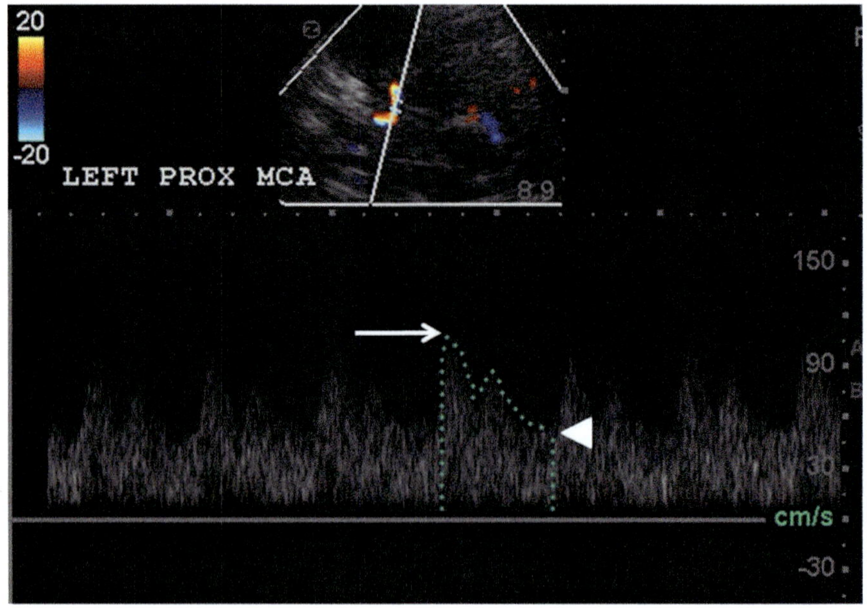

FIGURE 4.5: Normal TCD waveform of the left proximal MCA. The PSV (arrow) = 107.2 cm/s. EDV (arrow head) = 53.6 cm/s.

EDV, end diastolic velocity; MCA, middle cerebral artery; PSV, peak systolic velocity; TCD, transcranial Doppler ultrasound.

(Figure 4.6). Poor bone windows are more common in the elderly and women (18) and can cause significant error in velocity interpretation (19).

Another well-described ultrasound artifact is known as a twinkling artifact. A twinkling artifact is manifested by a rapidly changing mixture of red and blue Doppler signals, appearing as rapid changes in flow direction in relation to the TCD probe (20). Twinkling artifacts have been seen next to strongly reflecting structures such as parenchymal calcifications and cerebral aneurysm clips and coils (20,21). It is important to be aware of and recognize this artifact as aSAH patients typically have aneurysms secured by one of these devices, and many undergo routine TCD monitoring for VSP.

TCD is user dependent and only experienced ultrasonographers should perform the test for clinical assessment. A steady hand is required to both find and maintain arterial pulsations and appropriate wave forms. Even small, abrupt movements of the probe can cause small, abrupt changes in isonation, which may appear and sound like the short bursts of noise heard when microemboli travel through the arteries. An unsteady hand may create false-positive signs for cerebral microemboli, and should be avoided.

Brain Tissue Oxygen Monitoring

The goal of brain tissue oxygen monitoring is to prevent secondary brain injury after primary injury, such as traumatic brain injury, stroke, VSP, and status epilepticus. Brain tissue oxygen monitoring is expressed by the cerebral metabolic requirement of oxygen ($CMRO_2$), which is calculated by the product of CBF and the difference between arterial and jugular venous oxygen content: $CMRO_2 = CBF \times (CaO_2 - CjO_2)$. This equation can be rearranged such that $CaO_2 - CjO_2 = AJDO_2 = CMRO_2/CBF$.

Jugular Venous Bulb Oximetry

This technique requires placement of an oximeter into the jugular bulb to measure jugular venous oxygen saturation (SjO_2), which is proportional to CjO_2 (22). A decrease in SjO_2 less than 50% can be due to a decrease in SaO_2 (hypoxia, sepsis, and shock), a decrease in CBF (VSP, shock, and increased

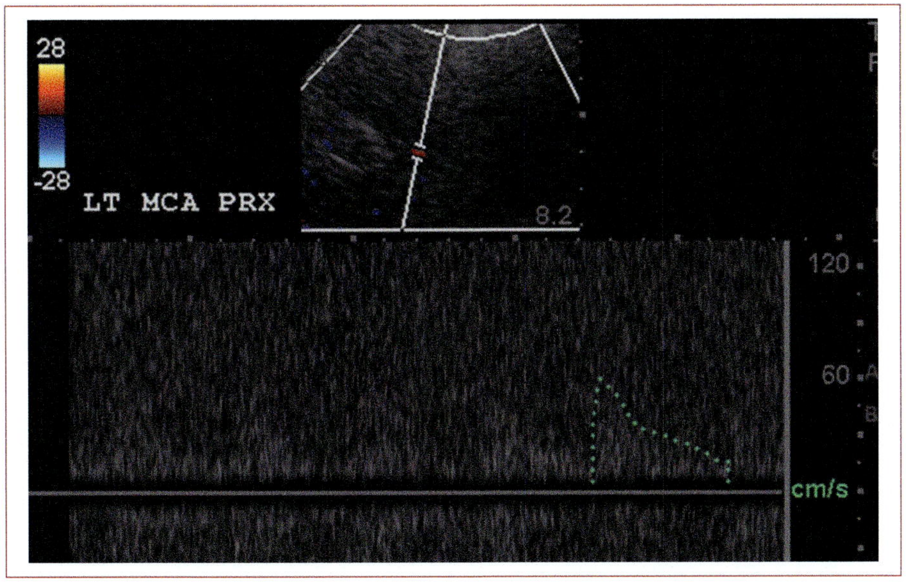

FIGURE 4.6: Due to poor bone windows, Doppler wave forms are less distinct, and the entire isonated field is more homogenous. Though in this case, a wave form may be outlined, it does not have the appropriate morphology to be considered adequate quality.

LT, left; MCA, middle cerebral artery; PRX, proximal.

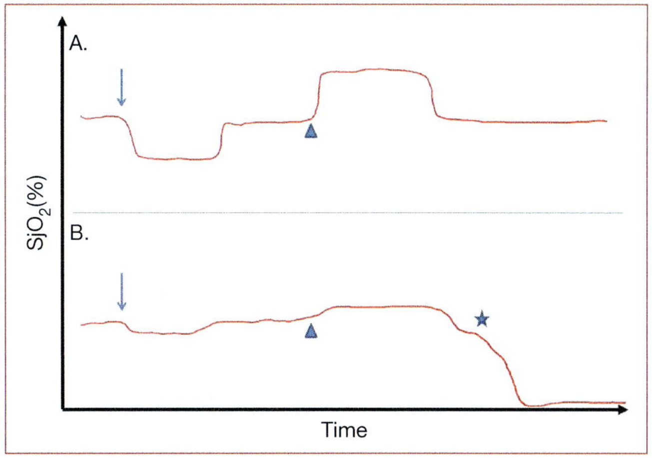

FIGURE 4.7: (A) Normal fiber optic continuous jugular bulb oxygenation tracing. (B) Continuous tracing of a jugular bulb oximetry catheter against venous wall, or with fibrin clot at tip. With the normal tracing, there is an appropriate decrease with SjO_2 in response to a decrease in SaO_2, an increase in (or in some cases a decrease in) $CMRO_2$ (arrow), and an appropriate increase in SjO_2 with an increased CBF or decreased $CMRO_2$ (arrow head). When the catheter becomes completely occluded (star), SjO_2 drops.

CBF, cerebral blood flow; $CMRO_2$, cerebral metabolic requirement of oxygen; SjO_2, jugular venous oxygen saturation.

ICP), or an increase in $CMRO_2$ (increased cerebral metabolism, fever, central nervous system infection, pain, inadequate sedation, and seizures). An increase in SjO_2 greater than 75% can be due to increased CBF (cerebral vasodilation, hypercapnia, and hypertension) or decreased $CMRO_2$ (deep sedation, coma, hypothermia, cerebral infarction, and brain death).

SjO_2 can be measured by serial samples, which are prone to error in a dynamic situation, or continuously via fiber optic monitoring (Figure 4.7A) (23). In either case, SjO_2 will be miscalculated if the catheter is malpositioned. The most common location of misplacement of the catheter is inferior to the jugular bulb. At this location, venous drainage from the head and neck will be included in the sampling. If the catheter is impinged against the wall of the jugular bulb or if there is occlusion (kinking or fibrin clot), the continuous monitor may be dampened or falsely low (Figure 4.7B) because the catheter will be less reactive to changes in true jugular venous flow and SjO_2. Furthermore, jugular venous oxygenation works well in determining global or hemispheric SjO_2, but has limitations on focal and posterior fossa lesions (24).

Near-Infrared Spectroscopy

Near-infrared spectroscopy (NIRS) uses the same supply and demand principles as jugular venous bulb oximetry (25). But instead of measuring the difference between SaO_2 and SjO_2, NIRS measures the difference between oxygenated and deoxygenated hemoglobin. NIRS delivers near-infrared light waves (680–1000 nm) through skin, bone, and brain tissue. Oxygenated hemoglobin has a maximum absorption of 900 nm and deoxygenated hemoglobin at about 760 nm (25). A forehead surface sensor measures the transmittance of the light, detecting mixed cerebral arterial–venous oxygen saturation. The factors that affect jugular venous bulb oximetry have the same effect on NIRS. Unlike jugular venous bulb oximetry, NIRS is more effective at localized changes in brain oxygenation, albeit limited to the frontal lobes.

The most common source of artifact for NIRS is surface contamination. Skin and skull variability will have an unpredictable effect on NIRS readings. NIRS optodes attach to the forehead like adhesive bandage. Diaphoresis and

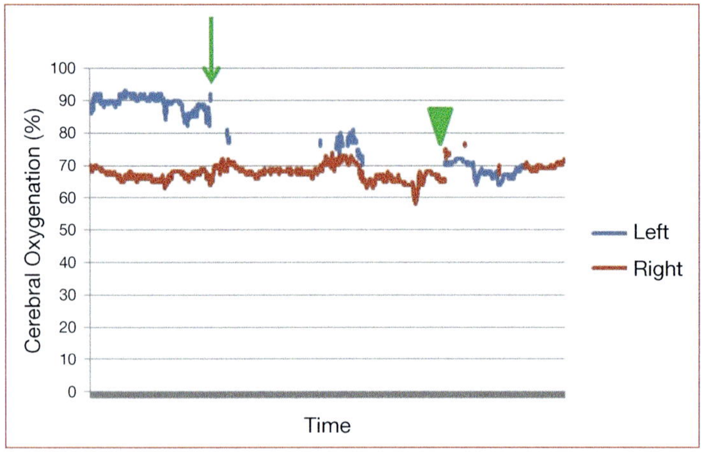

FIGURE 4.8: Continuous NIRS tracing showing a difference of approximately 20% in cerebral oxygenation, higher on the left side. This difference was due to increased venous oxyhemoglobin and decreased left hemispheric $CMRO_2$ due to steal phenomenon and ischemia. When the left carotid artery was sacrificed (arrow designates beginning of the procedure, arrow head designates post procedure), the left and right NIRS become symmetrical. The space between the arrow and the arrow head is the procedural period, a time where surface contamination becomes relevant, causing missing data during this time.

$CMRO_2$, cerebral metabolic requirement of oxygen; NIRS, near-infrared spectroscopy.

patient removal (as seen in encephalopathic or septic patients) limit NIRS use and provide for missing data and artifact.

Figure 4.8 demonstrates continuous NIRS tracing for a patient with left carotid-jugular fistula. The fistula created a steal phenomenon with left hemispheric ischemia (decreasing $CMRO_2$ on the left). In addition, the jugular venous blood had a higher concentration of oxyhemoglobin due to the fistula. As a result of decreased $CMRO_2$ and increased venous oxyhemoglobin, the NIRS tracing showed higher cerebral oxygenation on the left as compared to the right. After the left internal carotid artery was sacrificed with coiling, the left hemisphere received blood solely from the right carotid circulation. The left hemisphere then became adequately perfused and the NIRS tracing became symmetrical.

Direct Brain Tissue Oxygenation

Direct brain tissue oxygenation ($PbtO_2$) monitors are placed invasively, usually along with a bolt ICP monitor. When the probe is placed in normal white matter, it gives a sense of global brain oxygenation, but closer to a lesion will give more information regarding the local oxygen state. Artifact in this system is typically caused by misplacement of the probe into the wrong target (either normal or damaged brain) or caused by circuit and transducer malfunction.

Mobile Monitoring

The growth and expansion of technology and mobile health increases the ability to provide mobile NCCU monitoring. One route of mobile monitoring is via telehealth using wireless audio/visual carts connected securely to an intensivist's personal computer, laptop, or tablet. The benefits of such technology have already shown to be useful in the arena of acute stroke care (26). Artifacts related to this technology include slow network connection with audio and/or visual lag or choppiness, unfocused visualization, and visual obstruction. These artifact sources can impair the intensivist's ability to properly examine and analyze the patient's clinical condition.

Some quantitative EEG (QEEG) software packages send automatic email alerts to providers with updates or warnings, based on algorithm analysis of the QEEG. A full discussion of QEEG artifact is discussed separately in this text, but we will call attention to an example of how a QEEG artifact caused an email alert with incorrect analysis, and the diagnosis of the QEEG was sent to the clinician (Figure 4.9).

Somatosensory Evoked Potentials

Although there is a separate chapter devoted to somatosensory evoked potential (SSEP) monitoring, we will briefly discuss SSEPs artifact relative the NCCU. Two common uses for SSEP in the NCCU are for prognostication after cardiac arrest and brain death. Bilateral loss of the N20 responses is 100% predictive of a poor outcome: persistent coma, vegetative state, or death (27). Absent N20 responses are also compatible with brain death, as are missing P13 waves (28). However, SSEPs should be reserved only as an ancillary test in these conditions.

Although SSEPs are relatively unaffected by sedating medication (unlike EEGs), hypothermia can slow conduction velocities. Patients in the NCCU are often edematous, which can make it difficult to appropriately stimulate the median nerve, dampening the amplitude of all waves. Diaphoresis and poor electrode contact can cause artifacts as well (Figure 4.10).

CONCLUSION

The NCCU combines severely ill patients who can rapidly decompensate with a dynamic external environment. This combination creates a unique scenario where patients require a variety of neuromonitoring (dubbed multimodal monitoring [MMM]). All monitoring techniques are susceptible to artifact.

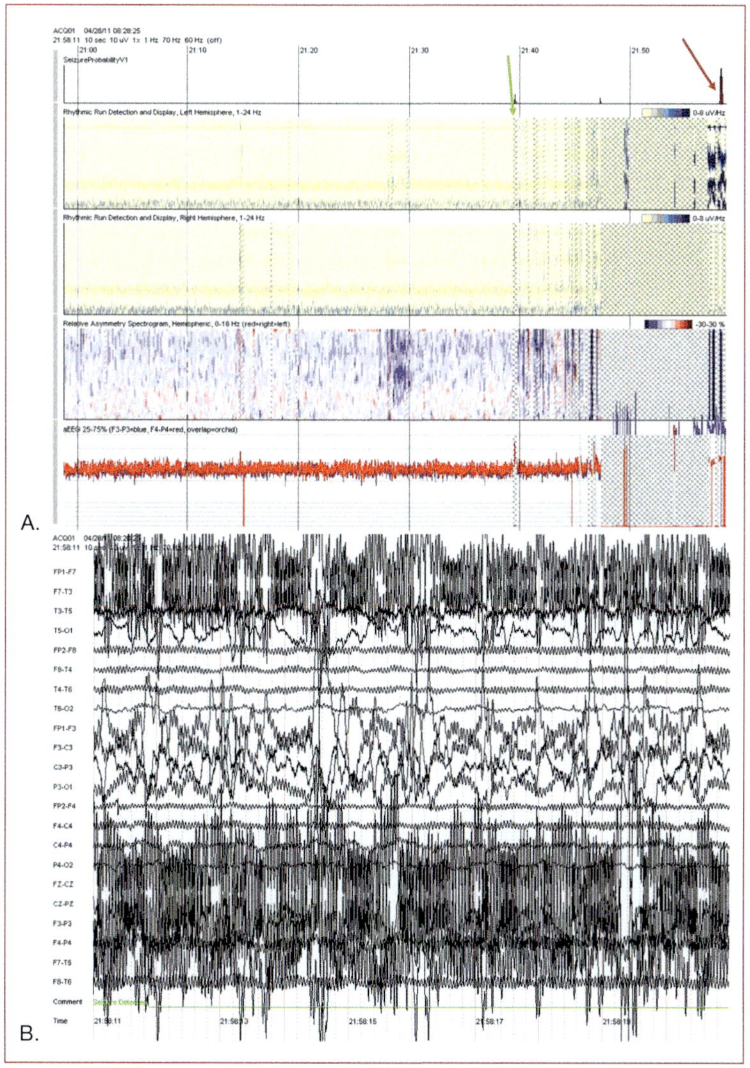

FIGURE 4.9: An email alert was sent to the neurointensivist with the subject line, "Seizure Detected @ 21:58:11," along with a clipping of the: (A) QEEG panel, and (B) the raw EEG tracing. This patient was put prone at 21:40 (green arrow) due to ARDS. The EEG became disconnected and several electrodes were removed (represented by the lattice overlay on the panel). The EEG was reconnected at 21:58:11, but there was still significant electrode, myogenic, and 60-Hz artifact. The software read this as seizure activity (red arrow), and emailed a seizure alert to the provider.

ARDS, acute respiratory distress syndrome; QEEG, quantitative EEG.

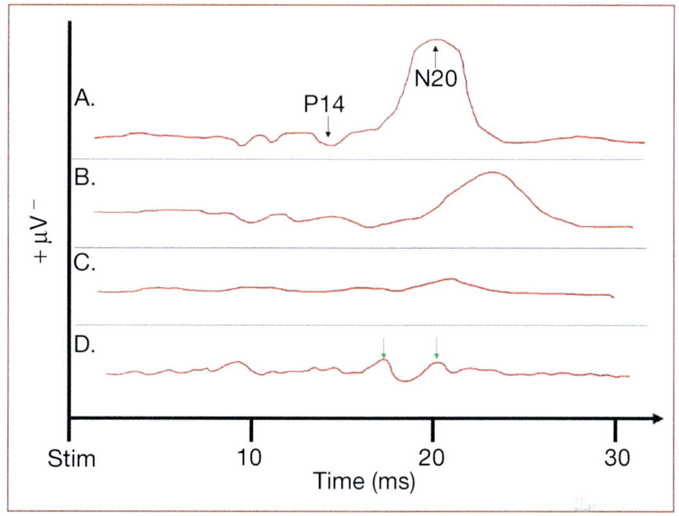

FIGURE 4.10: (A) Normal median nerve stimulated SSEP with P14 and N20 waves. (B) SSEP in a patient who is still hypothermic (e.g., post cardiac arrest). The N20 response is delayed. (C) Diffusely dampened wave forms due to poor median nerve stimulation in a patient with upper extremity edema from fluid overload in renal failure. (D) Poor electrode contact causing multiple, nonspecific wave forms (green arrows). These types of waves leave the technologist and neurophysiologist with the challenge of determining which, if either, is the correct N20 wave.

SSEP, somatosensory evoked potential.

This chapter addresses several sources of neuromonitoring artifact, including placement of the monitors, technique of the procedures, surface anatomy of the patient, and the patient's physical positioning. Though it is difficult to control for all of these factors in the NCCU, neurointensivists and neurophysiologists should be aware of these practical sources of artifact in critically ill patients as they interpret clinical neurophysiologic studies in the context of other sources of MMM employing nonelectrophysiologic measures.

REFERENCES

1. Freeman WD. Management of intracranial pressure. *Continuum (Minneap Minn)*. 2015;21(5 Neurocritical Care):1299-1323. doi:10.1212/CON.0000000000000235.

2. Chesnut RM, Marshall LF. Management of head injury. Treatment of abnormal intracranial pressure. *Neurosurg Clin N Am*. 1991;2(2):267-284. doi:10.1016/j.ncl.2008.02.003.

3. Muralidharan R. External ventricular drains: management and complications. *Surg Neurol Int*. 2015;6(suppl 6):S271-S274. doi:10.4103/2152-7806.157620.

4. Killer HE, Laeng HR, Flammer J, et al. Architecture of arachnoid trabeculae, pillars, and septa in the subarachnoid space of the human optic nerve: anatomy and clinical considerations. *Br J Ophthalmol*. 2003;87(6):777-781. doi:10.1136/bjo.87.6.777.

5. Hansen HC, Helmke K. The subarachnoid space surrounding the optic nerves. An ultrasound study of the optic nerve sheath. *Surg Radiol Anat*. 1996;18(4):323-328. doi:10.1007/BF01627611.

6. Kristiansson H, Nissborg E, Bartek J Jr., et al. Measuring elevated intracranial pressure through noninvasive methods: a review of the literature. *J Neurosurg Anesthesiol*. 2013;25(4):372-385. doi:10.1097/ANA.0b013e31829795ce.

7. Frumin E, Schlang J, Wiechmann W, et al. Prospective analysis of single operator sonographic optic nerve sheath diameter measurement for diagnosis of elevated intracranial pressure. *West J Emerg Med*. 2014;15(2):217-220. doi:10.5811/westjem.2013.9.16191.

8. Kimberly HH, Shah S, Marill K, et al. Correlation of optic nerve sheath diameter with direct measurement of intracranial pressure. *Acad Emerg Med*. 2008;15(2):201-204. doi:10.1111/j.1553-2712.2007.00031.x.

9. Major R, Girling S, Boyle A. Ultrasound measurement of optic nerve sheath diameter in patients with a clinical suspicion of raised intracranial pressure. *Emerg Med J*. 2011;28(8):679-681. doi:10.1136/emj.2009.087353.

10. Shah S, Kimberly H, Marill K, et al. Ultrasound techniques to measure the optic nerve sheath: is a specialized probe necessary? *Med Sci Monit*. 2009;15(5):MT63-MT68. PMID:19396044.

11. Copetti R, Cattarossi L. Optic nerve ultrasound: artifacts and real images. *Intensive Care Med*. 2009;35(8):1488-1489; author reply 1490-1481. doi:10.1007/s00134-009-1494-4.

12. Rajajee V, Fletcher JJ, Rochlen LR, et al. Comparison of accuracy of optic nerve ultrasound for the detection of intracranial hypertension in the setting of acutely fluctuating vs stable intracranial pressure: post-hoc analysis of data from a prospective, blinded single center study. *Crit Care*. 2012;16(3):R79. doi:10.1186/cc11336.

13. Naqvi J, Yap KH, Ahmad G, et al. Transcranial Doppler ultrasound: a review of the physical principles and major applications in critical care. *Int J Vasc Med*. 2013;2013:629378. doi:10.1155/2013/629378.

14. Gosling RG, King DH. Arterial assessment by Doppler-shift ultrasound. *Proc R Soc Med*. 1974;67(6 Pt 1):447-449. PMID:4850636.

15. Homburg AM, Jakobsen M, Enevoldsen E. Transcranial Doppler recordings in raised intracranial pressure. *Acta Neurol Scand*. 1993;87(6):488-493. doi:10.1111/j.1600-0404.1993.tb04142.x.

16. Nicoletto HA, Burkman MH. Transcranial Doppler series part II: performing a transcranial Doppler. *Am J Electroneurodiagnostic Technol*. 2009;49(1):14-27. doi:10.1155/2013/629378.

17. Kollar J, Schulte-Altedorneburg G, Sikula J, et al. Image quality of the temporal bone window examined by transcranial Doppler sonography and correlation with postmortem computed tomography measurements. *Cerebrovasc Dis*. 2004;17(1):61-65. doi:10.1159/000073899.

18. Tsivgoulis G, Alexandrov AV, Sloan MA. Advances in transcranial Doppler ultrasonography. *Curr Neurol Neurosci Rep*. 2009;9(1):46-54. PMID:19080753.

19. Lorenz MW, Loesel N, Thoelen N, et al. Effects of poor bone window on the assessment of cerebral autoregulation with transcranial Doppler sonography—a source of systematic bias and strategies to avoid it. *J Neurol Sci*. 2009;283(1-2):49-56. doi:10.1016/j.jns.2009.02.329.

20. Rahmouni A, Bargoin R, Herment A, et al. Color Doppler twinkling artifact in hyperechoic regions. *Radiology*. 1996;199(1):269-271. doi:10.1148/radiology.199.1.8633158.

21. Khan HG, Gailloud P, Martin JB, et al. Twinkling artifact on intracerebral color Doppler sonography. *Am J Neuroradiol*. 1999;20(2):246-247. PMID:10094345.

22. Stocchetti N, Le Roux P, Vespa P, et al. Clinical review: neuromonitoring—an update. *Crit Care*. 2013;17(1):201. doi:10.1186/cc11513.

23. Sheinberg M, Kanter MJ, Robertson CS, et al. Continuous monitoring of jugular venous oxygen saturation in head-injured patients. *J Neurosurg*. 1992;76(2):212-217. doi:10.3171/jns.1992.76.2.0212.

24. Gupta AK, Hutchinson PJ, Al-Rawi P. Measuring brain tissue oxygenation compared with jugular venous oxygen saturation for monitoring cerebral oxygenation after traumatic brain injury. *Anesth Analg*. 1999;88(3):549-553. doi:10.1097/00000539-199903000-00016.

25. Cyrous A, O'Neal B, Freeman WD. New approaches to bedside monitoring in stroke. *Expert Rev Neurother*. 2012;12(8):915-928. doi:10.1586/ern.12.85

26. Tatlisumak T, Soinila S, Kaste M. Telestroke networking offers multiple benefits beyond thrombolysis. *Cerebrovasc Dis*. 2009;27(suppl 4):21-27. doi:10.1159/000213055.

27. Zandbergen EG, Koelman JH, de Haan, et al. SSEPs and prognosis in postanoxic coma: only short or also long latency responses? *Neurology*. 2006;67(4):583-586. doi:10.1212/01.wnl.0000230162.35249.7f.

28. Wagner W. Scalp, earlobe and nasopharyngeal recordings of the median nerve somatosensory evoked P14 potential in coma and brain death. Detailed latency and amplitude analysis in 181 patients. *Brain*. 1996119(Pt 5): 1507-1521. PMID:8931576.

CHAPTER 5

Electroencephalography and Artifact in the Intensive Care Unit

Nishi Rampal, Carolina B. Maciel, and Lawrence J. Hirsch

INTRODUCTION

Monitoring the EEG in critically ill patients presents a unique set of challenges to the clinical neurophysiologist due to recording that takes place in an electrically "hostile" environment. Artifacts are numerous, occur commonly, may be generated from specialized types of machinery used in ICU, and arise from an abundance of electromechanical sources (1,2). Some artifacts are more easily identified, while others may closely mimic periodic patterns that resemble epileptiform activity or even rhythmic activity that resembles electrographic seizures. Additionally, ICU recordings often last for prolonged periods of time, increasing the likelihood that an artifact will be introduced into the recording. Therefore, there is occasionally the need for repeat continuous EEG (cEEG) monitoring. cEEG monitoring gives rise to progressive loss of electrode integrity as the duration of recording increases. This occurs in addition to concomitant exposure of the patient to procedures, treatments, and electronic machines during cEEG, all of which can create artifacts. An understanding of these pitfalls lies at the foundation of identifying electrical "fact from fiction" (3). Errors can occur at both ends of the spectrum, with artifacts causing loss of important information due to interference with interpretation and overinterpretation, resulting in adverse consequences (4–6). This chapter and its detailed figures aim to provide a framework to better identify common types of artifacts recorded in the ICU so patterns may be recognized to identify the common source of origin (Figure 5.1).

Artifacts in the ICU can be generated from three main sources: environmental, patient or patient care, and technical (6) (Tables 5.1–5.3). Environmental sources of artifacts in the ICU often result in readily identifiable artifacts (Table 5.1). These are often monomorphic oscillations that reflect their instrumental or mechanical origin. The appearance of 60-Hz artifact is a common artifact source in cEEG monitoring and is detailed in other chapters. In the ICU, unlike other recording environments, there are numerous electrical signal generators that warrant familiarity, such as bed oscillators (Figures 5.2 and 5.3), ventilators (Figures 5.4 and 5.5), temperature management devices (Figure 5.6), and hemodialysis and infusion pumps (7).

cEEG in the ICU is subject to artifacts common to all types of EEG recordings. The presence of eye movements (Figures 5.7 and 5.8), muscle activity generating a surface electromyogram (EMG) signal (Figures 5.9–5.12), ECG, and sweat artifact (Figures 5.13 and 5.14) are produced by the patient or derived from patient care (Table 5.2). Internal electric signals generated within a patient from implanted devices such as left ventricular assist devices and pacemakers (Figures 5.15 and 5.16) may also produce artifacts. There are a host of additional artifacts that are not unique to the critically

TABLE 5.1: EEG Artifact From Environmental Sources

50/60 Hz electromagnetic "main line" interference (60 Hz in North America)
Bed percussion (via bed oscillators, etc.)
Ventilator artifact–ventilator trigger, water oscillation
Extracorporeal membrane oxygenation
Hemodialysis
Warming/cooling blankets
Infusion pumps

ill patient but are more prevalent in the ICU environment. The critically ill patient often has an EEG that lends itself to interpreter uncertainty. With critical illness and its associated encephalopathy, the expected organization, frequencies, and state-dependent characteristics of normal EEG are often lost.

TABLE 5.2: EEG Artifacts From Patient or Patient Care

Stimulating procedures
Patting/shaking
Sternal rub
Sweating
Nursing or respiratory care
Bathing
Oral care/mouth swabbing
Suction
Chest physical therapy
Bed percussion
Eye movements
Eye rolling
Saccades
Nystagmus
Eyelid flutter
Electroretinogram
Tongue, mouth, palatal movements
Glossokinetic movements
Chewing
Coughing
Palatal myoclonus
Sucking on straw
Muscle and movement
Electromyogram
Shivering
Tremor
Myoclonus
Dystonia
Cardiovascular
ECG
Cardioballistic (head/body movement with each heartbeat/pulse)
Pulse
Pacemaker spikes
Left ventricular assist devices
Respiratory incursions/excursions

The resulting EEG obtained in the ICU is often chaotic, focal, or diffusely slowed background activity, with absent stages of sleep. Often, patient interaction can produce highly rhythmic, ictal-appearing patterns, particularly sternal rub (Figure 5.7) or chest percussion. At first look, identifying some types of artifact can be difficult to distinguish from true abnormality.

The EEG technologist is key to prevention, identification, and correction of artifacts, providing both routine maintenance of cEEG and technological expertise to "troubleshoot" artifact when technical sources are suspect (Table 5.3). The technologist–neurophysiologist team is crucial to interpreting ICU-EEG recordings. Entry of comments into the EEG recording by any care team member can also aid in artifact identification and source localizing information.

To further confound the issues, there is often an overlap of sources (Tables 5.1–5.3) producing artifacts, such as a patient placed on a cooling device (Figure 5.6) leading to shivering producing prominent EMG artifact and superimposed machine artifact. Add to this picture unexpected or abnormal movements, and it is easy to see how artifacts can build up to beguile and mislead the interpreter. When identified, the origin of the artifact can often be confirmed by video evaluation (an important reason to include video on all ICU recordings). This is especially true when the EEG is not attended by a technologist throughout the duration of recording to provide confirmatory steps such as moving or unplugging a device (Figure 5.6), clearing fluid from ventilator tubing (Figure 5.5), checking electrode impedances,

TABLE 5.3: EEG Artifacts From Technical Sources

Amplifier
Analysis/viewing errors
Filter selection: low pass, high pass, notch
Time base
Sensitivity
Jack box
Improper grounding or shielding
Lead secompensation
Unequal or high impedances
Contact bridging (gives flat channels on bipolar)
Poor electrode contact
Lead pop
Suboptimal lead placement
Due to injury, presence of surgical site, ventriculostomy/hardware placement
Wires

and making corrections when the integrity of the recording is compromised (Figures 5.17–5.24). This creates an opportunity not only to avoid erroneous interpretation but also to allow for interventions to improve the quality of the captured recording.

Some artifacts like 60/50 Hz are commonly encountered with or without additional types of artifact. Surprisingly, the effects of specific artifacts and the multiplicity of combinations can be seen to produce a varying array of patterns, as illustrated in Figures 5.1, 5.20, and 5.22. When approaching the spectrum of artifacts in the ICU-EEG produced by the patient, patient care, environment, or technically generated artifacts, a systematic approach is essential. In addition to the need for familiarity with common artifacts, it is essential when interpreting ICU-EEG and cEEG partially obscured by artifact to limit overuse of the digital filters. Both the use of low-frequency (high-pass) and high-frequency (low-pass) filters can adulterate the EEG and lead to misinterpretation (Figure 5.21). Similarly, use of the 60-Hz (or 50-Hz) "notch" filter, which is commonly employed, risks erroneous interpretations (Figure 5.20). Instead of relying on filters to clean up an ICU-EEG recording that is contaminated with artifact, eliminating the source by modifying technical, environmental, or patient-derived generators is always the best course of action when feasible.

Quantitative analysis (QEEG) or digital analysis, which uses algorithms to transform hours of raw EEG into single-page color images and graphs, is featured in numerous figures using digital analysis software from Persyst, Inc. (Prescott, Arizona) in this chapter. Digital analysis is useful for long-term trending of seizure detection and quantification (8–10). In addition, it has been used to detect ischemia (most commonly after subarachnoid hemorrhage), elevated intracranial pressure, rebleeding after intracerebral hemorrhage, hypoxemia, and other acute brain injuries (11,12). QEEG findings should always be corroborated by review of the underlying raw EEG data. This point cannot be overemphasized. Because QEEG uses raw EEG data, it is also subject to the same effects from artifacts. Artifacts such as the type generated by bed oscillation are easily identified on QEEG. This produces a very narrow frequency band in the spectral array derived from the fast Fourier transformation that starts and stops abruptly, unlike physiological activity. In this case, the QEEG helps to identify the artifactual nature of a rhythmic pattern (Figure 5.2D). Other commonly occurring artifacts like ventilator condensation can erroneously trigger the seizure probability index to rise (Figure 5.5B and D). These programs have attempted to combat artifact conflation by detecting specific artifacts and graphing their prominence (blinks, muscle, 60 Hz). This serves to indicate when an artifact is overwhelming the signals generated by the brain, beyond which graphic display may not be helpful, and artifact removal is required. Figure 5.12 demonstrates how artifact reduction software can produce the appearance of generalized periodic discharges (GPDs) with rhythmic delta activity (GPD+R) in EEG from widespread muscle artifact. Without reviewing the raw EEG and only assessing the QEEG, artifact might have been mistaken as a common abnormality of critical illness.

Intracortical EEG, or depth electrode placement in ICU-EEG monitoring, can provide essential information. The absence of electrographic seizures on scalp EEG does not exclude the possibility of seizures on intracortical EEG recording (13–15). Intracortical EEG is subject to a host of potential misinterpretations, as rhythms that are normally encountered on scalp EEG have a higher amplitude and sharper morphology. There is much less artifact on the intracortical EEG due to the much higher signal:noise ratio when bypassing the scalp and skull. This makes for an excellent method to detect changes in local field potentials including epileptiform activity and ischemia. However, there are still artifacts that may occur despite intracranial EEG recording. This is true due to the machinery and electrical connections (Table 5.3) that are related to movements of wires, plug-in connections, amplifiers, and even muscle artifact generated by patients, though to a lesser degree. Scalp EEG is also frequently performed in conjunction with invasive EEG, and likewise may also possess the tendency to manifest a unique type of artifact (Figure 5.22).

CONCLUSION

EEG interpretation often guides therapy in the ICU by providing real-time assessment in a critically ill population. Careful attention to artifact identification is paramount for correct interpretation of ICU-EEG and is directly tied to quality patient care. While artifacts in the ICU-EEG are numerous, they have a broad range of patterns that require a heightened index of suspicion as well as familiarity with the unique types that may occur. By using a stepwise approach to recognizing artifact focuses on identification of three main sources (environmental, patient or patient care, and technical); the EEG interpreter of ICU-EEG can safeguard against misinterpretation when elimination is not possible.

All EEG images were recorded with 21 leads with E1 (left lower canthus), E2 (right upper canthus) eye channels (blue), ECG1-ECG2 cardiac rhythm strip (red), with the following settings: LFF 1 Hz, HFF 70 Hz, Notch off, time base 30 mm/sec unless otherwise stated in the figure description. The recording reference was placed between Fz and Cz. Impedances were maintained at less than 10 kΩ, as established by the American Clinical Neurophysiology Society (ACNS) guidelines (16). New guidelines changed this from 5 to 10 kΩ to be more liberal. Many montages include one channel shown with a system reference (C3-ref, green). Most samples are shown using an anterior–posterior longitudinal bipolar montage; left hemisphere over midline and right hemisphere.

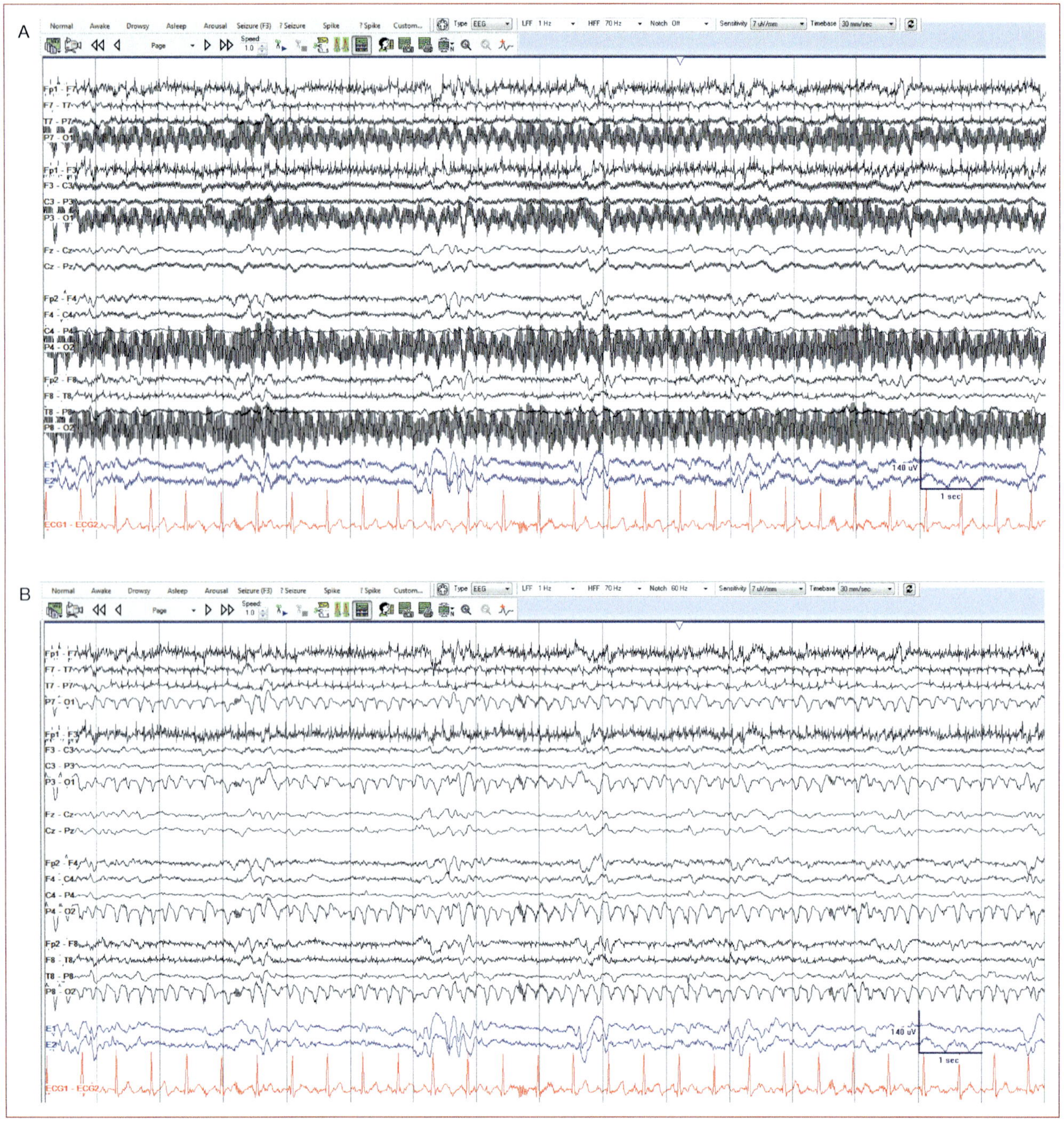

FIGURE 5.1: 60-Hz artifact. (A) Notch filter off. (B) Notch filter on revealing bioccipital rhythmic theta activity limited to O1/O2 derivations. **Figures 5.6**, **5.23**, and **5.24** also show additional examples of 60-Hz artifact demonstrating the broad array of patterns that may be visualized.

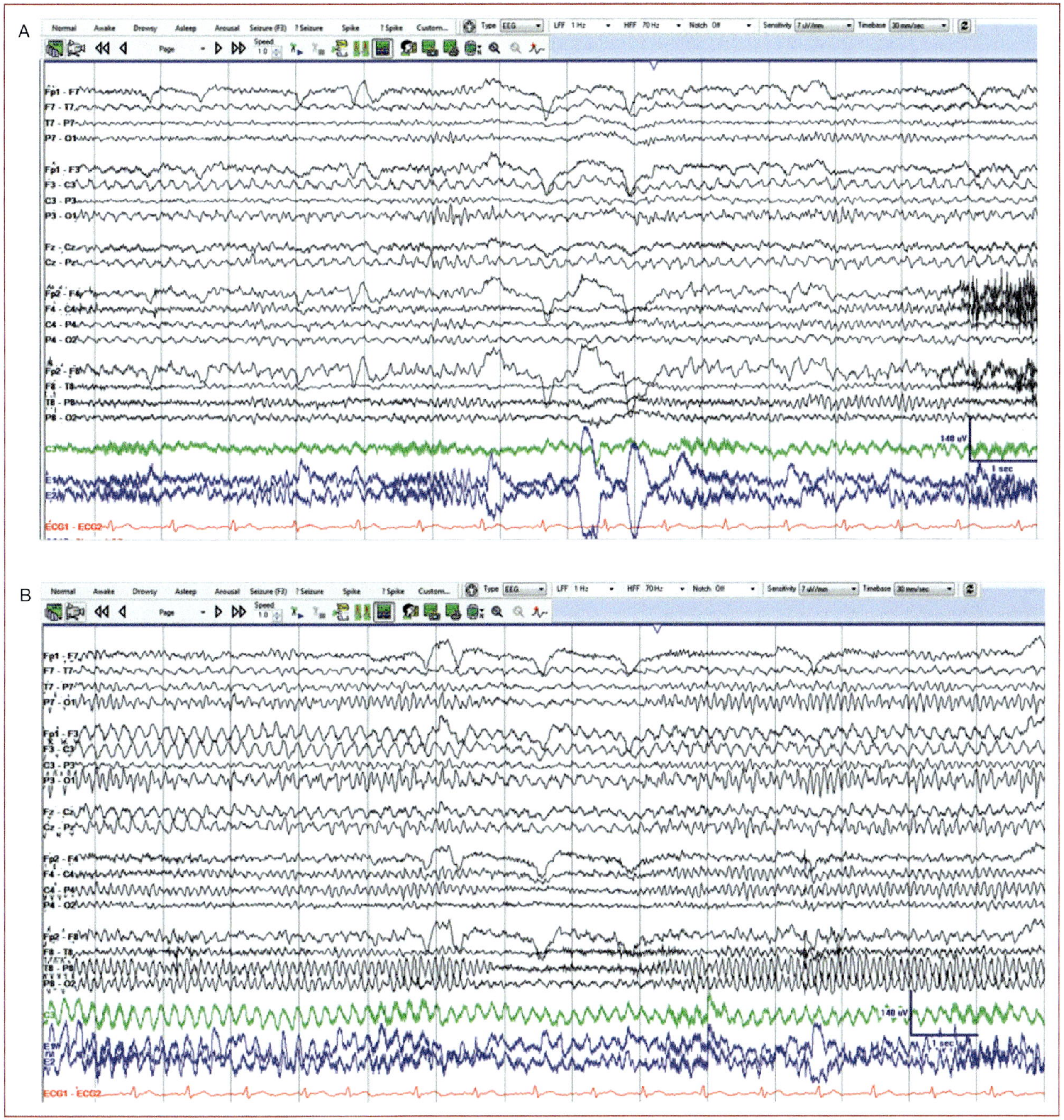

FIGURE 5.2: Bed percussion artifact mimicking an evolving ictal pattern on EEG. Three samples during an episode of apparent evolving rhythmicity lasting several minutes and ending abruptly. (A) Rhythmic theta and alpha activity at times appearing apiculate. (B) Further evolution of the pattern with apparent spread, faster frequencies, and increased voltages. (*continued*)

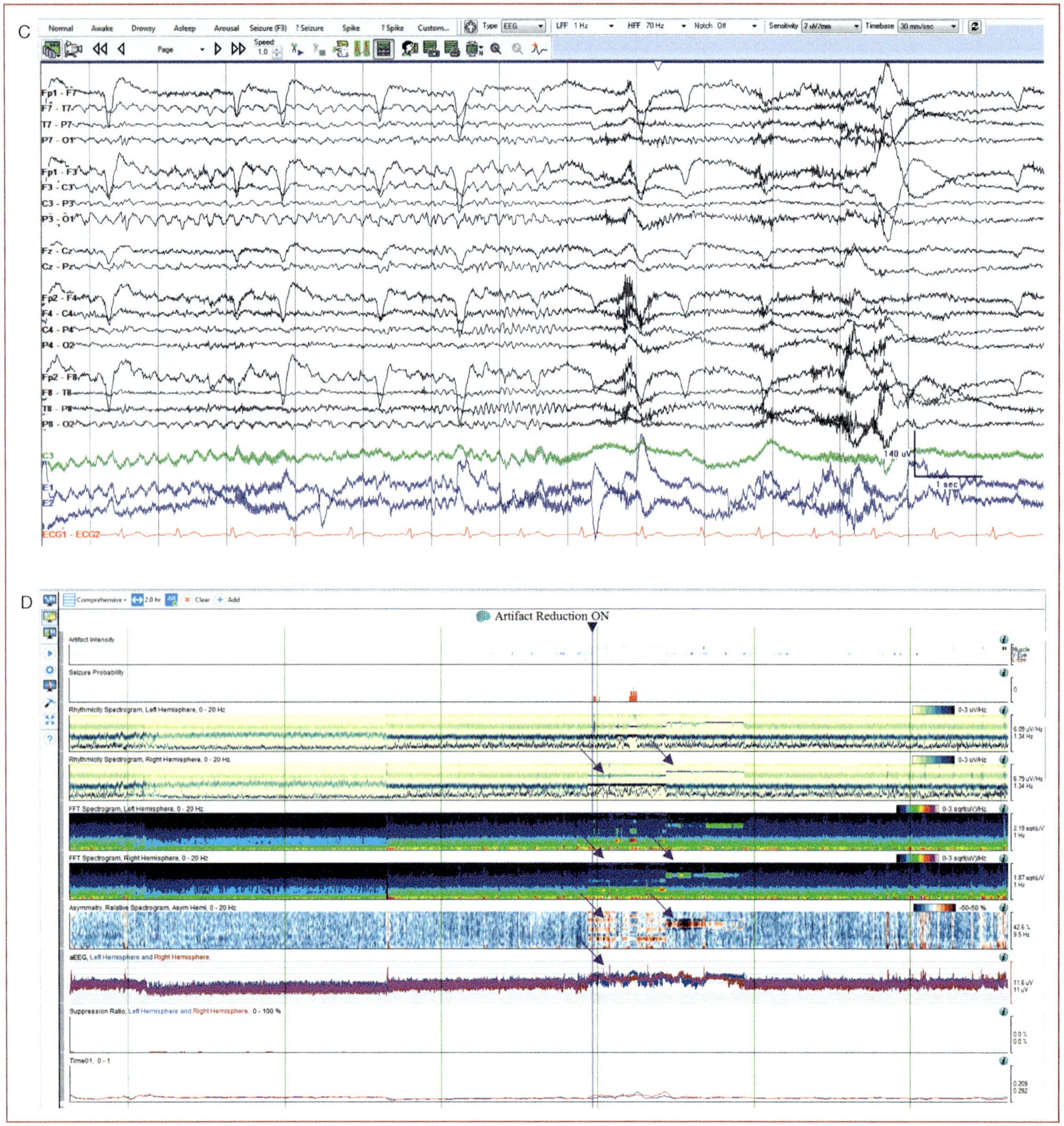

Figure 5.2: *(continued)* (C) The pattern seemed to slow with abrupt offset and resumption of background rhythms. (D) Digital analysis at this time (blue vertical line) reveals artifact with very narrow (one frequency only for a period of time) bars of high rhythmicity that start and stop. These are best seen on the rhythmicity spectrograms, FFT spectrogram, and asymmetry spectrogram (arrows).

FFT, fast Fourier transform.

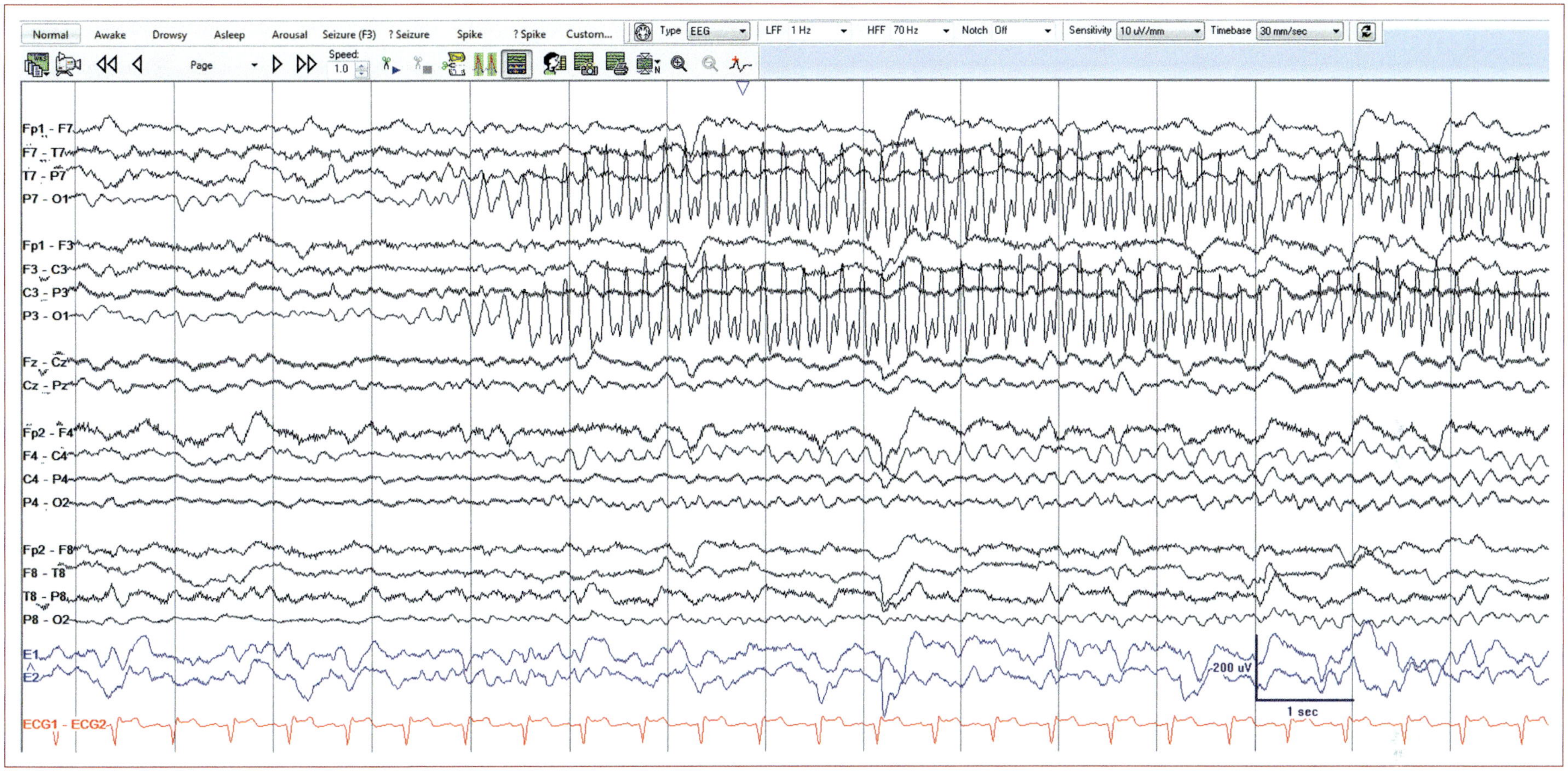

FIGURE 5.3: Bed percussion artifact. EEG with 5-Hz high-voltage spike-and-wave activity limited to O1 along with rhythmic 5-Hz theta activity, which appears to follow a second later. On video review, these artifacts were produced by bed percussion and varied with changes in percussion frequency, with a start-and-stop pattern that correlated to percussion initiation and termination. Sometimes this is trickier with more than one electrode involved, suggesting a believable spatial field of distribution (the electrodes contacting the pillow/bed). Having video can prevent misidentification of seizures in these cases. This type of artifact is challenging and common, especially in babies due to patting or rocking.

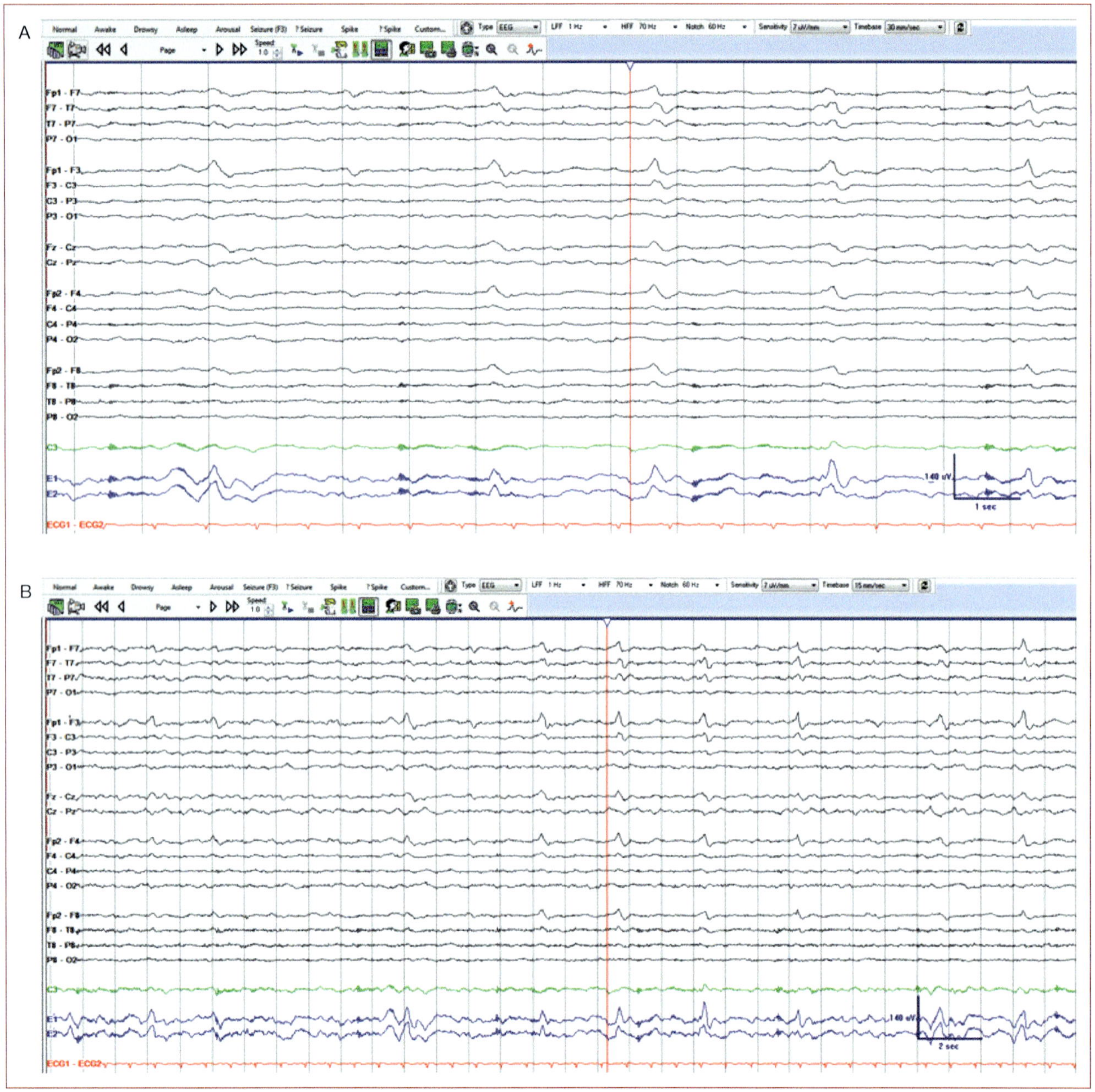

FIGURE 5.4: Ventilator-triggered artifact: (A) Typical time base of 30 mm/sec with periodic frontally dominant sharp waves. (B) Time base 15 mm/sec, allowing for compressed viewing of this artifact, which appears as slow, frontally maximal GPDs. These waveforms, on detailed video review, were produced by ventilator trigger and correlated with ventilator respiratory rate-setting changes and patient effort. The irregular interval was produced by the patient overbreathing the ventilator and triggering full breaths on his/her own.

GPD, generalized periodic discharge.

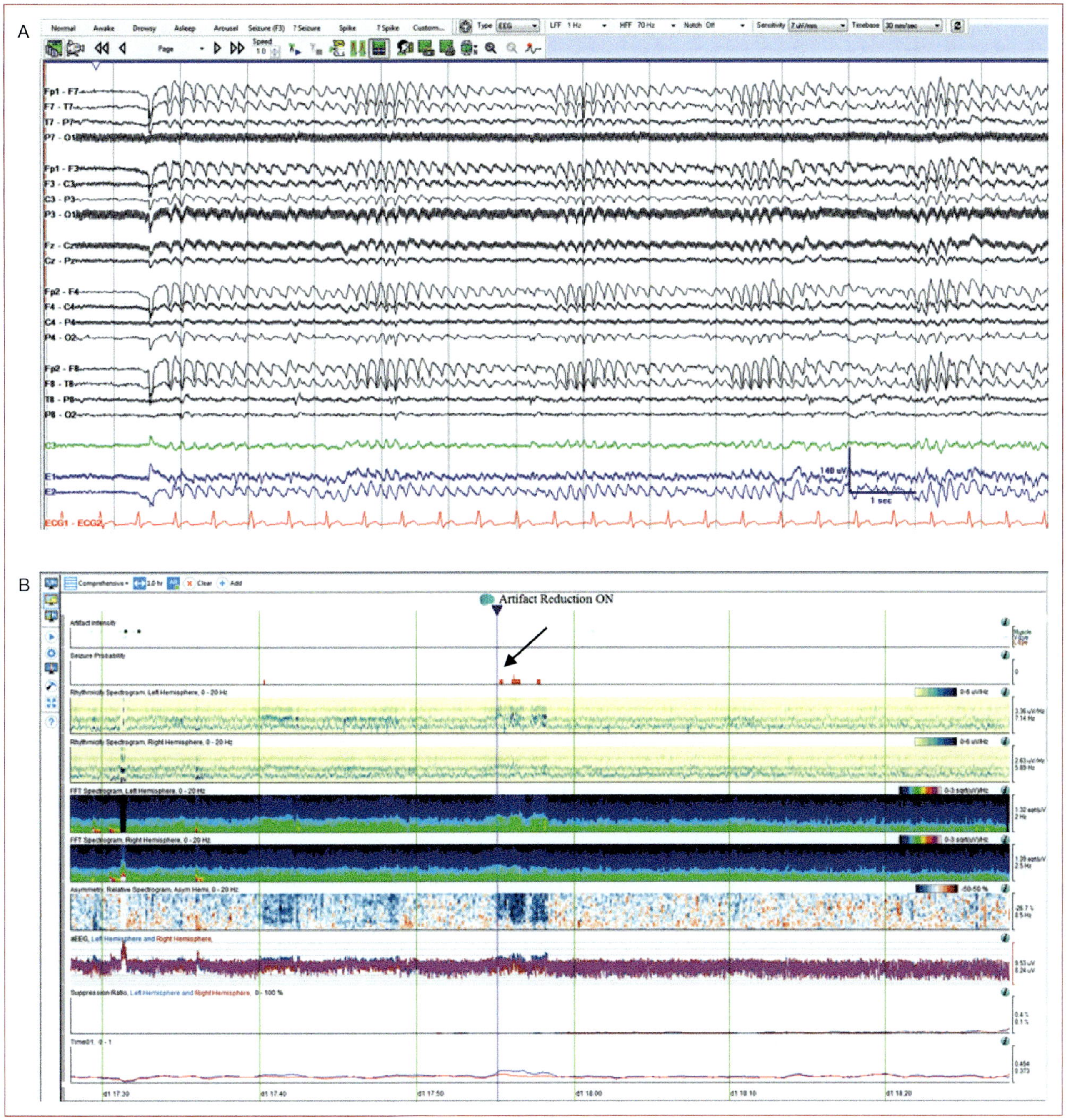

FIGURE 5.5: Fluid oscillating in ventilator tubing artifact. (A) EEG with diffuse rhythmic theta activity with a sinusoidal appearance, waxing, and waning. (B) Digital analysis of this time period (blue vertical line) reflects seizure identification within seizure probability index, increased rhythmicity on hemispheric rhythmicity spectrograms, and increased power on FFT spectrogram; all suspicious for epileptic seizures. (*continued*)

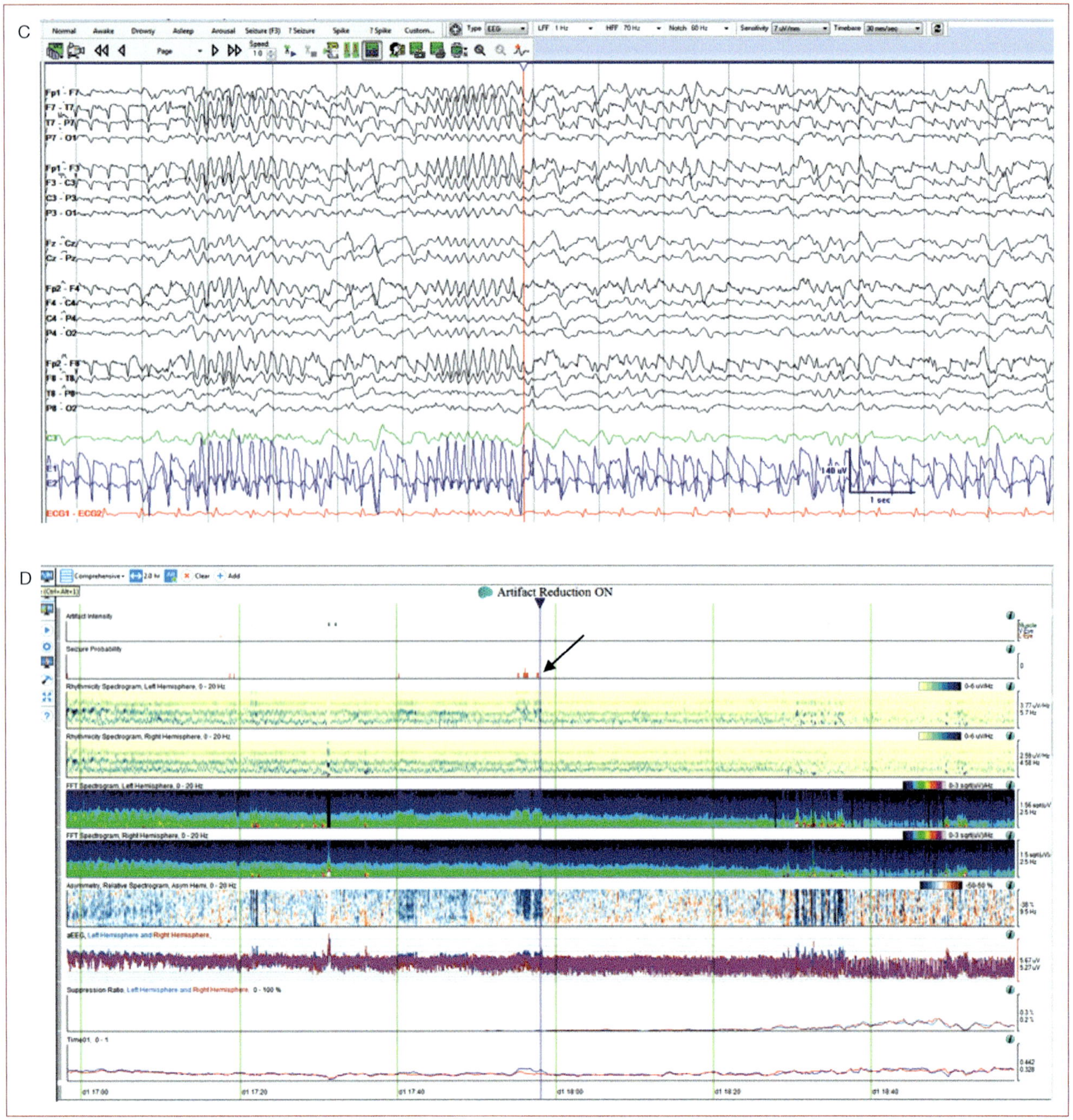

FIGURE 5.5: *(continued)* (C) Subsequent EEG showing clusters of very brief bursts of diffuse, frontally maximal, rhythmic theta activity with embedded sharp waves, which abruptly alternated with sharply contoured delta and theta rhythms. The red line marks the pattern transition, both artifactual in nature. (D) Digital analysis of this time period (blue vertical line) reflects seizure identification within the seizure probability index, increased rhythmicity on hemispheric rhythmicity spectrograms, and increased power on FFT spectrogram. These artifacts continued until the circuit was cleared of all fluid.

FFT, fast Fourier transform.

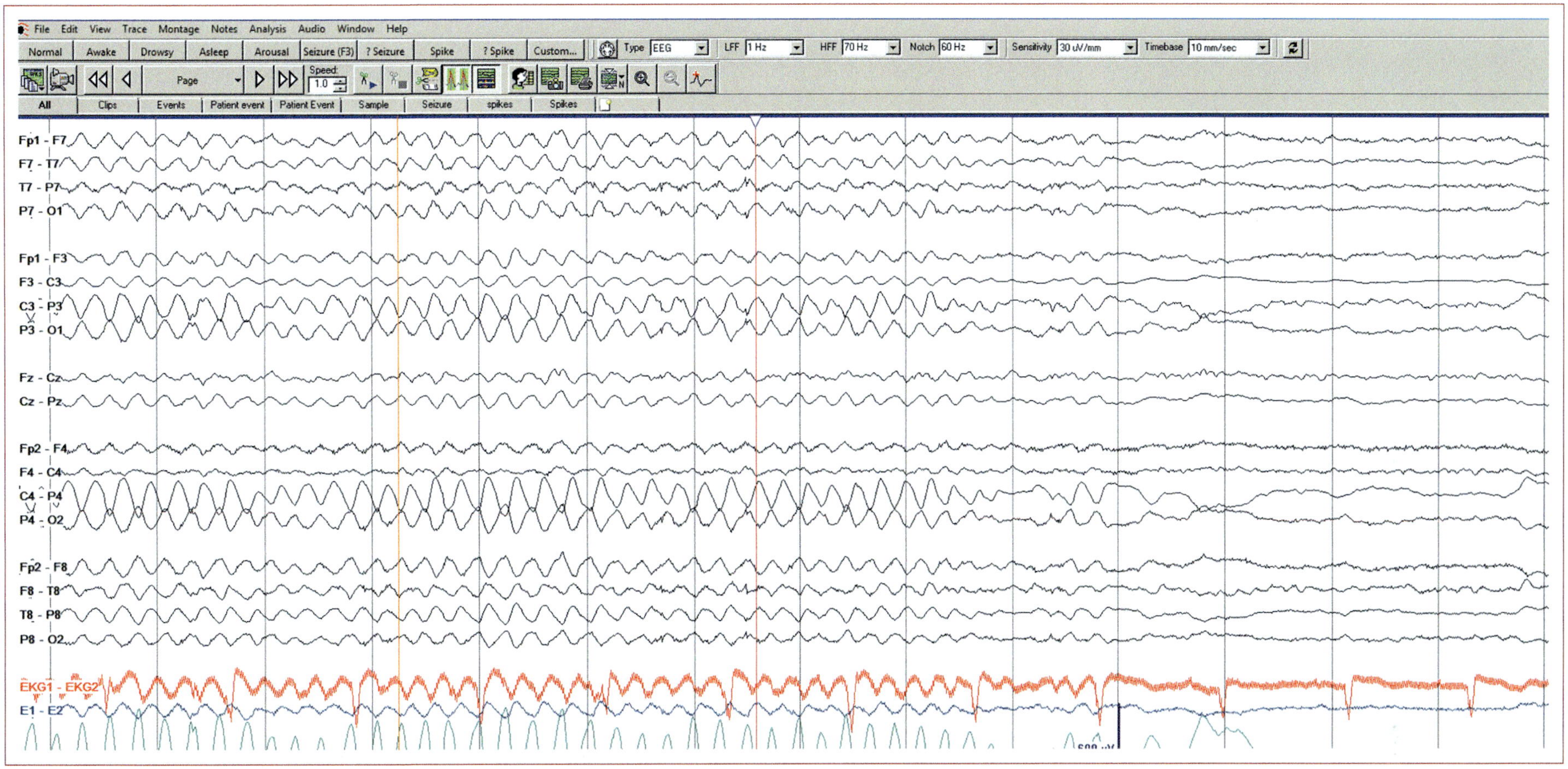

FIGURE 5.6: Cooling blanket artifact. EEG demonstrating artifact composed of rhythmic theta activity with a nonphysiological electrical field. Additionally, the artifact involves the ECG channel, which has two chest leads and no scalp leads, reflecting a noncerebral source. The origin of this artifact was confirmed by turning the cooling blanket device off at second 10 in this epoch.

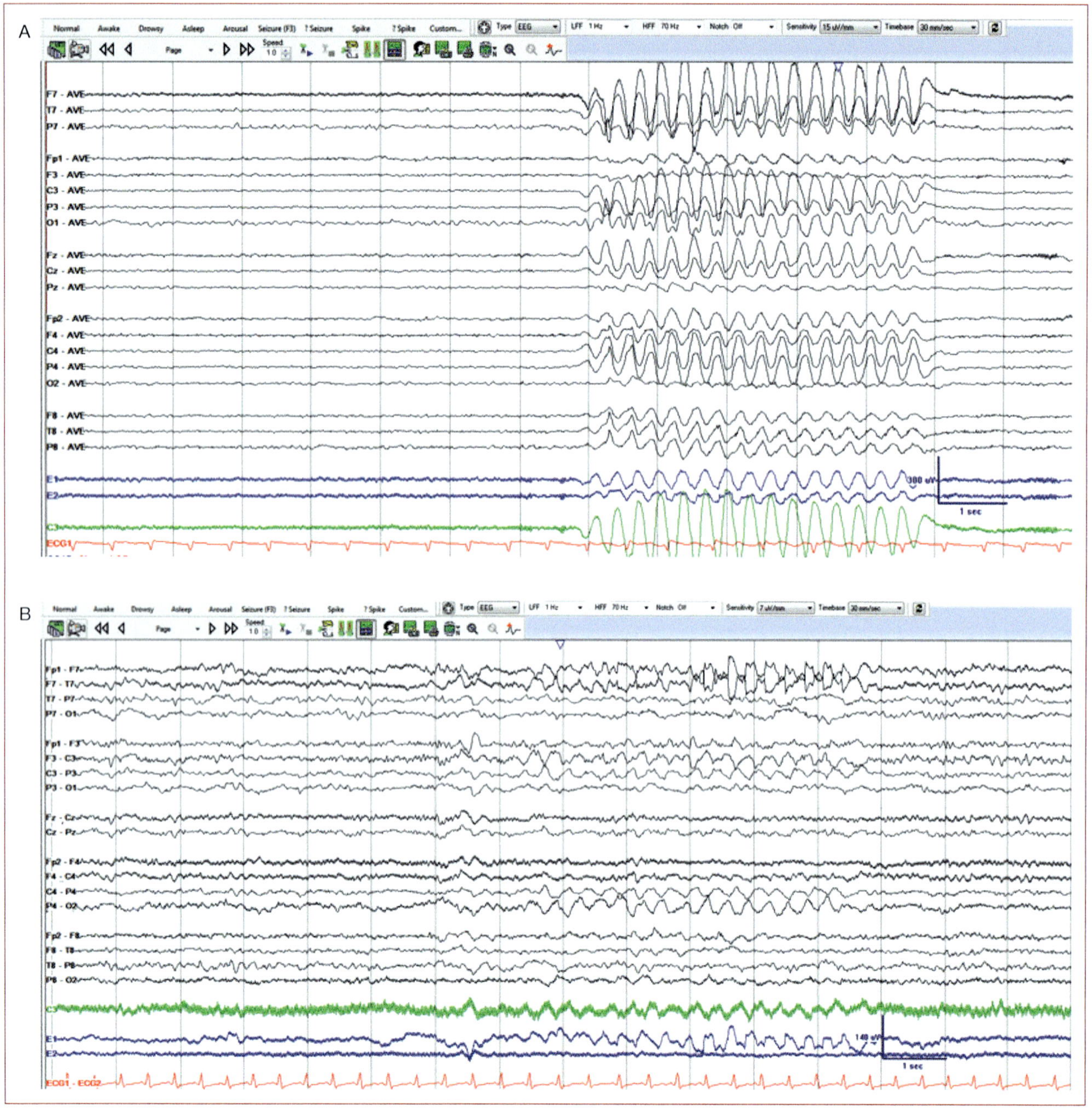

FIGURE 5.7: Alerting attempt artifacts: (A) Shaking patient produced generalized, rhythmic 3-Hz activity with abrupt onset and offset. (B) Sternal rub manifesting as episodes of very brief rhythmic delta activity. The origin of artifact was confirmed by video review. It showed attempts to arouse patient and achieve maximal stimulation. Note the relative sparing of the midline electrodes (Fz-Cz, Cz-Pz), a common phenomenon with most artifacts.

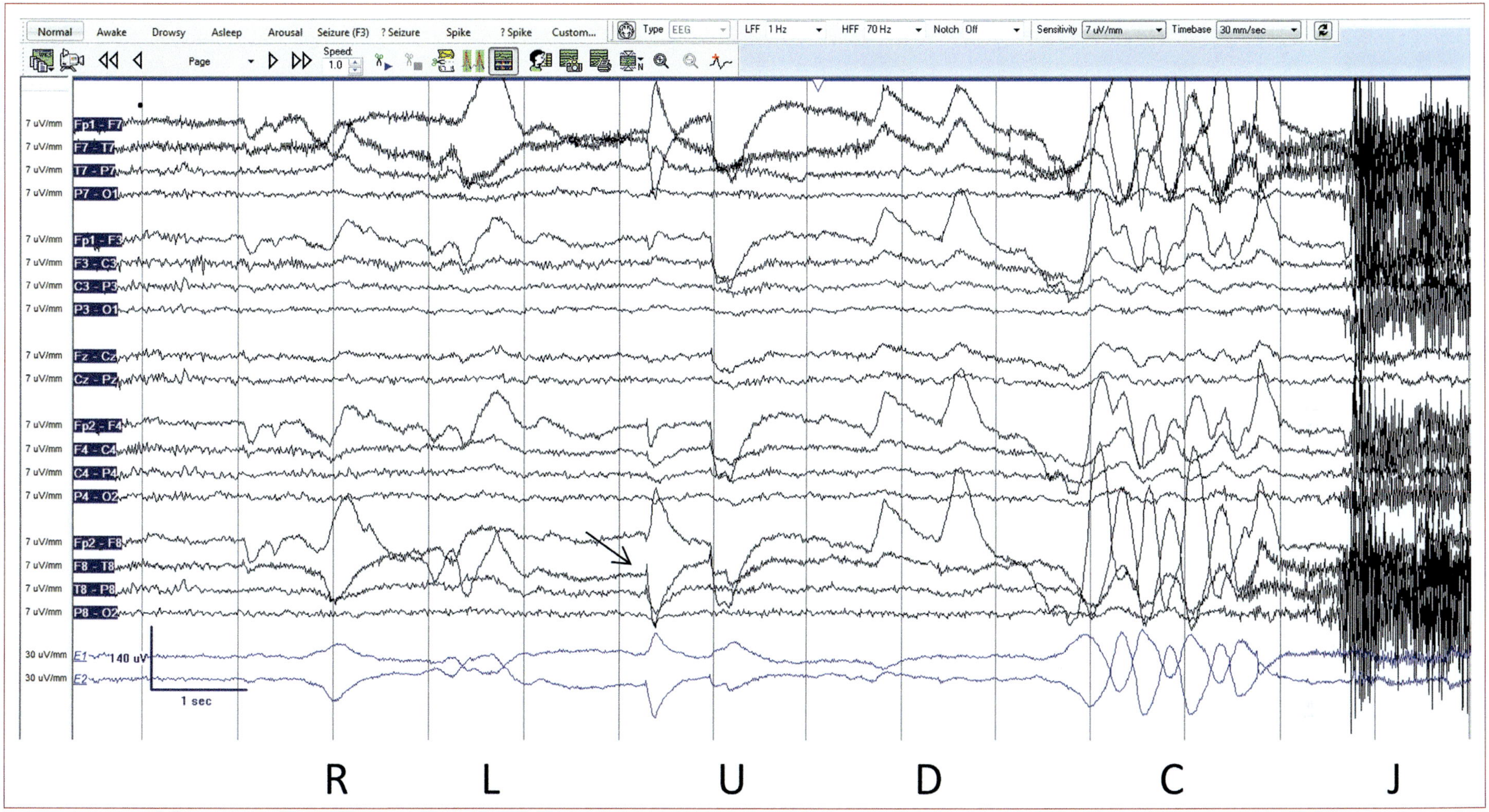

FIGURE 5.8: Eye movements and jaw clenching artifact. This figure demonstrates positive potentials seen ipsilateral to the direction of the eye movement (due to the corneal electropositivity moving toward this electrode; e.g., F8 on rightward eye movement). Negative potential seen contralateral to the direction of the eye movement. EMG artifact from the lateral rectus muscle is seen at F8-T8, ipsilateral to the direction of eye movement (lateral rectus "spike"; black arrow). R, right gaze; L, left gaze; U, up gaze; D, down gaze; C, chaotic eye movements; J, jaw clench with overwhelming EMG.

EMG, electromyogram.

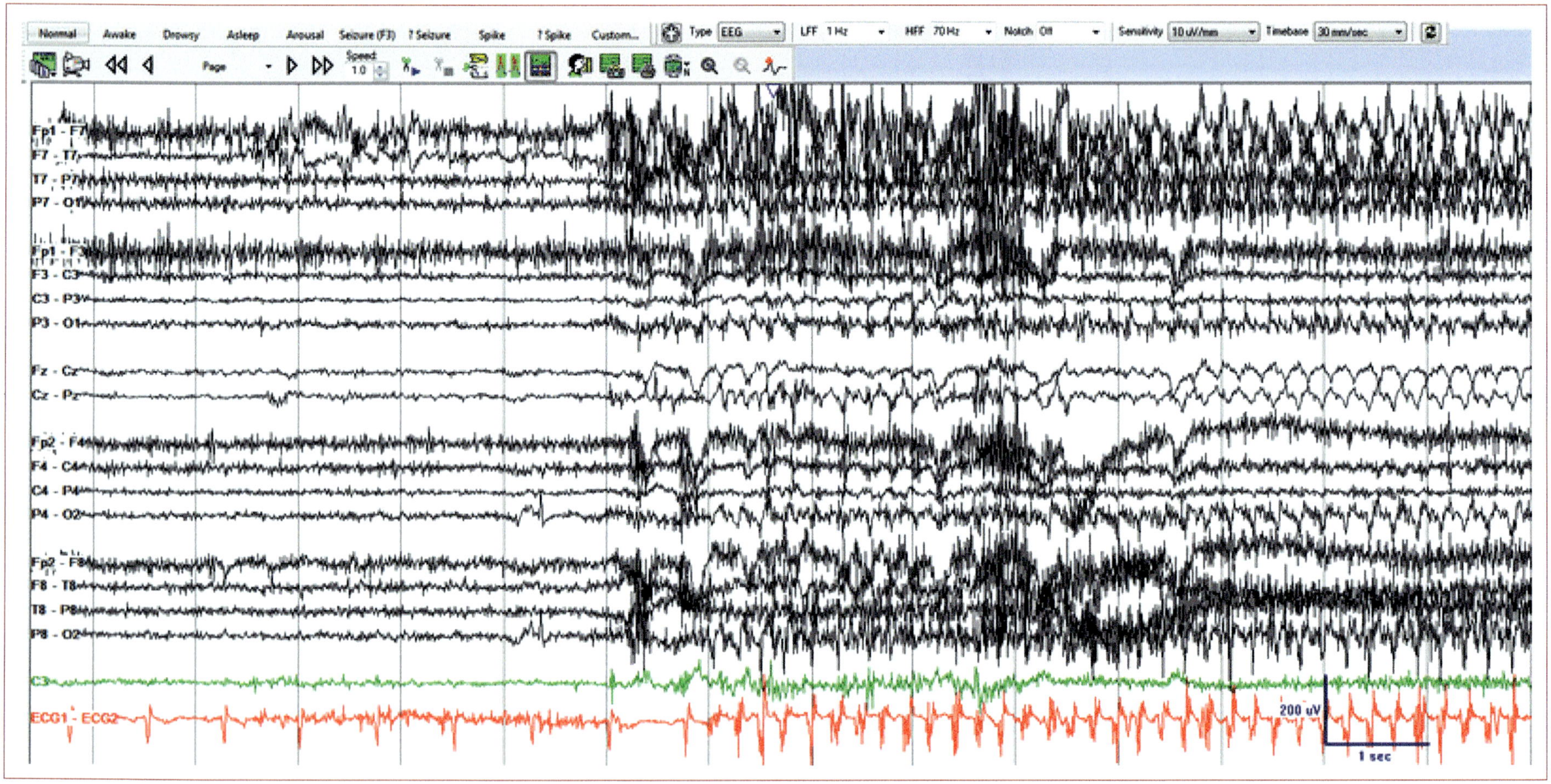

FIGURE 5.9: Oral hygiene artifact. EEG reflects diffuse rhythmic activity with abrupt onset and offset. Video review correlated EEG findings with oral hygiene care (tooth brushing). Note: this is a rare example of an artifact that is well developed in the midline. The muscle artifact is almost always absent or at least lowest amplitude there. This is likely due to electrical signals generated from the mouth, tongue, or dental work and projecting vertically.

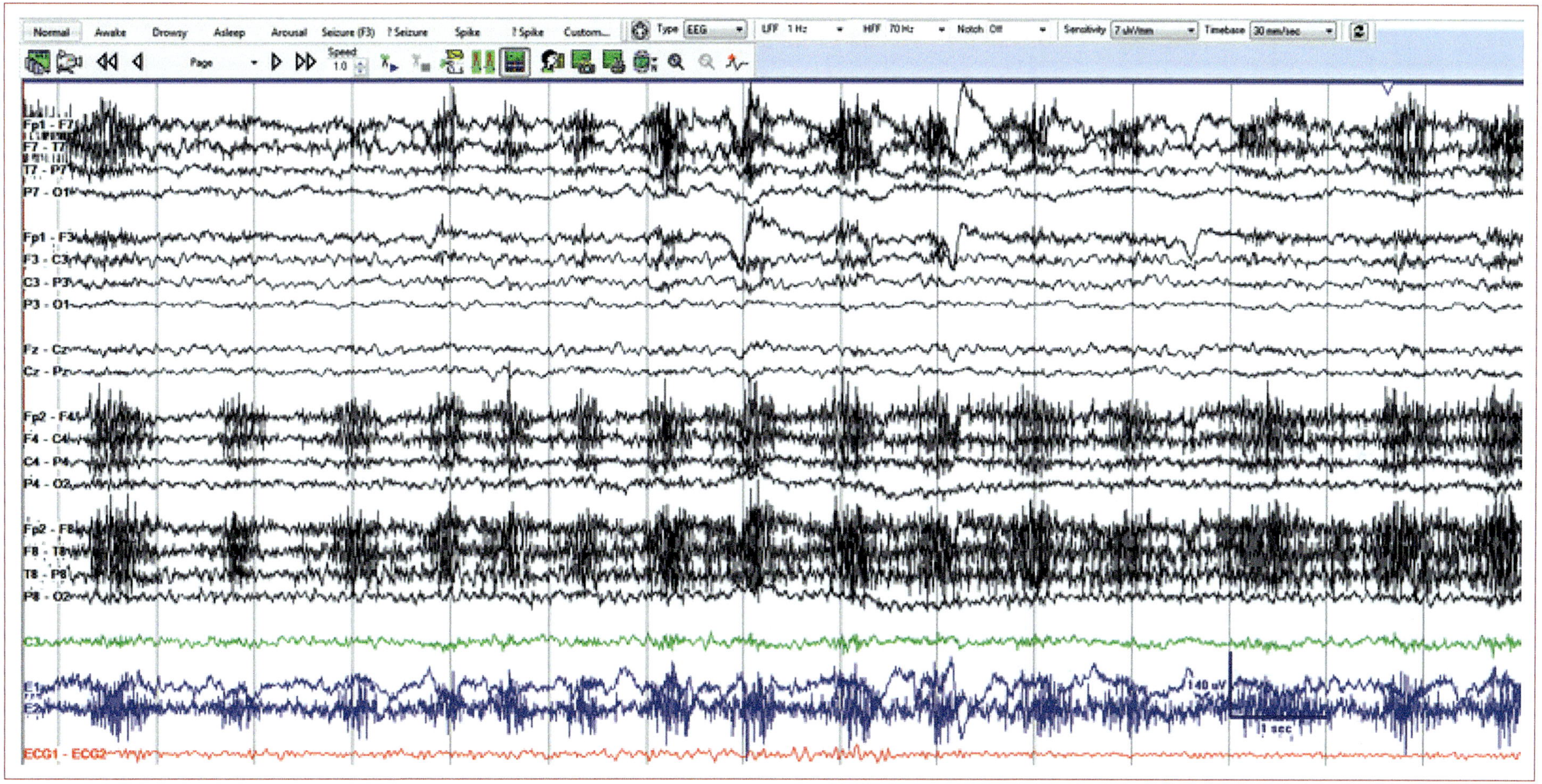

FIGURE 5.10: Chewing artifact. The presence of bilateral frontotemporal EMG artifacts correlates to patient chewing on the endotracheal tube. Similar artifact can be seen when patients are eating. Teeth grinding (bruxism) occurs with shifting EMG pattern that alternates sides, producing a "checkerboard pattern" on a left/right/left/right longitudinal, seen on the bipolar montage in the current example. Note that most of the muscle artifact is on the left. This could raise the possibility of either right facial hemiparesis or simply asymmetric chewing. Note the lack of artifact in the midline channels, as is typical for any muscle, oral, or glossokinetic artifact.

EMG, electromyogram.

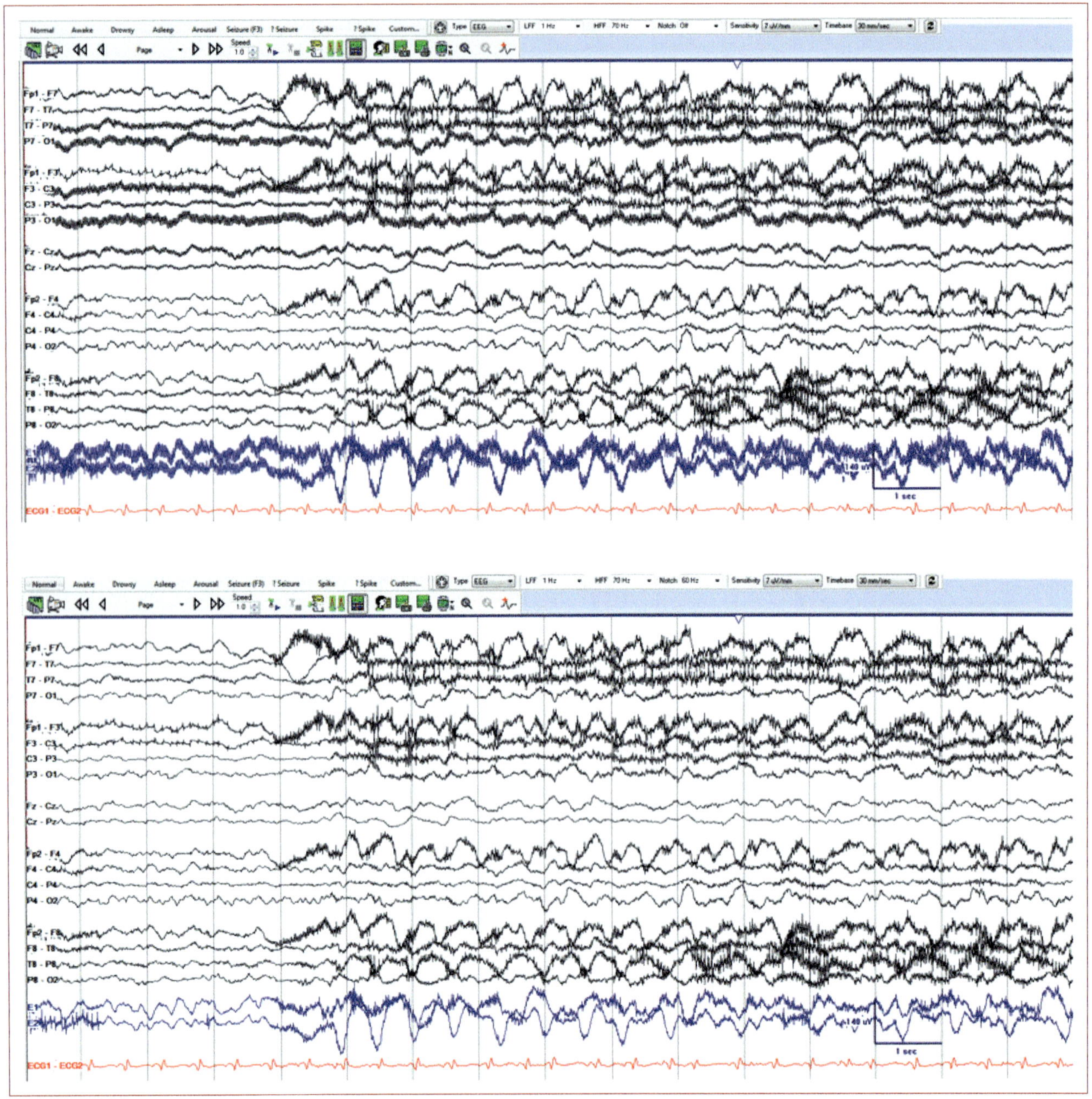

FIGURE 5.11: Coughing artifact. EEG with both glossokinetic and EMG artifact that correlated to bouts of patient coughing, which occurred spontaneously and after endotracheal tube suctioning. Again, note the lack of myogenic artifact in the midline channels.

EMG, electromyogram.

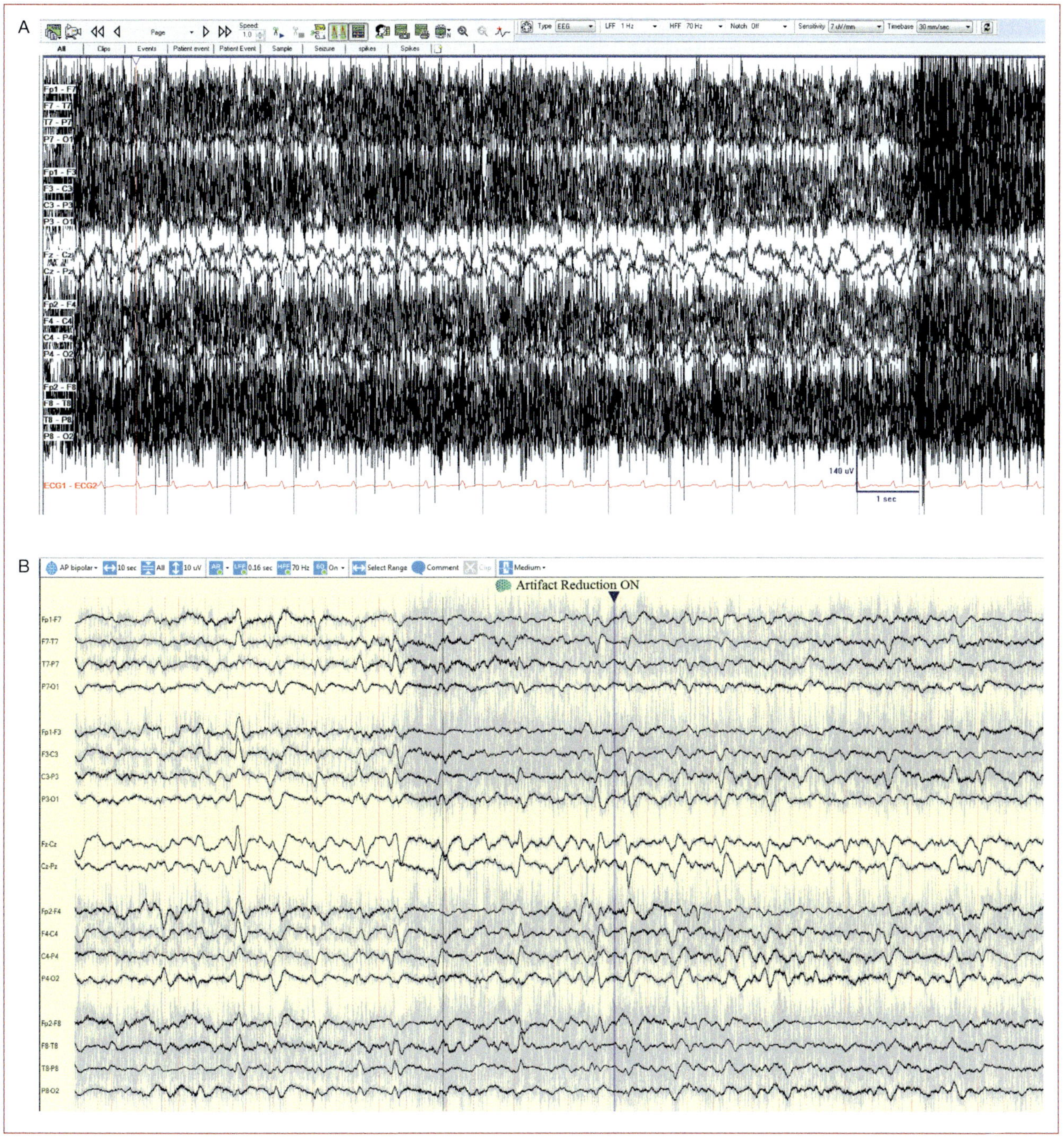

FIGURE 5.12: Overwhelming myogenic artifact from shivering. (A) Prominent myogenic artifact obscuring cerebral waveforms. Note the classic relative sparing of EMG artifact over the midline channels. The patient's presentation was highly suspicious for NCSE, yet the absence of mechanical ventilation precluded neuromuscular blockade. (B) Same EEG epoch using artifact reduction software (Persyst, Inc., Prescott, Arizona) revealed GPD+R. Red and blue lines demonstrate the same time point. Antiseizure drug trials including a bolus of 2 g levetiracetam were given. (*continued*)

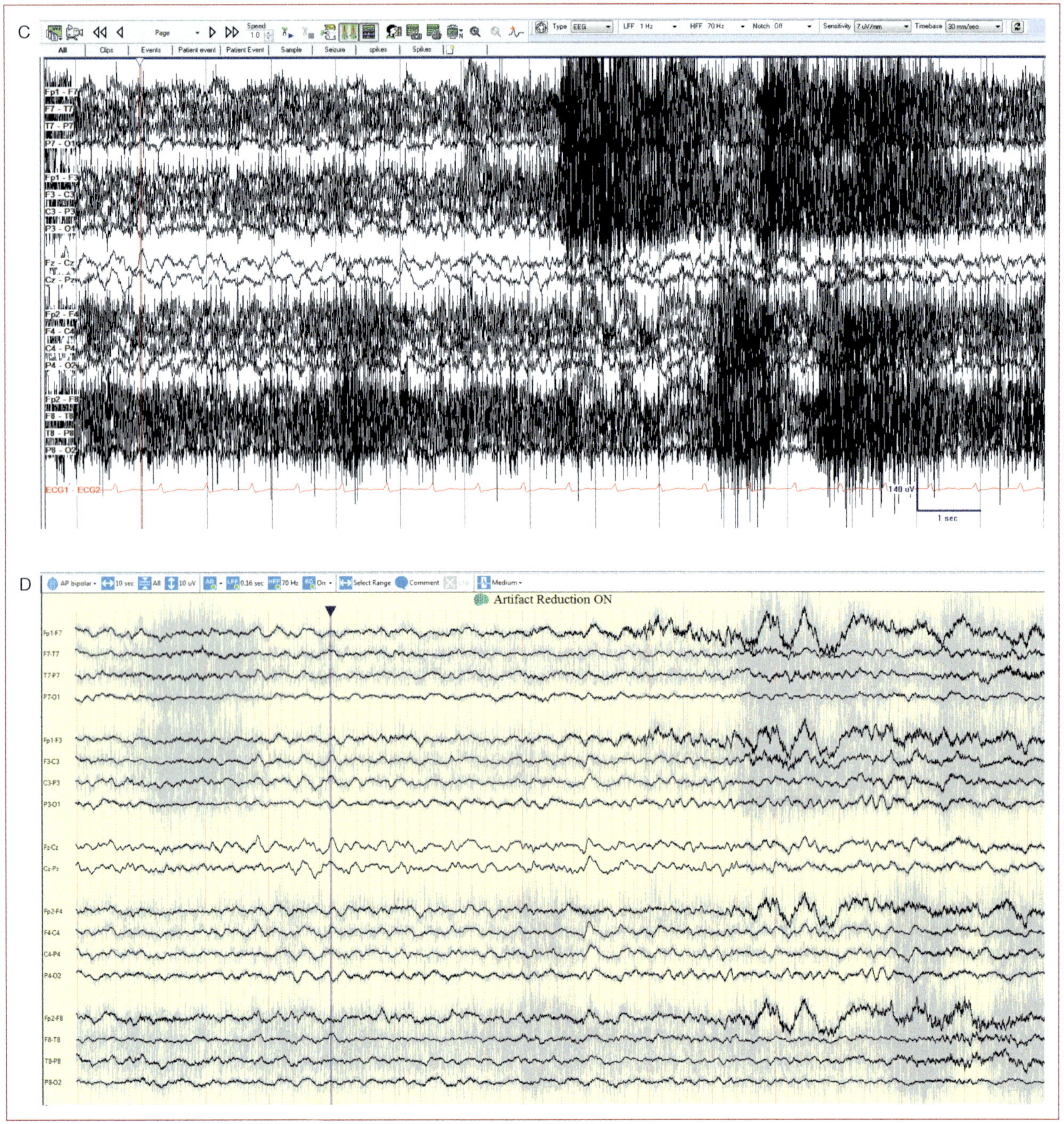

FIGURE 5.12: (*continued*) (C) Posttreatment epoch with continued prominent EMG artifact markedly limiting interpretation. (D) Same posttreatment epoch using artifact reduction revealed resolution of generalized periodic discharges and improved background frequencies. The clinical exam improved as well, following successful treatment for NCSE. Red and blue lines demonstrate the same time point.

EMG, electromyogram; GPD+R, generalized periodic discharges with rhythmic delta activity; NCSE, nonconvulsive status epilepticus.

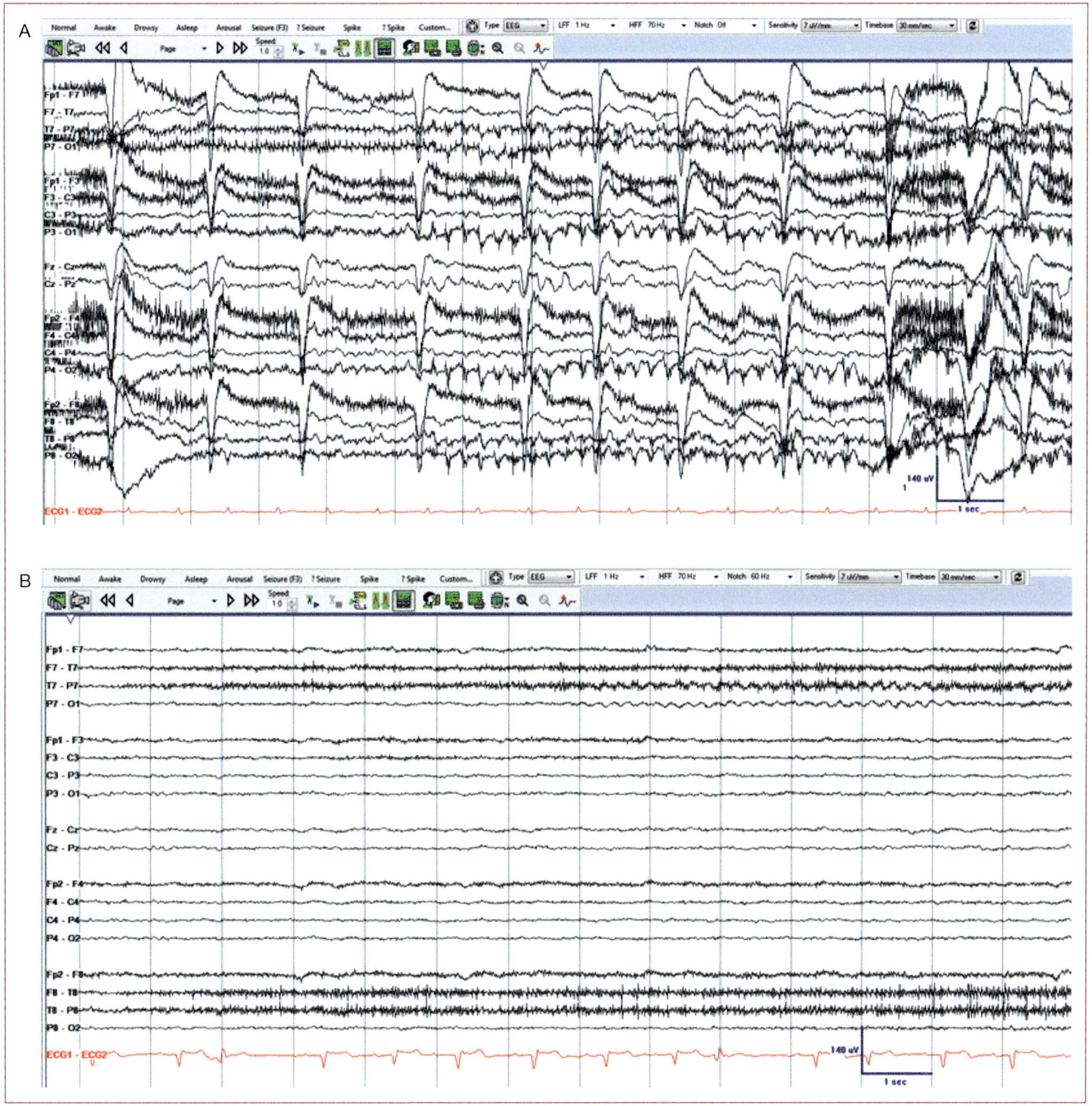

FIGURE 5.13: Tremor artifact. Patient with parkinsonism and bilateral hand tremors producing occasional, very brief to brief runs of rhythmic 4.0- to 5.0-Hz activity best seen over the posterior derivations that would change with head repositioning. (A) Tremor artifact with patient lying down with head midline during maximal wakefulness. (B) Same patient now drowsy with head turned to the left.

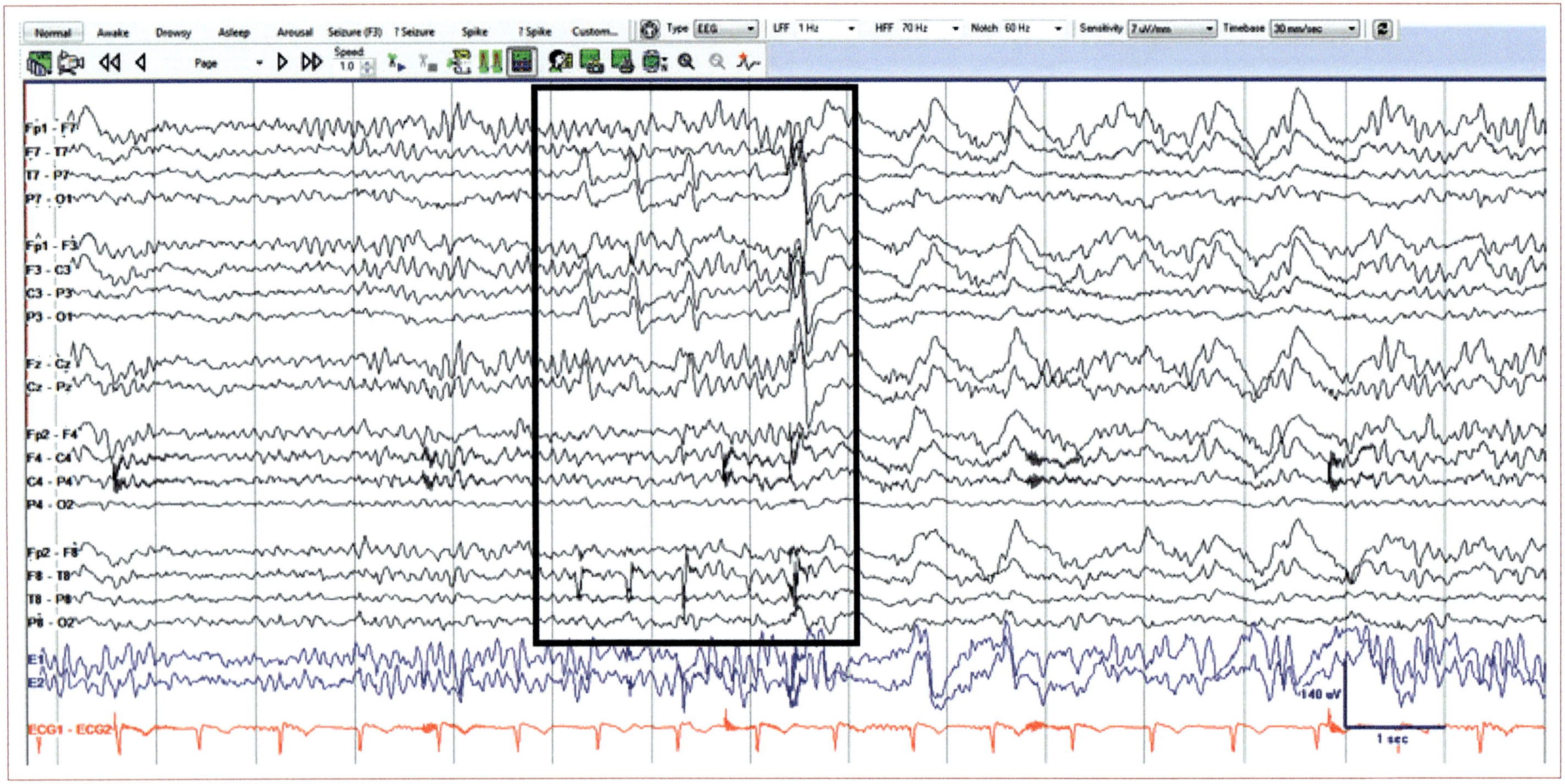

FIGURE 5.14: Myoclonic jaw movement artifact. Epoch with notch filter on captured four repetitive waveforms (black box) suspicious for sharp waves maximal over the left parietooccipital region. On video review, these waveforms correlated to myoclonic jaw jerking from an underlying movement disorder. This is an example where, without video, it may not be possible to appreciate "sharp waves" as artifacts.

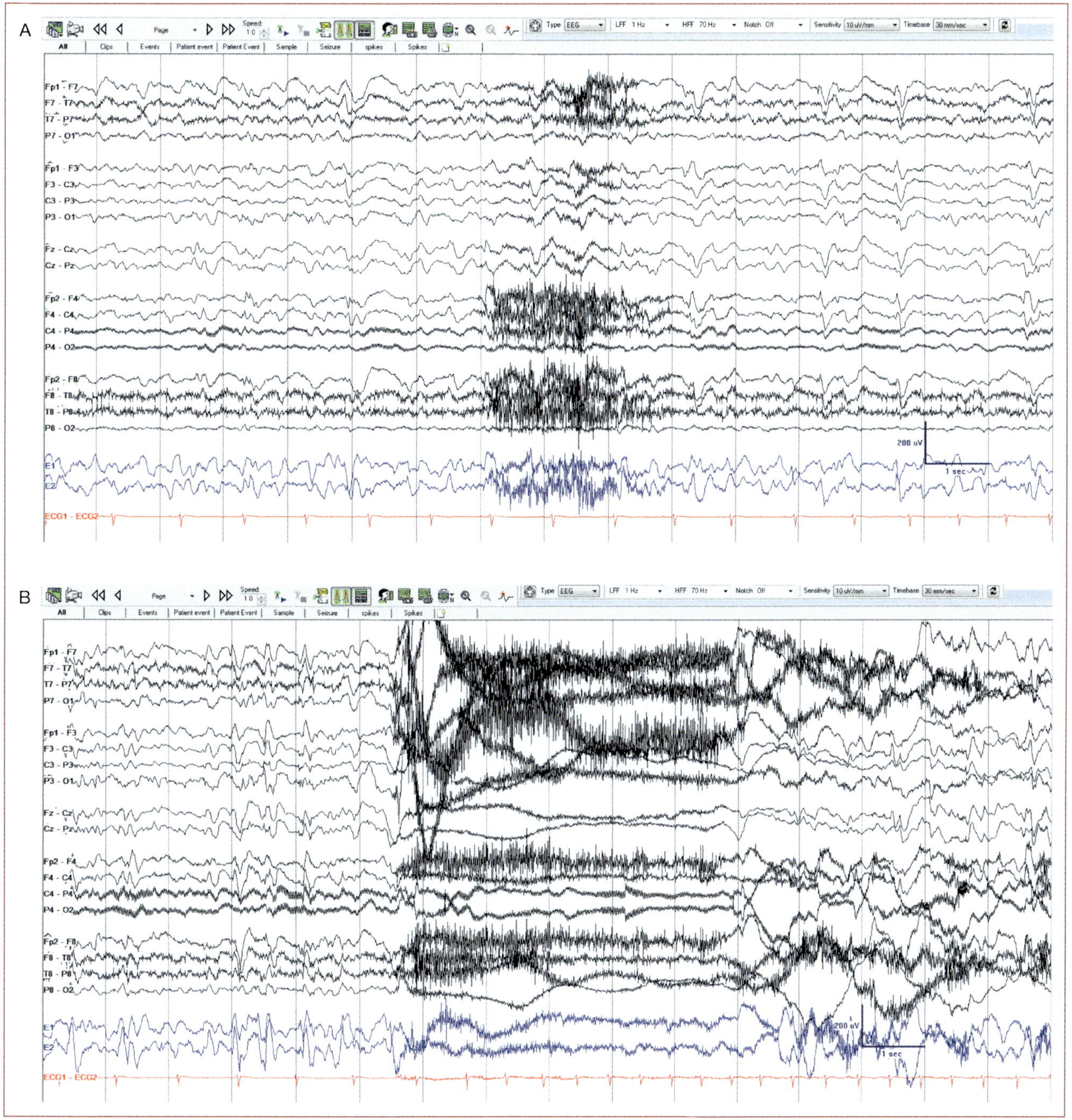

FIGURE 5.15: Dystonic movement artifact. This occurred in a patient with a movement disorder (nonepileptic dystonia) and dystonic seizures. (A) Epoch captures a dystonic movement of the right upper extremity, neck, and face, lasting several seconds. The EMG artifact is superimposed on the patient's background activity with multifocal epileptiform discharges. (B) During the same recording, a dystonic seizure was captured with diffuse myogenic artifact in addition to electrodecrement of the cerebral activity during a dystonic seizure. Postevent resumption of the interictal background is restored. EEG was the only reliable method for accurately distinguishing the movement disorder from a seizure.

EMG, electromyogram.

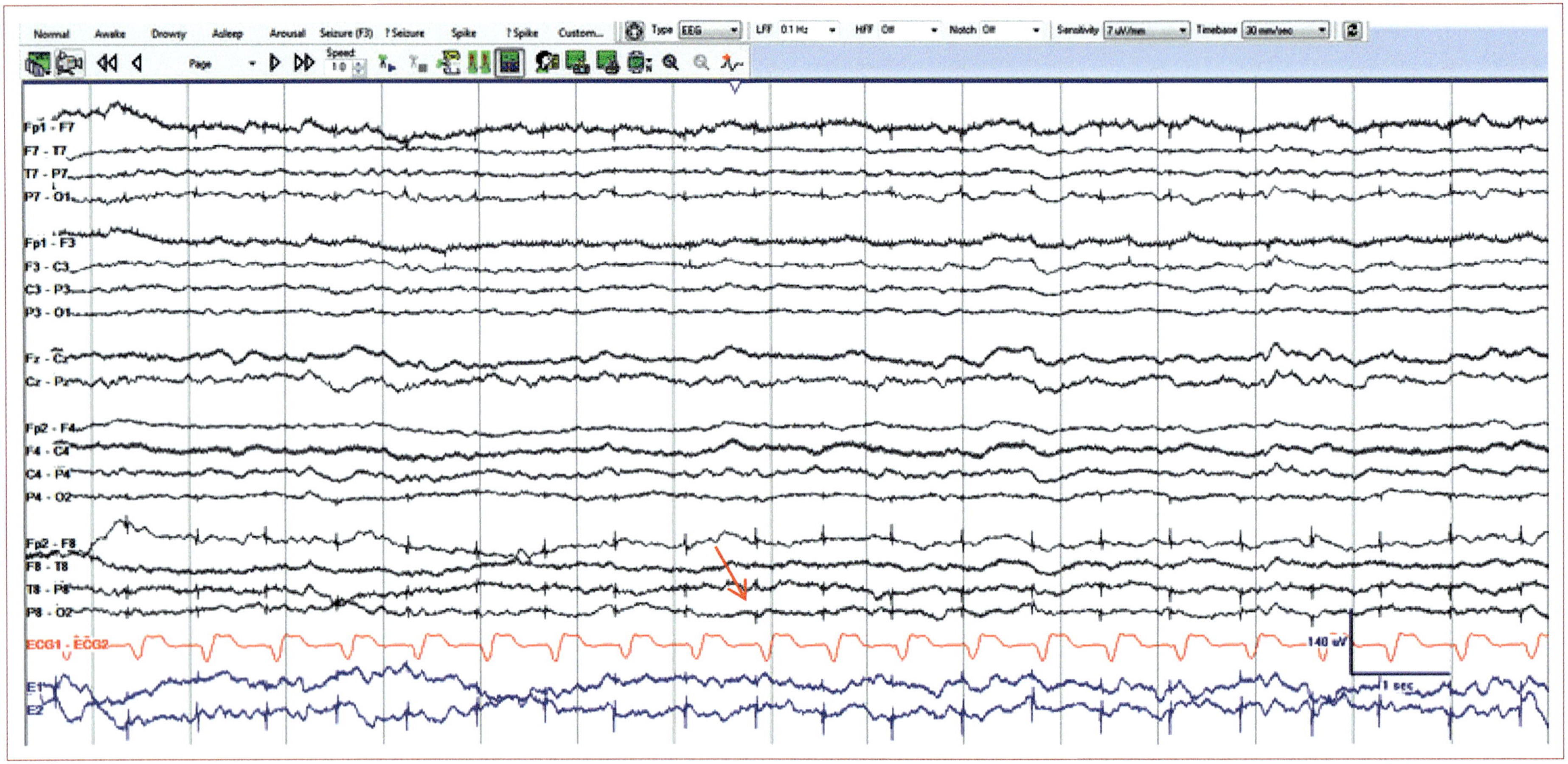

FIGURE 5.16: Pacemaker artifact and sweat artifact. Pacemaker spike (red arrow) occurring at regular intervals preceding the ventricular depolarization associated with the ECG. Additionally, this epoch shows very slow (1 Hz or less) activity due to sweat sway of the baseline that is best seen over the right temporal chain in the EEG.

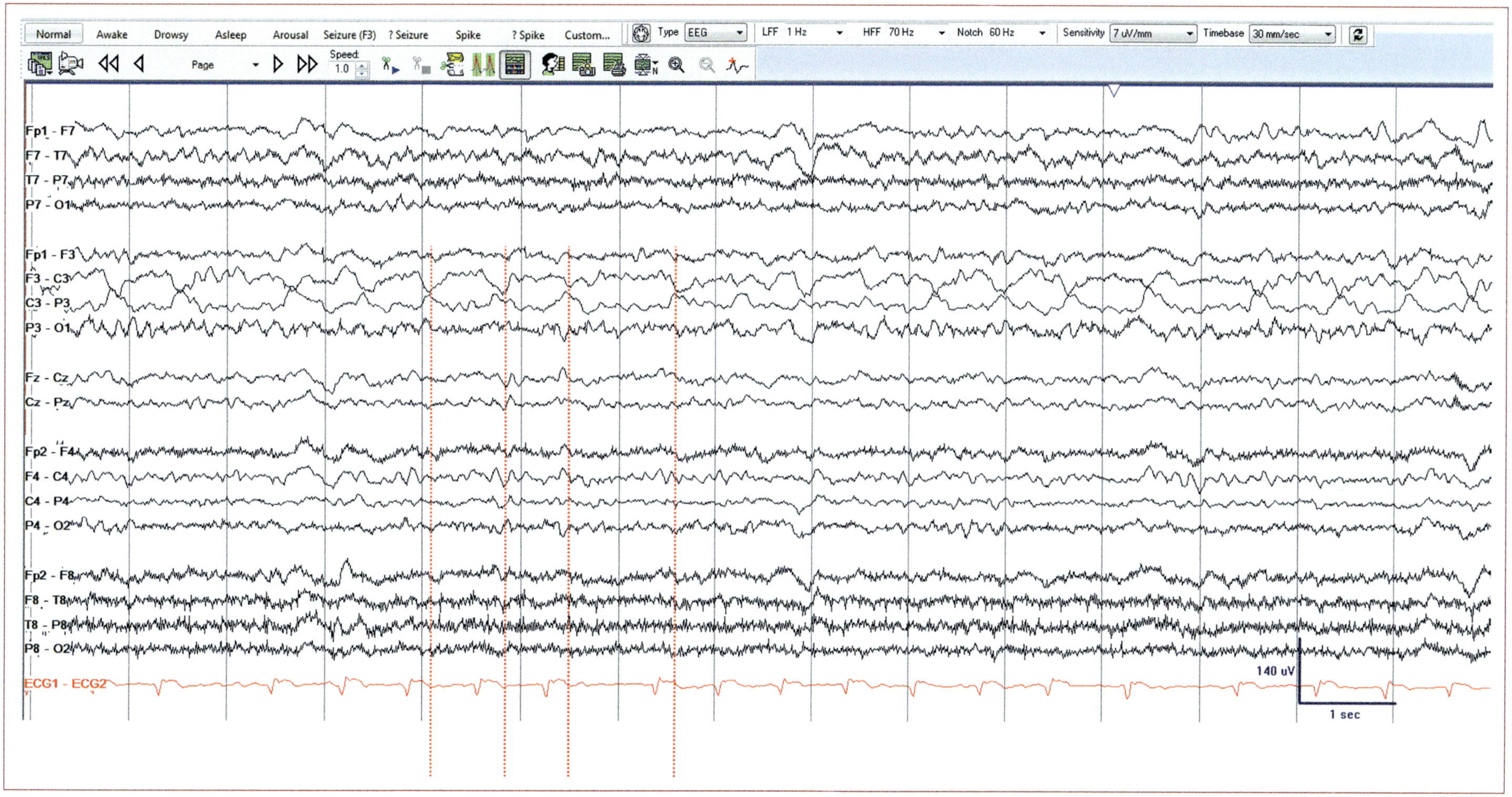

FIGURE 5.17: Pulse artifact. This is seen over the left frontocentral head region, most notable at the C3 derivation. Note that, while the heart rate changes, the artifact remains constant in relation to the QRS complex, marked with long red hashed line. This can be more easily appreciated by placing the ECG channel next to the channel with the pattern of interest or by increasing the gain on the ECG channel.

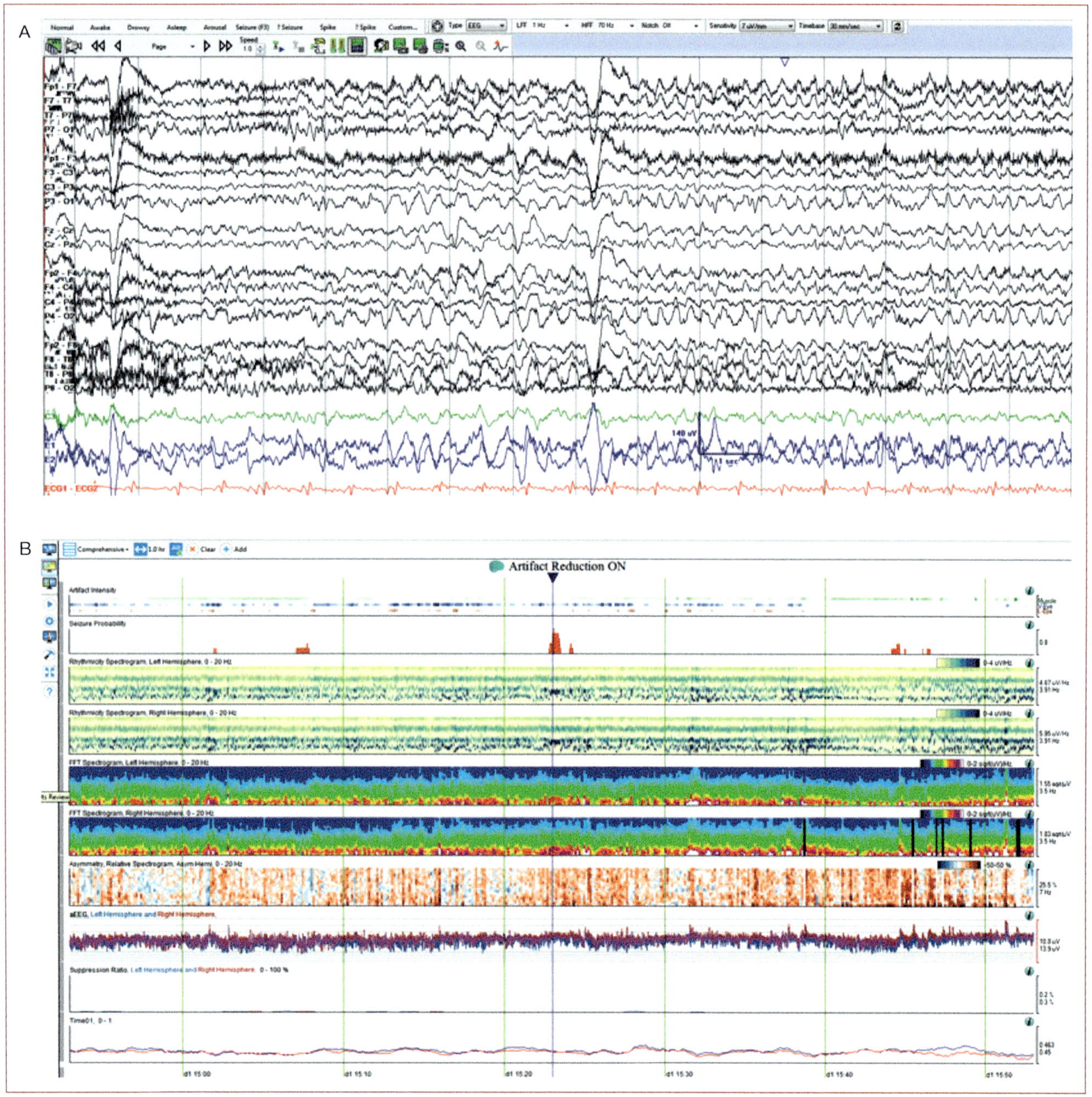

FIGURE 5.18: Drinking from a straw, causing an artifact. (A) EEG with diffuse rhythmic activity that appears to evolve in morphology and speed from 2.5 to 4 Hz, which correlated to the patient drinking from a straw on video. This was reproducible in the EEG of the patient and is an unusually prominent artifact during use of a straw. (B) Digital analysis of this time period (blue vertical line) reflects seizure identification as judged by the seizure probability index. It is also associated with increased rhythmicity on hemispheric rhythmicity spectrograms.

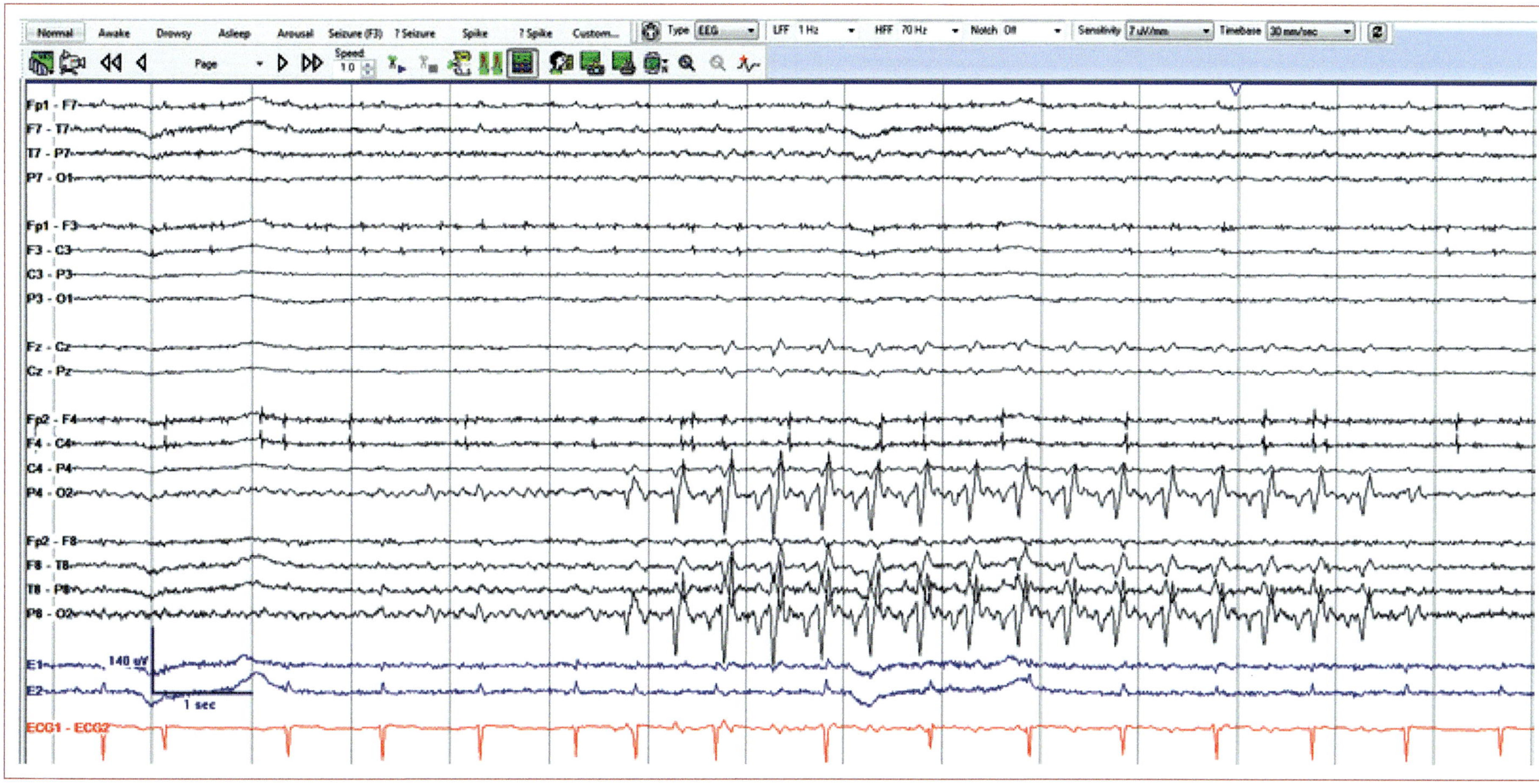

FIGURE 5.19: Open port amplifier artifact. Low-voltage fast activity and alpha activity best seen over the O2 derivations mimicking cerebral activity (repetitive polyspikes) maximal over the right posterior quadrant. This epoch actually captured electrical activity that was apparent even after the EEG leads were unplugged from the amplifier, resulting in open ports. Thus the patient was no longer connected to the EEG. The apparent polyspikes occurred when the amplifier was shaken. ECG recording continued to further add to the difficulty in artifact identification.

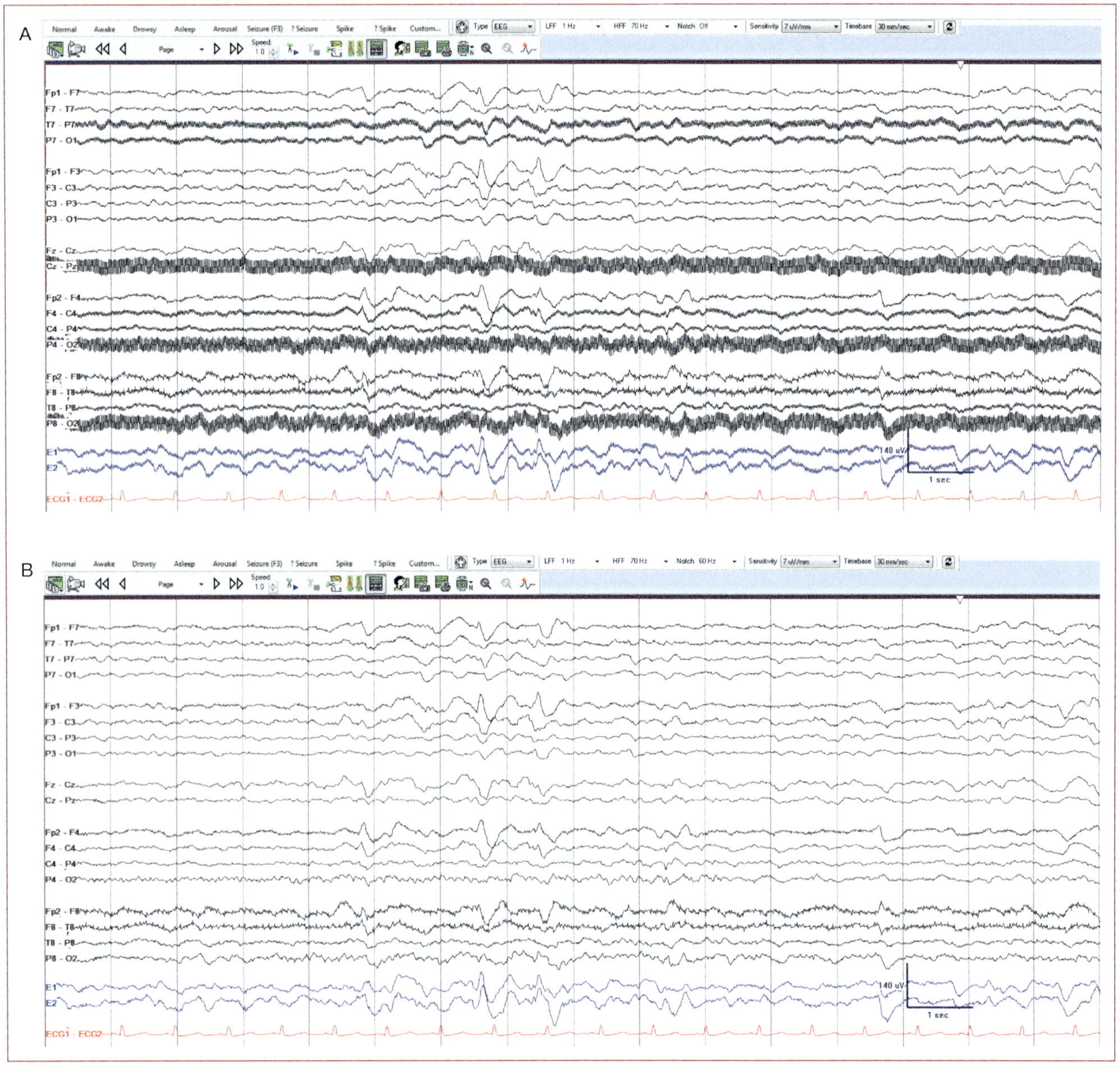

FIGURE 5.20: Analysis error, notch pitfall. (A) EEG with notch off with prominent 60-Hz artifact limited to O2–Pz. (B) Same epoch with the notch filter on, allowing for interpretation. Often subtle asymmetries in affected leads are discounted, like the 8-Hz activity seen at O2. This creates an anchor bias in which abnormalities in this region may be falsely overlooked. (*continued*)

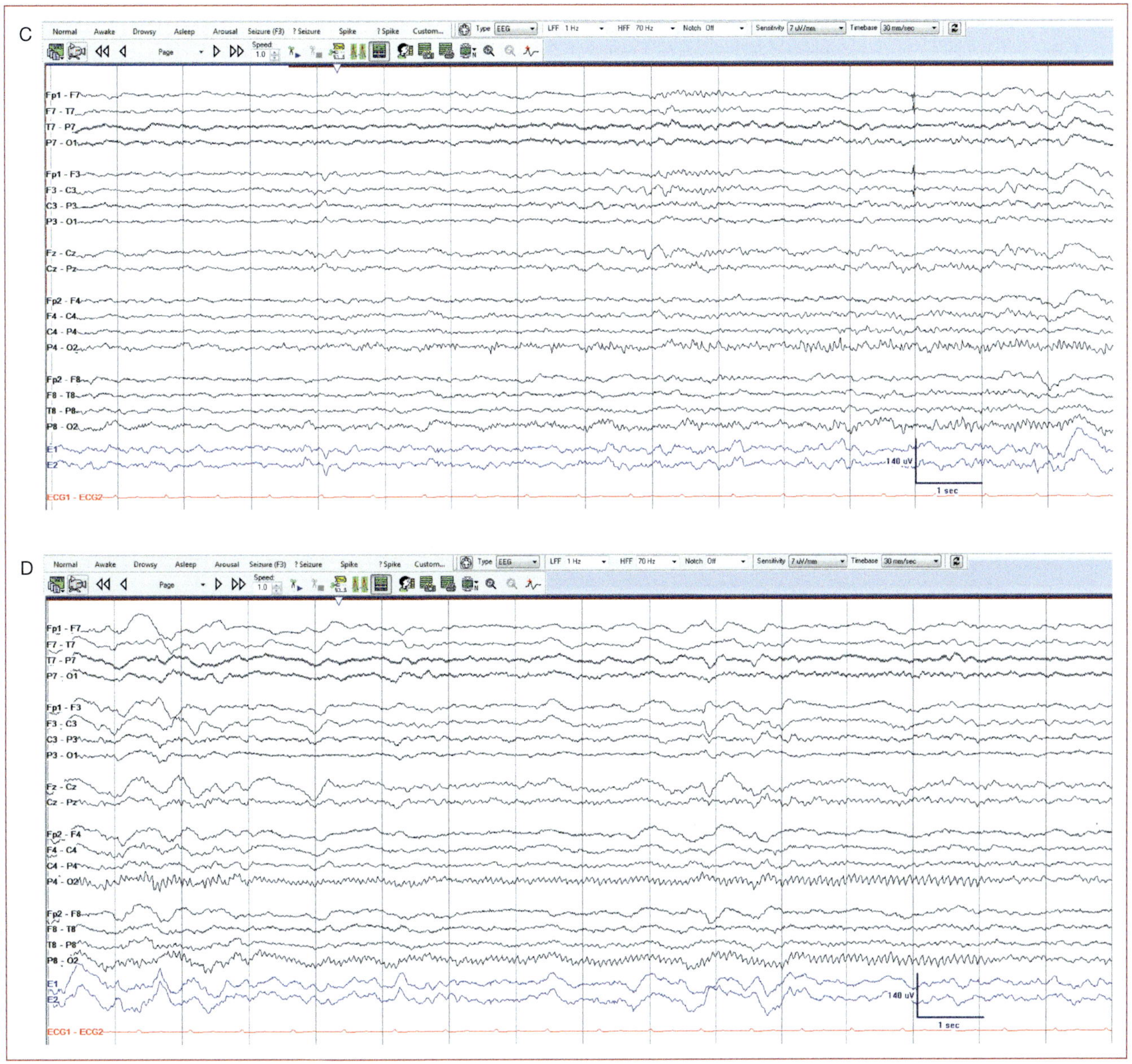

FIGURE 5.20: (*continued*) (C and D) Sequential epochs in the same patient after corrective measure (leads reapplied) with notch filter off, capturing a focal seizure at O2 spreading to involve Pz and O1. (*continued*)

E

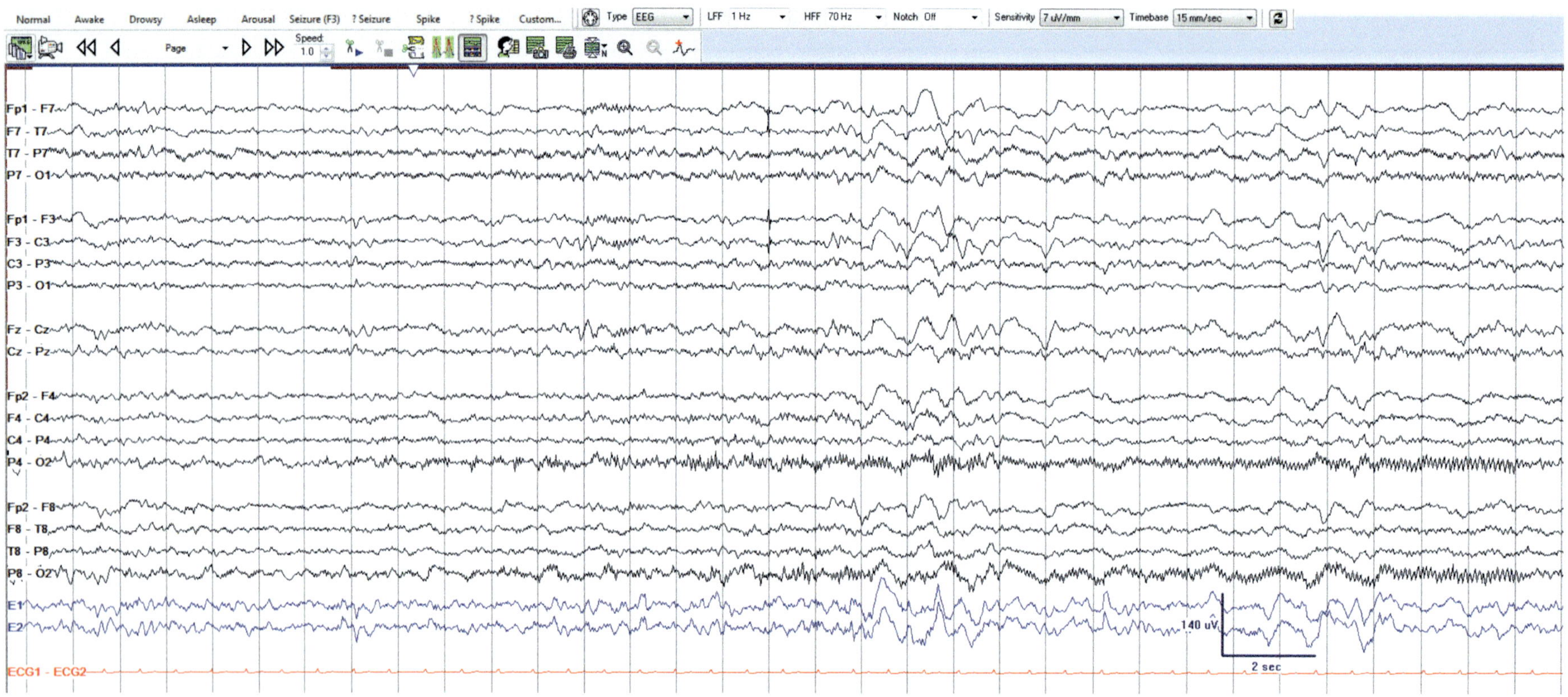

FIGURE 5.20: (*continued*) (E) Same two epochs with time base 15 mm/sec allowing for compressed view of the entire event. This highlights the need for lead maintenance as opposed to routine filtering. Undoubtedly, one should be very cautious about calling a focal seizure limited to channels with persistent 60-Hz artifact. In this case, there were indeed focal seizures in that region, proven by securing the electrodes to the scalp and continuing the EEG recording.

A

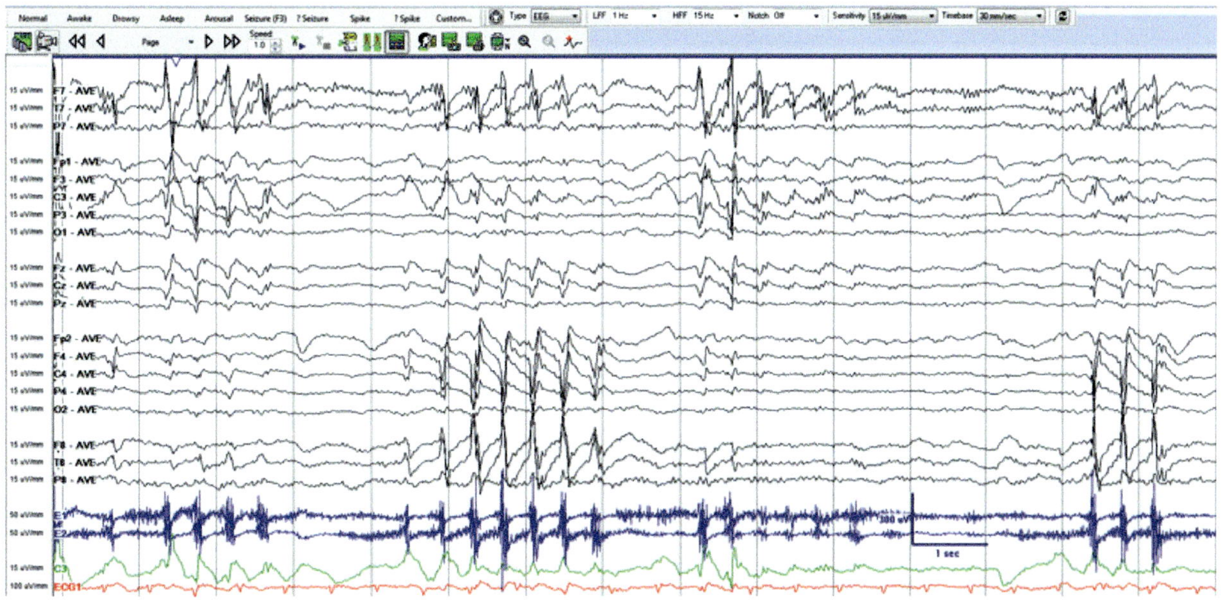

B

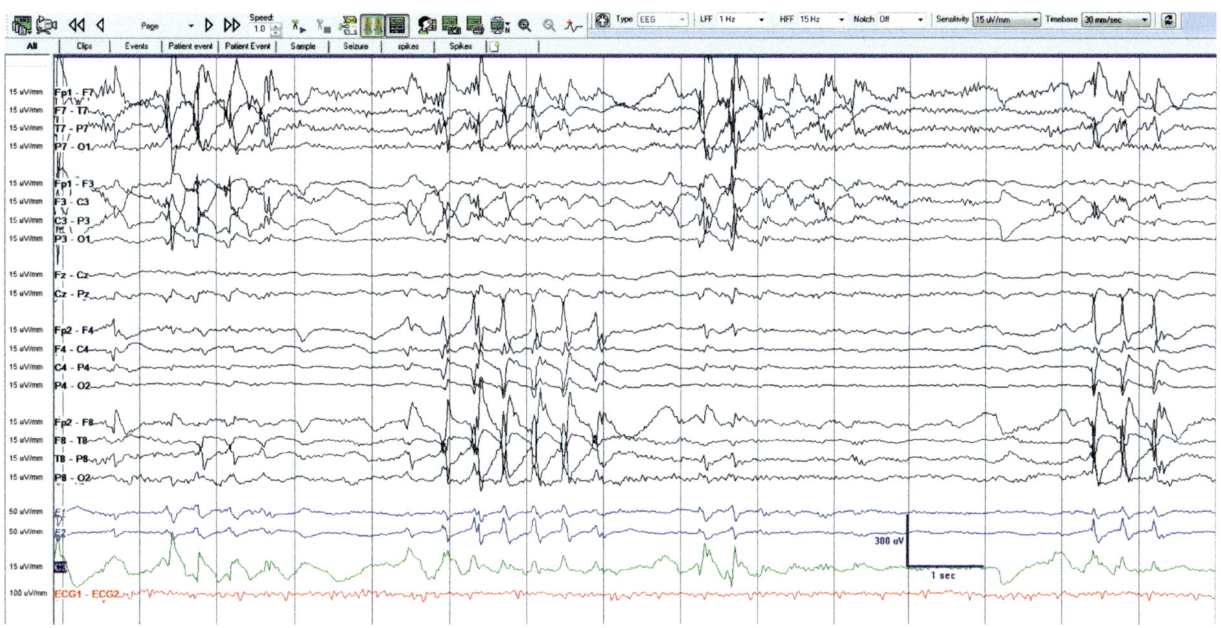

FIGURE 5.21: Analysis error, filter setting pitfall. (A) EEG viewed "as recorded" in an average reference with the high-frequency filter unexpectedly (and inappropriately) reduced to 15 Hz. (B) EEG viewed "as recorded" in a bipolar montage with the high-frequency filter unexpectedly (and inappropriately) reduced to 15 Hz. Both show repetitive polyspikes and slow wave complexes with overriding fast activity seen, with shifting maxima that mimics epileptiform discharges. (*continued*)

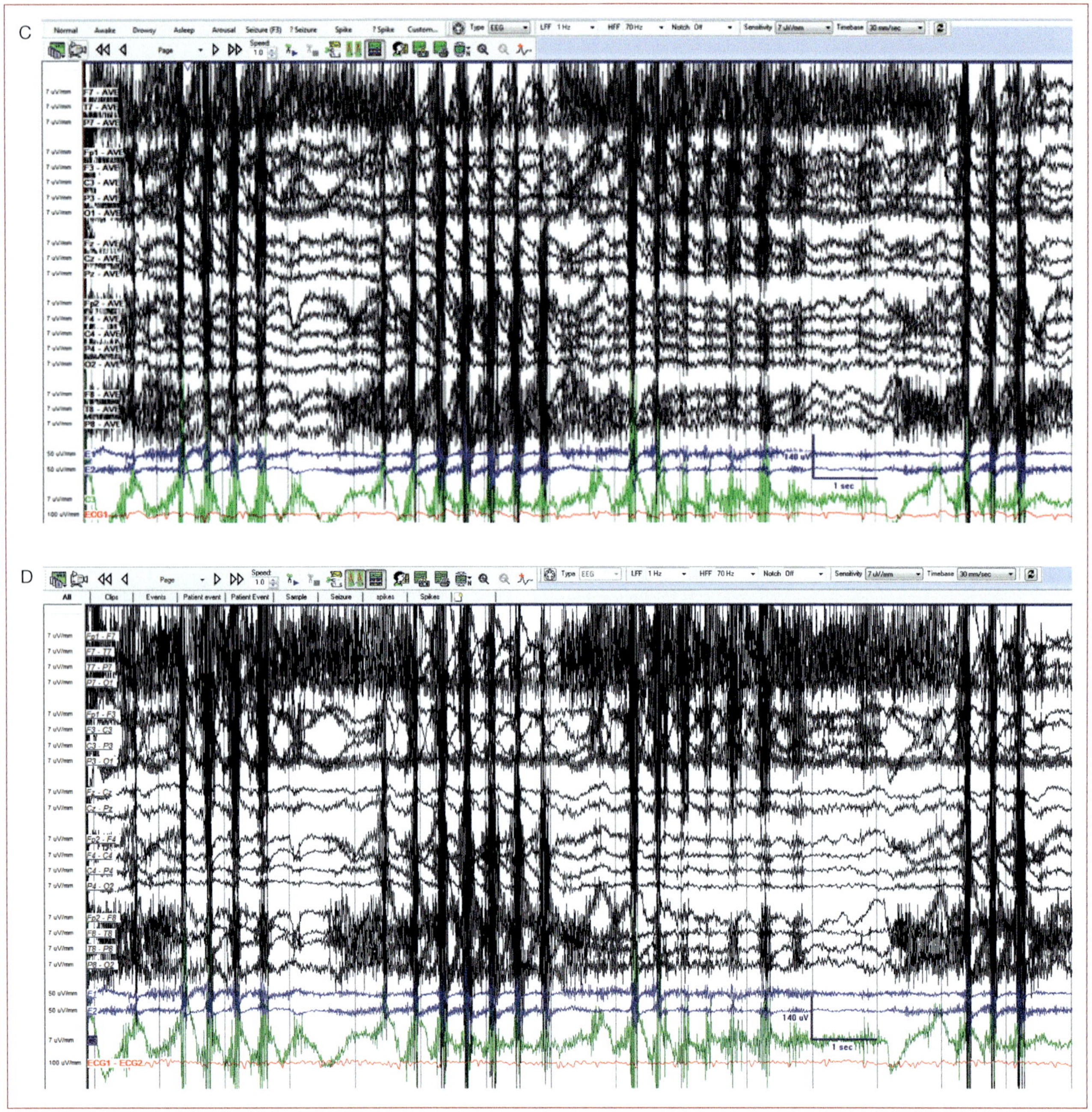

Figure 5.21: (*continued*) (C and D) Same epochs with corrected high-frequency filter setting at 70 Hz, reflecting EMG artifact while chewing.

EMG, electromyogram.

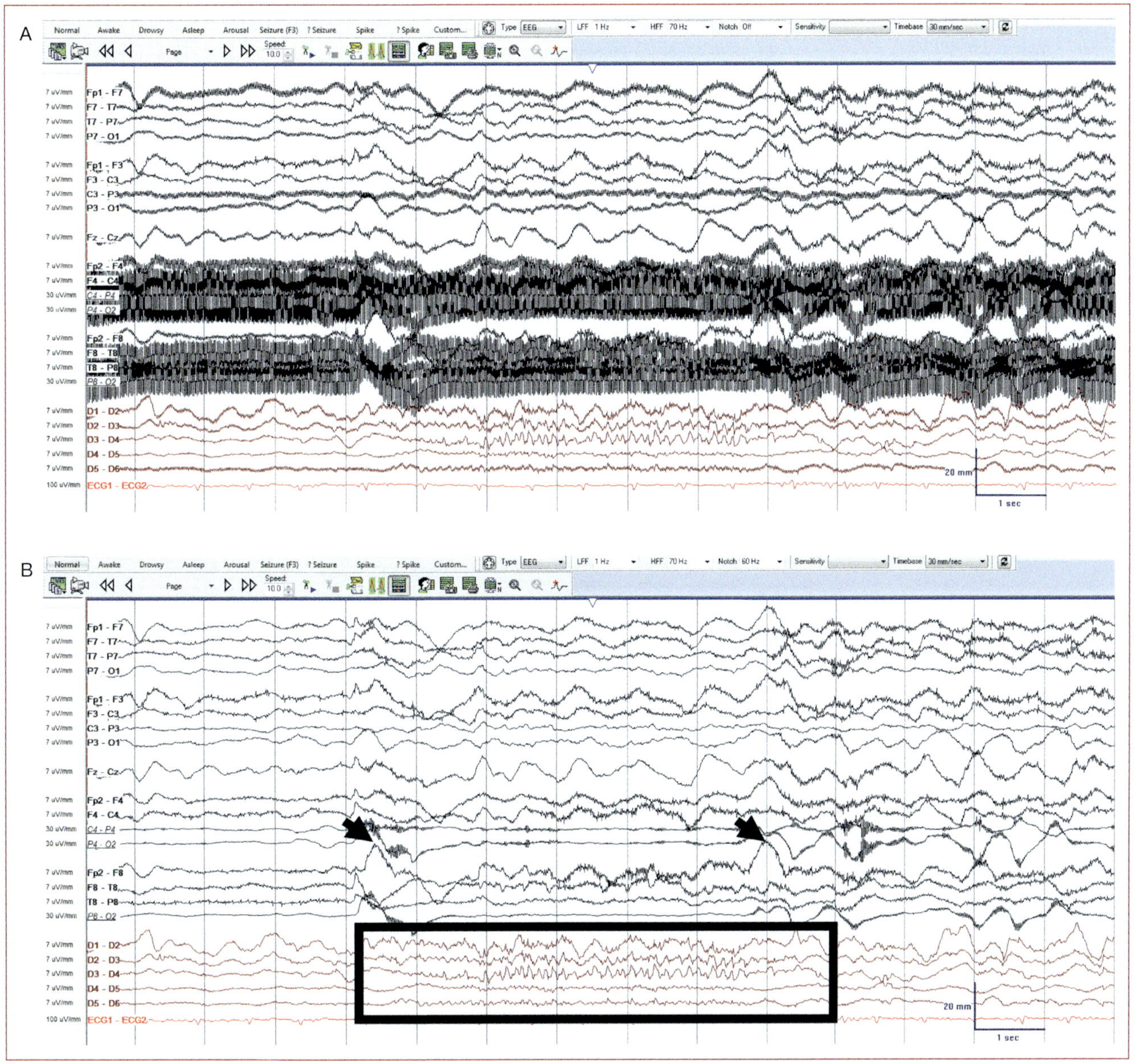

FIGURE 5.22: Scalp EEG with 60 Hz and suction artifact. Depth (intracranial) electrode strip artifact. (A) Notch filter off. (B) Notch filter on. Suction artifact on scalp EEG producing polymorphic delta waveforms with higher voltages than patient's cerebral activity suspicious for stimulation-induced GRDA. The box reveals sharply contoured alpha activity best seen at the depth electrode contacts D2D3/D3D4 corresponding to nursing care. The arrows reflect the onset and cessation of suction during patient care and repositioning. This sharply contoured alpha frequency at the depth electrode recurred during suctioning. Depth electrode artifact reflects a technical error in which the scalp system reference was inappropriately used for the depth electrode strip. This led to inadequate common mode rejection and was remedied by using a depth electrode reference for the depth electrode contacts.

GRDA, generalized rhythmic delta activity.

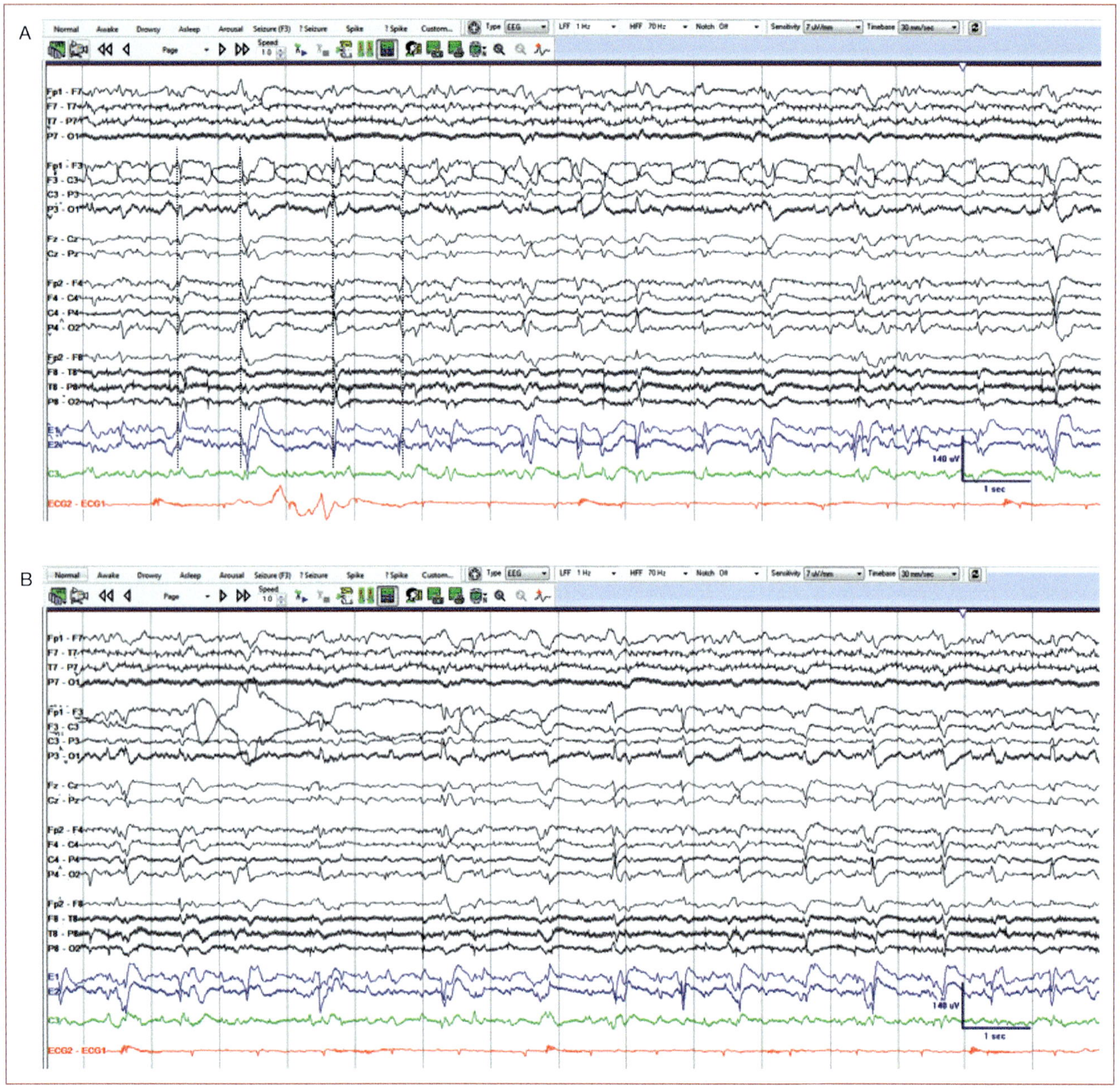

FIGURE 5.23: Lead pop artifact. (A) EEG appearing to capture bilateral, independent periodic discharges. The black line demonstrates right hemispheric lateralized periodic discharges with a broad field of distribution (LPDs, bilateral asymmetric) occurring at approximately 1 Hz. Independent to this pattern, left lateralized periodic discharges appear over Fp1/F3, F3/C3 at approximately 1.25 Hz. Note this can be fully explained by one electrode, F3. (B) Neighboring epoch with electrode pop affecting F3. Correcting the lead and attachment led to complete resolution of the F3 artifact that mimicked left LPDs. Persistent right hemispheric LPDs remained unmodified.

LPDs, lateralized periodic discharges

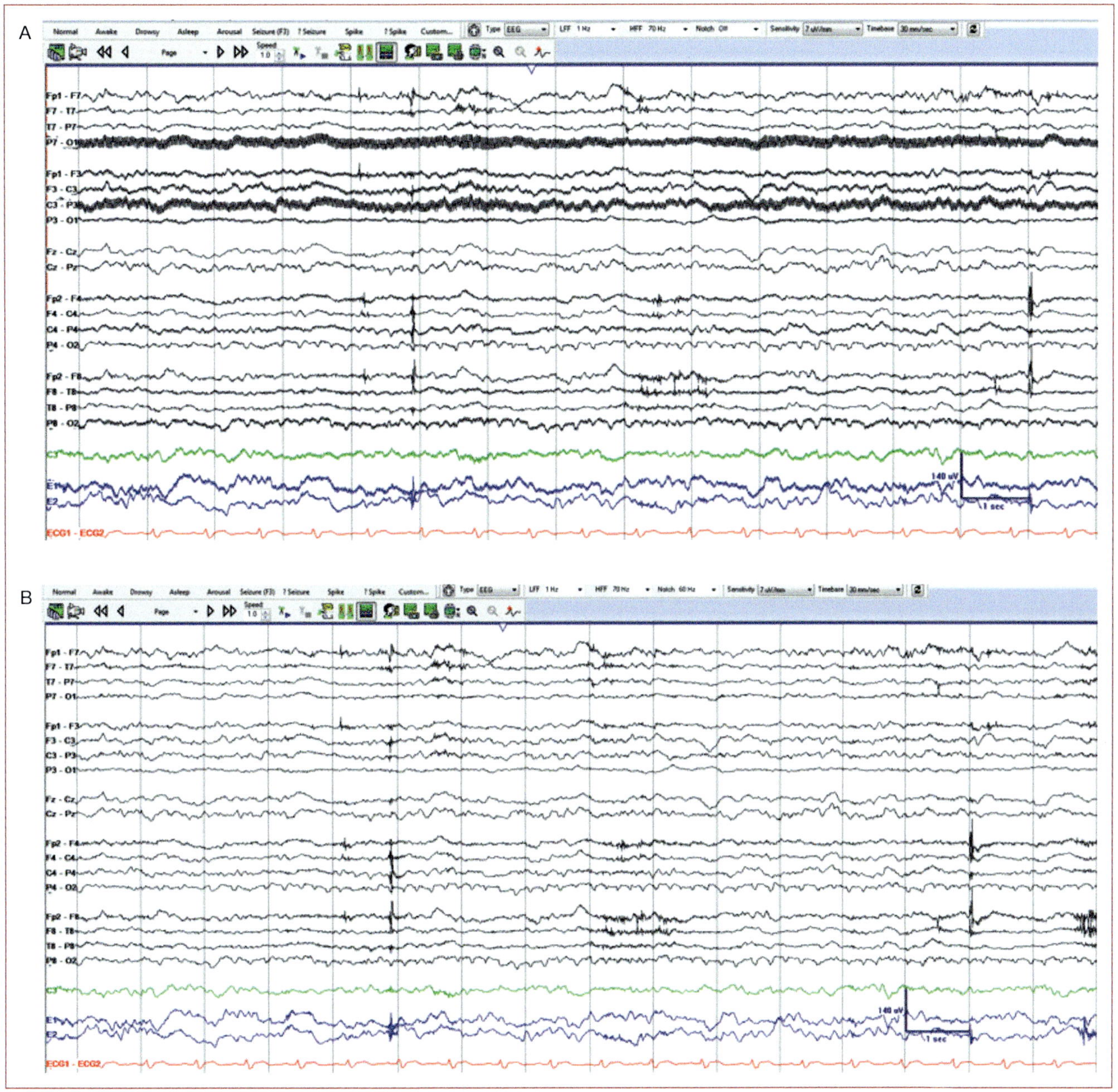

FIGURE 5.24: High-impedance artifact. (A) EEG with left parietooccipital 60-Hz artifact and rhythmic O2 activity maximal at 4.0 Hz with a notched appearance. This was concerning for a right occipital seizure. (B) The same epoch with the notch filter on, demonstrating resolution of the left parietal artifact but persistence of suspicious O2 rhythmicity and atypical waveform morphology. (*continued*)

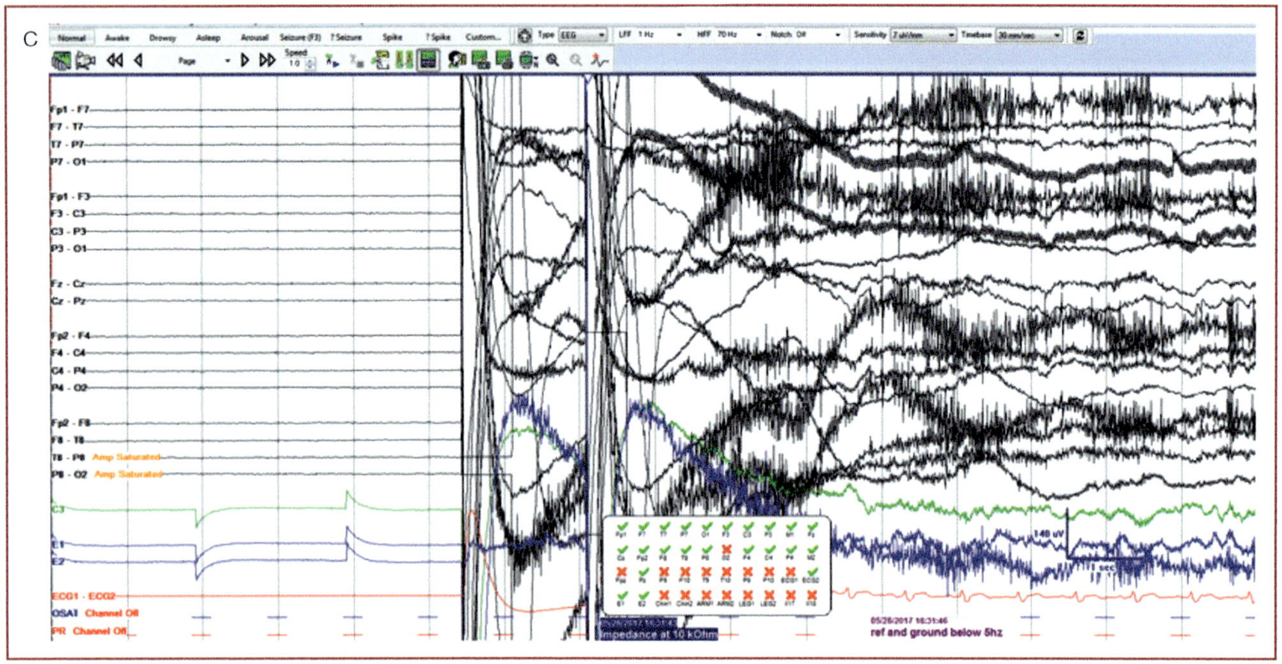

FIGURE 5.24: (*continued*) (C) Review of initial impedances revealed high O2 impedance. Correction of this electrode contact led to complete resolution of this pattern. This example highlights the importance of obtaining high-quality EEGs and the value of an experienced technologist.

REFERENCES

1. White DM, Van Cott AC. EEG artifacts in the intensive care unit setting. *Am J Electroneurodiagnostic Technol*. 2010;50(1):8-25. doi:10.1080/1086508X.2010.11079750.
2. Tatum WO, Dworetzky BA, Freeman WD, Schomer DL. Artifact: recording EEG in special care units. *J Clin Neurophysiol*. 2011;28(3):264-277. doi:10.1097/WNP.
3. Gaspard N, Hirsch LJ. Pitfalls in ictal EEG interpretation critical care and intracranial recordings. *Neurology*. 2013;80(suppl 1):S26-S42. doi:10.1212/WNL.0b013e31827974f8.
4. Hernandez-Frau PE, Benbadis SR. Pearls & oysters: errors in EEG interpretations: what is misinterpreted besides temporal sharp transients? *Neurology*. 2011;76:e57-e59. doi:10.1212/WNL.0b013e318211c1d.5.
5. Benbadis SR. Errors in EEGs and the misdiagnosis of epilepsy: importance, causes, consequences, and proposed remedies. *Epilepsy Behav*. 2007;11:257-262. doi:10.1016/j.yebeh.2007.05.013.
6. Alvarez V, Rossetti AO. Clinical use of EEG in the ICU: technical setting. *J Clin Neurophysiol*. 2015;32(6):481-485. doi:10.1097/WNP.0000000000000194.
7. Egol AB, Guntupalli KK. Intravenous infusion device artifact in the EEG-confusion in the diagnosis of electrocerebral silence. *Intensive Care Med*. 1983;9(1):29-32. doi:10.1007/BF01693703.
8. Haider HA, Esteller R, Hahn CD, et al. Sensitivity of quantitative EEG for seizure identification in the intensive care unit. *Neurology*. 2016 30;87(9):935-944. doi:10.1212/WNL.0000000000003034.
9. Swisher CB, White CR, Mace BE, et al. Diagnostic accuracy of electrographic seizure detection by neurophysiologists and non-neurophysiologists in the adult ICU using a panel of quantitative EEG trends. *J Clin Neurophysiol*. 2015;32(4):324-330. doi:10.1097/WNP.0000000000000144.
10. Stewart CP, Otsubo H, Ochi A, et al. Seizure identification in the ICU using quantitative EEG displays. *Neurology*. 2010;75(17):1501-1508. doi:10.1212/WNL.0b013e3181f9619e.
11. Gaspard N. Current clinical evidence supporting the use of continuous EEG monitoring for delayed cerebral ischemia detection. *J Clin Neurophysiol*. 2016;33(3):211-216. doi:10.1097/WNP.0000000000000279.
12. Muniz CF, Shenoy AV, O'Connor KL, et al. Clinical development and implementation of an institutional guideline for prospective EEG monitoring and reporting of delayed cerebral ischemia. *J Clin Neurophysiol*. 2016;33(3):217-226. doi:10.1097/WNP.0000000000000281.
13. Mikell CB, Dyster TG, Claassen J. Invasive seizure monitoring in the critically-Ill brain injury patient: current practices and a review of the literature. *Seizure*. 2016;41:201-205. doi:10.1016/j.seizure.2016.05.017.
14. Stuart RM, Waziri A, Weintraub D, et al. Intracortical EEG for the detection of vasospasm in patients with poor-grade subarachnoid hemorrhage. *Neurocrit Care*. 2010;13(3):355-358. doi:10.1007/s12028-010-9414-6.
15. Waziri A, Claassen J, Stuart RM, et al. Intracortical electroencephalography in acute brain injury. *Ann Neurol*. 2009;66(3):366-377. doi:10.1002/ana.21721.
16. Sinha SR, Sullivan L, Sabau D, et al. American Clinical Neurophysiology Society Guideline 1: minimal technical requirements for performing clinical electroencephalography. *J Clin Neurophysiol*. 2016;33:303-307. doi:10.1097/WNP.0000000000000308.

CHAPTER 6

Artifact in Pediatric Electroencephalography

Erika Takle Axeen and Phillip L. Pearl

INTRODUCTION

Surface recordings of electrophysiological brain activity are subject to artifact from a variety of sources (1). In an EEG recording, artifact is present in any tracing or changes in the tracing when it is attributed to a noncerebral source. Artifact can obscure a recording, rendering the electrocerebral activity unreadable. Familiarity with commonly seen patterns of artifact can help avoid misinterpretation, which when falsely attributed to cerebral sources, may have significant clinical implications. The pediatric EEG is subject to the same technical artifacts as seen in adults. Common examples include alternating current artifact (60 Hz) and vertical eye blink artifact during wakefulness. However, there are also artifacts that are unique to the pediatric population. Common examples of pediatric EEG artifacts are rhythmic patting and rocking artifact in the neonate and infant, which may be misinterpreted as an electrographic seizure without clinical signs. Therefore, video correlation of the EEG tracing may be indispensable to identify the potential source of artifact. This chapter includes common artifacts that are encountered in the EEG for a pediatric population. Specific pediatric patterns of artifact in the EEG that simulate seizures may be similar to those seen in an adult (see Chapter 7). Ictal mimics, ranging from benign epileptiform variants to induced cerebral activities, such as the texting rhythm (2-4), must be discriminated from common patterns associated with artifact.

PHYSIOLOGIC SOURCES OF ARTIFACT

Artifacts of physiologic or biologic origin are those arising from the patient's body, including eye movements, muscle activity (including glossokinetic), cardiac function, and sweat (Table 6.1).

Eye movements represent a common physiologic source of artifact seen in nearly every pediatric EEG tracing containing periods of wakefulness. This common artifact emanates from the frontal head regions and is best seen in the frontopolar and frontal electrodes (Figure 6.1). The inherent dipole in the eye is the generator of this artifact with the retina being relatively electronegative and the cornea electropositive. A useful mnemonic is "pupil positive, nerve negative." Attention to eye movements may be informative regarding the patient's state of alertness, with eye blink artifact signifying wakefulness and slow-roving eye movements suggesting drowsiness. Lateral rectus spikes can commonly be seen with lateral visual scanning. With rapid eye movement, the artifact producing the "spikes" from contraction of the lateral rectus muscles signifies a motor unit potential.

In the active child, muscle artifact is a pervasive feature that can obscure the EEG tracing. This is identified as high-frequency activity most prominently seen over the bilateral temporal and frontal regions. Predictable rhythmic patterns such as chewing or tongue movements can be identified based on their rhythmicity (Figures 6.2 and 6.3). Close attention to the timing of muscle artifact with event analysis can help discern whether movements are related to a seizure discharge.

TABLE 6.1: Common Sources of Physiologic Artifact

• Eye movements
• Muscles
• Tongue movements
• Cardiac
• Sweat

TABLE 6.2: Common Sources of Nonphysiologic Artifact

• Electrodes and lead wires
• Machines (e.g., ventilator)
• Environment (e.g., 60 Hz)
• Behavior (patient or caregiver)
• Other devices (e.g., pacemakers)

A frequently encountered artifact in all ages is the electrocardiogram. Pulse artifact can also be seen depending on positioning and can be mistaken for rhythmic slowing (Figure 6.4). Hiccups can also produce potentially confusing rhythmic artifacts requiring clinical correlation (Figure 6.5). The phenomenon known as sweat sway, with low-voltage undulating delta usually seen diffusely, is another example of an endogenous artifact from a physiologic but extracerebral source.

NONPHYSIOLOGIC SOURCES OF ARTIFACT

As in adults, commonly encountered nonphysiologic artifacts, such as electrode artifacts, are related to the technique and recording process of obtaining an EEG (Table 6.2).

In the inpatient setting, particularly where surrounding machines and equipment are abundant, such as in intensive care units or the operating room, 60-Hz artifact is frequently seen. A 60-Hz notch filter may be necessary to eliminate this artifact despite the potential loss of detecting underlying epileptiform activity. Figures 6.6A and B show 60-Hz artifact in an infant, which is attenuated utilizing the notch filter, after which electrode artifact remains. Figure 6.7 shows a periodic discharge attributable to the movement of the ventilator in a child who otherwise has electrocerebral inactivity on EEG. Nebulized respiratory therapy can serve as an exogenous source of artifact as well (Figure 6.8).

Electromagnetic disturbances can similarly occur in the outpatient setting, whether in the EEG laboratory or during ambulatory studies. A prominent EEG artifact simulating generalized spike-and-wave may be associated with ringing from a cellular telephone. In this case, proper grounding is needed to reduce these machine-related artifacts (5).

Rhythmic movement artifacts are commonly seen in the newborn, infant, and young child associated with patting and other soothing behaviors provided by caregivers (Figure 6.9). The rhythmicity, polarity, and location of the artifact can look suspiciously like an electrographic seizure. This is especially true for neonates who are prone to focal seizures that may be seen in only a single electrode. Use of video to identify movement patterns is critical in these situations as is close observation of the EEG for patterns of evolution and propagation, which are less likely to be seen in a purely artifactual pattern. Chest physical therapy introduces another artifact in the EEG produced by the exogenous repetitive behavior (Figure 6.10) (6,7).

Video 6.1 demonstrates very prominent EEG waveforms during which the video confirms the source as the child playing with a balloon! The active child will create frequent movement artifacts. This is seen as a myogenic artifact (surface electromyogram [EMG]) on the EEG recording. Occasionally, these behaviors may appear rhythmic, creating an unusual artifact (Figure 6.11).

ROLE OF ARTIFACT IN EVENT ANALYSIS AND SPECIALIZED RECORDING TECHNIQUES

EEG artifact is often frustrating in that it can obscure the cerebral recording, with loss of valuable electroclinical and localizing information. Alternatively, close correlation with video may be instrumental in identifying the source of the artifact as a psychogenic, nonepileptic seizure (**Video 6.2**). In addition, there are circumstances where an epileptic seizure can be initially detected by a stereotypical artifact. Examples include a rhythmic artifact in the frontopolar region caused by nystagmoid eye movements. Similarly, an extracerebral artifact may demonstrate characteristic patterns associated with EMG, electrocardiographic, or electrooculographic activity in an evolving fashion despite the absence of an electrocerebral change (**Figure 6.12**).

Specialized pediatric EEG recordings require meticulous attention to artifacts and may pose particular challenges. Ambulatory EEG recordings may produce a bewildering array of artifacts that may be especially difficult to explain or verify, and corresponding videography may be too obscure or unavailable for analysis. Unrestricted activity during ambulatory recordings and relative absence of observer information compounds the problem. Although many artifacts on ambulatory recordings are similar to those seen in conventional EEG (e.g., smiling, chewing, swallowing, eye and head movements, cable movement, coughing, startling, and talking), there are other artifacts that are relatively unique to ambulatory recordings (8). These include movements throughout sleep such as turning the head on a pillow, movements of others near the patient, walking, and poor connections at the preamplifier input. These have been mitigated by performing the initial portion of ambulatory EEGs in a controlled laboratory, documenting the appearance of common movements and other sources of artifact, in addition to verifying the integrity of the connections between the input electrode cables and recording unit.

The feasibility of novel, highly compact, wireless multichannel EEG in NICU has been challenging to interpret due to the prominent artifact. Also known as micro-EEG, this is a miniature, wireless recording device that digitizes the EEG signals for wireless transmission and represents an attempt to record EEG from an electrode cap. This method is used to achieve full-channel recordings with user-friendly application, enhanced portability, and ease of use. In a study of preterm newborns between 24 and 33 weeks gestational age with a postnatal age less than 30 days and at least two episodes of apnea, bradycardia, or oxygen desaturation within a 12-hour period, over half of the recordings were uninterpretable due to artifact in patients with a corrected gestational age of 35 weeks (9). Yet only 10% were uninterpretable due to artifacts in infants prior to 35 weeks corrected age. Negative predictors adversely affecting accurate interpretation included infants that were older and heavier and those with a large head circumference, but the primary reason for low interpretability was disconnection of the cap from the scalp. Another form of EEG recording that has gained increasing acceptance in the NICU is that of amplitude-integrated EEG (aEEG), which is highly practical although limited to 2 to 4 electrodes and is thus poorly representative of the scalp EEG and less informative for detecting focal epileptiform discharges (10–12). A higher rate of artifacts has been reported in aEEG recordings compared with scalp EEG recordings due to the presence of muscle activity, suboptimal electrode positioning, and unstandardized electrode application (13,14).

CONCLUSIONS

Artifacts of EEG recording are pervasive in pediatric recordings similar to adults; however, some are unique to this age period. Accurate discrimination of an artifact from cerebral sources is a critical skill for the encephalographer. Knowledge of common patterns of artifact is a useful tool that ensures appropriate interpretation of the pediatric EEG. Use of concurrent, time-locked video is indispensable for determining the source of some artifacts and differentiating them from interictal epileptiform discharges and electrographic seizures, particularly in the active child. Additionally, use of known artifact patterns can prove useful for determining the state of the patient (e.g., vertical eye blink artifact reflecting wakefulness) as well as the analysis of patterns during event monitoring, separating epileptic from nonepileptic seizures.

VIDEOS

Video 6.1: Artifact from a balloon near the EEG equipment. Note that the artifact changes frequency and amplitude depending on how the balloon is moved.

Video 6.2: A psychogenic nonepileptic spell can be diagnosed by careful analysis of artifact. In this video, note the muscle artifact is time-locked with the movements. Other features such as abrupt onset/offset (clinically and electrographically) and spell semiology are suggestive of a nonepileptic spell.

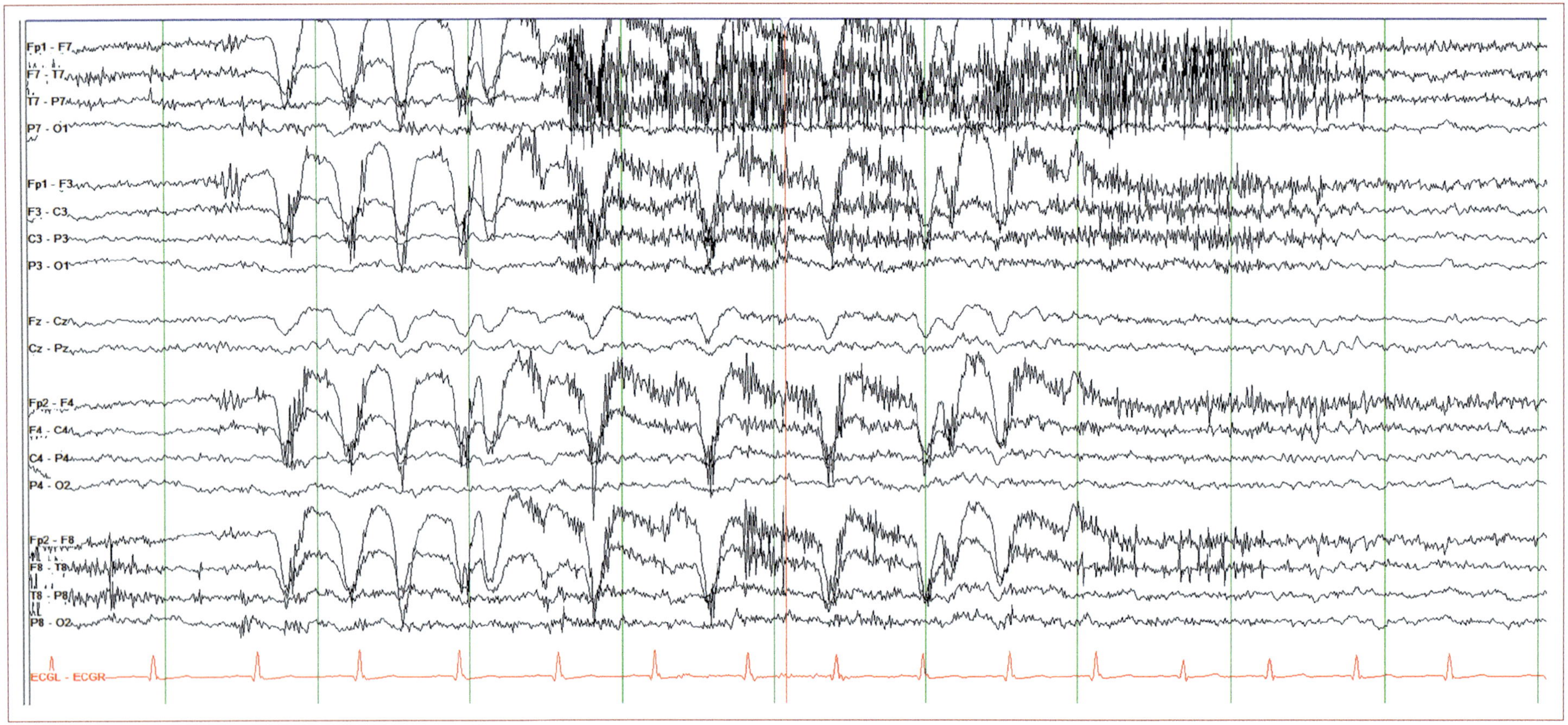

FIGURE 6.1: This EEG of a 13-year-old patient shows rhythmic eye blink artifact seen most prominently in the bilateral frontopolar leads as well as prominent muscle artifact especially obscuring the left temporal chain.

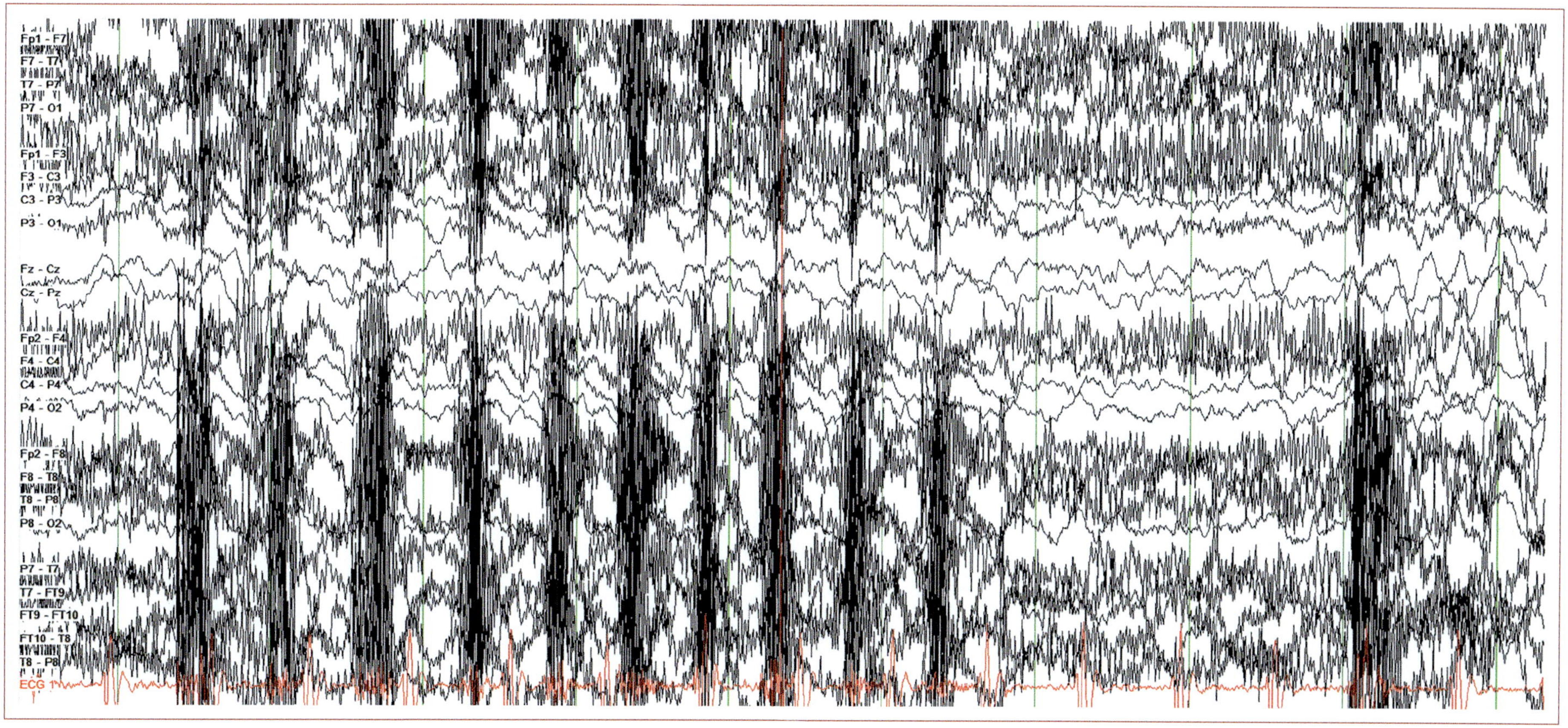

FIGURE 6.2: Prominent chewing artifact with the typical rhythmic and diffuse, but bitemporal, predominant distribution.

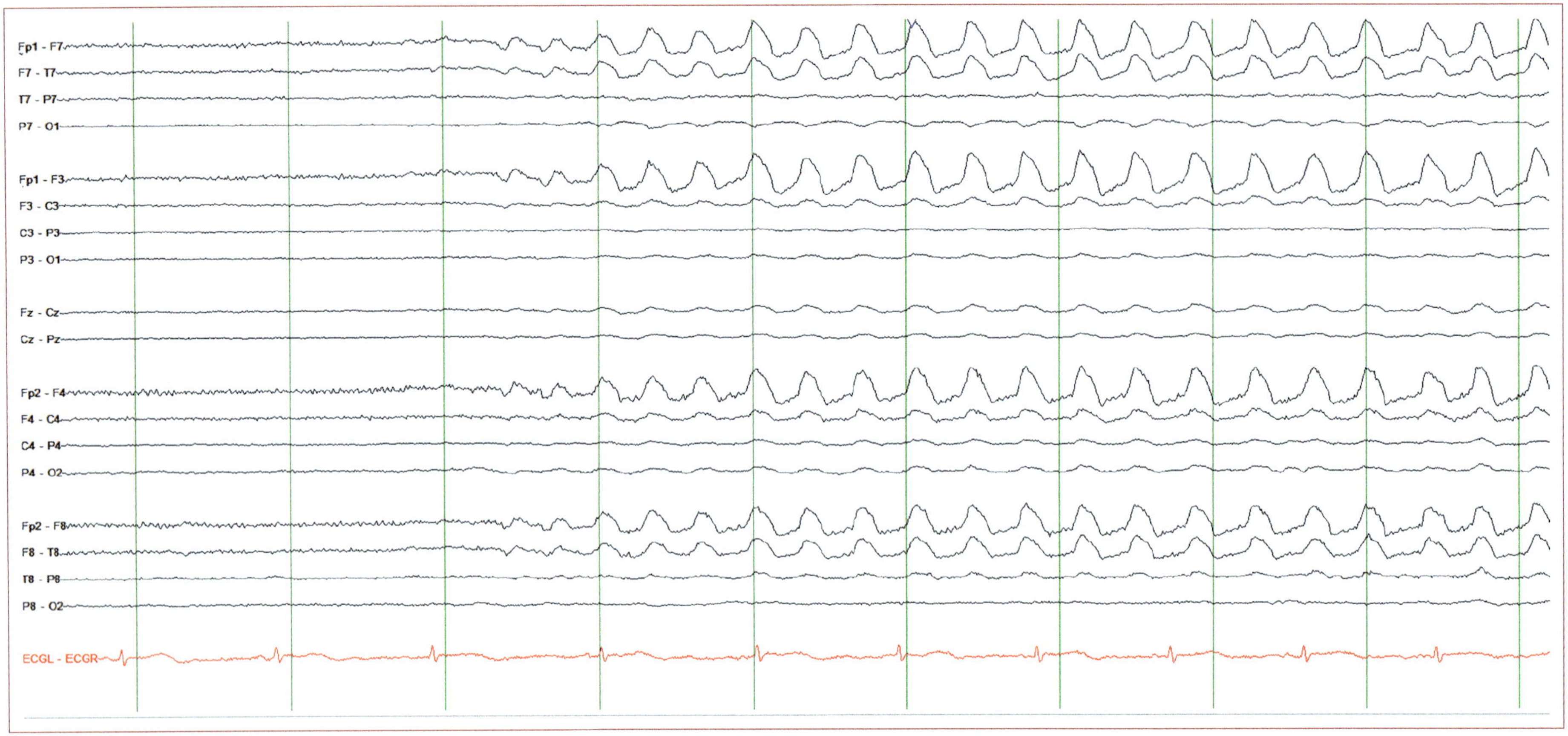

FIGURE 6.3: Glossokinetic artifact on EEG of a child with endotracheal intubation. EEG shows repetitive tongue movements against the endotracheal tube.

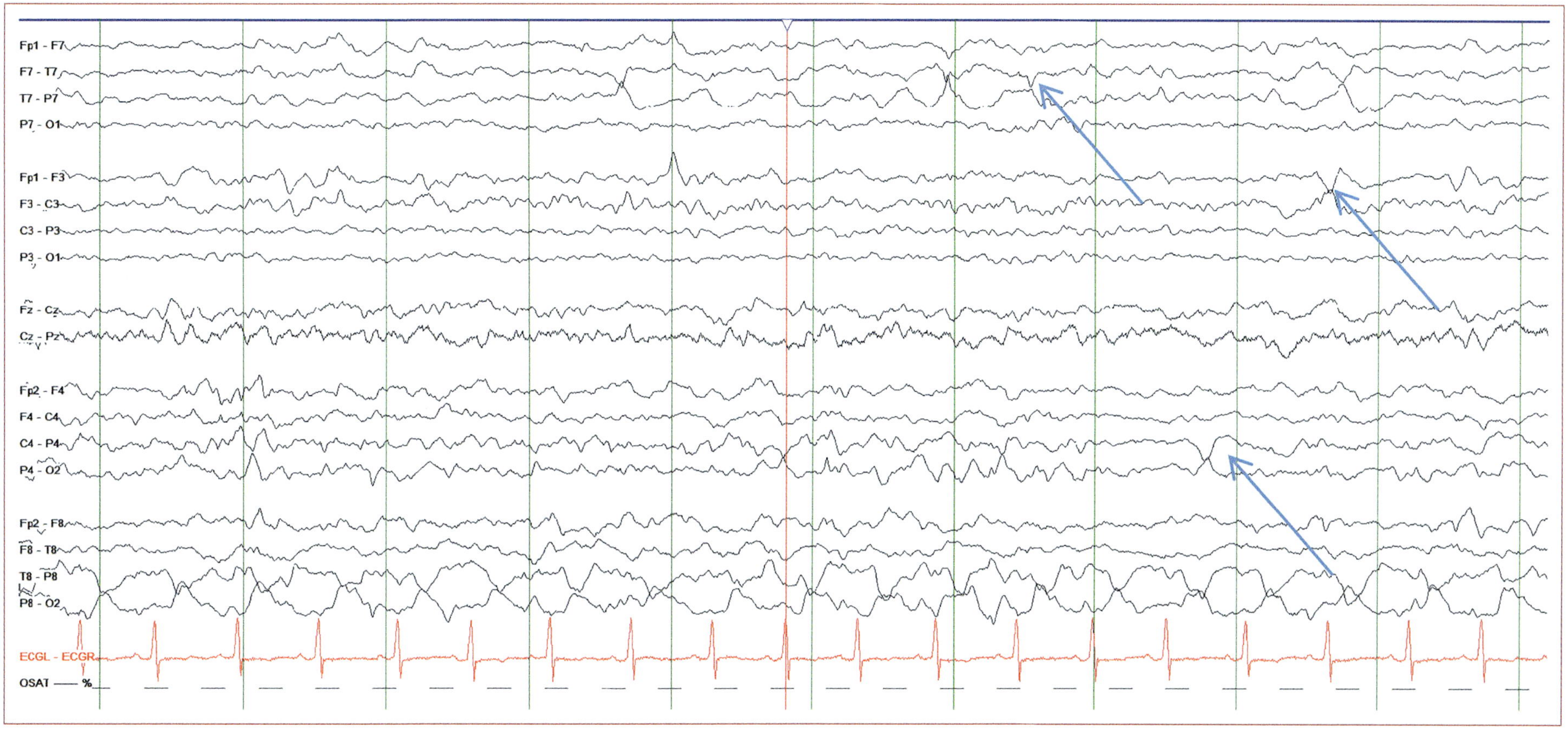

FIGURE 6.4: Pulse artifact shown in the EEG of a 1-month-old baby with multifocal sharp waves resulting from hypoxic ischemic injuries and a history of seizures. There is a pulse artifact in P8 that is persistently time locked with the EEG in this page (bottom two EEG channels). This continued invariantly for 40 minutes until the child was repositioned.

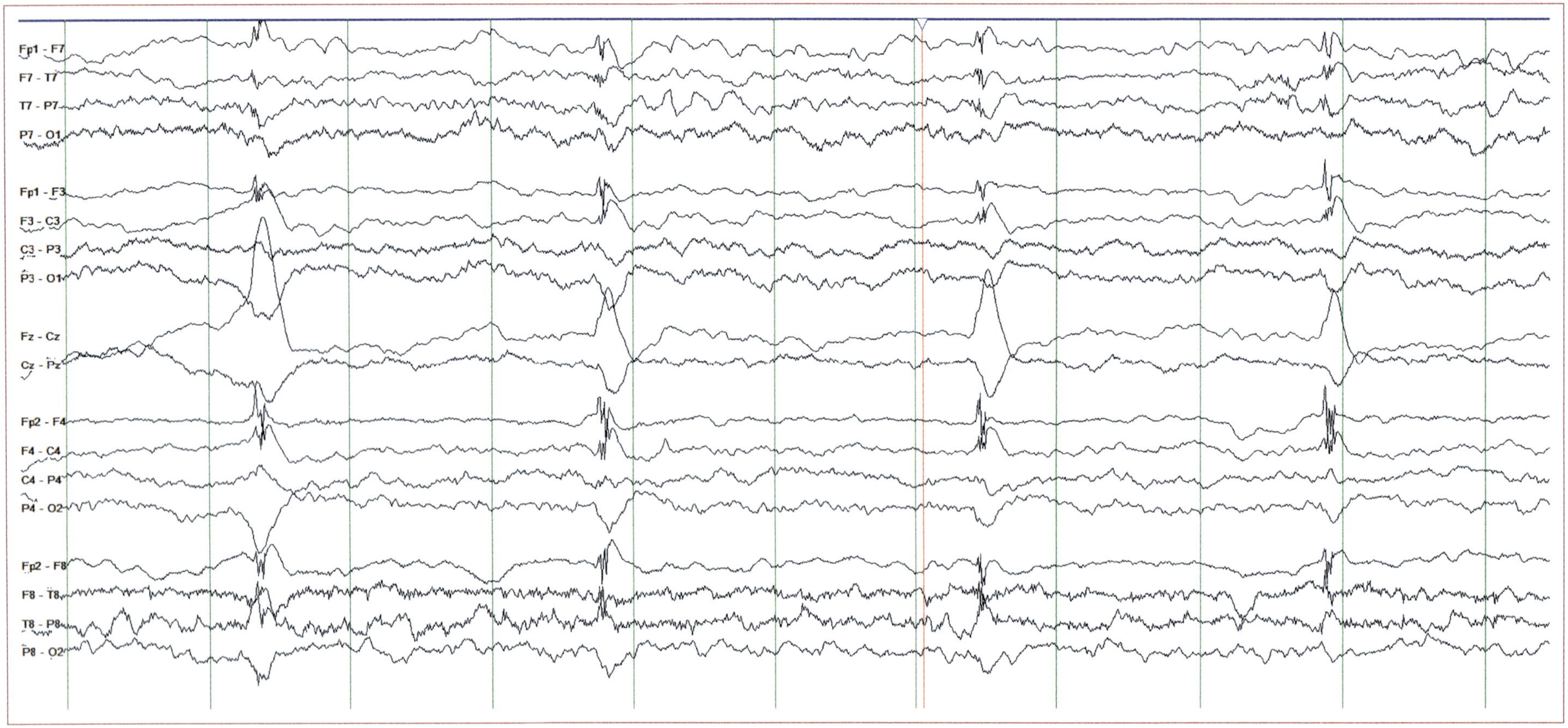

FIGURE 6.5: Hiccup artifact. This EEG shows a 4-month-old, former 27-week premature infant with periodic hiccup artifact. LFF 1 Hz, HFF 70 Hz, Sensitivity 7 uV/mm.

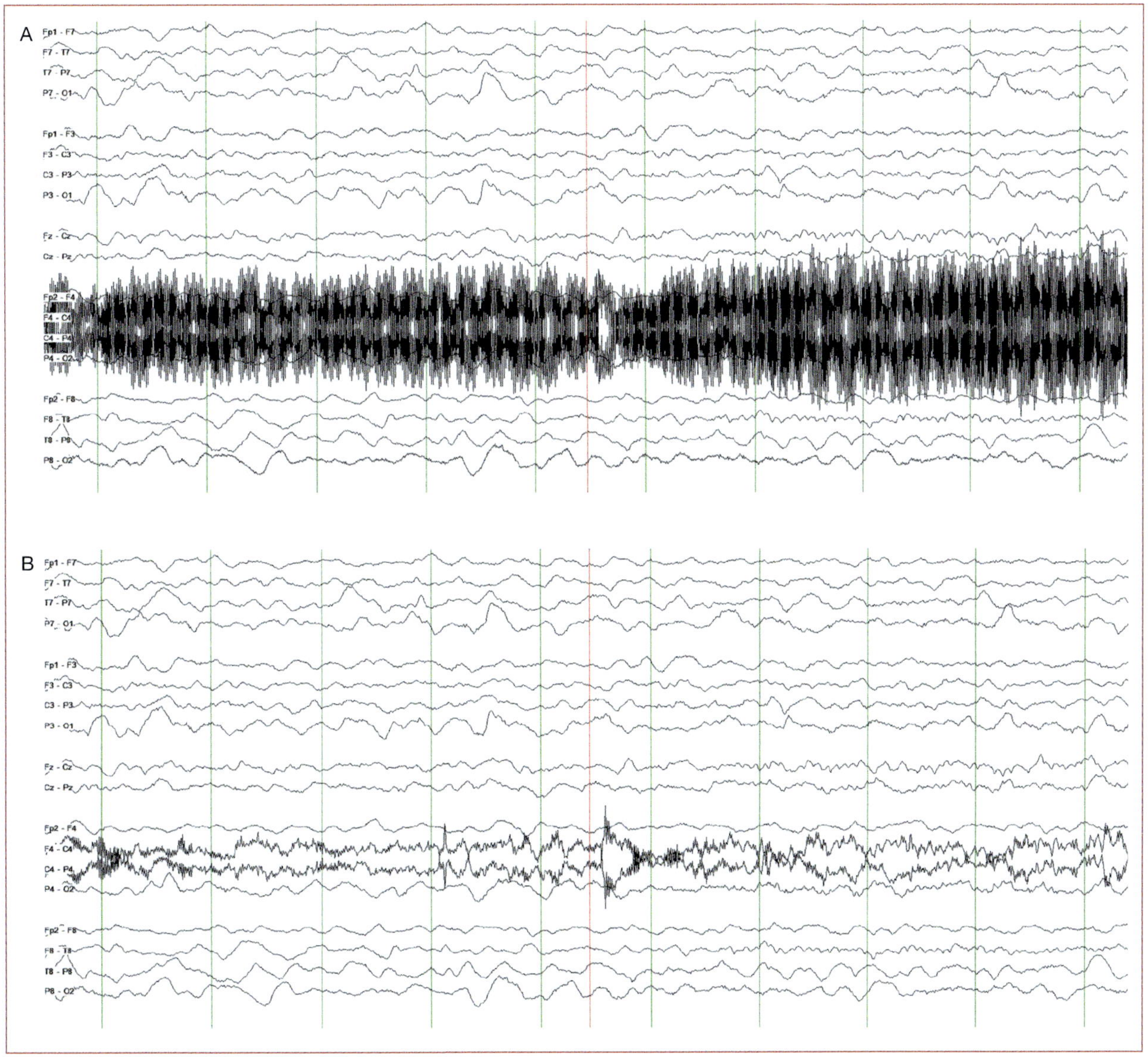

FIGURE 6.6: (A) 60-Hz artifact is prominent in this EEG of a 3-month-old infant during quiet sleep over the right parasagittal chain. (B) This is the same EEG with a 60-Hz notch filter in place that removes the high-voltage prominent fast activity. Note that C4 has persistent artifact and electrode "pop," suggesting this electrode is not working properly and needs to be regelled.

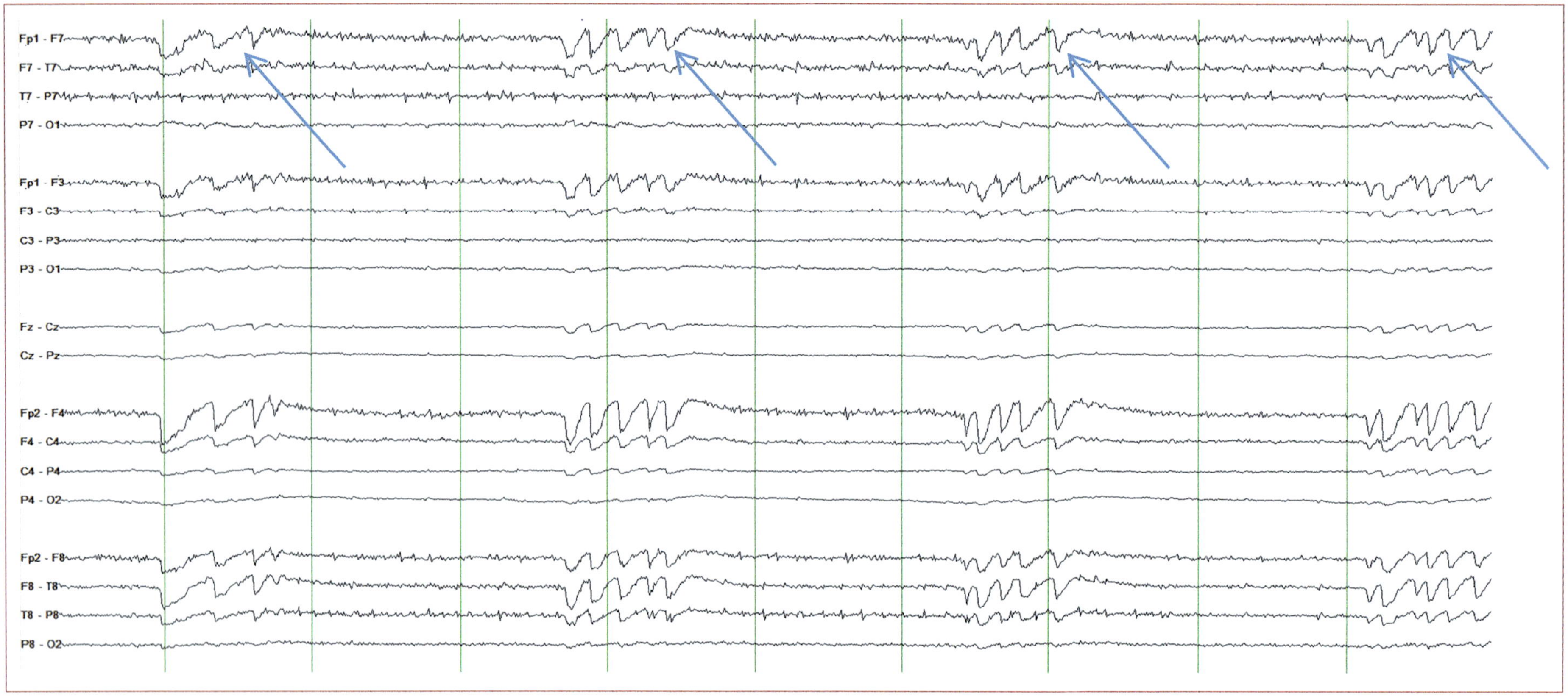

FIGURE 6.7: Ventilator artifact. This EEG is from a child with a significant brain injury resulting in electrocerebral silence. There is periodic ventilator artifact from the mechanical breath. Sensitivity is 7 uV/mm.

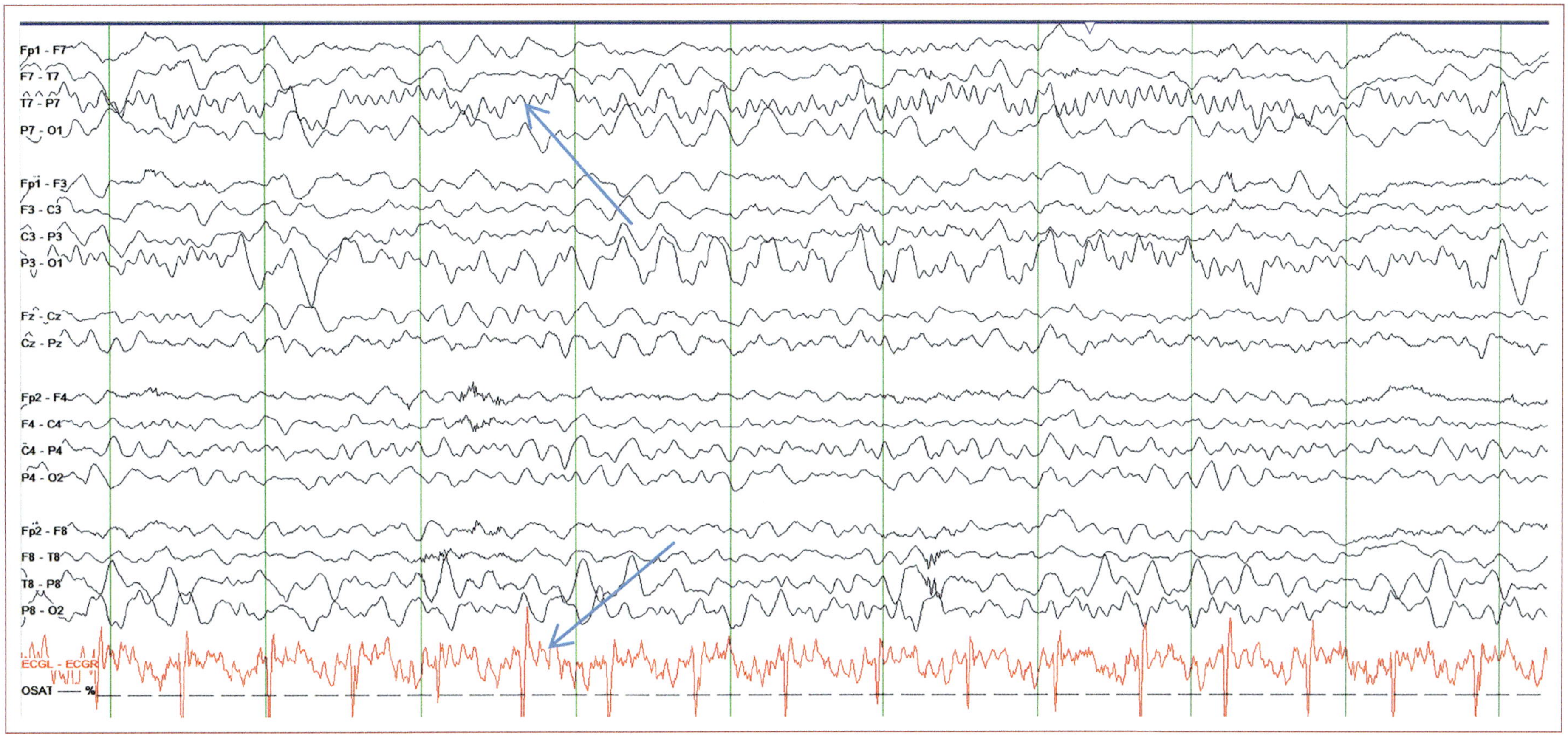

FIGURE 6.8: Nebulizer artifact. This artifact is from a young boy receiving a nebulizer treatment, which is seen as 12-Hz rhythmic activity in the ECG electrode as well as multiple EEG leads.

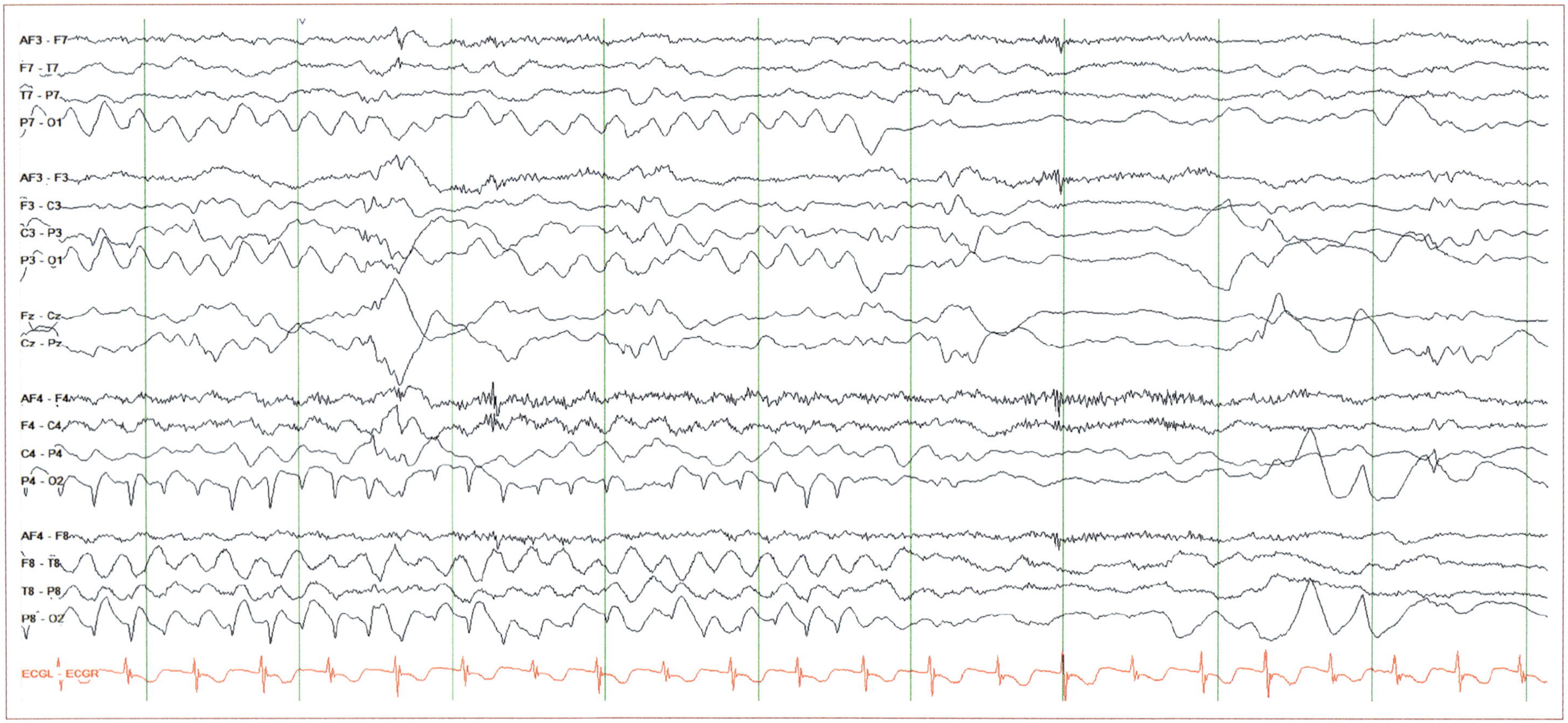

FIGURE 6.9: Patting artifact seen on the EEG of a 2-month-old baby. Note the abrupt cessation of rhythmic activity, distinct from the slowing of frequencies, regional distribution, and devolution that might be expected with ictal rhythmic activity.

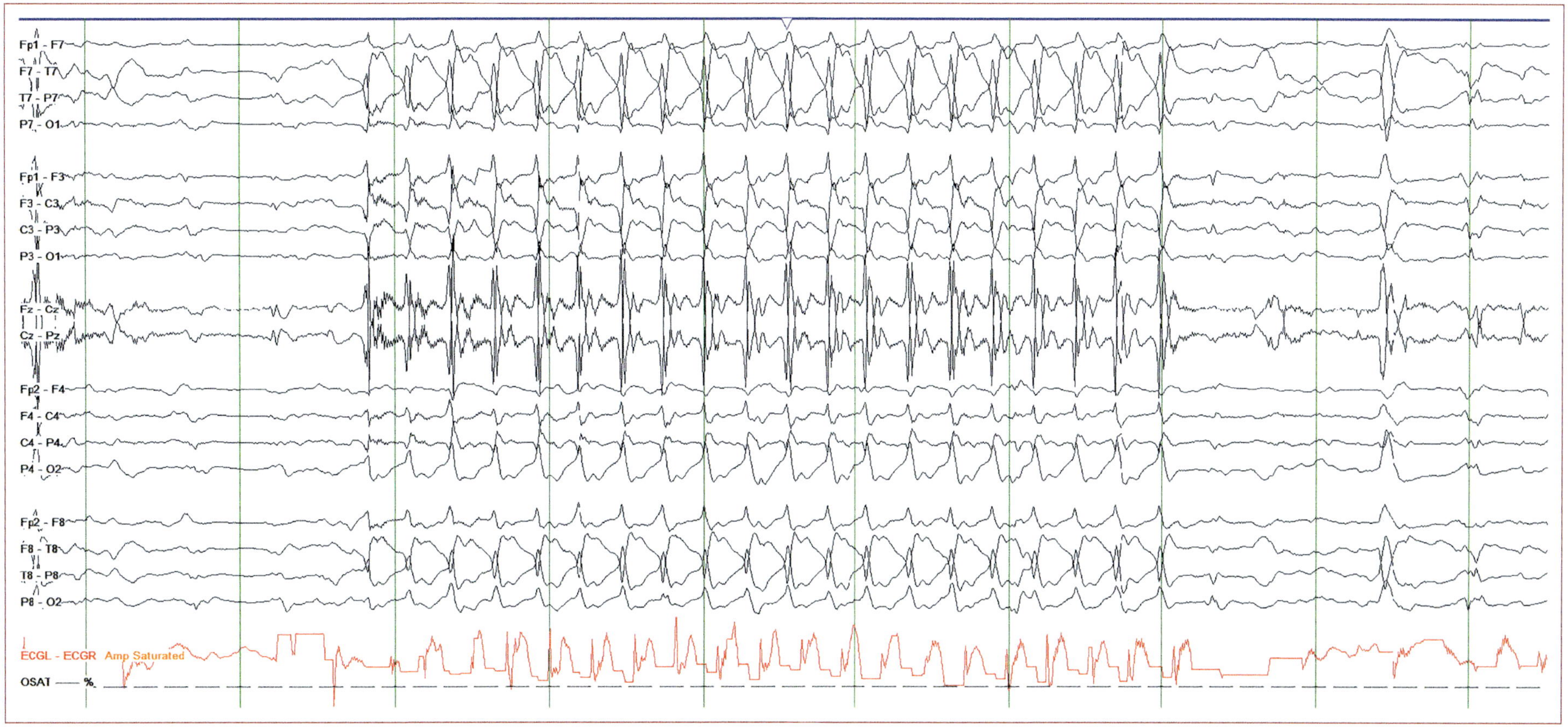

FIGURE 6.10: Chest physical therapy artifact. This EEG tracing is from a 13-year-old boy with generalized seizures in the ICU for superrefractory status epilepticus. This EEG tracing shows a rhythmic pattern electrographically distinct from the appearance of his seizures that is concordant with chest physical therapy.

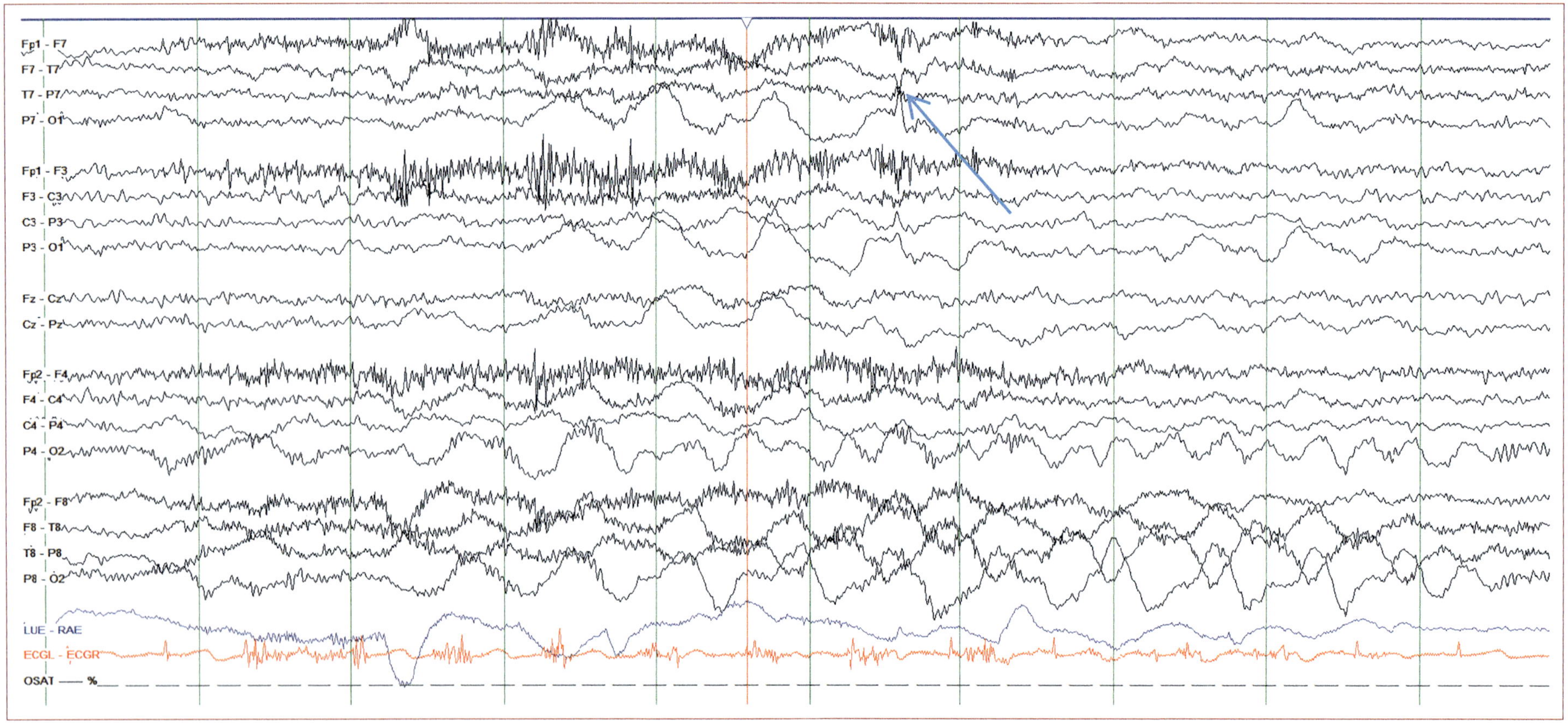

FIGURE 6.11: Kicking artifact. This EEG is from an active 6-year-old boy during a routine EEG. Rhythmic activity from the child's kicking resulted in an artifact prominent in the posterior leads and the right temporal region. There is a T7/P7 spike, which is characteristic of this child's background.

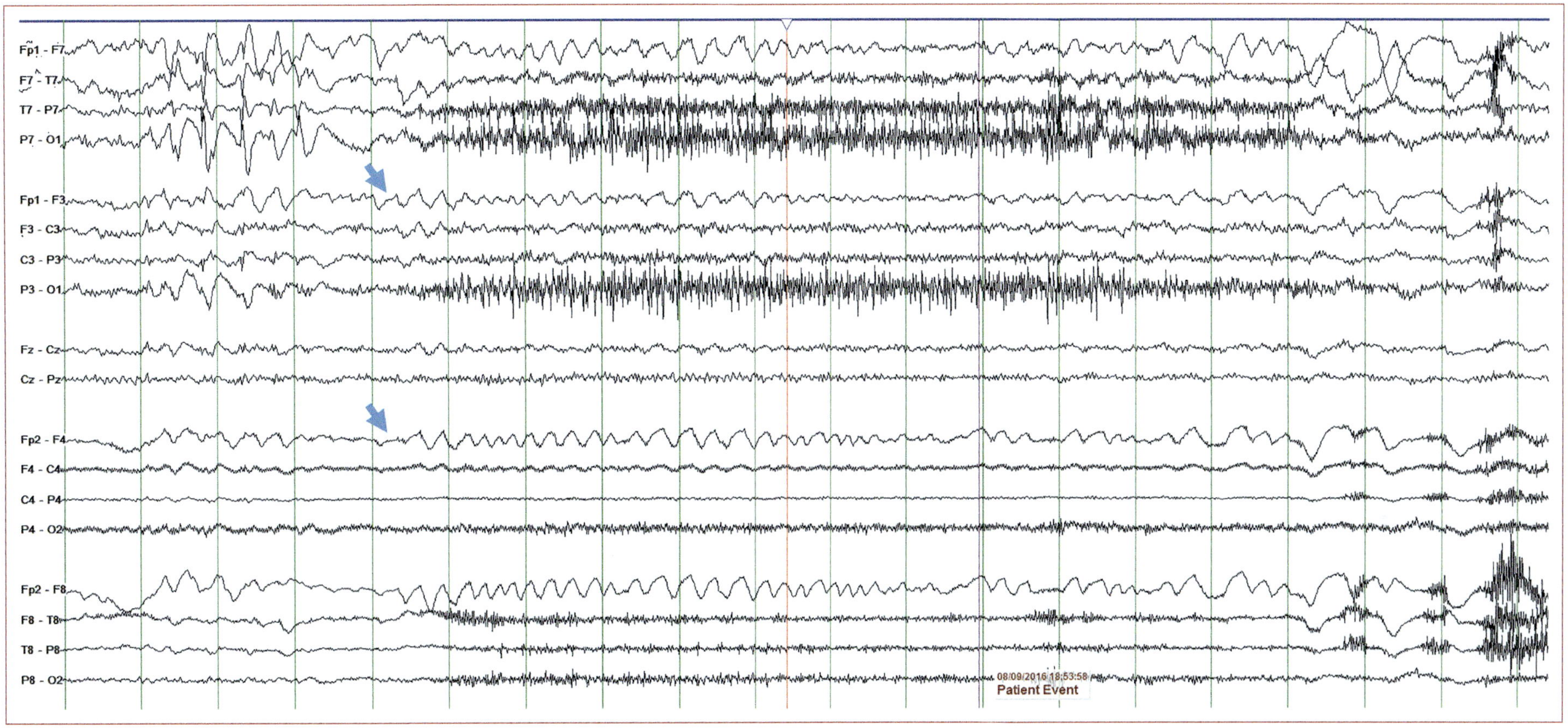

FIGURE 6.12: Artifact signaling ictal onset. This EEG tracing shows a seizure in a 22-year-old young woman with Aicardi syndrome and long-standing history of medically refractor epilepsy being monitored in the ICU for status epilepticus. She had many similar seizures electrographically seen as attenuation over the left temporal and parasagittal chains, followed by fast activity. A rhythmic monomorphic delta pattern is seen in the frontopolar regions (arrows) confirmed on video and at bedside as corresponding with ocular flutter artifact, which consistently accompanied the seizure discharge. The left temporal discharges preceding the seizure were interictal discharges seen frequently in the EEG background.

REFERENCES

1. Dworetzky B, Herman S, Tatum WO. Artifacts of recording. In: Schomer DL, Lopes da Silva FH, eds. *Niedermeyer's Electroencephalography*. 6th ed. Philadelphia, PA: Wolters Kluwer/Lippincott Williams & Wilkins; 2011:239-266.
2. Westmoreland BF. Benign electroencephalographic variants and patterns of uncertain clinical significance. In: Ebersole JS, Pedley TA, eds. *Current Practice of Clinical Electroencephalography*. 3rd ed. Philadelphia, PA: Lippincott Williams & Wilkins, Philadelphia; 2003:235-245.
3. Tatum WO, DiCiaccio B, Kipta JA, et al. The texting rhythm: a novel EEG waveform using smartphones. *J Clin Neurophysiol*. 2016;33:359-366. doi:10.1097/WNP.0000000000000250.
4. Tomko S, Loddenkemper T, Pearl PL. Texting rhythm with temporal predominance. *J Clin Neurophysiol*. 2016;33:570. doi:10.1097/WNP.0000000000000353.
5. Sethi PK, Sethi NK, Torgovnick J. Mobile phone artifact. *Clin Neurophysiol*. 2006;117:1876-1883. doi:10.1016/j.clinph.2006.05.001.
6. Sethi NK, Torgovnick J, Sethi PK. Chest percussion artifact. *Clin Neurophysiol*. 2007;118:475-476. doi:10.1016/j.clinph.2006.10.016.
7. Young B, Raihan S, Ladak H, et al. Rhythmic artifact of physiotherapy in intensive care unit EEG recordings. *J Clin Neurophysiol*. 2007;24:252-256. doi:10.1097/WNP.0b013e318053e6af.
8. Jayakar PB, Patrick JP, Sill J, et al. Artifacts in ambulatory cassette electroencephalograms. *Electroencephalogr Clin Neurophysiol*. 1985;61:440-443. doi:10.1016/0013-4694(85)91036-3.
9. Ibrahim ZH, Chari G, Abdel Baki S, et al. Wireless multichannel electroencephalography in the newborn. *J Neonatal Perinatal Med*. 2016;9:341-348. doi:10.3233/NPM-161643.
10. Bourez-Swart MD, van Rooij L, Rizzo C, et al. Detection of subclinical electroencephalographic seizure patterns with multichannel amplitude-integrated EEG in full-term neonates. *Clin Neurophysiol*. 2009;120:1916-1922. doi:10.1016/j.clinph.2009.08.015.
11. Wusthoff CJ, Shellhaas RA, Clancy RR. Limitations of single-channel EEG on the forehead for neonatal seizure detection. *J Perinatol*. 2009;29:237-242. doi:10.1038/jp.2008.195.
12. Toet MC, van der Meij W, de Vries LS, et al. Comparison between simultaneously recorded amplitude integrated electroencephalogram (cerebral function monitor) and standard electroencephalogram in neonates. *Pediatrics*. 2002;109:772-779. doi:10.1542/peds.109.5.772.
13. Suk D, Krauss AN, Engel M, et al. Amplitude-integrated electroencephalography in the NICU: frequent artifacts in premature infants may limit its utility as a monitoring device. *Pediatrics*. 2009;123:e328-e332. doi:10.1542/peds.2008-2850.
14. Hagmann CF, Robertson NJ, Azzopardi D. Artifacts on electroencephalograms may influence the amplitude-integrated EEG classification: a qualitative analysis in neonatal encephalopathy. *Pediatrics*. 2006;118:2552-2554. doi:10.1542/peds.2006-2519.

CHAPTER 7

Adult Electroencephalography Artifact

William O. Tatum, IV

INTRODUCTION

The scalp EEG is composed of a signal that is generated by a pool of cerebral neurons. It may be modified by the conductive properties of an electrode, the dipole orientation of the cortical generator, and properties conducting electrophysiological potentials from the brain to the recording electrode on the scalp (1). Artifact is an especially important feature to recognize in the adult EEG as it is present in virtually every recording. The ability to distinguish an artifact is subject to human interpretation. Artifact is identifiable when waveforms that do not conform to an expected electrophysiological field are generated by the brain (2). However, while artifact may produce "interference" of identifying the underlying electrocerebral activity, it is also an essential part of the recording to aid in identifying the levels of consciousness and sleep stages. Oftentimes however, artifact is a limiting feature that interferes with the interpreter's ability to render a confident diagnosis to fully characterize the EEG (**Figure 7.1**). When present, artifact may act as a "contaminant" that interferes with proper interpretation of the EEG recording. Excessive artifact is quickly and readily apparent during review of the EEG when waveforms are obscured by movement or myogenic artifact sufficient to interfere with useful interpretation. Judging how much artifact is excessive remains a common problem and is subject to individual determination (3). Without guidelines to identify when and why excessive artifact is present, the author uses a cutoff of greater than 50% of the recording in more than 50% of the EEG channels before interpreting a "limited EEG" recording (patient factor). When technical issues are involved that are uncorrected (e.g., high electrode impedances), a "technically limited EEG" recording (technical factor) is reasonable to distinguish the different conditions. Quantifying the amount of artifact using a computer-based scoring system may become more advantageous in future applications of digital EEG reporting to overcome the subjectivity involved, for both clinical and research purposes (4).

The sheer prevalence of artifact underscores its potential to serve as a pitfall to EEG interpretation. Both physiological and nonphysiological sources of artifact may occur to fool the interpreter into believing an abnormality exists. The presence of many "suspicious" spiky waveforms exist (**Figure 7.2**) in the normal adult EEG (5). Maulsby noted almost 50 years ago, "Every spiky-looking wave is an artifact unless there are one or more good reasons for suspecting otherwise" (6). Spiky waveforms become problematic when normal features of the EEG are interpreted as abnormal interictal epileptiform discharges (IEDs) (7,8). Artifact is much more prevalent than benign (normal) variants of uncertain significance, yet the latter are commonly misinterpreted, leading to an epilepsy diagnosis (7). Early definitions of a spike (20–70 ms) and sharp wave (70–200 ms) identify the potential morphology but do not indicate whether it is a normal or pathological waveform, nor identify the source. Some artifact closely mimics abnormal IEDs and challenges the interpreter to separate artifact from abnormal features of the EEG (**Figure 7.3**). When the EEG is misinterpreted as abnormal, overinterpretation of pathological IEDs may lead to a misdiagnosis of epilepsy and result in mistreatment of patients with antiseizure drugs (ASDs) and miss the treatment of the true underlying condition (9,10). In a survey of 47 clinical neurophysiologists, 97.9% reported encountering an EEG read as an abnormal recording based upon artifact (10). Uncorrected and unrecognized misinterpretation of artifact may lead to inappropriate treatment with ASDs and potentially compromise patient care and overall quality of life (11).

Difficulty recognizing artifact in the EEG stems from several factors. Waveform interpretation involves identifying brain signals derived from a three-dimensional source in the brain that is translated into two-dimensional EEG recordings. Pattern recognition alone, when applied to EEG, may serve as a pitfall to proper interpretation unless the principles of artifact recognition are applied (Table 7.1). Recognizing undesirable signals such as artifacts requires a basic understanding of polarity and localization in the orderly approach to EEG interpretation (12). Furthermore, standards for digital recording necessitate an inherent understanding of digital systems and technology before artifactual waveforms can be identified. Recognizing artifacts and identifying the source is a skill learned through familiarity of the interpreter provided by experience and exposure to expert teaching during residency or fellowship.

Most standard adult EEG artifact encountered is scalp-based. Ensuring the EEG signal reflects an electrophysiological potential or series of potentials derived from a cerebral source as opposed to artifact is required for determining an accurate interpretation for clinical purposes. However, artifact may intervene in any form of EEG recording including ambulatory EEG (aEEG) monitoring, video-EEG monitoring (VEM), intracranial EEG (iEEG) recording, and EEG recorded in the operating room (OR) (Table 7.2). All forms of EEG recording share similar susceptibility to artifact, though with increasing use of long-term EEG monitoring (LTM), a greater predisposition to artifact exists. Video recording as an adjunct to EEG has helped interpreters confirm artifact. Time-locked frequencies of a possible abnormality on the EEG linked to a specific clinical behavior with a similar frequency on the video recording increases the likelihood of identifying artifact. During VEM in epilepsy to characterize seizures during a presurgical evaluation, artifact may impair the ability to localize seizure onset (Figure 7.4).

A team approach is essential. By applying basic concepts of recording, manipulating instrument parameters post hoc, and having an experienced technologist modify the environment during the recording, the technologist and clinical neurophysiologist serve as crucial members of the team to obtain an interpretable record. Ensuring the minimum technical requirements are met, standards for electrode position and montages are used, and guidelines for recording EEG are adhered to, help ensure an optimal outcome for interpretation (13). When these standards are met, interpretation of the EEG reduces the risk of overinterpretation and facilitates proper management of patients (7,11). Dr. Chadwick noted the "Routine interictal EEG recording is one of the most abused investigations in clinical medicine and is unquestionably responsible for great human suffering" (14). In this chapter, we highlight common and uncommon examples of EEG artifact obtained during routine clinical practice to highlight the impact it may have on patient management.

TABLE 7.1: Electrophysiological Domains in the EEG That Are Suggesting Artifact

Feature	Concept	Corrective Action
1. Location	Single-channel activity	Test impedance, regel, or replace the electrode until resolved.
2. Field	End-of-chain activity	If the above action is ineffective, extra electrodes applied around the eyes/ mouth may reveal the generator.
3. Spatial distribution	Noncontinuous activity and nonepileptiform generalized potentials	Eliminate extraneous movement and electromagnetic fields that could lead to nonphysiological distribution.
4. Polarity	Adjacent double/ triple phase reversals	Reapplication of electrodes involved in the affected region.
5. Morphology	Complex waveforms or discrete periodicity	Troubleshoot for an extracerebral source (e.g., pumps, ventilator, tubing).
6. Frequency	Very fast (>30 Hz) and very slow (<1 Hz)	Unless iEEG is used, these frequencies require troubleshooting for a source.

iEEG, intracranial EEG.

TABLE 7.2: Common Types of Artifacts Encountered Include Physiological and Nonphysiological

Physiological	Nonphysiological

Eye
Muscle
Tongue
Heart
Bone
Skin
Movement
	Extrinsic
	  Environment
	    60 Hz
	    Movement/devices
	  Equipment
	    Electrodes/connections
	    EEG machine
	Intrinsic
	  Implanted electrical devices

PRINCIPLES OF ARTIFACT

The principles of artifact recognition apply to virtually every EEG recording (15). EEG interpretation is based upon the inverse problem of localizing a three-dimensional generator from a two-dimensional graphic projection (16). Current flow through the tissues is volume conducted from deep and surface-based generators recording EEG at the scalp–electrode interface. The principles of artifact are predicated on the same principles involved in localizing a physiological source. Extracerebral artifact must be recognized before the cerebral source is identified. Artifacts from overfiltering, electrode pops, and myogenic artifact are common types of artifact during standard EEG recording. Elimination of artifact is attempted when the waveforms disrupt an accurate interpretation of the underlying EEG. Principles involved in identifying artifact are essential rules to arrive at an accurate interpretation of the EEG recording (see Table 7.1). Artifact is present when extracerebral electrophysiological potentials are recorded. Identifying the mismatch between potentials, which are generated by the brain from potentials that are not generated by the brain, form the basis of artifact recognition (8). Some simple concepts for recognizing artifact are important to understand for both the EEG technologist and the electoencephalographer alike before considering a waveform abnormal. Activity that is confined to a single electrode (Figure 7.5) with a restricted spatial distribution should be considered artifact until proven otherwise. To this end, when a technologist is recording the EEG and single-channel potentials are encountered, especially if they are in question, an electrode test may reveal a high impedance, demonstrating a predisposition to artifact. Another concept involved with artifact occurs when EEG activity is present at the end of an electrode chain within a montage (Figure 7.6). This limits the ability to appreciate an electrophysiological field of a waveform or series of waveforms that is generated by the brain. Changing montages may help delineate a restricted field of artifact. Alternatively, application of a movement monitor (e.g., ocular or perioral electrodes) may be the electrical source as artifact generated by ocular or glossopharyngeal movement. Artifact should also be considered when a noncontinuous or nonphysiological spatial distribution or atypical generalized potentials are encountered (Figure 7.7). Intravenous (IV) mechanical pumps, feeding tube delivery systems, electrical beds, and so on should be sought by the technologist to look for any extraneous movement or interference from electrical generators in an effort to resolve the artifact. Diffuse artifact involving all channels of the EEG occurs when a common reference (Figure 7.8), the ground, or cable connections between the patient and machine have compromised integrity. Similarly, when periodic patterns are precise without variation (Figure 7.9) this suggests a mechanical as opposed to a biological source. Identifying a competing electrical source for EEG waveforms may lead to quick resolution by transiently unplugging nonessential equipment. Additionally, when periodicity is present in the EEG, using a slow display speed (e.g., 10–15 mm/sec) may help demonstrate the precision necessary to recognize artifact. Adjacent double- and triple-phase reversals are also common manifestations of artifact (Figure 7.10). In this case, a negative phase reversal lies immediately adjacent to a positive phase reversal (double-phase reversal) in an electrode chain of a montage. This is best seen in a bipolar montage and results from repetitive movement. The nonphysiological origin is evident when negative–positive–negative (triple) phase reversals appear. The field speaks for artifact and becomes increasingly likely over time as the scalp–electrode interface deteriorates. It is the responsibility of the technologist during the recording to recognize and identify whether a waveform is due to an artifact, and eliminate it from the recording when it is possible (17).

SCALP EEG

The vast majority of adult EEG interpretation is based upon standard scalp EEG recorded in the "Berger band" for clinical purposes. The bandwidth for interpreting clinical EEG focuses on a range of frequencies between 1 and 30 Hz with digital filtering between 1 and 70 Hz. Frequencies that appear outside this bandwidth suggest artifact (e.g., very slow; sweat, very high; myogenic or 60 Hz) (Figure 7.11). The cause of an artifact is subdivided into physiological and nonphysiological sources (Table 7.2). Physiological artifacts arise from active bioelectric properties generated by tissue other than the brain. Physiological artifacts such as eye movement and myogenic artifact may facilitate interpretation of the EEG and does not require elimination. Nonphysiological artifacts may be extrinsic arising from electrodes, equipment, and those within the environment or intrinsic and arise from internal electrical devices (e.g., pacemakers, stimulators). Nonphysiological morphology, polarity, or spatial field of distribution may be recognized as artifact, but defy identification of the source or isolation to attempt elimination of its presence in the EEG (Figure 7.12).

PHYSIOLOGICAL ARTIFACT

Physiological sources of artifact present during routine EEG recording occur from biological generators that produce an electrical dipole. Some are routinely present in the adult EEG. Eye movements, myogenic and body movements, and cardiac sources are among the most common types of artifact that are frequently encountered by clinical electroencephalographers during interpretation of the EEG. Factors that underlie electrical fields and polarities derived from the brain and living tissue define a physiological source of artifact (18). Common physiological sources of artifact are listed as follows.

Eyes

Eye movement artifact is perhaps the most common physiological form of artifact identified in the adult EEG. It occurs in essentially every waking individual during standard EEG recording. The artifact produced by yoked movement of the eyes is detected because of an inherent corneal–retinal resting electrophysiological potential (Figure 7.13). The cornea is relatively electropositive compared with the electronegativity present in the retina, generating a DC potential difference measurable by EEG. The potential difference is easily measured in the vertical (Figure 7.14) and horizontal (Figure 7.15) plane. The benefit of recognizing eye movement artifact lies in the ability to correlate the clinical level of arousal and of consciousness. In the normal waking individual, vertical eyeblink artifact is present. Upon closing the eyelid, there is a concomitant upturning of the eyeball (Bell's phenomenon). Slow, rolling eye movements are characteristic of drowsiness (Figure 7.16), while rapid eye movement (REM) artifact defines REM sleep. Sleep cycling is more obvious during prolonged recordings (and those who are sleep-deprived). Unless eye movements are monitored (see Figure 7.14), they may mimic abnormalities such as frontal intermittent rhythmic delta activity (Figure 7.17), or combine with other forms of artifact to provide the false appearance of an epileptiform abnormality (see Figure 7.3).

Eye movements are differentiated from cerebral waveforms with the use of an external occulogram (or electrooculogram [EOG]). An EOG requires application of surface electrodes above and below the eye (referred to a reference or each other). The EOG is an essential means of recording eye movement artifact during EEG as well as to delineate the level of arousal in polysomnography (19). In-phase deflections with a surrounding electrophysiological field are characteristic of a cerebral dipole. The exception is when the generator lies below the EOG electrodes. Out-of-phase deflections characterize a generator that lies between the recording EOG electrodes typical of an eye movement (see Figure 7.17). Horizontal and skew eye movements are identified using a bipolar montage if opposite polarities occur in homologous anterior temporal derivations of the EEG (e.g., F7/F8). Phase reversals that are "positive" (i.e., out of phase) reflect the location of the eyes closest to the cornea. The "negative" phase reversal reflects the polarity associated with the retina in the contralateral eye during a lateral eye deviation.

Muscle

Muscles are another common source of artifact in the EEG capable of producing "spikes" that may be mistaken for IEDs. The temporalis and frontalis muscles are the principal myogenic sources of artifact on EEG that produce a characteristic temporal (Figure 7.18) or frontal predominance (see Figure 7.3). Chewing is a common source for myogenic artifact (Figure 7.19). Unless the principles of artifact recognition are followed, chewing artifact may mimic the appearance of polyspike-and-waves. Myogenic spikes, also referred to as "muscle spikes," are high-frequency signals with a duration less than 20 milliseconds. The technologist may ask the patient to relax their jaw when jaw clenching occurs or request the patient open their mouth during the recording to eliminate bitemporal artifact, which occurs with tonic or phasic muscle contraction from the masseter and muscles of mastication. The presence of spikes may also occur from movement of the eye muscles of the globe, such as the lateral rectus muscles (Figure 7.20). These are differentiated from pathological spikes due to the intimate association with REMs. They represent motor unit potentials best seen in the F7 and F8 derivations of the scalp EEG. Frontalis muscle contraction during eye movement may produce a superimposition of frequencies to mimic a generalized periodic discharge (see Figure 7.3). When this occurs during intermittent photic stimulation, vertical eyeblink or eye flutter artifact, in combination with frontalis myogenic spikes, can produce a response that may be mistaken for a photoparoxysmal response. A high index of suspicion is required in this case to prevent overinterpretation. Eliminating myogenic artifact may occur by restricting appropriate movement, though this may necessitate medication promoting muscle relaxation when significant enough to interfere with interpretation.

Tongue

Similar to the artifact generated by eye movement, artifact generated by the tongue is based on the principal of a bioelectric dipole. The tip of the tongue is relatively electronegative compared with the root, which is electropositive. Glossokinetic artifact may occur during tongue and oropharyngeal movements due to the DC potential produced. By elevating and depressing the tongue during swallowing or speaking, motions are generated that often produce a brief series of diffuse, frontally distributed waveforms that appear abnormal due to the presence of intermittent bursts of delta on the EEG (Figure 7.21). The spatial distribution of the electrophysiological field produced by the tongue is a frontaloccipital broad-based artifact compared with artifact produced by eye movements. A simple bedside technique used by technologists to identify glossokinetic artifact is simulated by asking the patient to repeat "Tom Thumb" or "lilt." This action uses tongue and glossopharyngeal muscles to recreate the artifactual pattern when intermittent bursts are in question as an abnormal finding in the EEG. Like eye movements, motions of the mouth may also be monitored. Similarly, validation is obtainable by applying an electrode above the upper lip, and below the lower lip around the mouth. Using bipolar EEG recording, a tongue movement monitor will identify artifact with deflection of the waveforms that are out of phase. During movement of the mouth such as speaking, teeth may touch one another. When the teeth contain metallic implants or amalgam to fill dental caries, brief spikes may be produced due to electrical properties generated. The field of dental artifact is typically diffusely distributed, and the single spikes are very rapid (Figure 7.22).

Heart

Monitoring cardiac function is performed during EEG using a rhythm strip recording the ECG. Due to the unique information incorporated during EEG, it is arguably the single most important channel recorded but, like EEG, may be prone to artifact (Figure 7.23). There are multiple EEG channels dedicated to recording brain function, but there is only one used to represent the heart. However, cardiac function may significantly influence artifact that appears in the EEG (Figure 7.24). Contamination of the EEG by the ECG is more likely to occur when referential montages use ear references. The A1 and A2 electrode derivations accentuate ECG artifact. This is augmented in patients with short necks, those who are overweight, and when higher sensitivity or long interelectrode distances are used. These conditions facilitate recording electrophysiological signals from the left ventricle to override the EEG signals during the process of amplification. Left lateralization of ECG artifact may occur due to the direction of the QRS vector associated with ventricular contraction. The QRS complex reflects the spread of electrical current through the myocardium. When distributed over a broad field, ECG artifact may mimic periodic discharges. These may have a lateralized or generalized distribution (Figure 7.25). When present, ECG artifact may demonstrate opposite polarities of the R-wave in the left and right hemispheres when an ear reference montage is used. The left ear reference may transmit an electronegative potential, while the right ear electrodes appear as an electropositive deflection. When periodic potentials are visible in the EEG and time-locked to the QRS complex, the precise intervals make ECG artifact readily recognizable and the source easily identifiable. Eliminating ECG artifact can be accomplished by repositioning the patient's head and neck to alter detection of the cardiac signal, or by changing the montage (e.g., using an average reference or linking the ear reference). Eliminating or reducing ECG artifact can help optimize interpretation when it obscures the EEG.

Pulse artifact occurs as a periodic waveform that is synchronized to the QRS complex of the ECG. Unlike ECG artifact, the mechanical pulsation of blood produces artifact that involves a single channel (Figure 7.24). Like ECG artifact, pulse artifact may be identified as periodic waveforms set in time-locked fashion to the ECG 200 to 300 ms following the QRS complex. Elimination of pulse artifact requires moving the electrode to a distance away from a scalp arterial source. The contraction of the myocardium can also produce a forceful mechanical movement of the head to produce a ballistocardiographic artifact that appears as though the patient is repetitively rocking his head, resulting in a regional or lateralized slow wave component. Elimination may require stabilizing the head with towels to minimize head movement.

Bone

Bone is inactive compared with other soft tissues in the body; however, the skull may create the appearance of artifact when a breach rhythm is encountered. This is due to the high frequencies that appear in a focal or region of the EEG following head trauma or neurosurgery (Figure 7.26). A bipolar montage is the best recording technique to recognize a breach effect. Recording EEG this way accentuates the spatial contrast of voltage differences between beta frequencies normally attenuated by the skull to make a breach rhythm more obvious. Myogenic artifact may also occur when electrodes for recording EEG are applied adjacent to a skull defect. The patterns of myogenic artifact may exist as a repetitive motor unit potential (similar to lateral rectus spikes) or as a continuous pattern. Recording surface electromyogram (EMG) produces similar patterns created without a skull breach by the temporalis and frontalis muscles. Individual motor unit potentials (Figure 7.6) or continuous musculoskeletal artifact surrounding a breach rhythm may be reduced by sleep or when muscles are relaxed.

Skin

The skin acts as an electrical source with measurable electrodermal–electrophysiological activity. When the skin produces sweat, sodium chloride and lactic acid may react with the metallic component of the EEG electrodes to produce ultraslow frequency artifact (e.g., 0.25–0.5 Hz). When the electrode impedance is greater than 10 kΩ, this provides the foundation for artifact at the electrode sites responsible for sweat artifact. These are typically maximal in the front of the head (over the forehead), where sweat tends to occur, and deteriorate the scalp–electrode interface. The alternating polarity when bilaterally distributed is without a physiological spatial field of distribution. The sweat produces a sway of the baseline, which produces a notable waveform that can interfere with an interpretable recording (Figure 7.27).

A "salt bridge" is formed when adjacent channels are connected by a smear of electrolytic gel. It is recognized when a single channel lacks similar electrocerebral activity to other nearby electrode derivations, producing an artifact with the appearance of a near isoelectric or low-amplitude EEG signal (Figure 7.28). The formation of a salt bridge occurs because similar or undetectable voltage differences are identified by the differential amplifier of the EEG machine. The result is that there is cancellation of the electrophysiological potentials from the two sites to result in the false appearance of a focal, near-isoelectric EEG present in the affected channel.

Movement

Movements of respiration may produce a physiological respiratory artifact (Figure 7.29). Respiration artifact is common in the ICU during mechanical ventilation. Periodic potentials may be identified as respiratory artifact if the technologist annotates the record when respiration is synchronizing with body movement. Very slow synchronous frequencies are characteristic during the thoracic movements of respiration at approximately 0.5 Hz. This regularity creates an artifact that appears rhythmic, periodic (e.g., 20 breaths/minute), and occipital-predominant. Faster frequencies during rapid inspiration and exhalation during hyperventilation may produce movement-induced periodic potentials, which are especially prominent in high-impedance electrodes in the standard EEG (Figure 7.30). Additional respiratory monitors may be applied with uncertainty. Artifact may be monitored using a chest belt or nasal thermistor to help determine sleep stages, though application of a movement monitor over the site of involvement may also be performed to discern artifact when breathing compromises the interpretability of EEG. Sleep-related movements such as snoring, periodic limb movements, myoclonic jerks, or arousal patterns may be suggested by the pattern of myogenic or movement artifact that appears on the EEG (20).

Movement artifact in the EEG is time-locked to patient movements and may be evident on video recording. Certain movement disorders produce unique patterns of movement-induced artifact on the surface EMG. For example, characteristic patterns of artifact may help identify disorders such as essential tremor and Parkinson's disease based upon frequency, similar to actigraphy. For example, essential tremor-precipitated artifact may appear as a bilateral, 7- to 11-Hz frequency in the EEG when compared with a unilateral, fluctuating, higher amplitude 4- to 7-Hz tremor artifact often encountered in Parkinson's disease (Figure 7.31). On the other hand, rhythmic sinusoidal tremor artifact may be confused with electrocerebral activity. The artifact may appear rhythmic, intermittent or continuous, and lateralized or generalized depending upon the source of movement. The movement itself may create an artifact with a field involving opposite polarity in adjacent channels (Figure 7.32) including double- and triple-phase reversals. Regardless of the pattern, the presence of a nonphysiological field should suggest artifact (Figure 7.33). Monitors will have higher amplitudes compared to the scalp EEG unless the sensitivity of the recording channel is adjusted (Figure 7.34).

Some movements are complex and may require simultaneous monitoring of several functions (Figure 7.35). Video recording may be helpful in these cases. Spontaneous movement, as well as interactions with a medical examination, nursing assessment, or other health care professional may produce complex movement artifacts. By applying extra electrodes on or nearby a suspected source, muscle/movement artifact that is present in electrodes placed to monitor motion can characterize certain movements when they occur.

NONPHYSIOLOGICAL ARTIFACT

Extrinsic

The majority of adult EEG artifact is generated by sources and electrical fields that are external to the patient. External artifact usually arises from extrinsic sources in the environmental nonphysiological generators. Often, this is produced by the EEG equipment with the most unstable connection associated with the electrode interfacing with the patient. Extrinsic artifact may be associated with simple (Figure 7.36) and complex (Figure 7.37) waveforms. When activity is confined to a single channel without an electrical field, electrode artifact should be suspected irrespective of its complexity (see Figure 7.36). Activity that is generated in the brain has a field of distribution that radiates to neighboring electrodes (21). Eliminating single-electrode artifact first requires assessment of electrode impedances. Securing or replacing the involved electrode may be necessary without resolution. Electric motors in nearby machines produce electromagnetic fields that may intermittently create "noise" in the EEG or become continuous depending upon the type of machine. The ubiquitous nature of artifact is such that it may arise from multiple electrical generators and "contaminate" the EEG at any place between the patient's scalp and the EEG machine. Nonphysiological artifact that is recognized as extrinsic to the patient requires isolating the source and eliminating it from the environment, modifying the EEG parameters, or annotating and monitoring the source during the recording. Some extrinsic artifacts are difficult to eliminate despite isolating the source due to necessity (e.g., medication pumps). A technologist experienced in artifact detection is crucial when called to "troubleshoot" and eliminate or minimize the source. A heightened awareness should be maintained with repeat impedance checks if the integrity of EEG becomes compromised (22).

Environment

Environmental artifacts produced outside an EEG laboratory are common. Medication infusion pumps, mechanical beds, feeding delivery systems, and electrical monitoring devices produce electromechanical and electromagnetic sources of interference with EEG recording. Nearby telephones (Figure 7.38), portable computers and tablets, and gaming devices can also produce artifacts in the adult EEG. Electrostatic, capacitive, and inductive artifacts may occur. IV machines are commonly used in the hospital setting outside the EEG laboratory. A transient electrostatic force is produced when a drop of fluid or medication is conducted to nearby electrodes and wires. This creates an intermittent nonphysiological potential in the EEG that may lead to the appearance of a spiky artifact. However, the precise periodicity and generalized spatial distribution distinguishes the potentials as IV drip artifact (see Figure 7.9). Similarly, static electricity may be introduced into the nearby wiring or recording electrode. The cables from the patient to the EEG machine containing electrode wires can produce capacitance artifact because the cable acts like a capacitor. Multiple insulated wires in the cable are capable of generating conductive artifactual waveforms due to movement or compression of the cable (Figure 7.39). Sometimes the appearance of a paroxysmal or epileptiform discharge may result, underscoring the importance of the technologist's role in annotating the record during recording. As a general rule, the polarity and nonphysiological field will be evident to suggest artifact.

Environmental artifact due to alternating current (AC) is one of the most common environmental artifacts encountered during EEG recording. Magnetic fields generated by electrical motors near the EEG recording can result in electrical potentials visible as artifact. This may interfere with the identification of the brain's biological signals. Artifact in the EEG due to AC current is induced by nearby power mains and electrical outlets introducing electrical interference. This is often produced by the equipment used in recording EEG.

Equipment

The most common artifact encountered in the EEG is due to an insecure connection between the electrodes and the patient scalp or connections to the machine (23). Artifact in the EEG may arise from many different combinations of electrode types and configurations (Table 7.3). Scalp EEG is performed most frequently. During standard EEG recording, electrodes must be secured to the patient's scalp to limit artifact. This is accomplished by applying an adhesive compound to the electrode to conduct the EEG. High impedances of electrode pairs greater than 10 kΩ increase the risk for electrode artifact.

TABLE 7.3: Electrode Types and Configurations Used in Recording EEG

Electrode Types	Electrode Configurations
• Standard noninvasive - Cup (10-20 system) - Other (e.g., nasoethmoidal, nasopharyngeal) • Invasive - Needle (ICU and OR) - Sphenoidal (EMU) - Foramen ovale (OR) - Intracranial (OR) ∘ Subdural ∘ Depths	• Noninvasive plus - 10-10 system - Caps - High density • Special uses (combinations) - Subdural strips/grids (stereo-EEG) - Intracortical depths • Research - High density - Hybrid grids/depths - Microwires

EMU, epilepsy monitoring unit; OR, operating room.

During LTM, collodion provides a more secure and longer-lasting contact of the electrode to the patient's scalp. Electrodes are composed of conductive metals such as silver, silver–silver chloride, and gold plating, though nonferromagnetic or plastic electrodes are available for MRI compatibility. Abrading the skin enhances the contact with the scalp. The epidermis has high electrical impedance. Use of an electrolyte gel enhances electrical conductance and reduces the scalp–electrode biological resistance (impedance). High-impedance electrodes predispose to artifact, which may be evident during intermittent photic stimulation. When activation with photic stimulation is performed, an artifact known as the photoelectric (or photovoltaic) effect may be present (Figure 7.40). This occurs when photic flashes produce a transitory electrochemical response to the light in susceptible electrodes. The morphology may appear as a train of brief, spiky potentials time-locked to the flash frequency. The photoelectric effect can be eliminated by covering the involved electrodes with a cloth or piece of paper to block the reaction produced by light. Electrode artifacts are usually easy to recognize, though complex discharges should raise the suspicion of artifact (Figure 7.41).

When an electrode mismatch of greater than 5 kΩ is present or when poor electrode contact with the scalp exists, this facilitates a greater risk for 60-Hz artifact. When artifact is unresponsive to simple troubleshooting techniques such as securing or replacing the electrode, changing to a referential montage may prove a cerebral source is present when more than a single electrode is involved. When electrode artifact remains in question, switching the involved electrode pin to another site on the jack box supports a cerebral source when the abnormality remains. A very focal abnormality will not switch to the new electrode derivation with a properly functioning jack box. Similar to high-impedance electrodes, electrical noise caused by EEG amplifiers are also capable of producing 60-Hz artifact (50 Hz in Europe). This is due to the internal electronic components and is easily eliminated when a 60-Hz notch filter is applied during the EEG recording (Figure 7.42).

When diffuse 60-Hz artifact is encountered (Figure 7.43A), then the integrity of the ground should be reassessed. In addition, ensuring proper patient–machine connections ensures that the integrity of patient safety has not been compromised. Supplemental use of filters, including a 60-Hz notch filter (Figure 7.43B), can be applied during postacquisition review. One earth ground is important for patient safety. The ground electrode directs the flow of electrical current through the EEG machine instead of conducting current to the patient. A ground loop recording (Figure 7.44) can also be seen when unsecured electrodes default to the ground electrode instead of the normal electrode derivation. Occipital electrodes are particularly vulnerable to this type of artifact due to their location. Like the frontopolar electrodes, occipital electrodes may become dislodged. When this occurs, the resultant morphology is due to the electrode–ground comparison of the differential amplifier.

Intrinsic

Intrinsic electrical nonphysiological potentials may also occur during EEG. Intrinsic artifact caused by electromagnetic generators may produce recognizable artifacts in the adult EEG (Figure 7.45). Subcutaneous, implanted electrical devices may produce artifact in patients during EEG recording when an electrical signal produced by the device is recorded. The internal electronic circuitry generates the electrical signal that is detected by the EEG electrodes. The electrodes function like an antenna to detect stimulator-induced electrical currents. Similar to the effect observed when 60-Hz artifact is present in the EEG, internal power sources from devices depolarize EEG electrodes through magnetic fields created by electrical current flow (24). Intrinsic artifact due to both cardiac (Figure 7.46) and neurological devices, such as the vagus nerve stimulator (Figure 7.47), may be encountered during EEG recording. Permanent cardiac pacemakers and implantable cardiac defibrillators are common medical devices that produce intermittent artifact in the EEG. Intermittent artifactual potentials are composed of a similar morphology and precise periodicity, and strongly suggest artifact. Newer implantable electrical devices such as the responsive neurostimulator may also produce intrinsic artifact during EEG recording, recognizable as a brief series of spiky potentials (Figure 7.48). The internal electronics of the battery-operated stimulator can be detected when a seizure is detected, and the device discharges a burst of electrical stimulations.

LONG-TERM EEG MONITORING

There are many different techniques to record adult EEG (Table 7.4). When standard scalp EEG is unrevealing and diagnostic concerns exist, LTM may be considered. LTM refers to a prolonged duration of EEG recording

TABLE 7.4: Techniques Used in Recording Adult EEG

- Standard scalp (routine) clinical EEG
- Ambulatory EEG
- Video-EEG monitoring
- Critical care continuous EEG monitoring
- Quantitative EEG/trend analysis
- Intracranial EEG
  - Wideband intracranial EEG
  - Electrocorticography

beyond the standard recording time of 20 to 30 minutes. Otherwise known as continuous EEG (cEEG) monitoring, it typically refers to VEM of a patient for days during hospitalization. VEM and cEEG monitoring are routinely performed in patients when extending EEG recording to detect, quantify, or characterize seizures is desirable (25). Extending the EEG recording time may also be performed outside the hospital while the patient is ambulatory and identify unexpected findings (**Figure 7.49**). Either form has a higher recovery rate of interictal and ictal abnormalities, but also introduces a greater likelihood of artifact contaminating interpretable EEG (26).

Computer-assisted LTM systems that record, analyze, process, and store data digitally are widely available to clinical practitioners both in the hospital as well as when the patient is in an outpatient ambulatory setting (27). An experienced technologist is essential to ensure LTM is not limited by artifact. The American Board of Registration for EEG Technologists and Evoked Potentials has standards set by examination to provide credentials reflecting competency for technical performance of EEG (www.abret.org). The American Clinical Neurophysiology Society (www.acns.org), in conjunction with the American Board of Clinical Neurophysiology (www.abcn.org), has established minimum standards and guidelines to aid physician interpretation and reporting. When excessive artifact intervenes in the EEG, a technologist who is able to "troubleshoot" and eliminate the source of artifact to facilitate interpretation of a recording is critical. Applying additional extracerebral monitors, obtaining control of patient position, noting IV drip and the medication delivery system, or temporarily disabling nearby electrical generators help identify the source and can often lead to elimination of artifact that would otherwise impair interpretation.

Ambulatory EEG

Prolonging outpatient LTM offers a distinct advantage in recording signals of interest when compared with routine scalp EEG (28). Monitoring aEEG typically occurs over 1 to 3 days depending upon the indications for use (29). Advantages of AEEG include diagnostic use when the clinical history and routine EEG are nondiagnostic. Spike and seizure detection software may be helpful but may capture artifact mimicking an epileptiform discharge (**Figure 7.50**). Recording paroxysmal neurological events and seizures is much more likely to occur when aEEG recordings are performed compared with routine scalp EEG, though artifact increases relative to the length of the recording (30). In addition, quantifying recurrent seizures and monitoring other physiological parameters are important uses of aEEG, which may also incur artifact. aEEG may be an alternative to definitive diagnosis in the epilepsy monitoring unit (EMU) (**Table 7.5**). It may also bridge VEG when seizure capture fails to occur in the EMU to extend recording after discharge from the hospital (31). aEEG monitoring is portable and records episodic behaviors in one's "natural" environment where multiple sources of artifact exist.

TABLE 7.5: Indications for Outpatient Versus Inpatient Long-Term EEG Monitoring

Outpatient	Inpatient
• Very young or very old • Diagnosis in a patient with frequent events • Hospital-based LTM has been ineffective • Barriers exist for hospitalization	• Medication withdrawal • Ancillary testing (e.g., ictal SPECT*) necessary • Presurgical evaluation and invasive EEG used • Outpatient LTM has been ineffective

LTM, long-term monitoring.

Adapted from Tatum WO. Artifact and ambulatory EEG. In: Tatum WO, ed. *Ambulatory EEG Monitoring*. New York, NY: Demos Medical; 2017:41-73.

The primary disadvantage of aEEG is the inherent tendency for movement and routine activities of daily living to introduce artifact into the recording. Artifact becomes increasingly obscured by artifact in parallel with the duration of the recording. In addition, there is limited technical support to ensure proper ongoing integrity of the recording system. It may be inconclusive for patients requiring differential diagnostic evaluation. It is inappropriate for safety reasons to withdraw ASDs and is therefore limited for detailed behavioral analysis associated with a presurgical evaluation. Despite improvements in technology with increasing memory capability and artifact reduction algorithms, instrumental problems occur that defy correction of artifact until the technologist is able to physically interact with the patient (32). Some artifact correction and reduction is able to be performed by some aEEG companies when real-time monitoring is able to intervene. Greater convenience, lower cost, improved access, and greater sampling of natural sleep and assessment of normal circadian rhythms are key advantages of aEEG (26).

Epilepsy Monitoring Unit

Certain artifacts have a distinctive appearance that helps in identification and elimination, whereas others may be unavoidable and limit interpretation of the EEG. Movement artifact, common during LTM, is able to be determined using the same principles used to identify IEDs (see Table 7.1). The lack of an electrophysiological spatial distribution and polarity, such as the presence of double- and triple-phase reversal in a bipolar montage in conjunction with video analysis of the semiology, will often suggest artifact. While artifact may serve as a contaminant (Figure 7.1), artifact may also be an important component that could add to the common problem of a failed diagnosis (33). When rhythmic movements produced by the patient occur in nonepileptic conditions such as psychogenic nonepileptic attacks (PNEAs), resultant EEG artifact can mimic a seizure and lead to misdiagnosis (34) (Figure 7.51). With movement-induced artifact in the EEG, the movement frequency is identical to the artifactual frequency. Another clue to movement artifact is, oftentimes, ipsilateral location of the artifact in relation to the movement. However, lateralization is dependent upon associated head movement that may at times be in a different plane than the primary visible movement of the patient. The combination of EEG with video analysis increases the yield of EEG and helps separate artifact when analysis of the EEG alone is inadequate (35). If the technologist is present during the recording, they will be able to identify movement artifact by annotating the record. Certain standards are necessary to assist the interpreter to avoid misinterpretation due to artifact in the EMU (36). When technical challenges arise, an experienced LTM technologist will be able to minimize artifact by ensuring appropriate parameters (Figure 7.52) and integrity of the recording system is appropriate and intact. Scalp-EEG-based seizure monitoring is often contaminated by myogenic artifact with high-frequency discharges in the range of 30 to 100 Hz and even higher when vigorous movement is involved, and may interfere with a presurgical evaluation as a result (Figure 7.53). However, artifact has also been helpful in monitoring epilepsy. The spatiotemporal evolution of movement and myogenic artifact may also impart diagnostic information. It has been used to successfully differentiate epileptic seizures from PNEA (37). For example, time–frequency mapping using the fast Fourier transform assessing the dominant ictal frequency with a coefficient of variation was successfully used to differentiate an epileptic convulsion from a nonepileptic event (38). Variation was greater with epileptic seizures due to the evolving frequencies absent in patients with PNEA despite a similarity of the median frequencies involved. This dissimilarity has been successfully utilized in seizure detection software algorithms to provide monitoring systems that use non-EEG-based signal detection in diagnosis of patients with paroxysmal behavioral events (39).

Intracranial Recording

Invasive EEG recordings are produced from surgically placed intracranial electrodes. There is a wide array of contact configurations (e.g., strips, grids, and depths) which may be implanted in the brain parenchyma or placed on the cortical surface. The electrodes connect to a cable through a stab wound in the scalp to attach to the EEG equipment. Digital standards for EEG recording systems exist to ensure optimal acquisition, analysis, management, transfer, and storage of information. Visual inspection is the gold standard in iEEG interpretation, which emphasizes the importance of ictal recording. Human screening is the standard to rely on artifact recognition, identification, and elimination. Seizure monitoring has diagnostic implications when a clear ictal recording on iEEG is present, though it may be similar to scalp EEG also containing artifact (Figure 7.54). During invasive, `EEG-based seizure monitoring, high-frequency waveforms representing surface-based motor unit potentials are typically absent unless a contaminated, extracerebral reference (e.g., mastoid) is utilized. However, external to the invasive electrodes outside the skull, inductive and capacitance artifact is still possible (Figure 7.55). Despite the differences between scalp EEG and iEEG, the principles of artifact in EEG recording continue to apply (see Table 7.1).

Identification of high-frequency oscillations (HFOs) greater than 30 Hz present in epileptogenic tissue has been a major discovery in the surgical treatment of epilepsy (40). When brief intermittent high-frequency artifact is present during iEEG, it may appear similar to HFOs. HFOs have been recorded using commercially available equipment and, similar to scalp EEG artifact, may interfere with interpretation in the iEEG (Figure 7.56). When surgical resection of normal-appearing brain tissue is performed for drug-resistant epilepsy based upon HFOs, it is critical to separate artifact from HFOs generated by the brain (41).

Operating Room

The OR is an area in the hospital that is electrically complex (hostile environments) and is predisposed to forming artifacts (42). In the OR, nonphysiological artifacts are common. Multiple sources are encountered that introduce AC from nearby electromechanical devices. This produces 60-Hz artifact in the EEG from multiple sources requiring an electrical outlet and power supply. Like 60-Hz artifact, some forms of artifact are easily recognizable due to the pattern (Figure 7.57). Multiple machines with electrical motors are present in the OR. Motors produce magnetic fields and generate artifact that limits visualization of the underlying brain signals in the EEG (20). Furthermore, artifact may be present in the EEG to mimic electrophysiological activity (Figure 7.58). Physiologic artifacts are infrequent due to the anesthesia and neuromuscular blocking medication routinely utilized. However, when an awake craniotomy is performed during electrocorticography, a mixture of environmental and instrumental artifact may coexist (**Figure 7.59**). In this case, low-voltage, high-frequency components that are not normally seen in scalp EEG become visible in the electrocorticogram, requiring separation from other high-frequency sources such as myogenic artifact.

In the OR, highly unusual artifacts may be encountered. During surgery, the technologist must exert supervisory control of essential life-support machinery to perform an artifact-free recording. When elimination is not feasible, the relationship to the source generating the artifact may be identified by application of additional monitors or annotating the chart to delineate the generator. When intervention is possible (e.g., through suction of nasal respiratory passage and repositioning of head), this may lead to resolution of the artifact. Some highly complex waveforms with unusual morphologies from artifactual patterns may be encountered in the OR (43). In this case, the possibility of artifact requires a high index of suspicion to guide the dialogue between the surgeon, the anesthesiologist, and the neurophysiologist.

Automated Artifact Elimination

Artifact reduction techniques include several methods. *Artifact removal* manually extracts artifact from the EEG. Technologists identify and eliminate artifacts during visual review of the EEG recording. This method is good for detecting multiple and complex artifacts. However, it is performed after the EEG has been recorded, is time-consuming, cost-ineffective, and impractical for LTM. Furthermore, subjectivity and human bias for artifact rejection is present to create variability in quality and reliability of its use. If a segment of EEG contains artifact, it is then eliminated from final analysis. Therefore, a limited representation of the entire EEG recording results, potentially eliminating useful information from final interpretation. Automated *artifact rejection* is another artifact rejection technique. This is able to identify most artifacts. Filtering, montage selection, adjustment in sensitivity, and alteration of the display speeds are methods to eliminate the source of artifact. However, digital filters alter the amount of artifact visible to the interpreter, distorting waveforms that may lead to misdiagnosis (**Figure 7.52**). There can be a significant loss of physiological signal that is lost using automated artifact rejection software. Automated *artifact subtraction* uses software algorithms to reject short segments of EEG when certain segments exceed preset parameter thresholds. These sections are then eliminated from the EEG. Some techniques use additional extracerebral channels (e.g., EOG, EMG, ECG) to monitor artifact. When these channels exceed preset thresholds, EEG containing the artifact will be rejected. *Artifact regression* is another technique to limit the appearance of artifact in the EEG. It is a computerized, software-based method that selectively subtracts artifact based upon a temporal or frequency-based domain "regressing" common sources of artifact from the final EEG recording. Similar to rejection and subtraction techniques, artifact regression includes subtracting physiological signals from the EEG. Common sources of artifacts (e.g., eye movements and ECG) are most amenable to reduction techniques (44). Multiple artifacts and complex artifacts often associated with movement frequently are not amenable to reduction method isolation and elimination.

Improved software algorithms are being designed for artifact reduction involving the most common types of artifacts generated by the eye, skeletal muscles, and ECG (45). Methods of artifact reduction that separate electrical sources increasingly use independent component analysis and methods based upon principal component analysis (46). Breaking down the EEG into individual frequency components can identify, preselect, and selectively eliminate artifact present in scalp EEG (47). Blind source separation is a new technique (48) that separates the original signals detected from various sources and subsequently eliminates common types of artifact, such as eye movements, myogenic potentials, single-electrode artifact, and ECG (49). Eliminating several simultaneous sources of artifact is the goal for artifact reduction techniques, and as a result limit associated interpretive error that may lead to patient harm (50).

CONCLUSIONS

The adult EEG recording contains a variety of physiological and nonphysiological artifacts that may challenge the interpreter's expertise (2), and visualizing the patterns may be a helpful learning tool (51,52). Some artifacts in the adult EEG reflect physiological function that is essential for proper interpretation of EEG. However, many nonphysiological sources obscure the EEG and limit interpretation. Worse yet, some artifact can mimic abnormality, leading to EEG misdiagnosis and subsequently to mistreatment of patients. Qualitative interobserver agreement in EEG interpretation has been only moderate according to some studies (4). LTM increases the yield in seizure monitoring yet so does the risk of artifacts. Some are simple and easy to recognize; however, others are more complex and difficult to discern. It is impossible to eliminate all diagnostic errors from the decision-making process (52, 53). However, certain principles are available to help recognize artifact though recognition should be followed by source identification in an effort to eliminate it from the EEG recording when it interferes with interpretation. Specific inpatient and outpatient characteristics of recording exist, though artifact is omnipresent and some site-sensitive specificity can be present for "hostile environments." Performance and interpretation of EEG is a large component of clinical neurophysiological procedures performed by neurologists and neurophysiologists. It is through understanding these patterns that optimal patient management will be achieved.

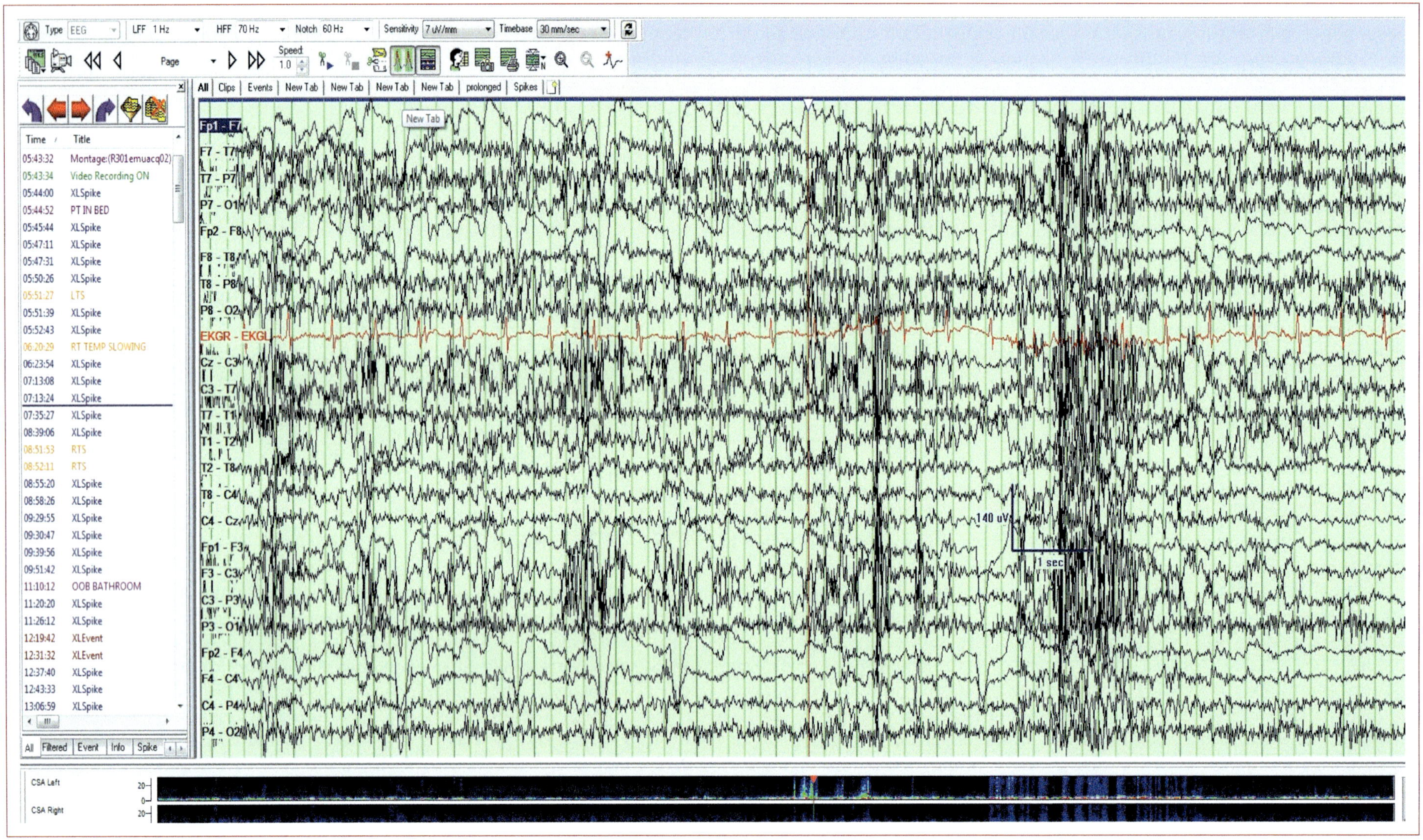

FIGURE 7.1: Excessive artifact limiting interpretation of the interictal EEG in a patient with temporal lobe epilepsy during epilepsy monitoring. Note the multiple types of artifact present and the corresponding bursts on compressed spectral array, reflecting a high-frequency power increase (note the increase/burst in power of high frequencies associated with artifact in the second half of the trend analysis).

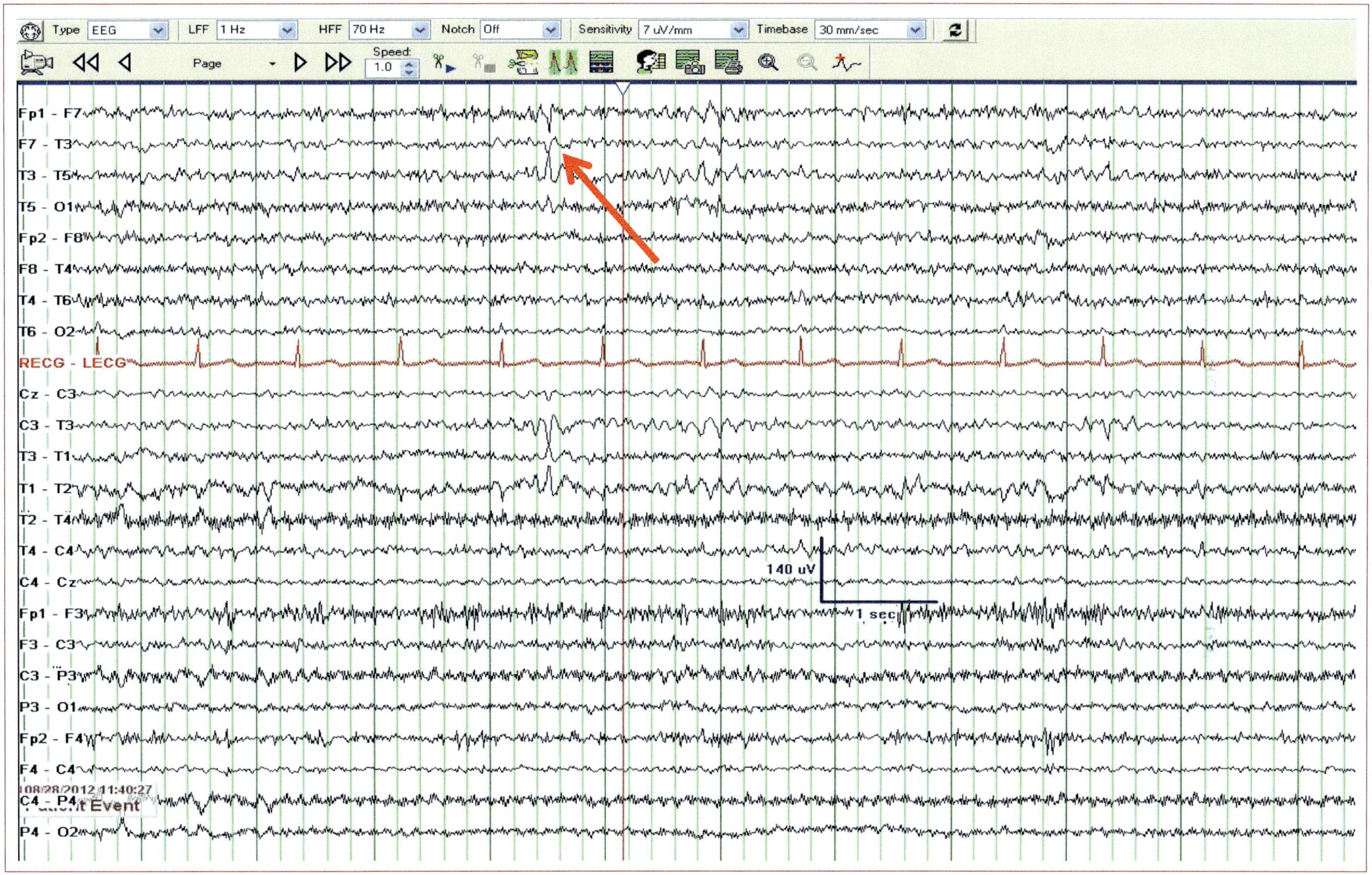

FIGURE 7.2: EEG with a left mid-temporal isolated wicket spike (arrow) during scalp recording. Note the increased artifact present in the double-distance T1-T2 electrode derivation.

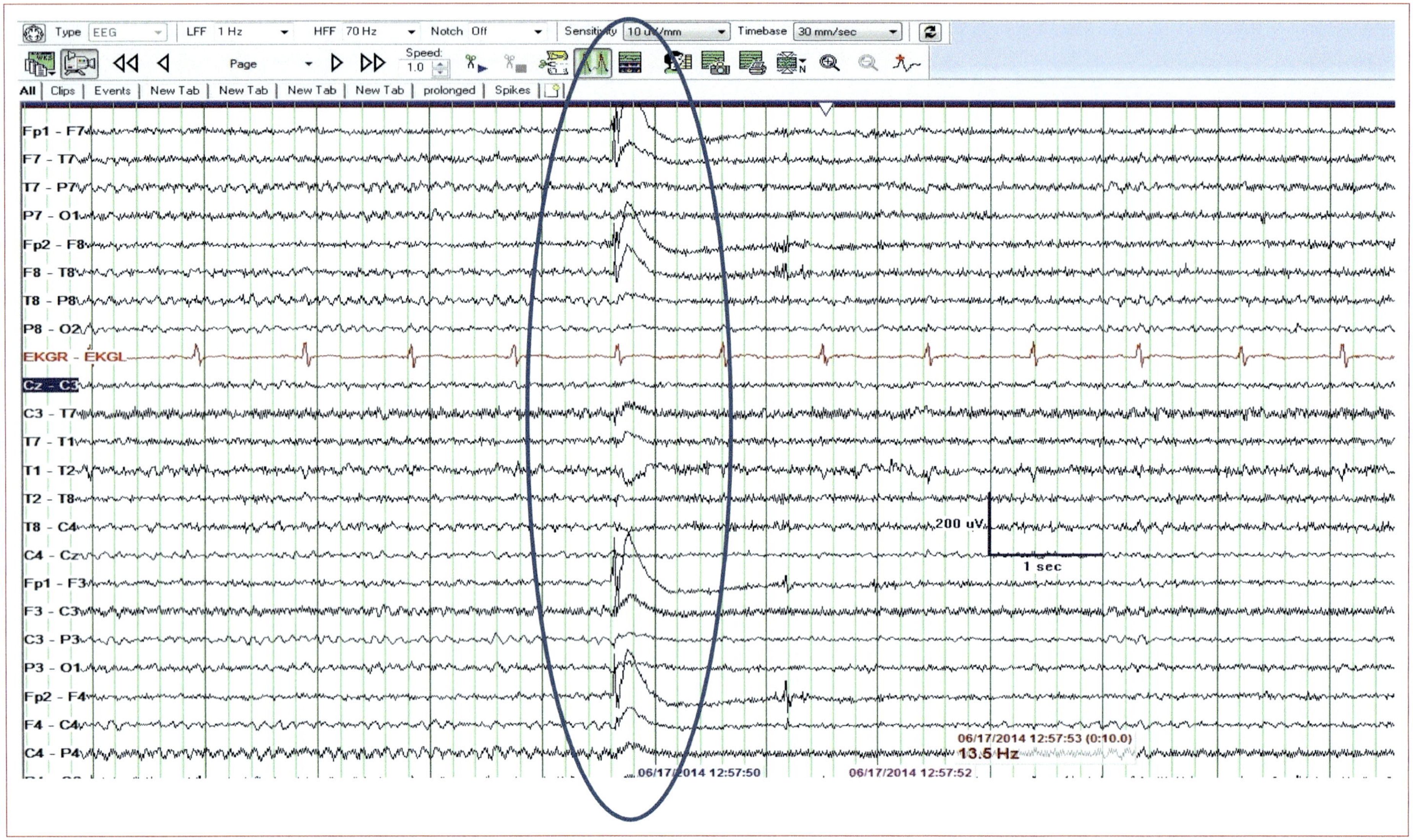

FIGURE 7.3: Combined artifacts mimicking an abnormal interictal epileptiform discharge. The frontalis myogenic "spike" coincides with the eye movement to create a pseudogeneralized spike-and-slow wave.

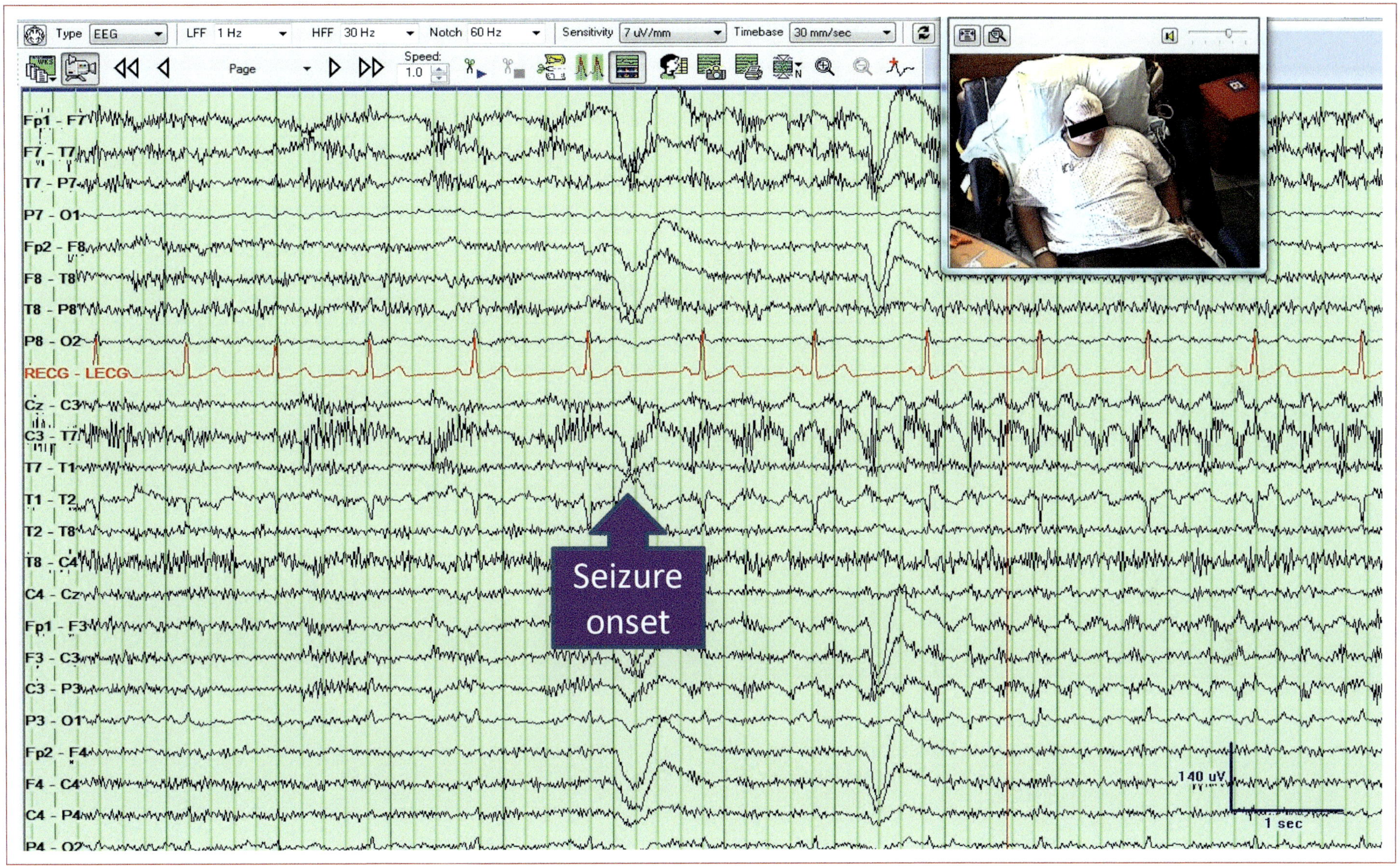

FIGURE 7.4: Artifact due to unilateral bruxism at the onset of the clinical seizure obscuring the ictal EEG onset. Clinical features occurred prior to EEG onset of low-voltage fast activity later localized with depth iEEG prior to left temporal laser ablation.

iEEG, intracranial EEG.

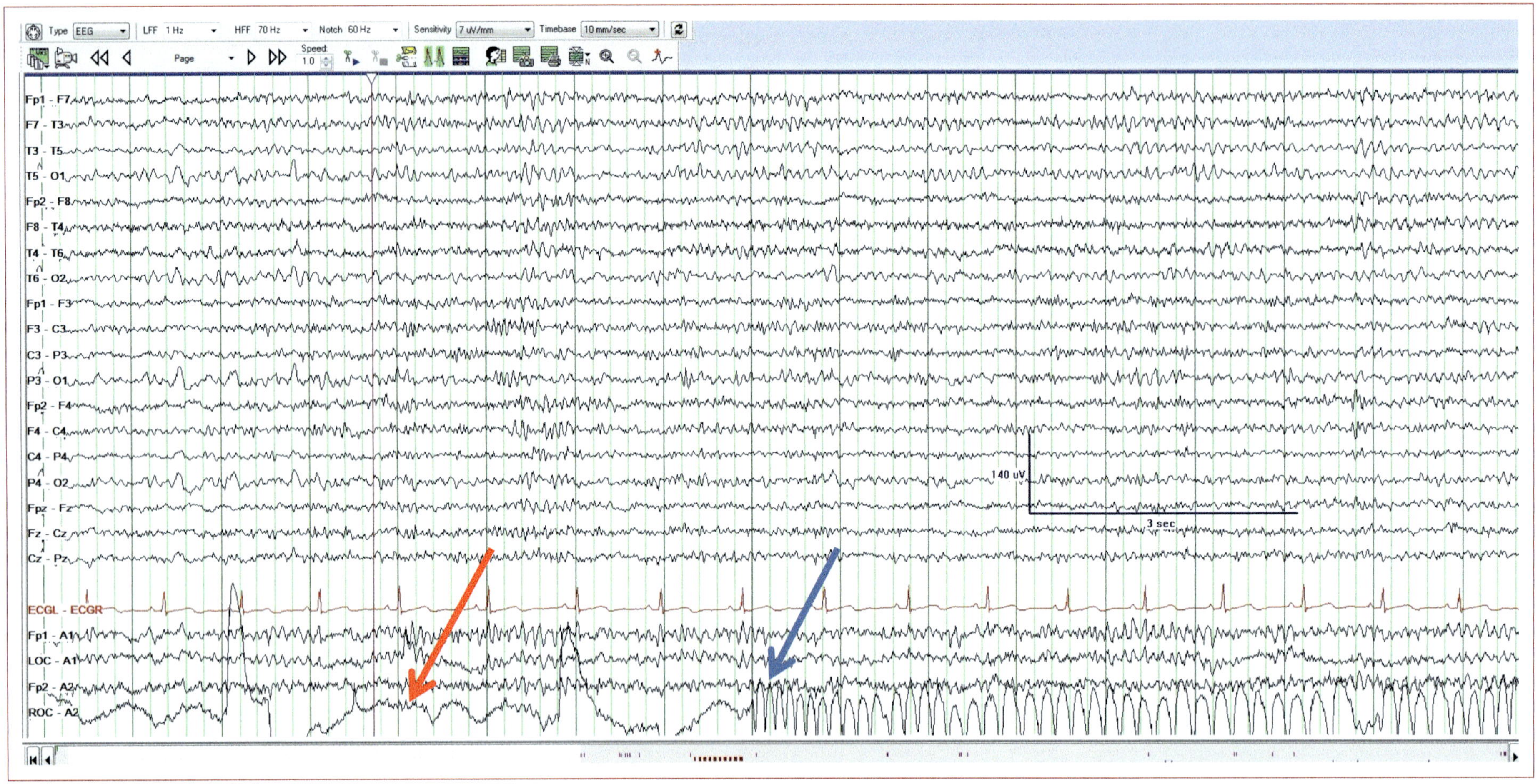

FIGURE 7.5: Single-electrode artifact in the right occulogram demonstrating slow (red arrow) and fast (blue arrow) patterns that may occur. Securing the electrode led to resolution.

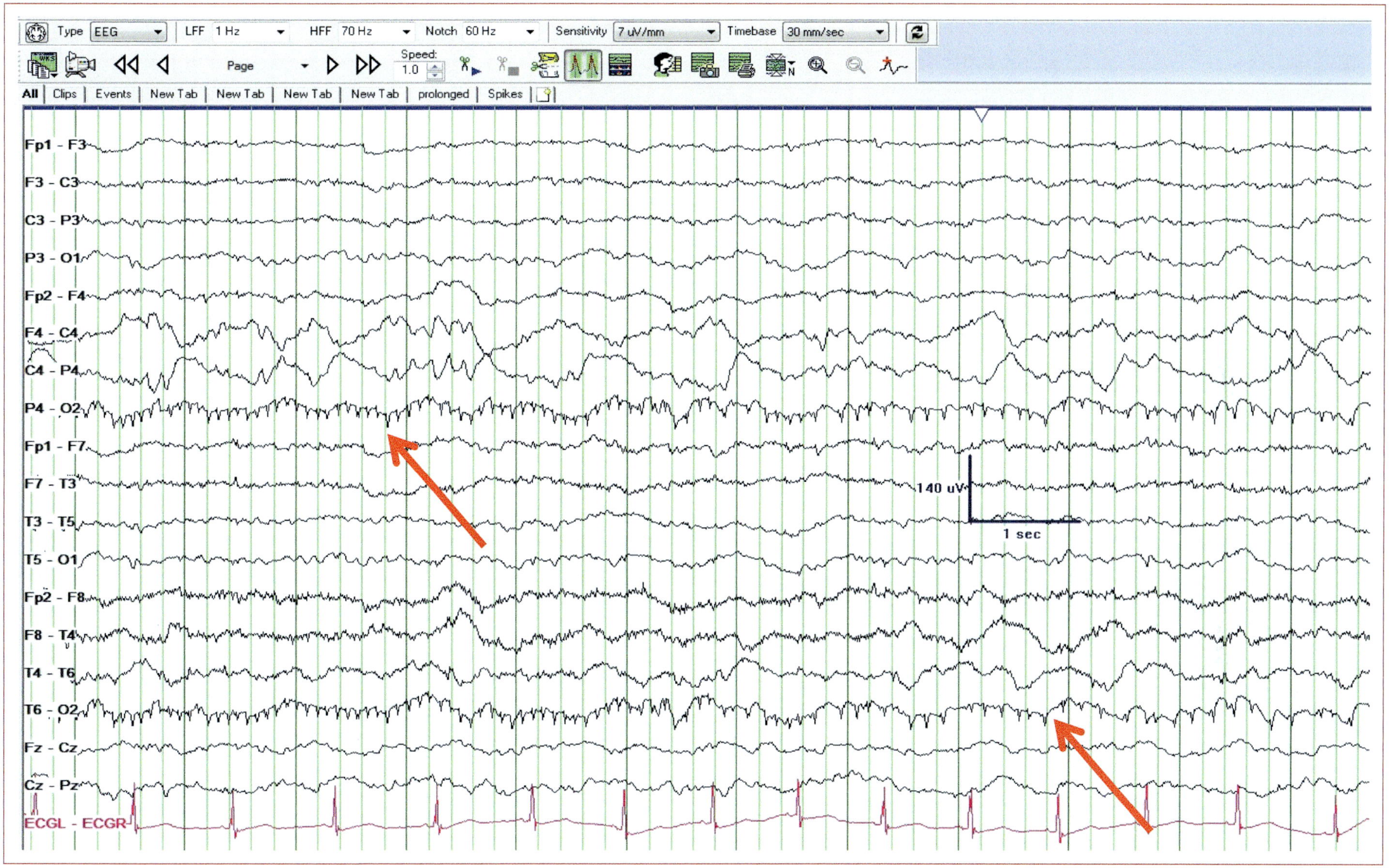

FIGURE 7.6: O_2 myogenic artifact (arrows) at the end of an electrode chain manifest as repetitive low-amplitude motor unit potentials. Regelling was ineffective, and replacing the lead wire lead to artifact resolution. Note the right hemispheric centrotemporal slowing from prior craniotomy.

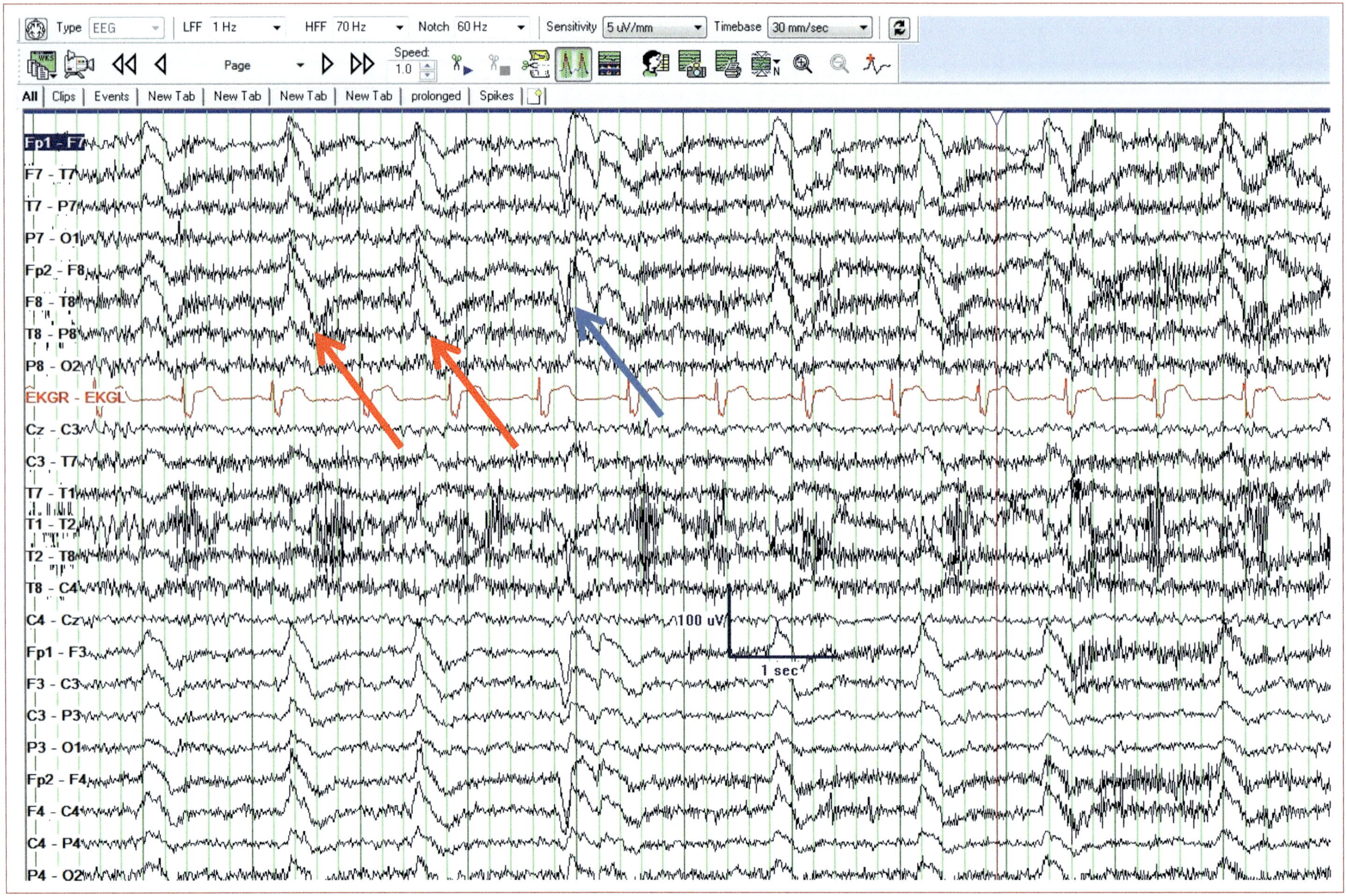

Figure 7.7: Generalized, atypical periodic discharges due to artifact (red arrows) caused by tongue clicking. Note the vertical eyeblink artifact in second 5 (blue arrow).

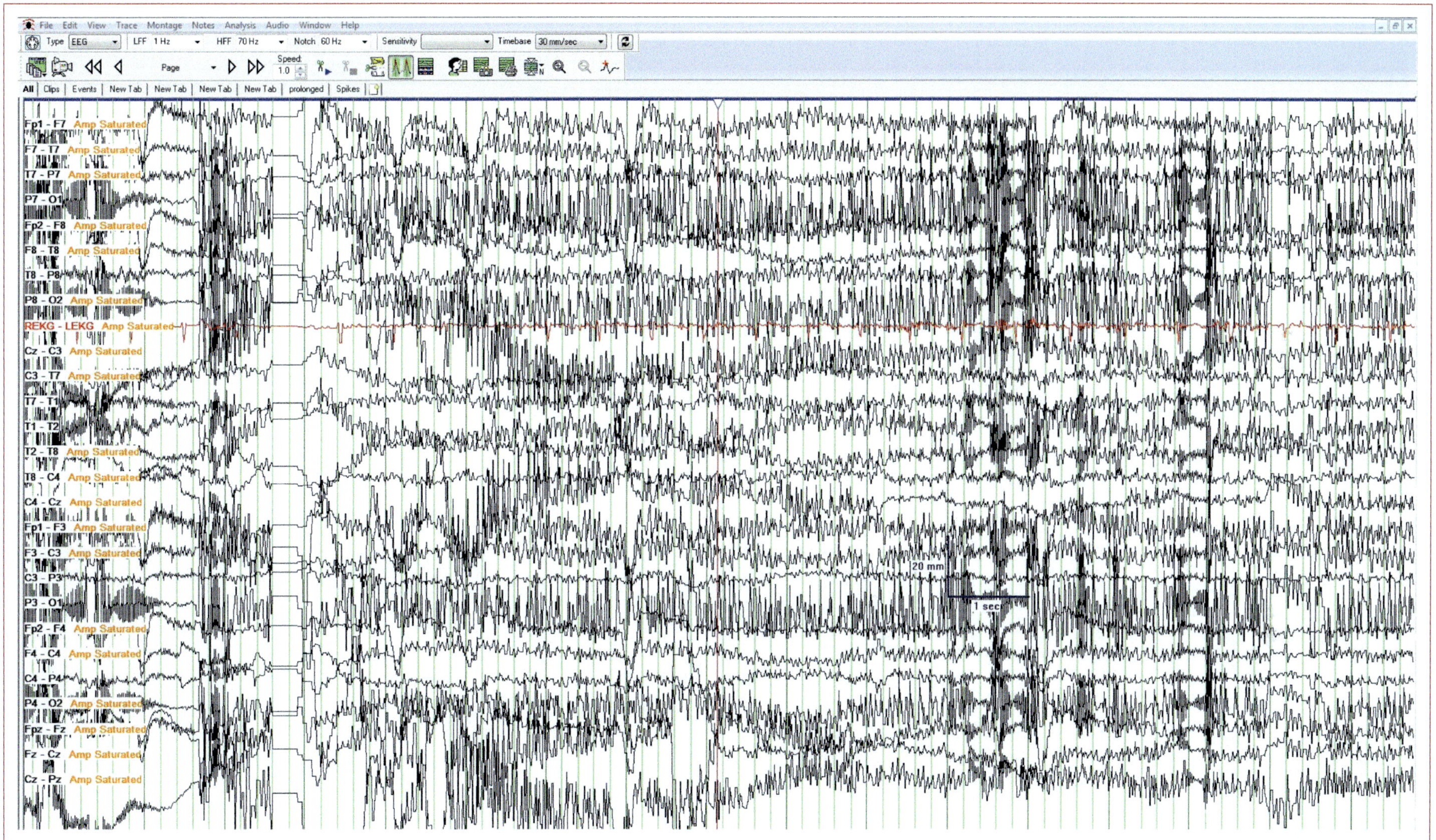

FIGURE 7.8: Artifact present in every channel due to the reference electrode being dislodged during LTM.

LTM, long-term monitoring.

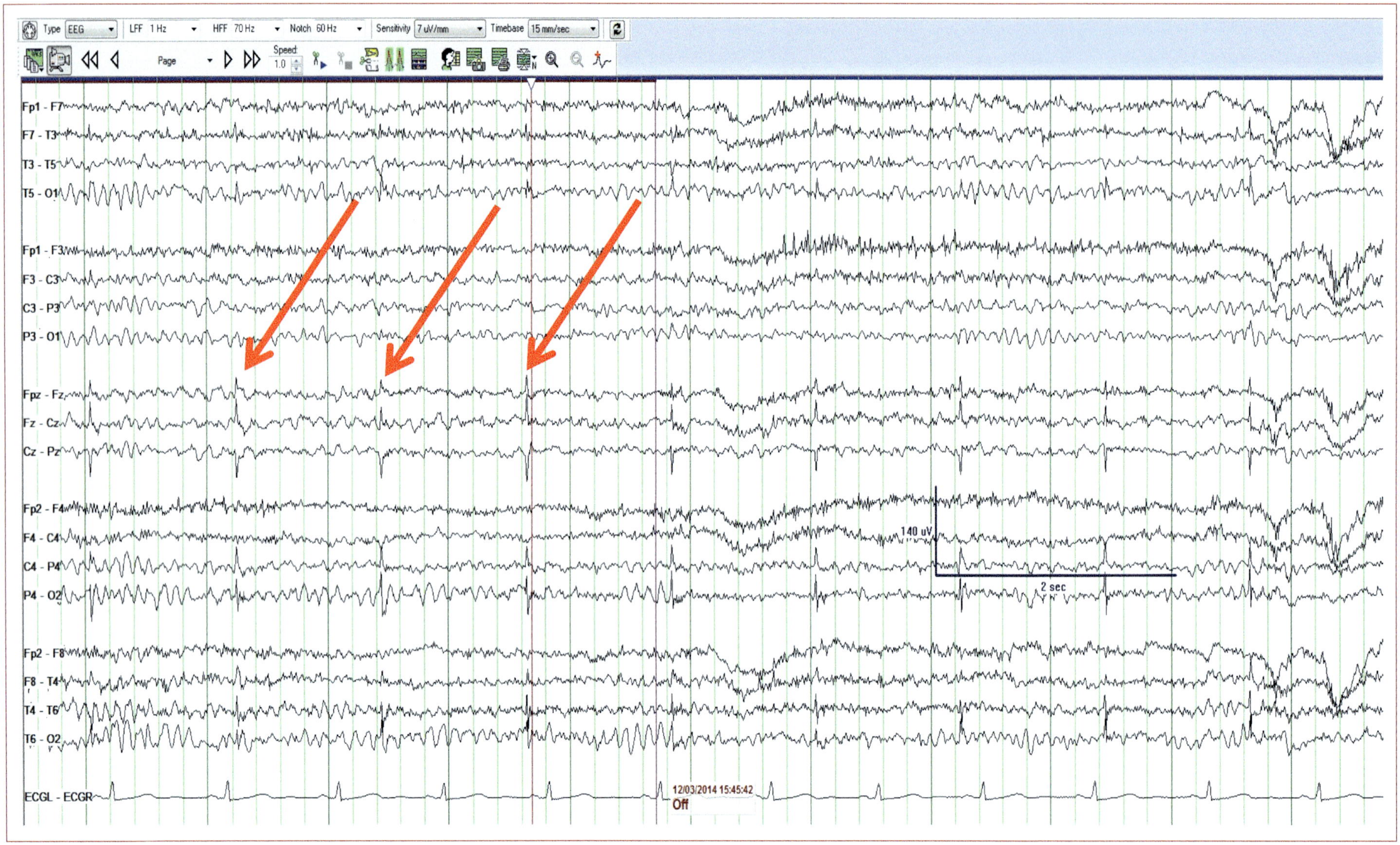

FIGURE 7.9: Intravenous drip artifact. Notice the precise intervals (arrows), brevity of potential (<20 ms), positive polarity, and nonphysiological spatial distribution.

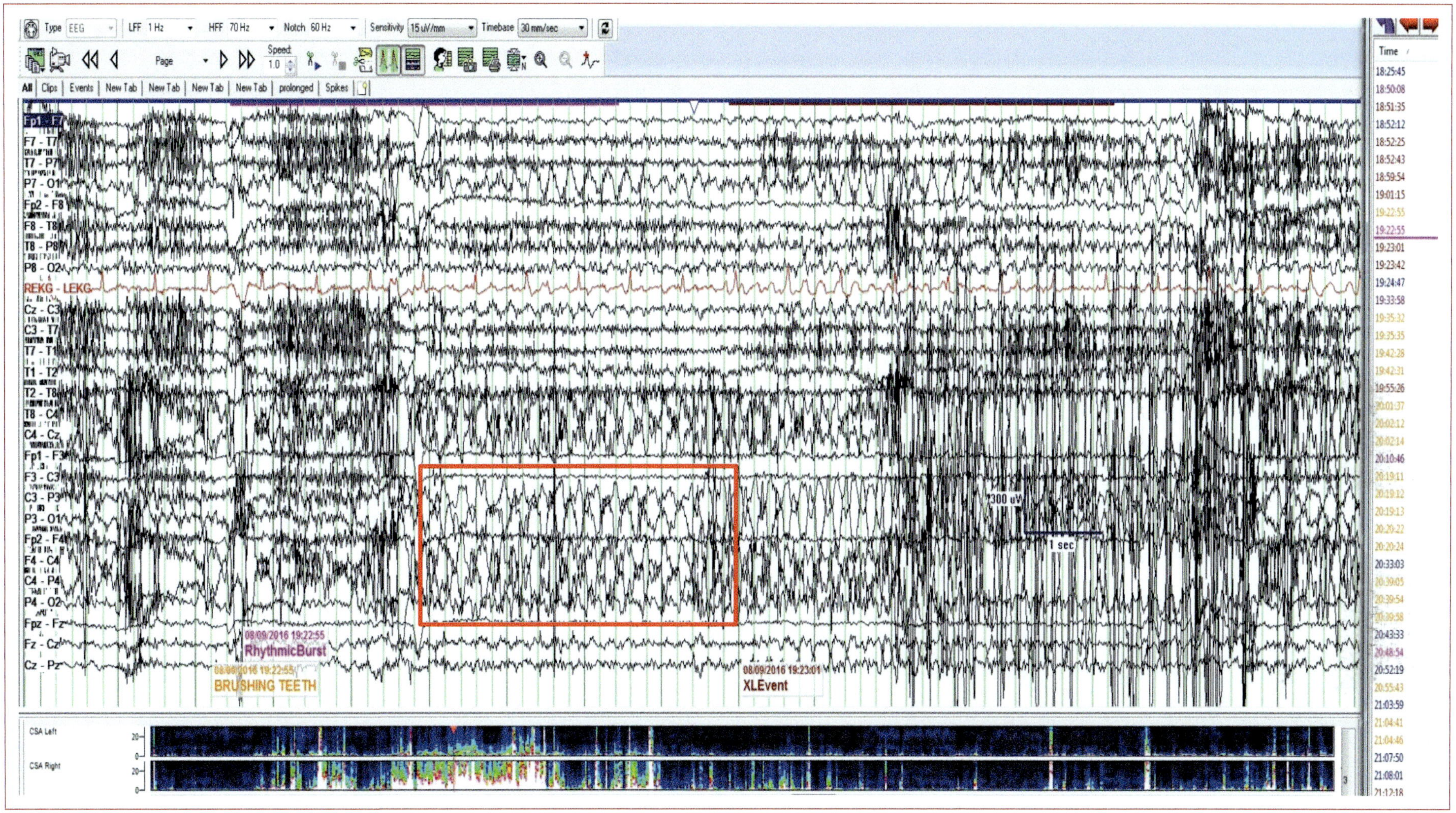

FIGURE 7.10: Toothbrushing artifact. Note the adjacent double- and triple-phase reversals (red square) on the EEG. Rhythmic movement may be deceiving and simulate a seizure when toothbrushing fluctuates in frequency and amplitude (see the CSA trend in the QEEG).

CSA, compressed spectral array; QEEG, quantitative EEG.

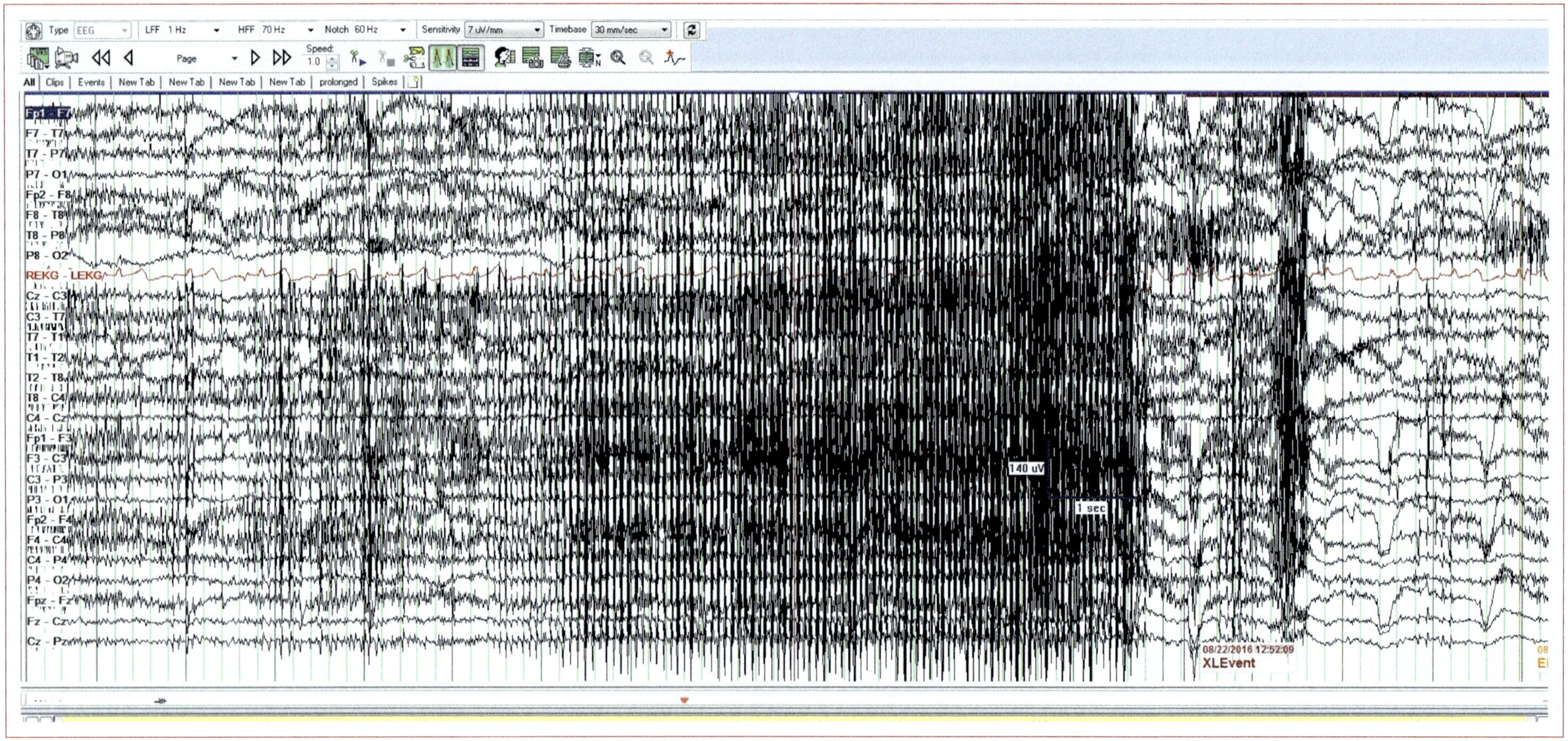

FIGURE 7.11: Shiver artifact with high frequencies characteristic of myogenic artifact. Note the brief crescendo buildup and abrupt offset that mimics the evolution of a focal seizure.

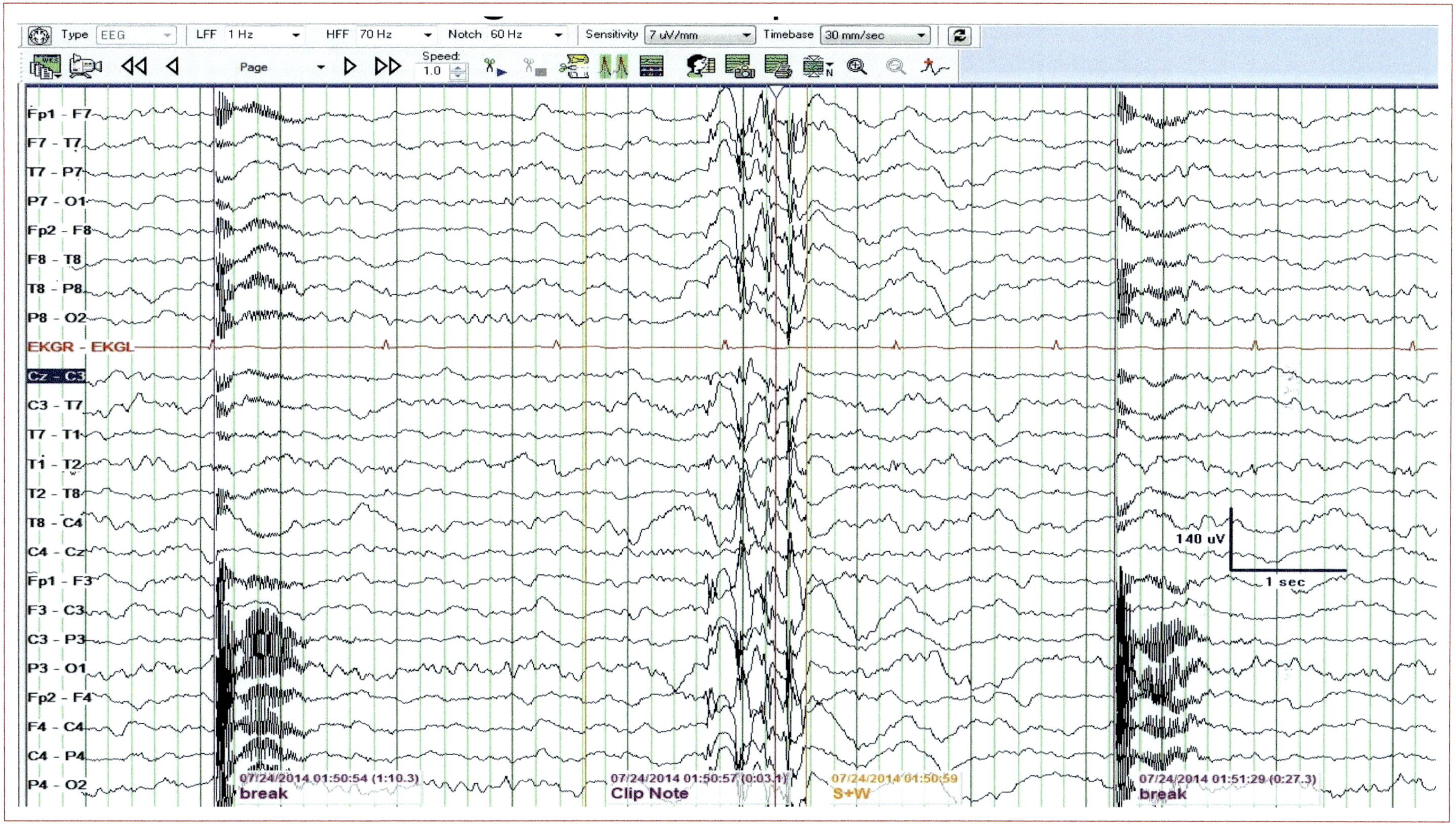

FIGURE 7.12: Artifact during initiation of EEG after sampling. The exact mechanism in the EEG machine was unable to be determined by the technologist and could not be eliminated. Note the burst of generalized spike-and-wave in the second 5.

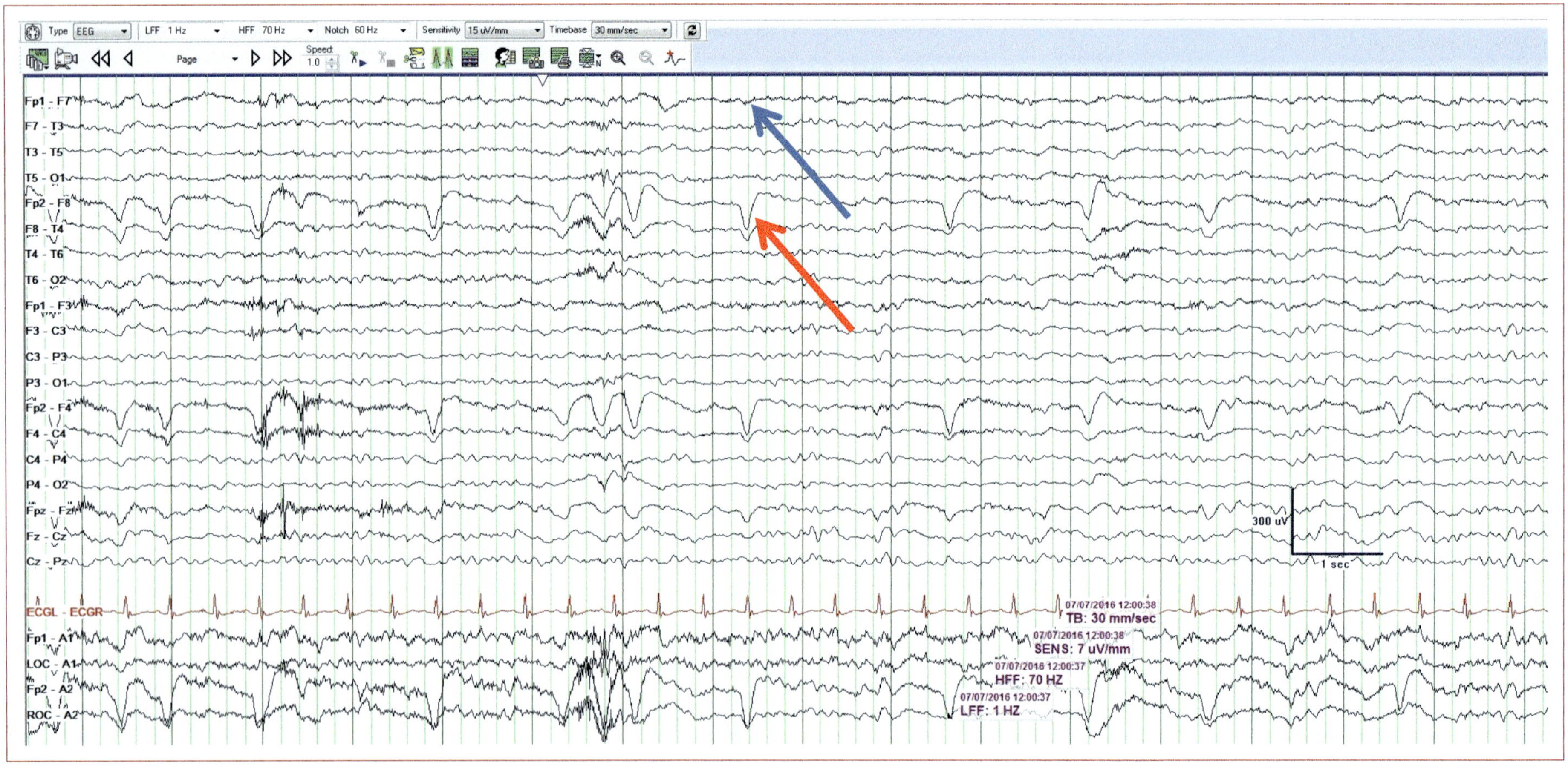

FIGURE 7.13: Unilateral eyeblink artifact (red arrow). This was due to a left enucleated eye for melanoma with absent similar artifact on the opposite side of the head (blue arrow).

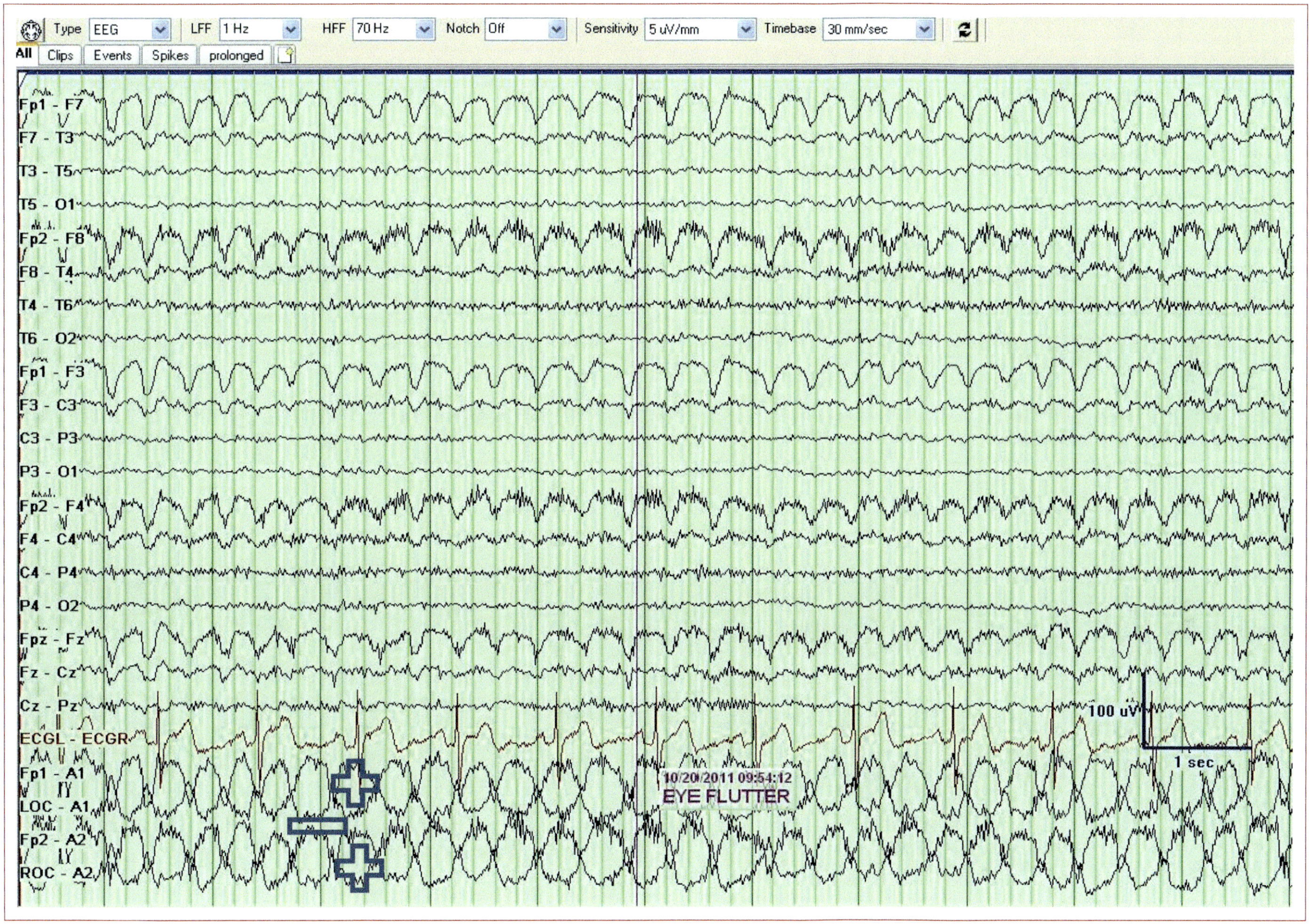

FIGURE 7.14: Continuous vertical eye flutter artifact. Note the "out-of-phase" polarity in the eye movement monitors (lower four channels) to identify the eye as the generator as opposed to the brain.

Source: From Tatum WO. *Handbook of EEG Interpretation*. New York, NY: Demos Medical Publishing; 2014:14.

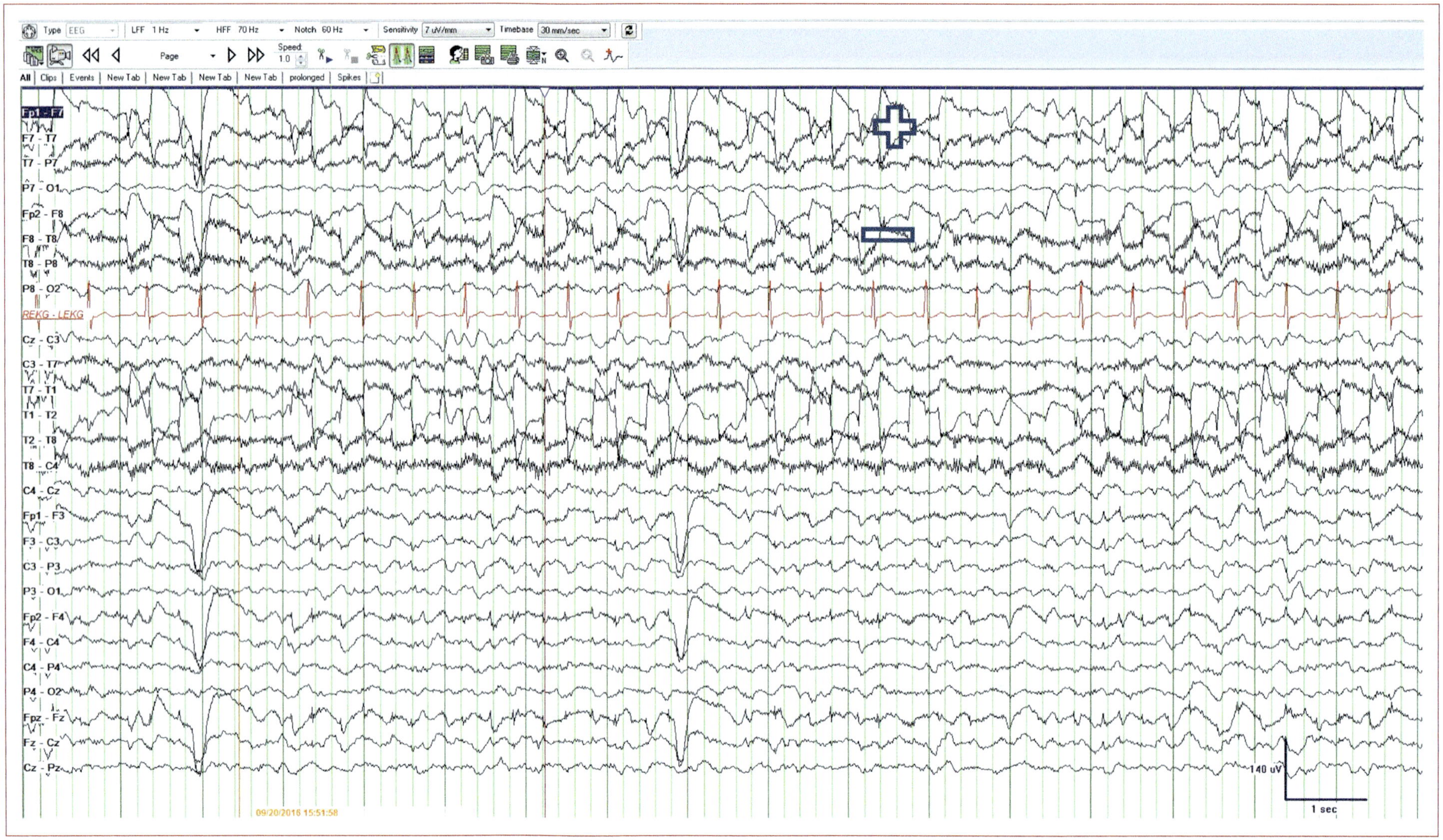

Figure 7.15: Rapid horizontal eye movements back and forth produce a complex artifactual field in a patient with autism spectrum disorder. Note the opposite polarity (positive and negative) in homologous channels.

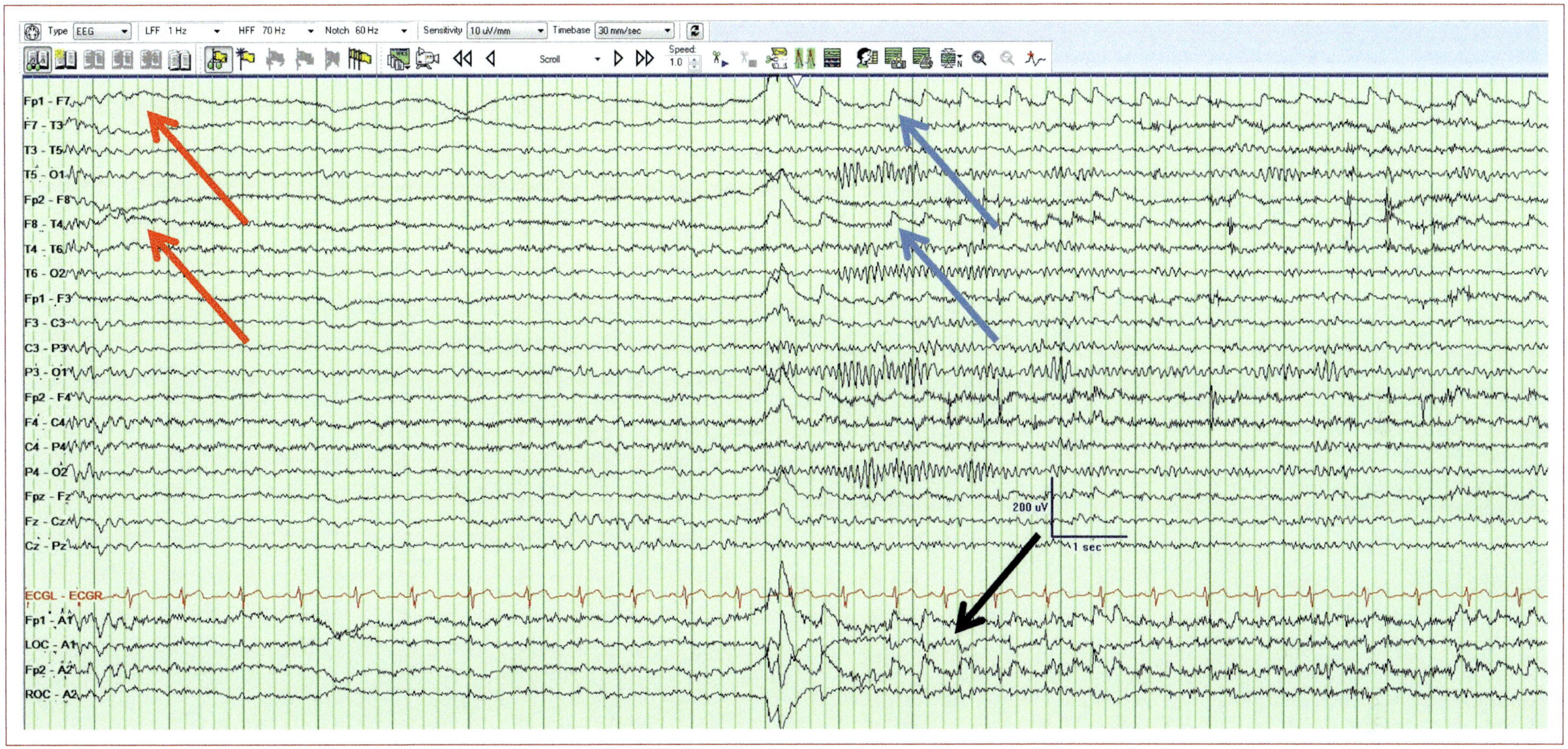

FIGURE 7.16: Slow rolling eye movements of drowsiness (red arrows) and subsequent nystagmoid artifact during wakefulness (blue arrows). Note the out-of-phase deflection present in the monitors during eye movement (black arrow).

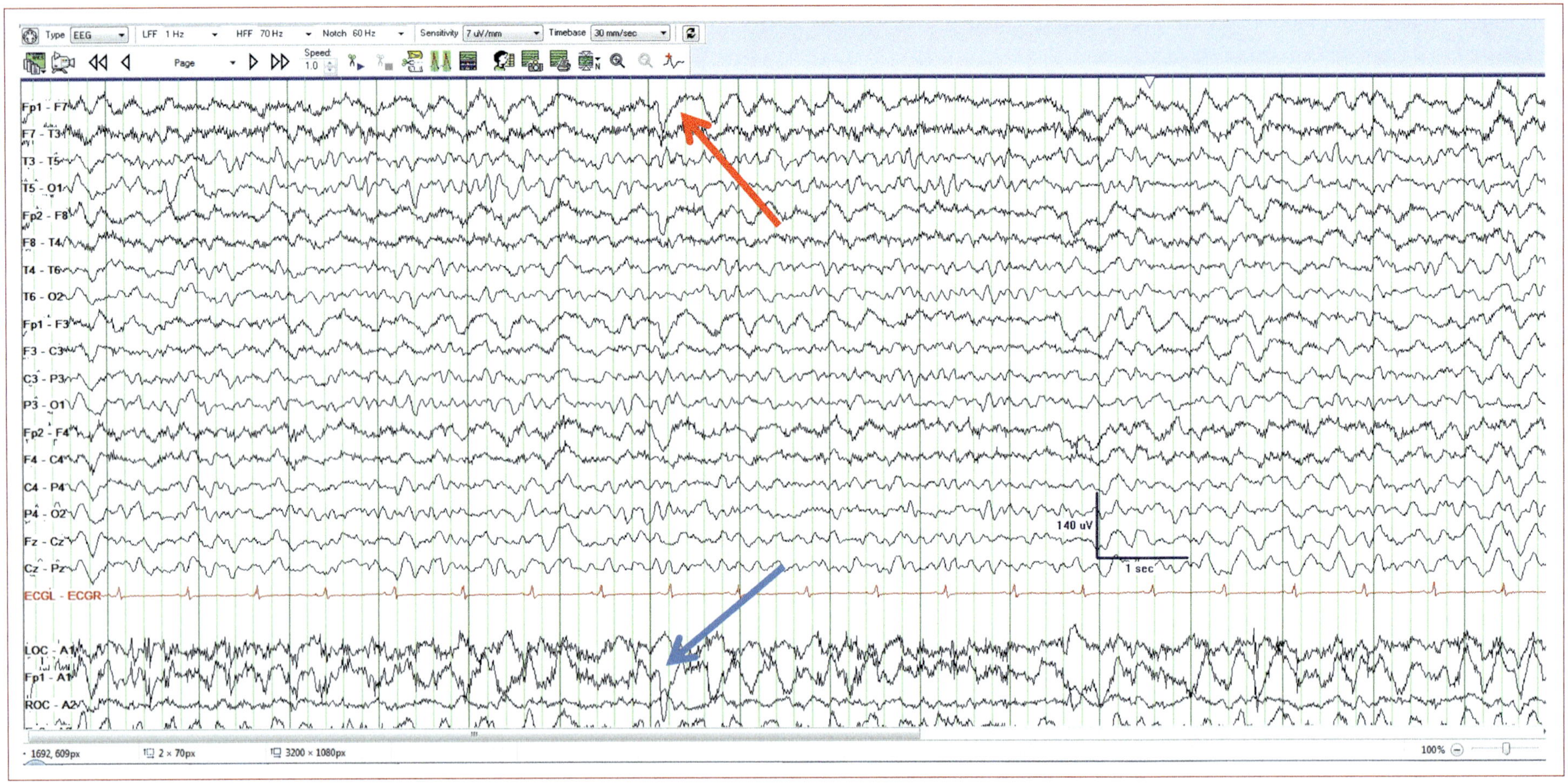

FIGURE 7.17: Triphasiform frontal slow waves (red arrow) due to low-amplitude vertical eyeblink artifact that may appear rhythmical and even mimic frontal intermittent rhythmic delta activity. Note the delineation of the ocular generator by the movement monitors showing out-of-phase deflections (blue arrows).

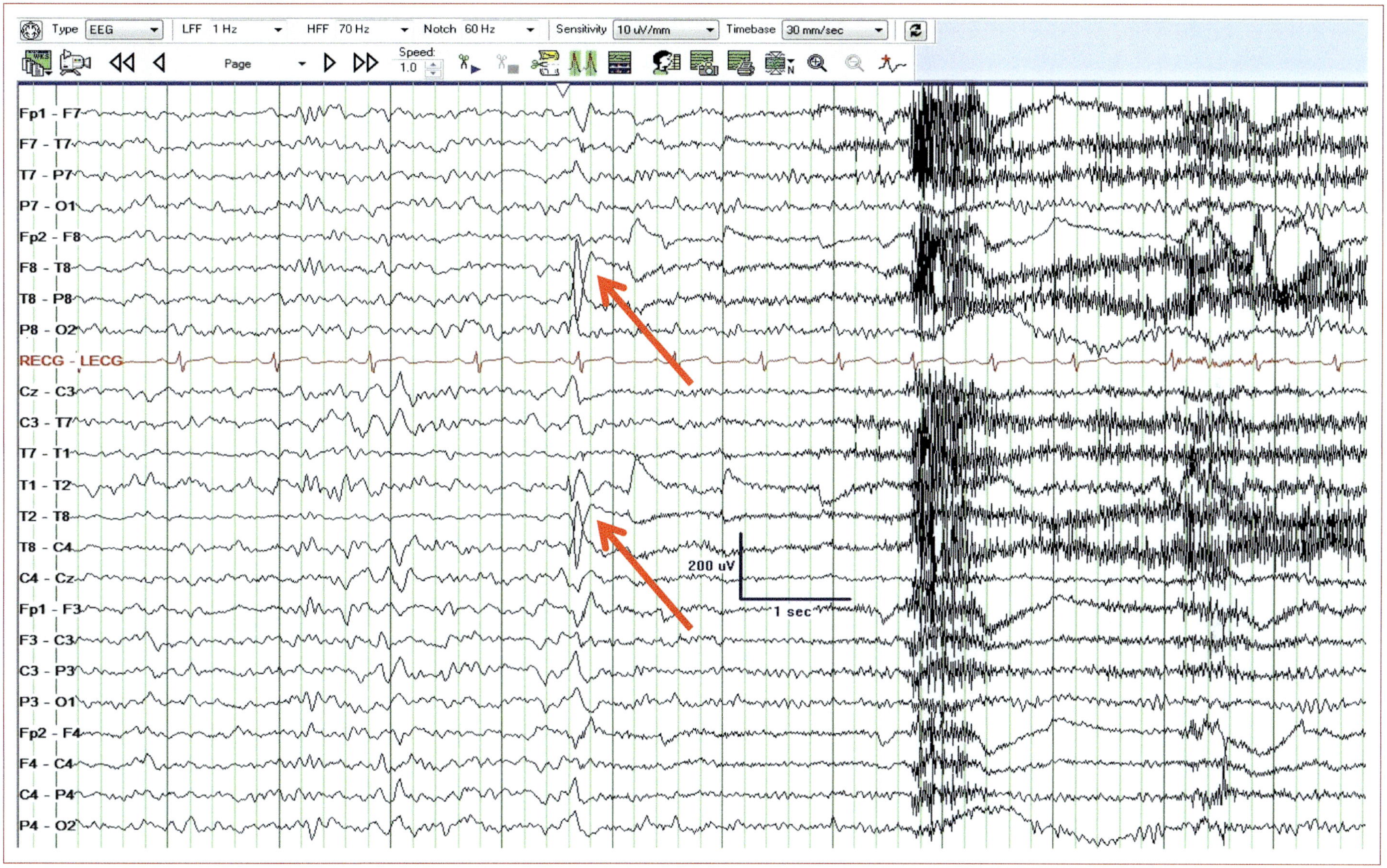

FIGURE 7.18: Pseudospike in the right temporal region (T8) due to artifact (red arrows). This is followed by a generalized burst of "muscle artifact" 2 seconds later.

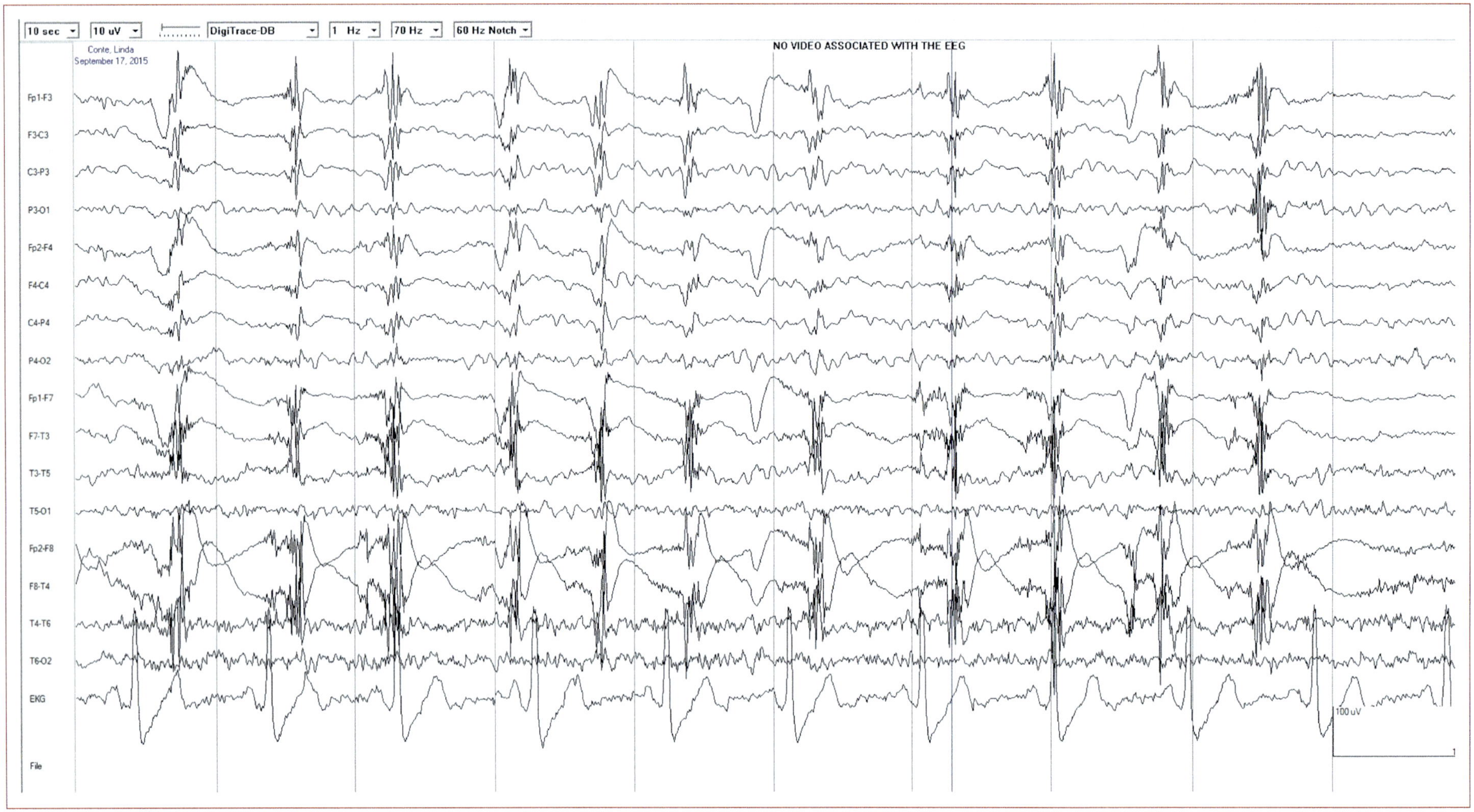

FIGURE 7.19: Chewing artifact in a patient with GGE. Note the bitemporal phasic polyspike morphology, nonphysiological positive temporal polarity, and frontotemporal field characteristic of myogenic artifact.

GGE, genetic generalized epilepsy.

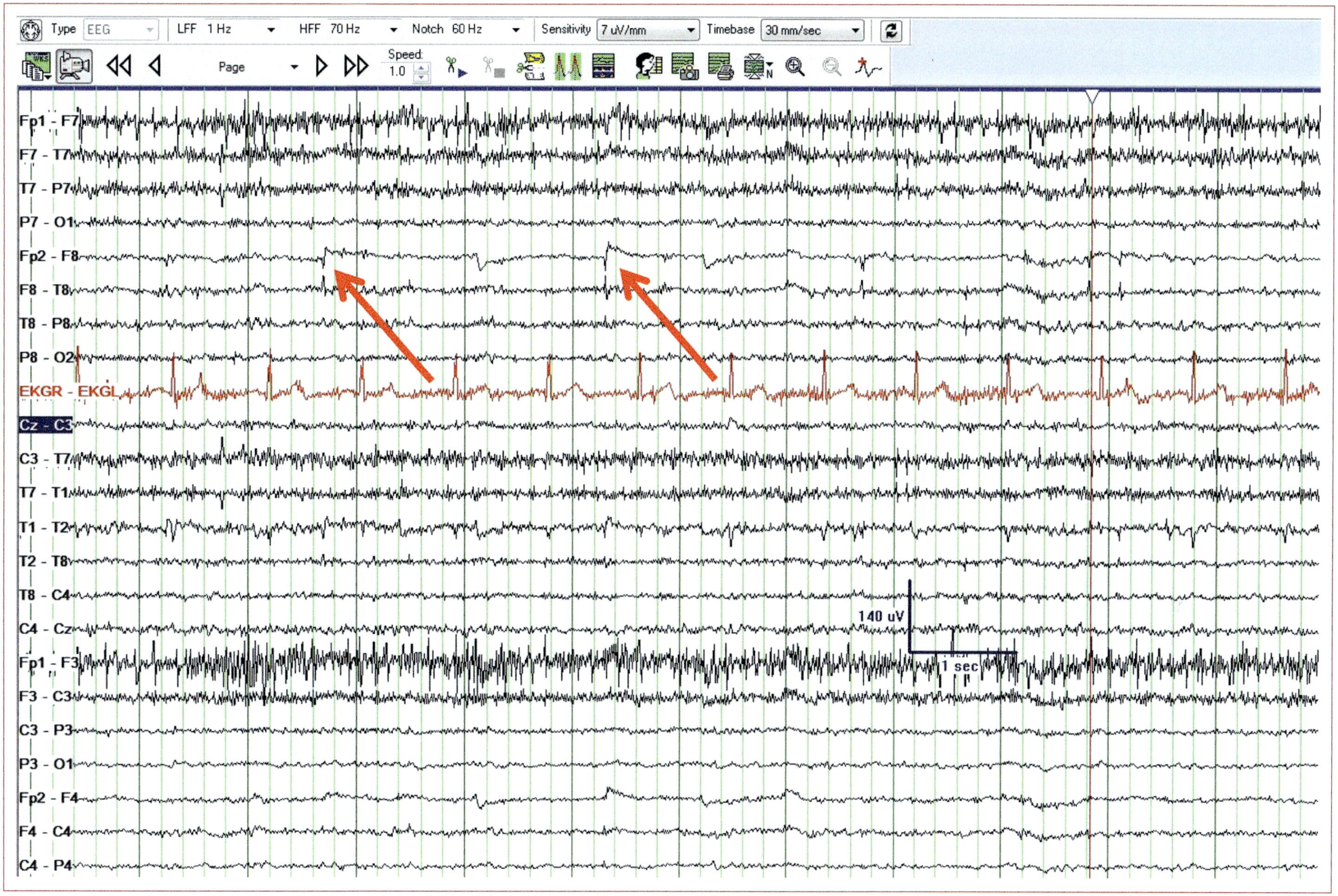

FIGURE 7.20: Lateral rectus spikes (arrows) produced during rapid horizontal eye movements. Note the apparent unilateral field due to continuous contralateral myogenic artifact in the homologous electrodes to give the appearance of right anterior temporal spikes.

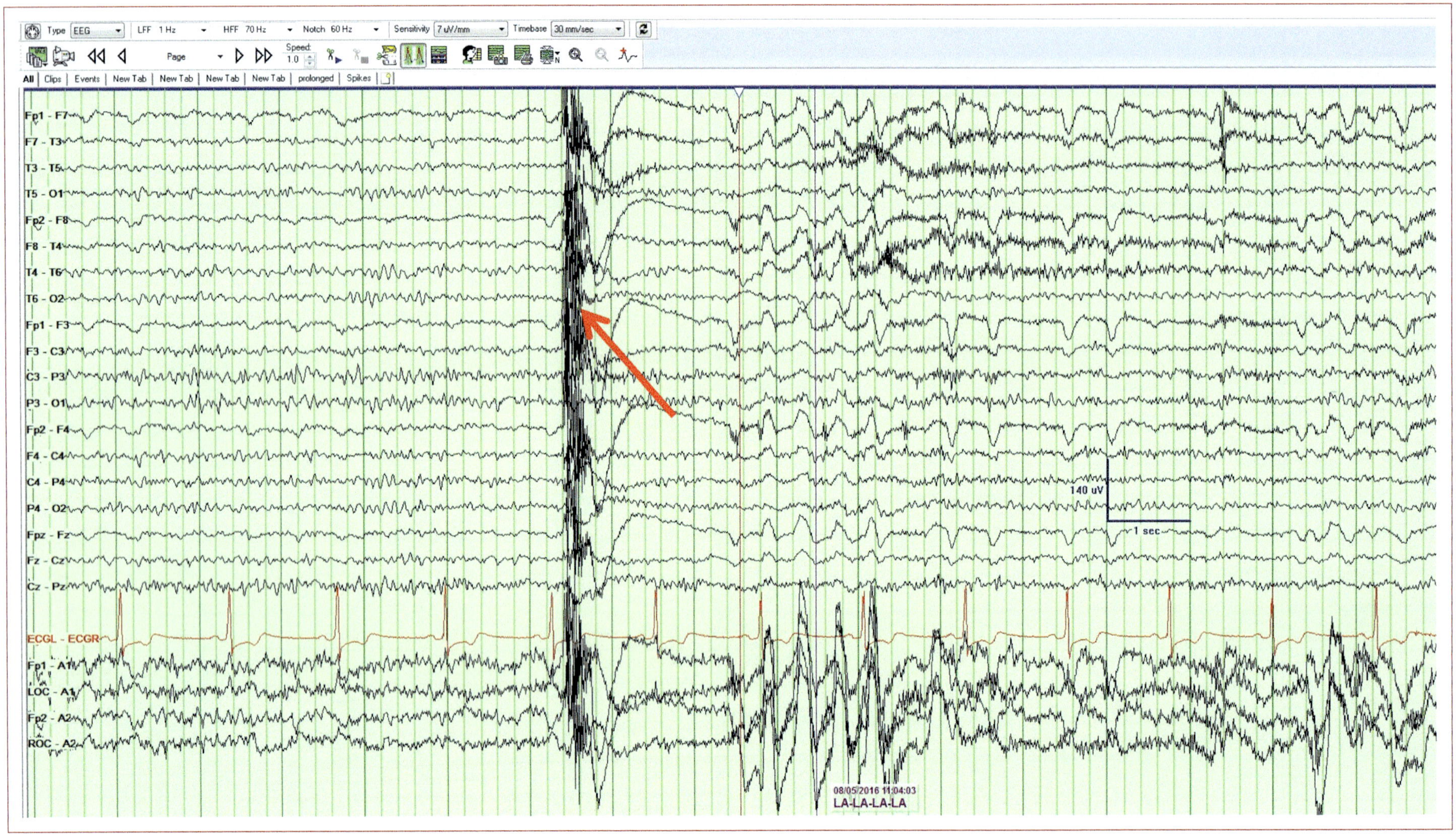

FIGURE 7.21: Glossokinetic artifact manifesting as a single swallow (arrow) followed 1½ seconds later by an artifact reproduced when asking the patient to repeat "lalala." Note the in-phase deflections in the eye movement monitors due to the lingual-pharyngeal generator arising inferior to the electrodes.

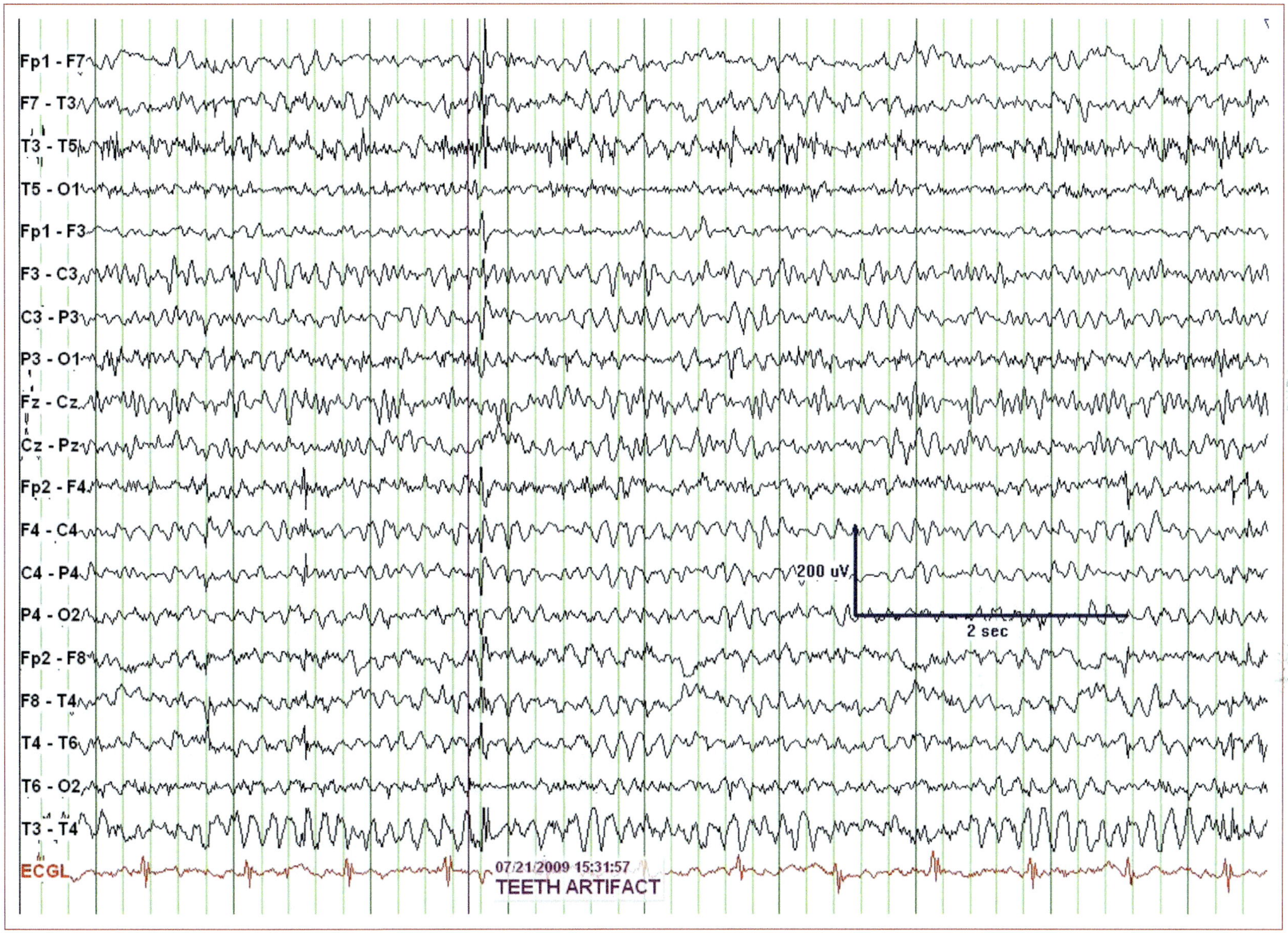

FIGURE 7.22: Dental artifact in second 3 labeled "Teeth Artifact." Note the brief spiky appearance and nonphysiological field.

Source: From Tatum WO, Reinsberger C, Dworetzky B. Artifacts of recording. In: Schomer DL, Lopes da Silva FH, eds. *Niedermeyer's Electroencephalography: Basic Principles, Clinical Applications, and Related Fields*. 7th ed. New York, NY: Oxford University Press; 2018, with permission.

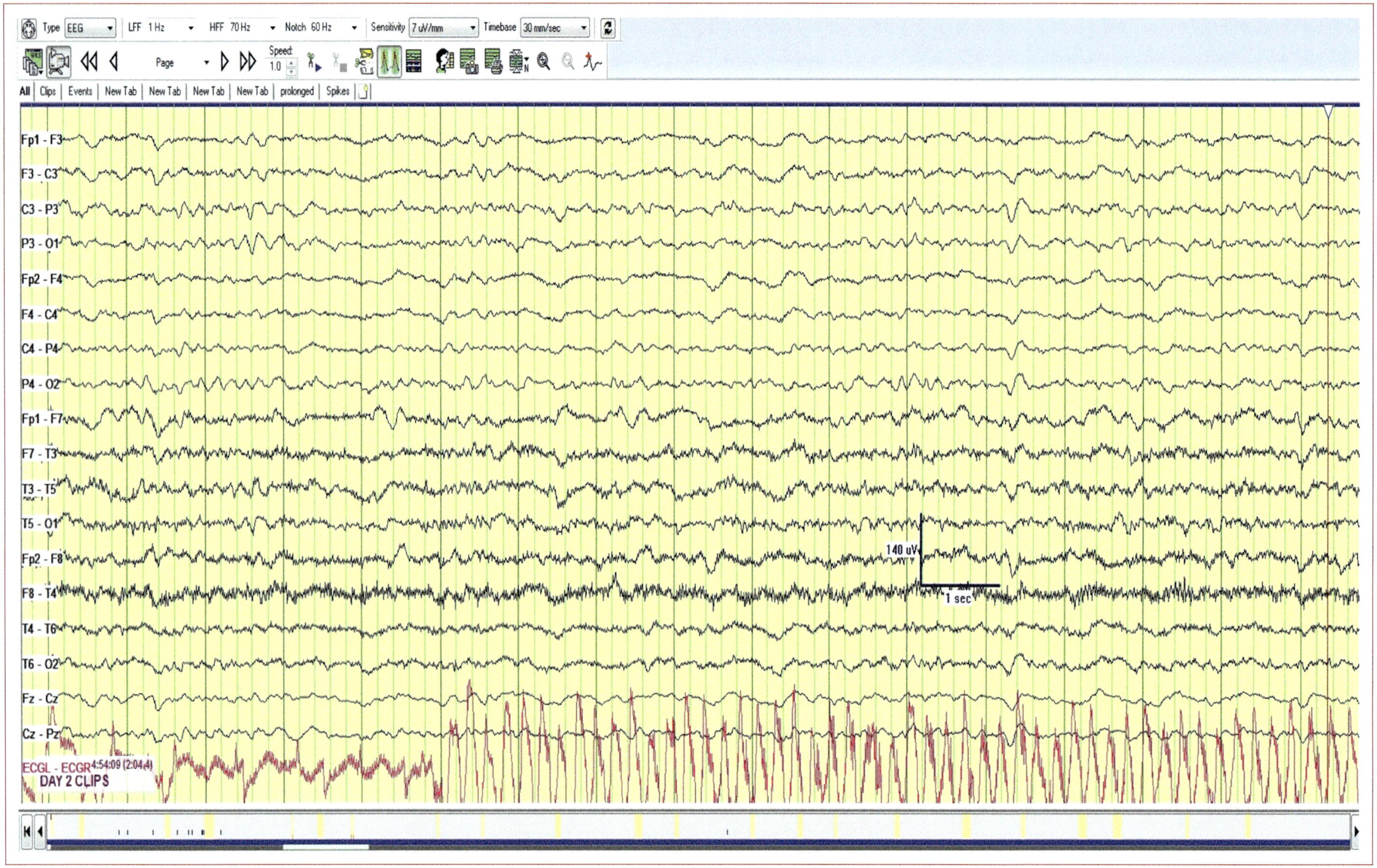

FIGURE 7.23: ECG lead with rhythmical artifact that simulates ventricular tachycardia when the electrode becomes unglued from the chest. Note the presence of 60-Hz artifact in the ECG preceding it and the presence in multiple EEG channels as well.

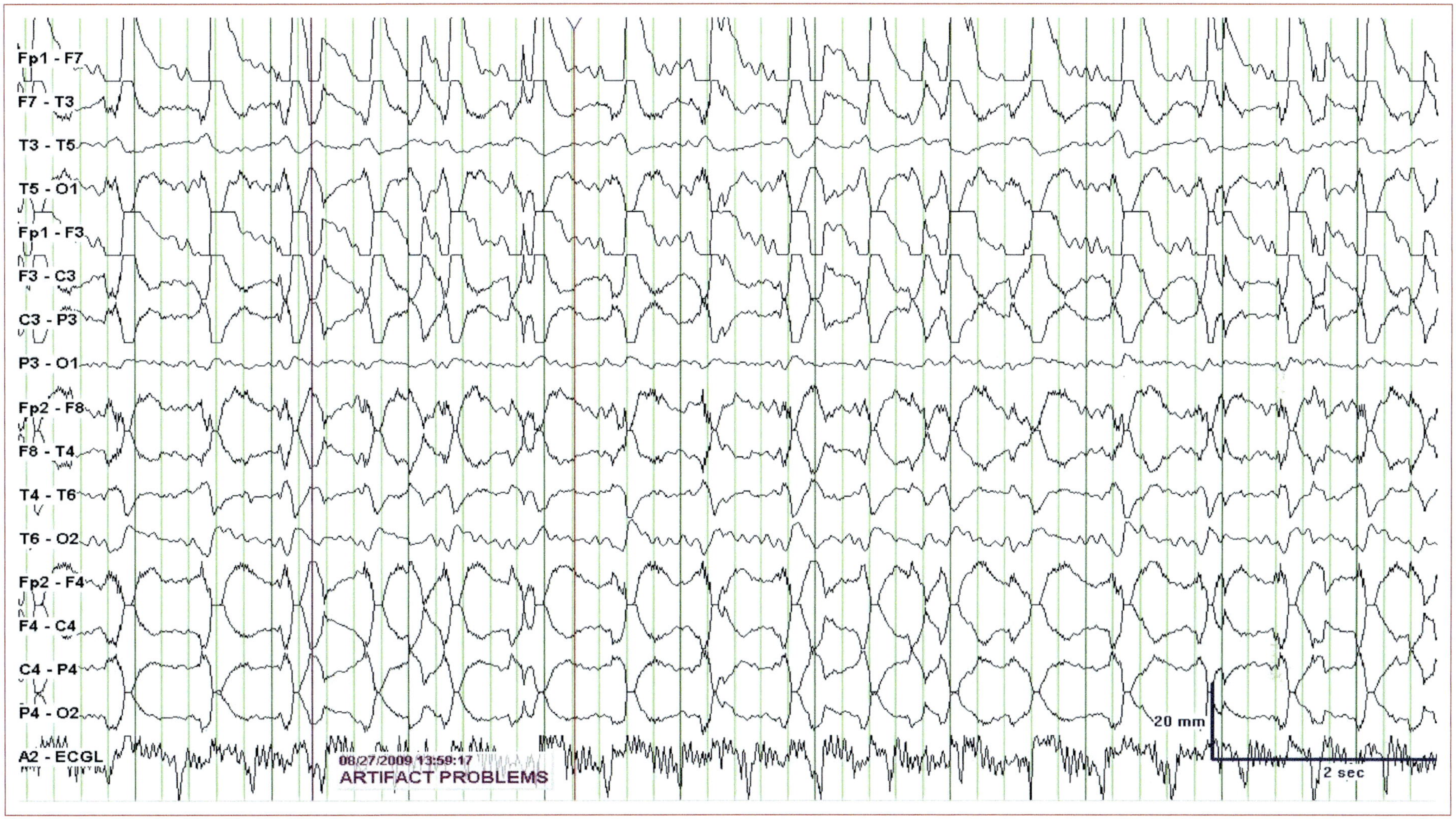

FIGURE 7.24: Diffuse mechanical artifact during EEG caused by a left ventricular assist device in a patient with heart failure awaiting transplantation.

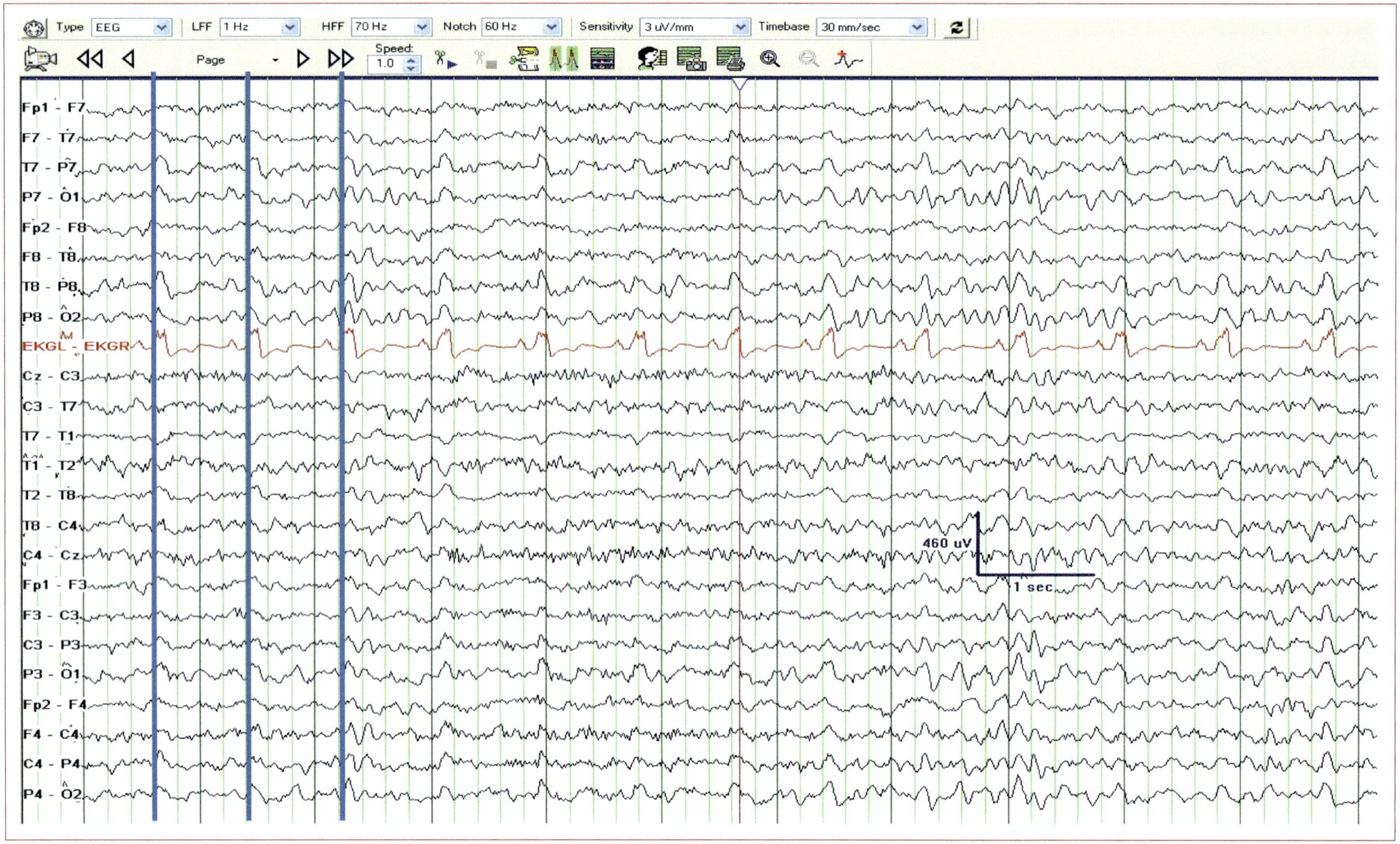

FIGURE 7.25: Artifact due to ECG producing generalized periodic discharges in the EEG (blue lines).

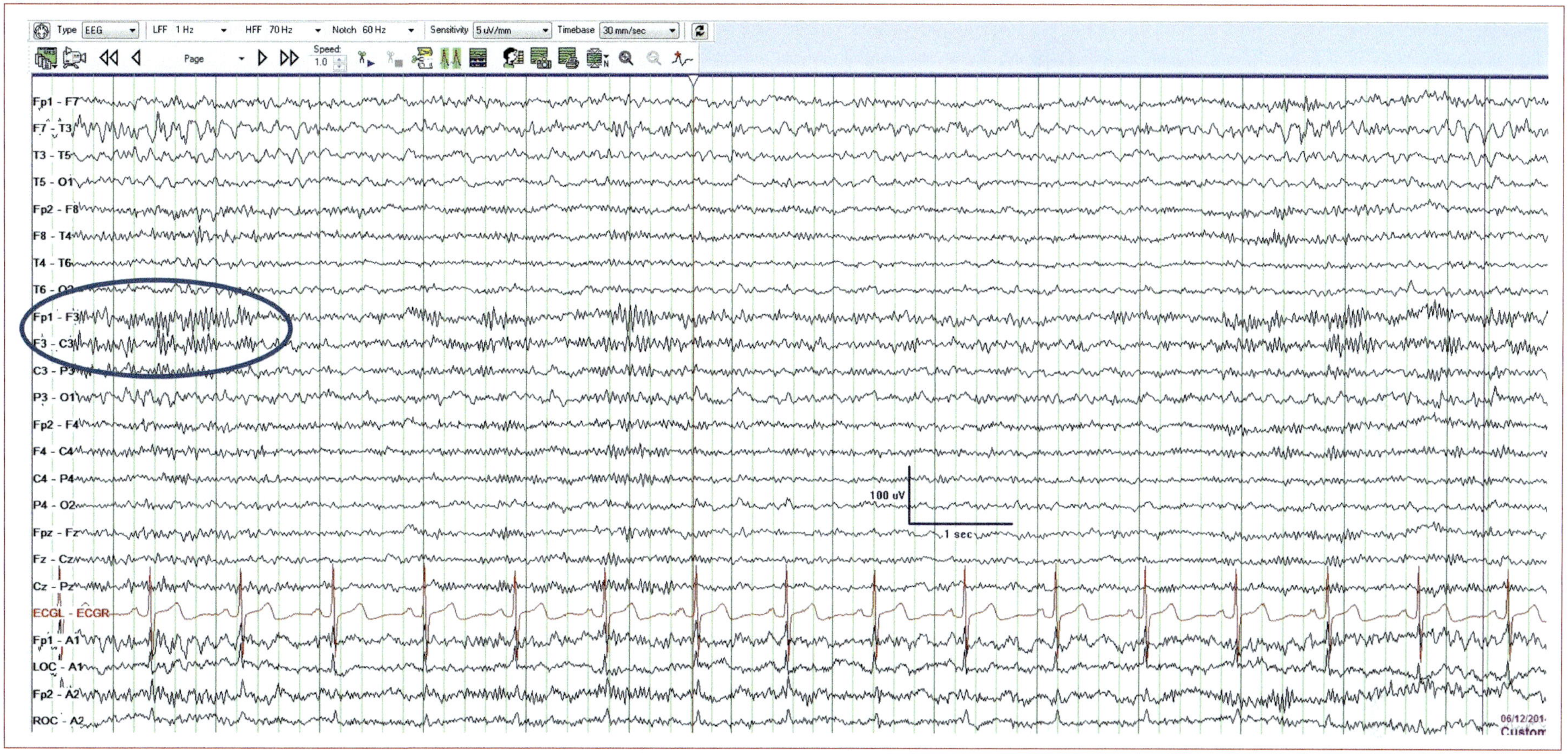

FIGURE 7.26: Left frontal breach (oval) with focal, high-frequency fast activity simulating myogenic artifact.

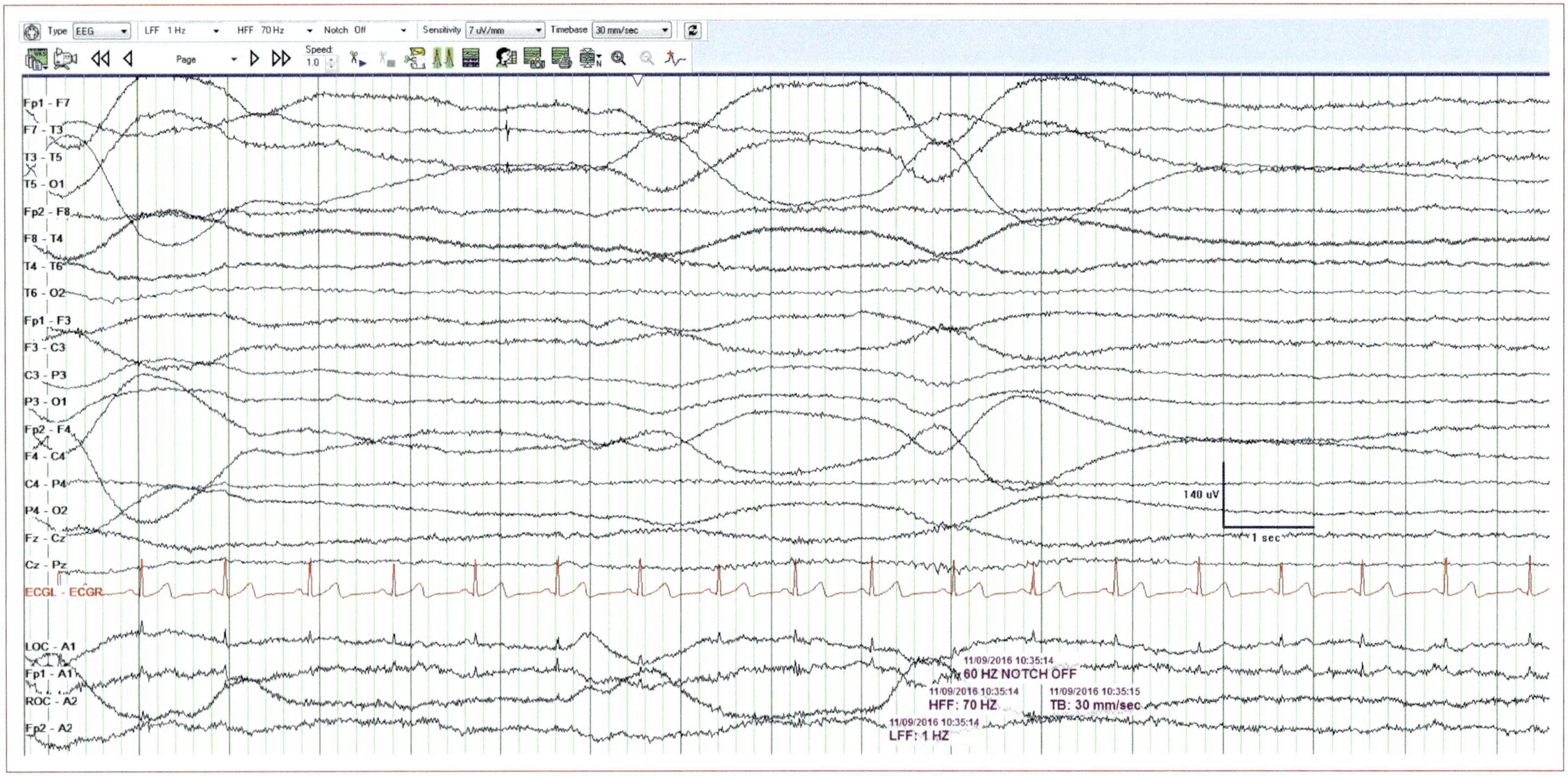

FIGURE 7.27: Sweat artifact manifesting as slow, wavering potentials without a physiological field; often frontally dominant within areas of perspiration accumulation.

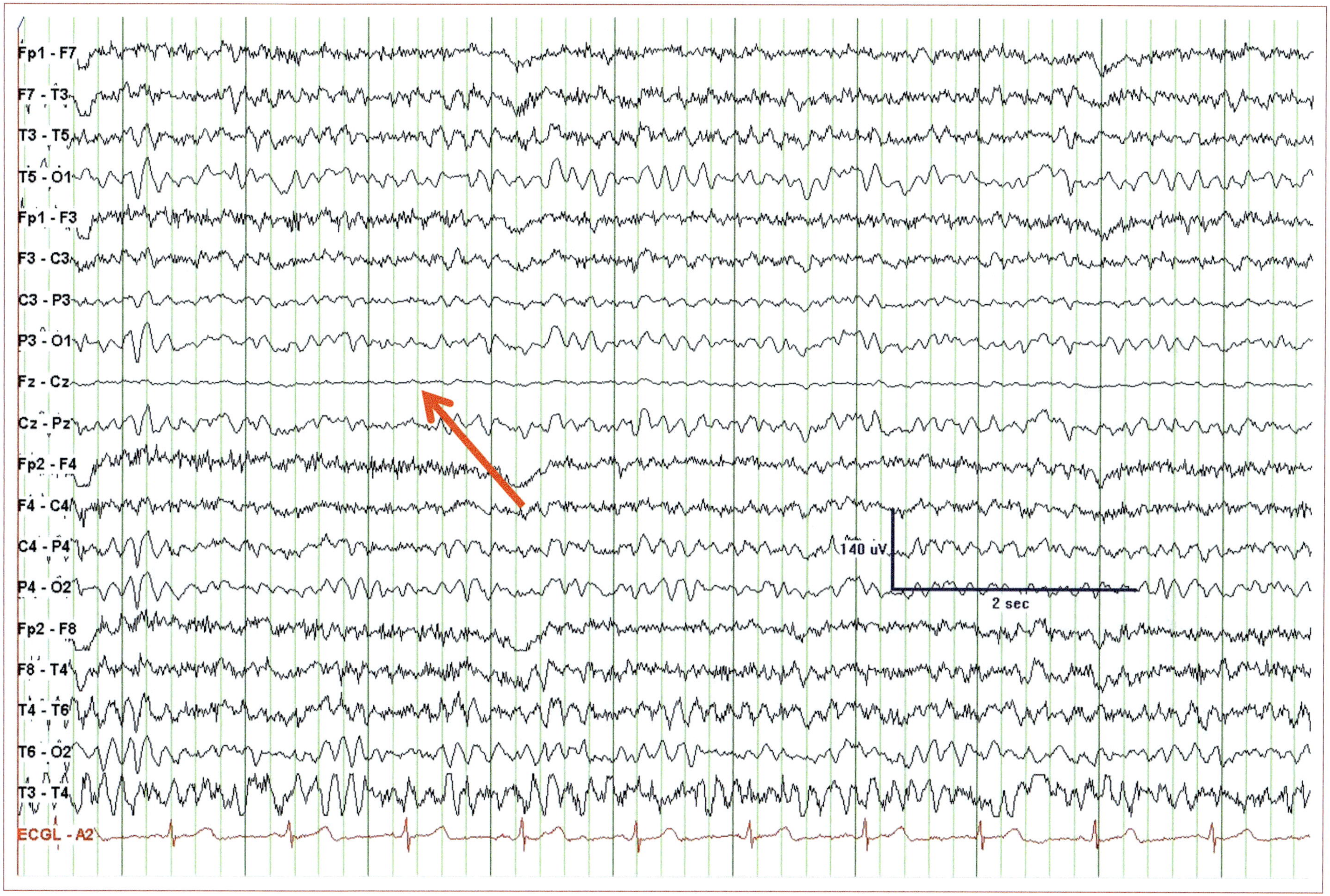

FIGURE 7.28: Salt bridge at Fz-Cz (arrow).

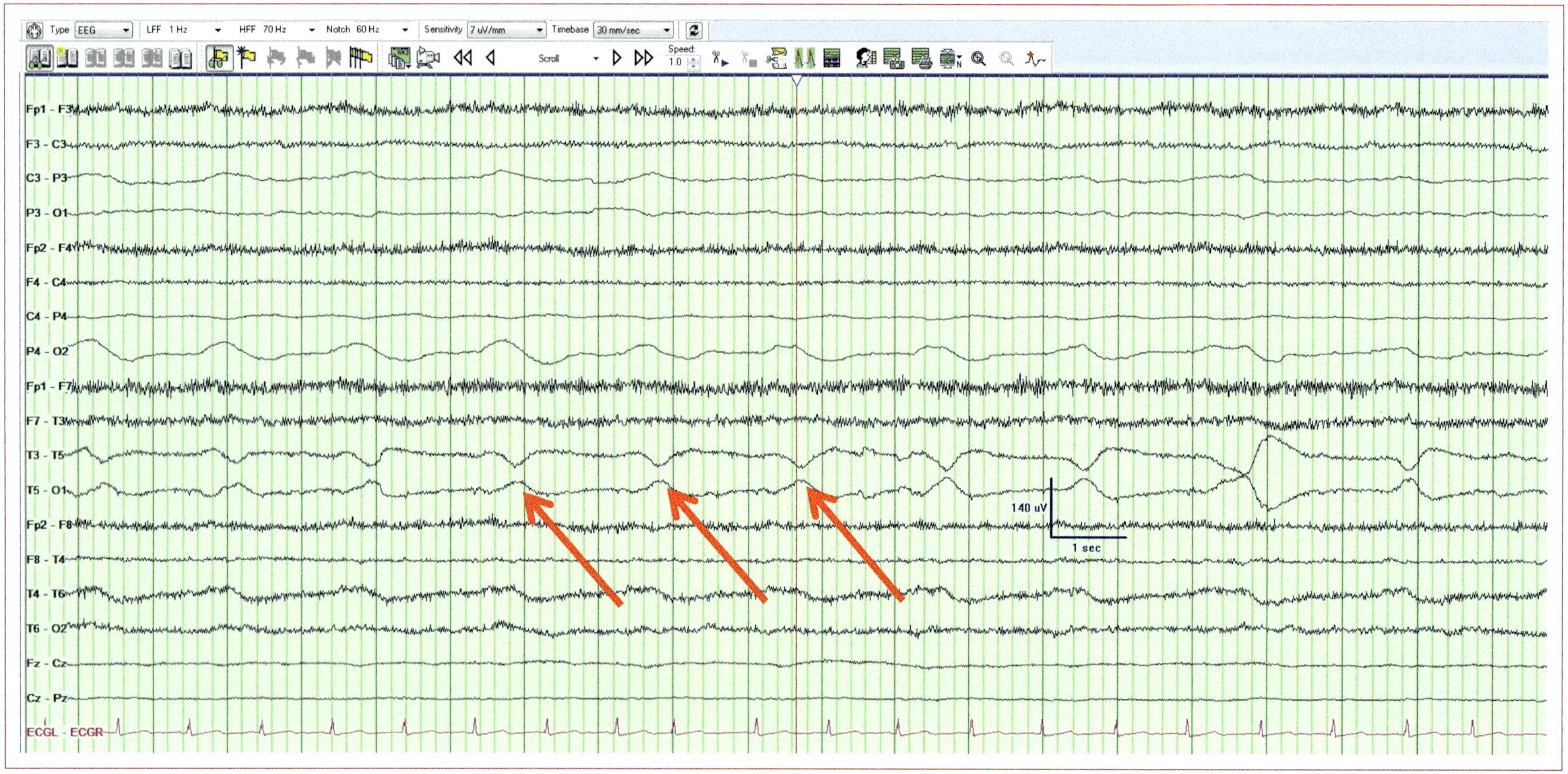

FIGURE 7.29: Respiration artifact during mechanical ventilation following termination of status epilepticus. Note the precise periodicity due to the machine-initiated inspiration (arrows).

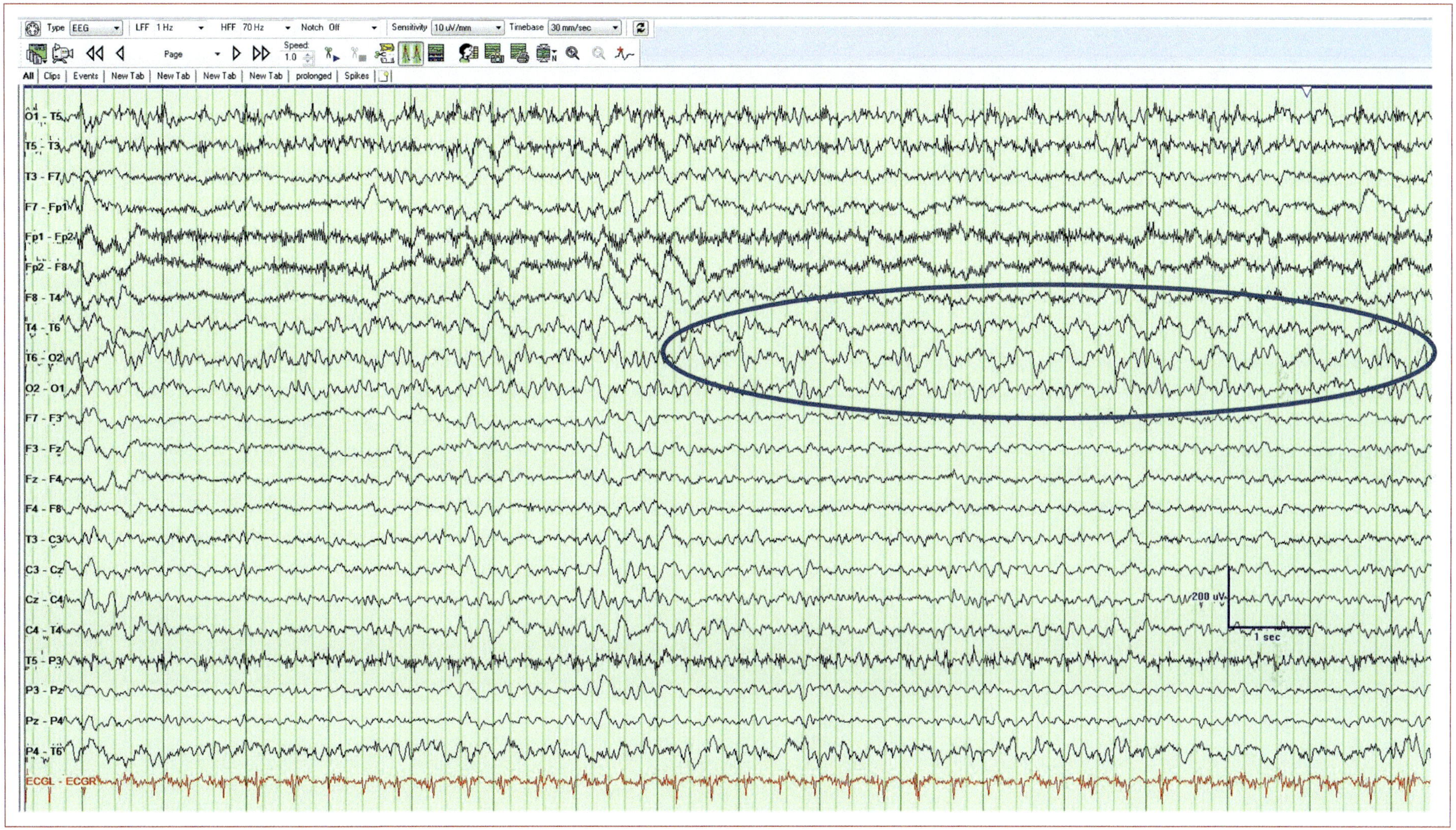

FIGURE 7.30: Pseudoslowing observed by head-rocking artifact (oval) during hyperventilation. This is readily identified by the nonphysiological polarity in T6-O2 on a circle montage. Note the bursts of frontal intermittent rhythmic delta activity in seconds 5 and 7.

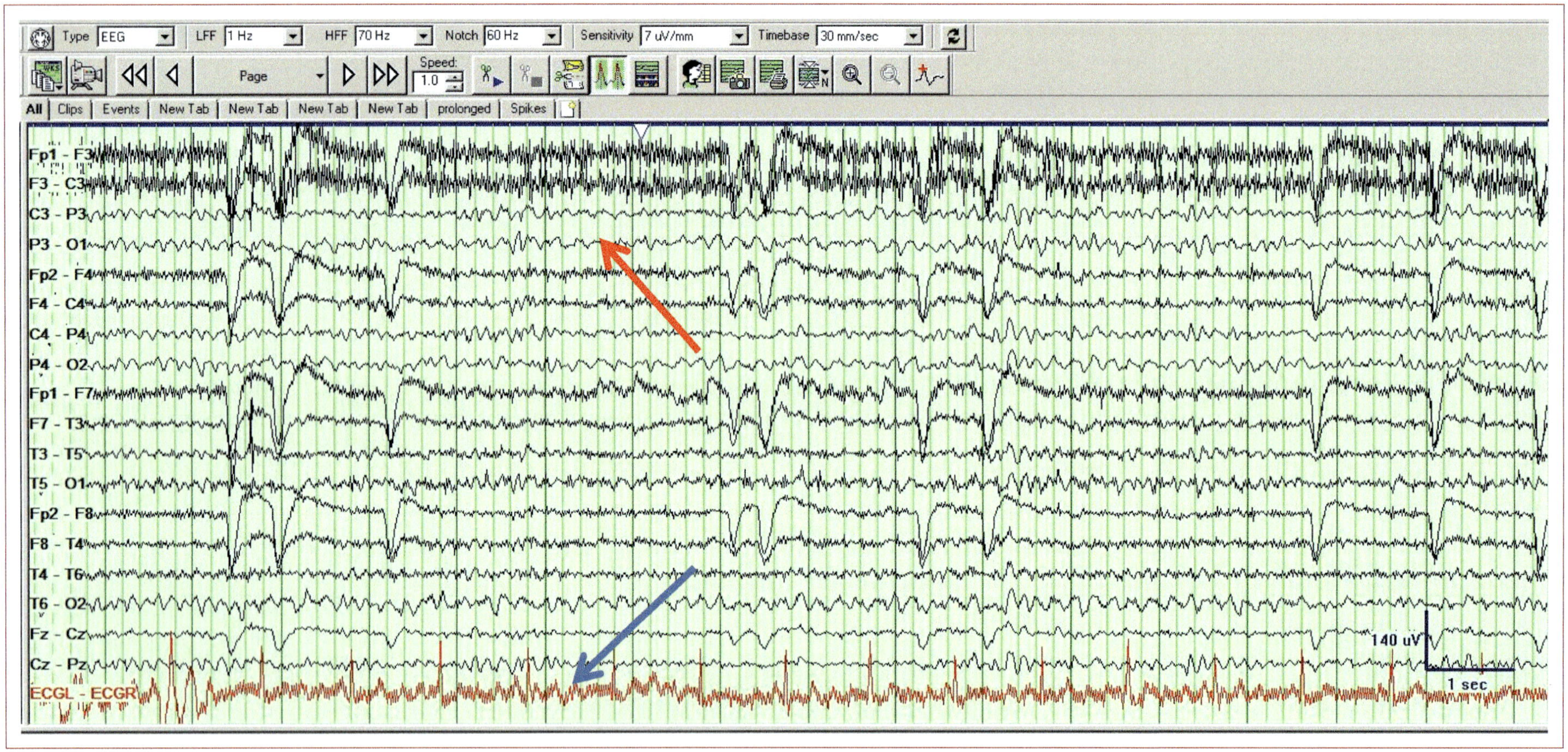

Figure 7.31: Parkinsonian tremor at 4 to 5 Hz distributed diffusely in the EEG (red arrow). Note the same frequency in the ECG (blue arrow).

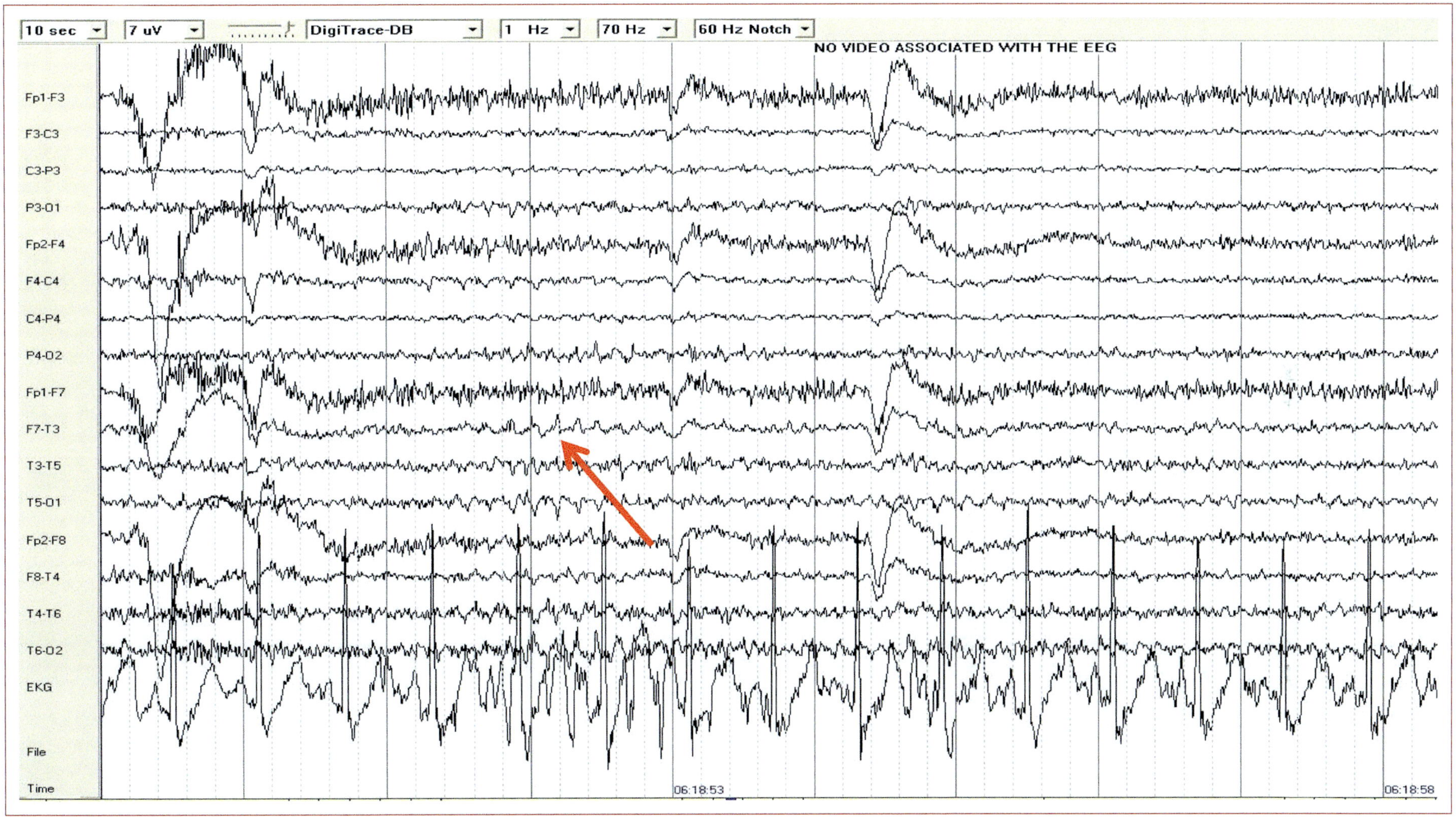

FIGURE 7.32: Artifact during rhythmic hand movement. Note the positive polarity (arrow) and bitemporal field (lower eight channels) as well as involvement of the ECG with the movement.

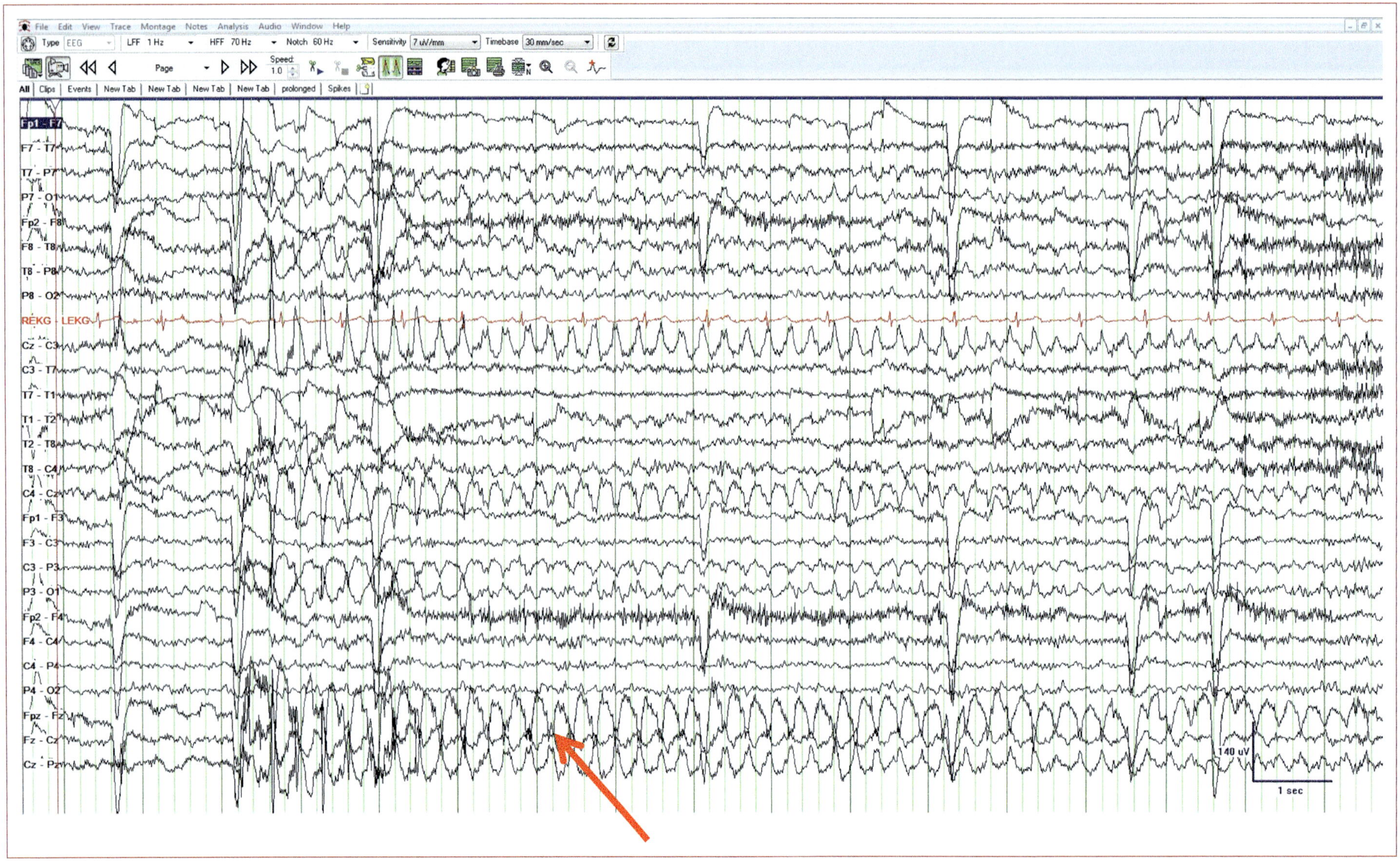

FIGURE 7.33: Movement artifact created by foot tapping by the patient. Note the rhythmic, nonphysiological electric field produced by the pattern that simulates a focal seizure (arrow).

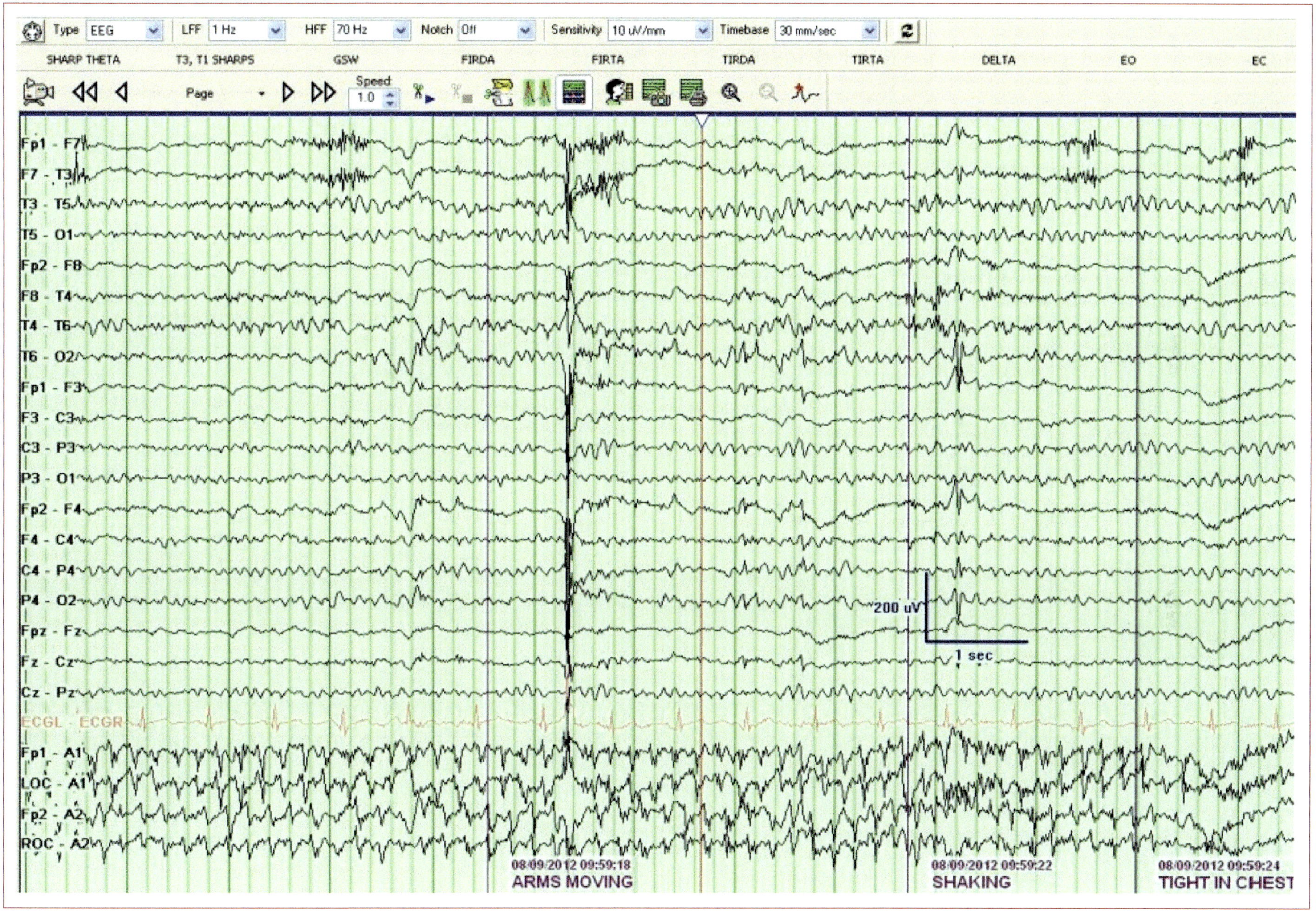

FIGURE 7.34: Tremor ("shaking") artifact in the periocular leads due to source localization and the lower sensitivity setting of the EOG.

EOG, electrooculogram.

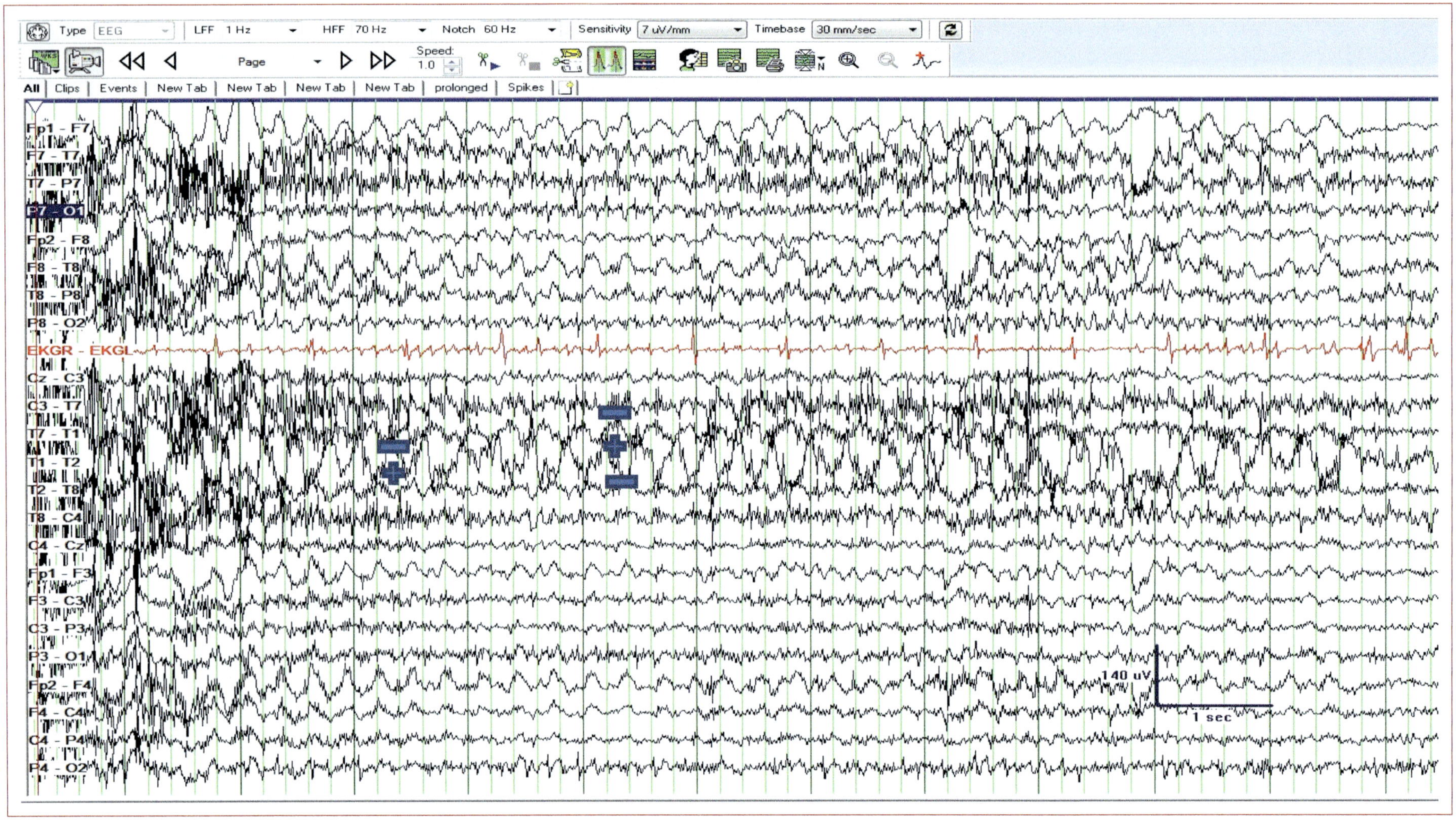

FIGURE 7.35: Complex artifact produced by a patient brushing his teeth. Note adjacent triple-phase reversals (blue signs) reflecting alternating polarity inconsistent with the spatial distribution of an electrophysiological generator.

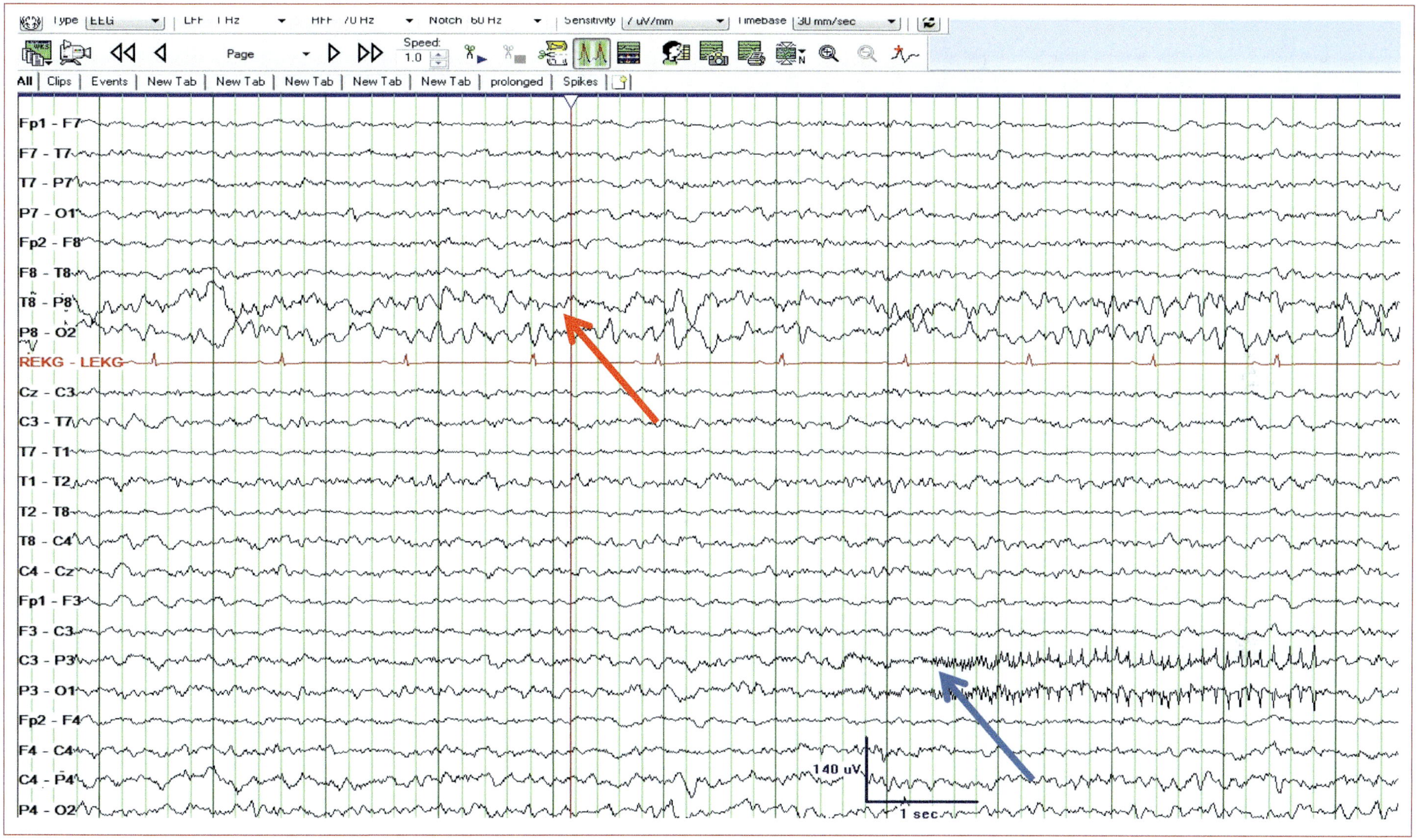

FIGURE 7.36: Complex repetitive discharge at P3 (blue arrow) mimicking a subclinical seizure. More typical single-electrode artifact is present at P8 (red arrow). Note positive polarity at P3 in a single electrode despite the paroxysmal evolving frequencies and amplitude.

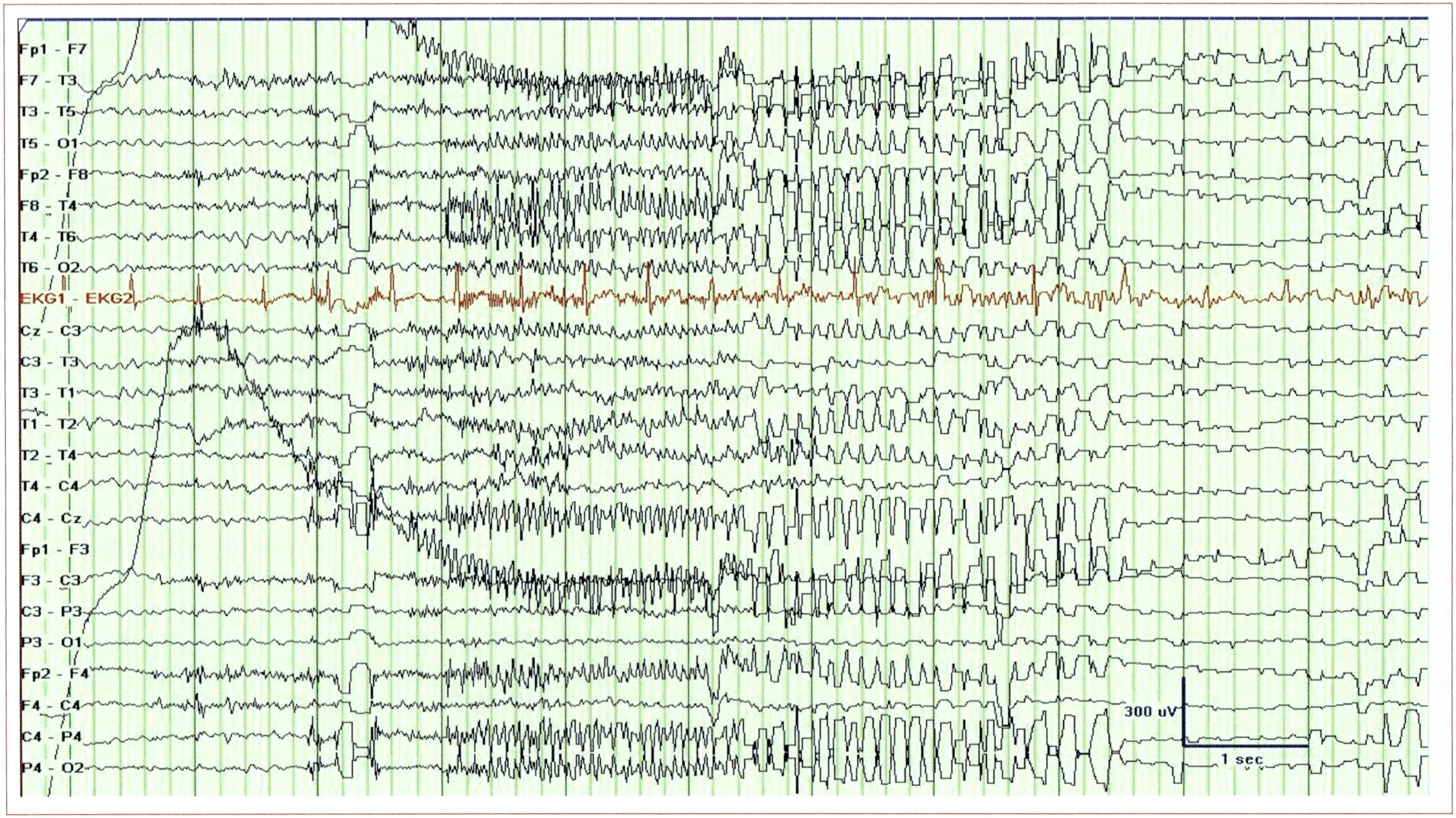

FIGURE 7.37: Multiplexing artifact in second 6 when a laptop is brought close to the cable during video-EEG monitoring.

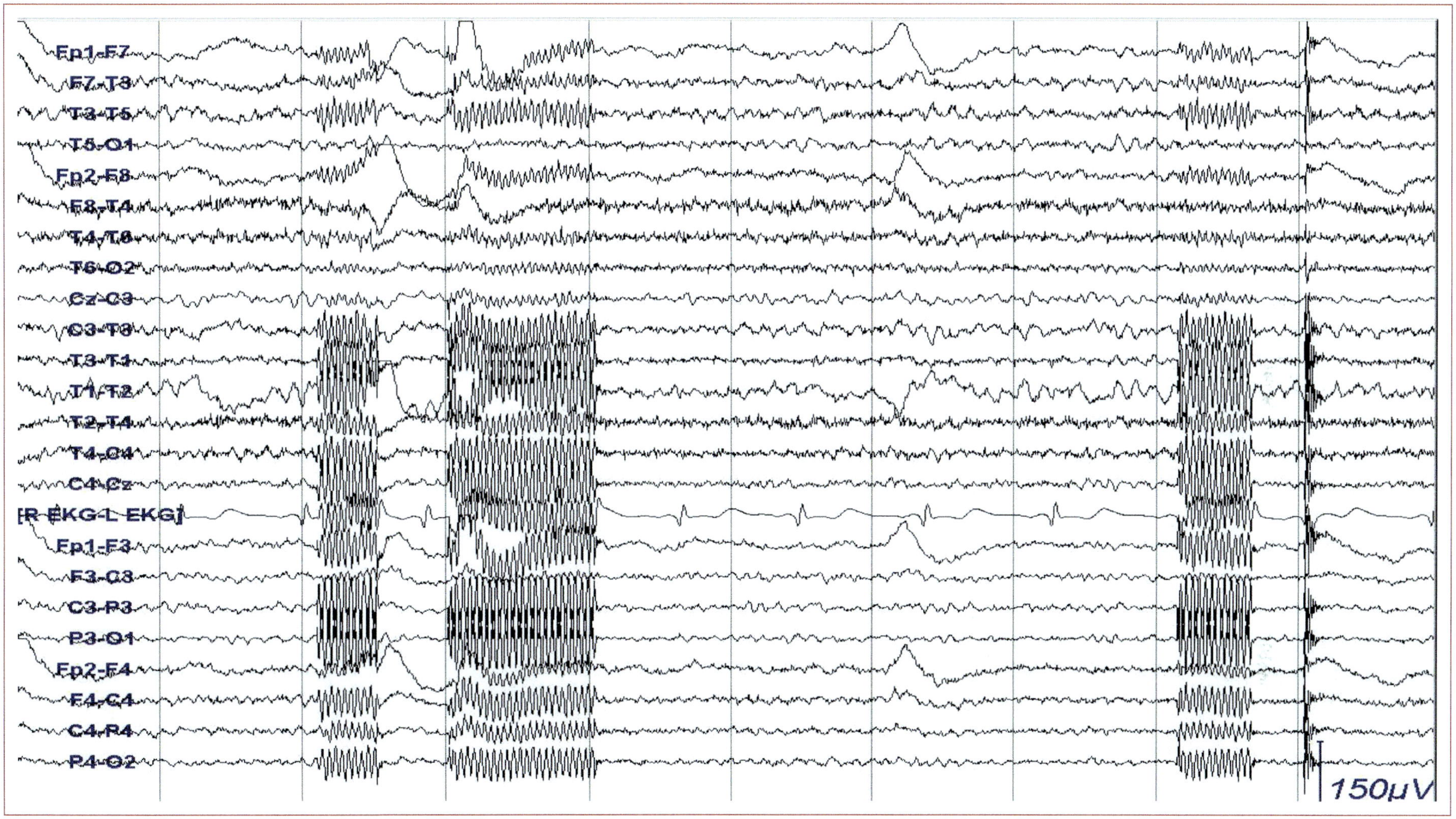

FIGURE 7.38: Artifact generated during telephone ringing.

Source: From Tatum WO. *Handbook of EEG Interpretation*. New York, NY: Demos Medical Publishing; 2014:14.

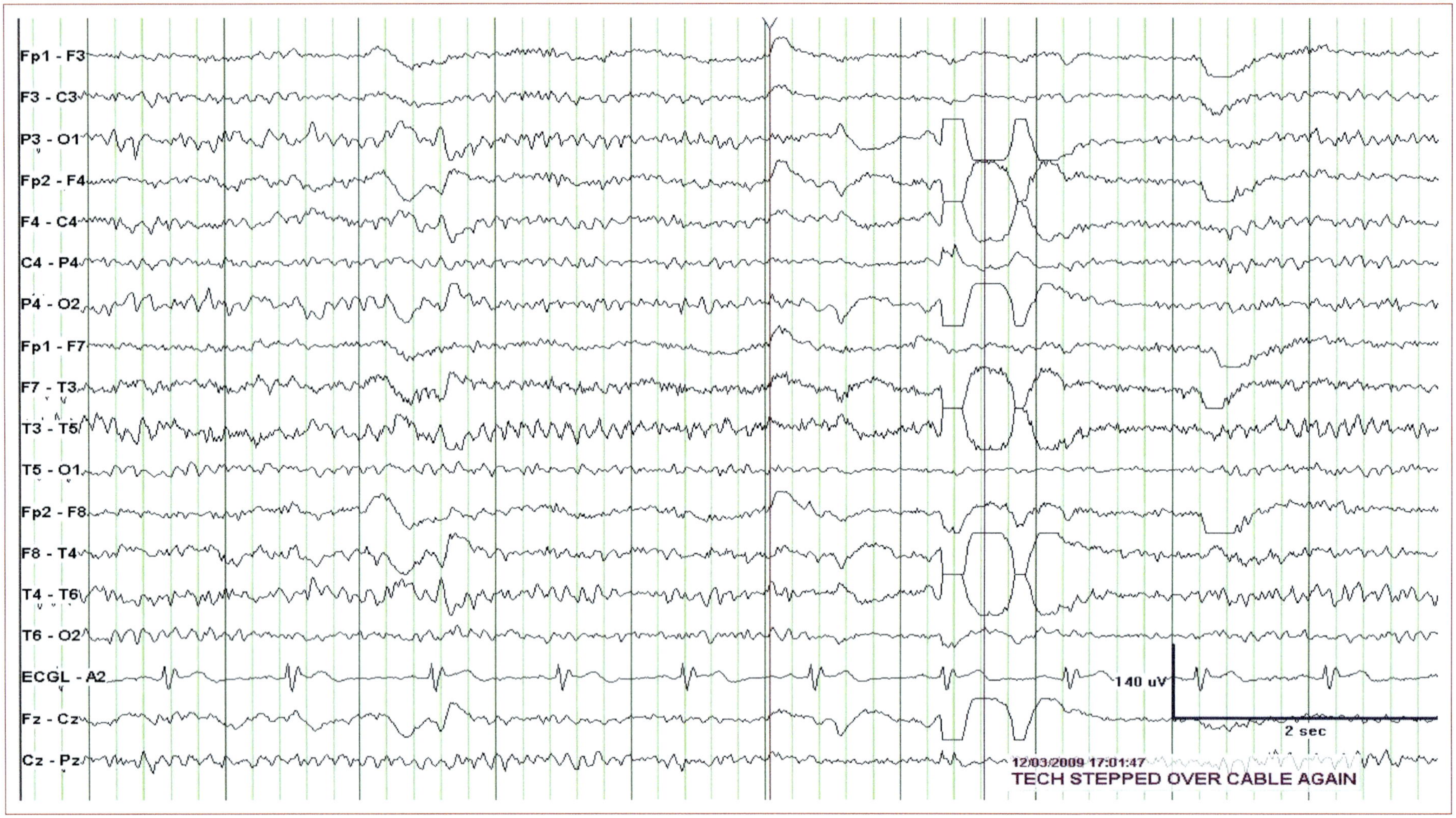

FIGURE 7.39: Capacitance artifact in second 7 caused by compression of the cable when it is accidentally stepped on by the technologist.

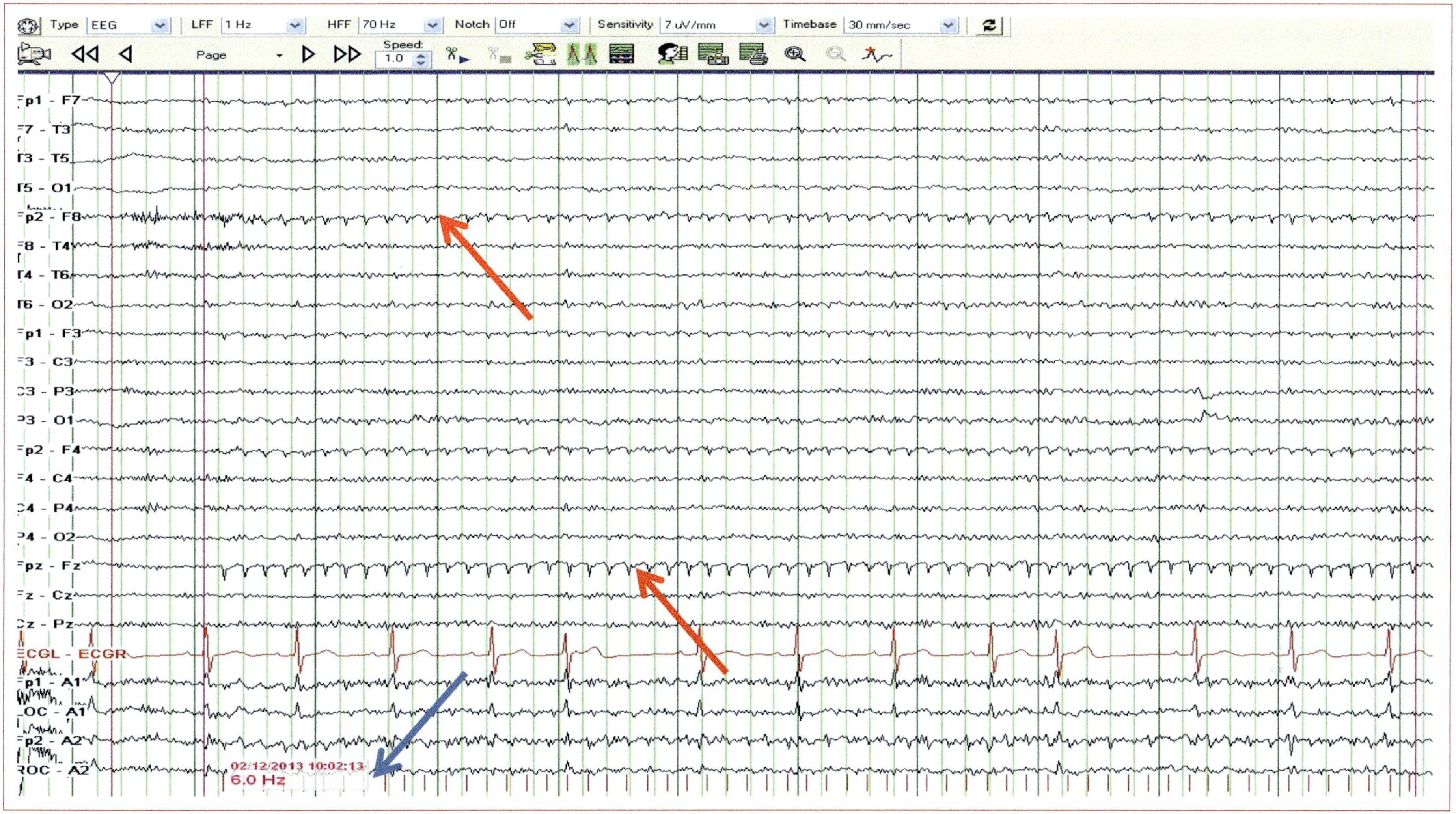

FIGURE 7.40: Photoelectric effect in the frontopolar electrodes (red arrows) during intermittent photic stimulation at 6.0 Hz (blue arrow). Note the asymmetry with greater representation over the right frontopolar head regions due to positioning (head turned left).

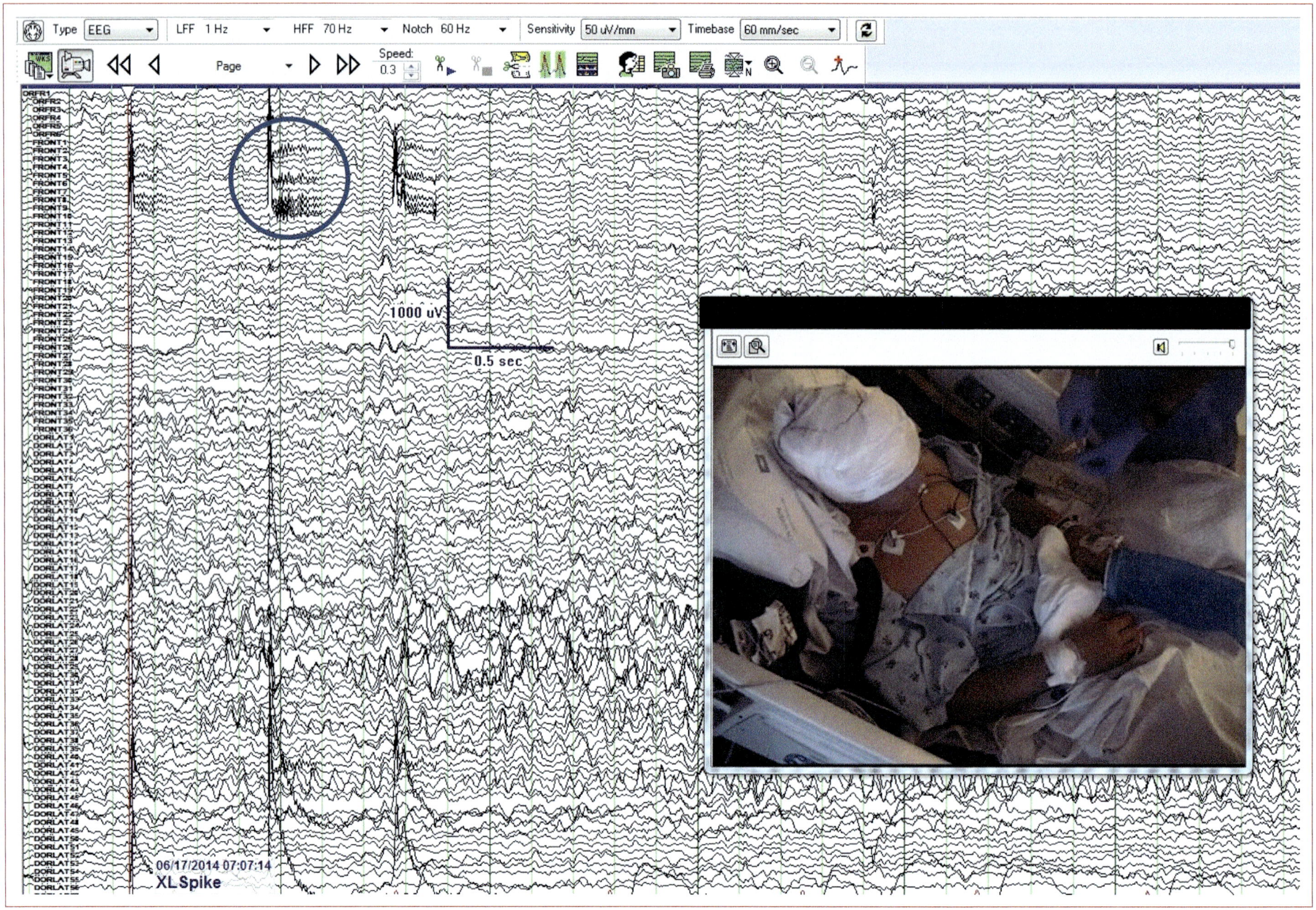

FIGURE 7.41: Complex focal high-frequency artifact (circle) during transitioning recording by the machine. Note the software detection as a "spike."

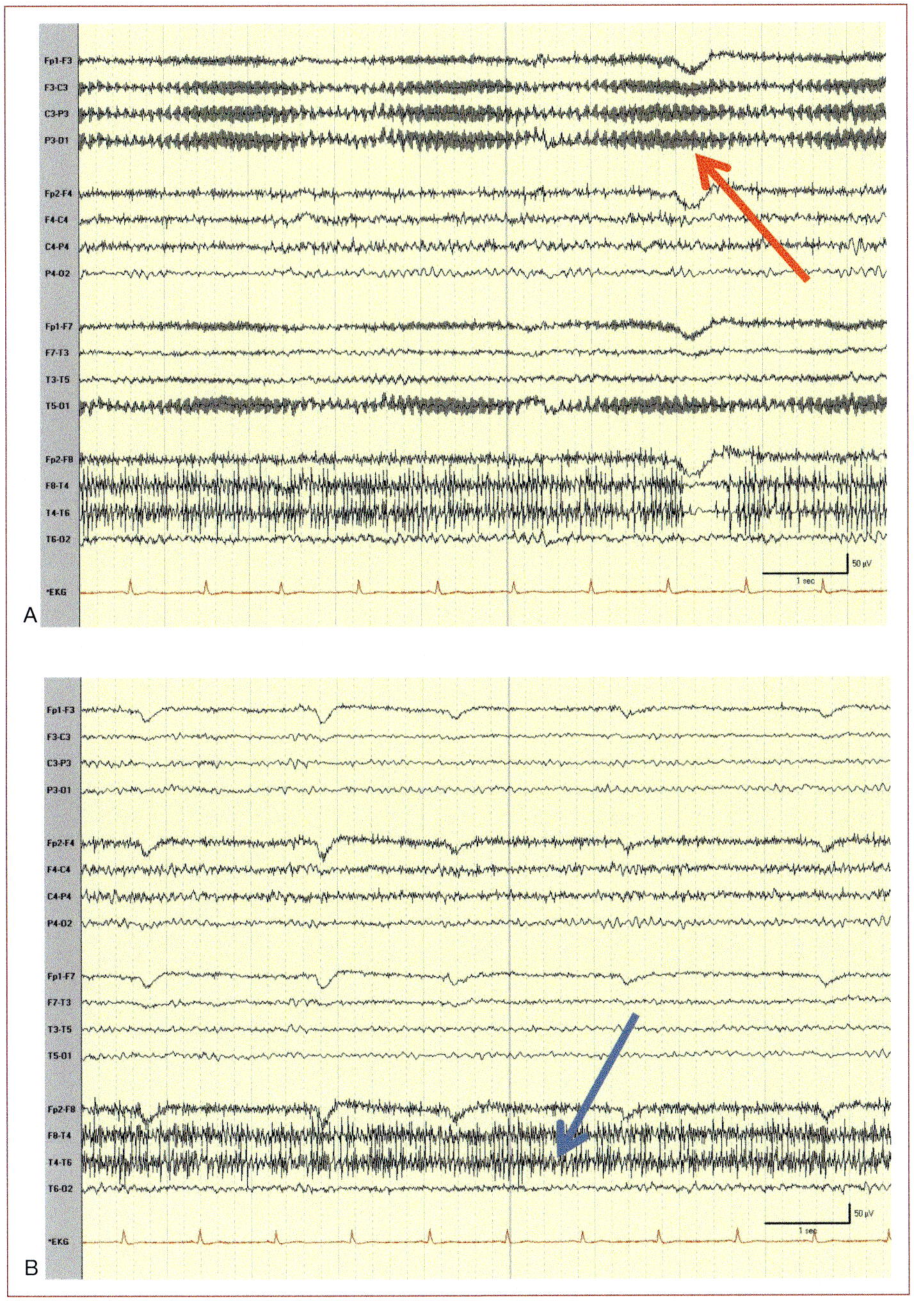

FIGURE 7.42: EEG demonstrating a combination of high-frequency artifacts. (A) 60-Hz artifact obscures the EEG. (B) 60-Hz artifact is eliminated after application of the notch filter (red arrow). Note the presence of myogenic artifact is unaffected due to a frequency that is not produced at 60 Hz (blue arrow).

Source: From Tatum WO. *Handbook of EEG Interpretation*. New York, NY: Demos Medical Publishing; 2014:25-26.

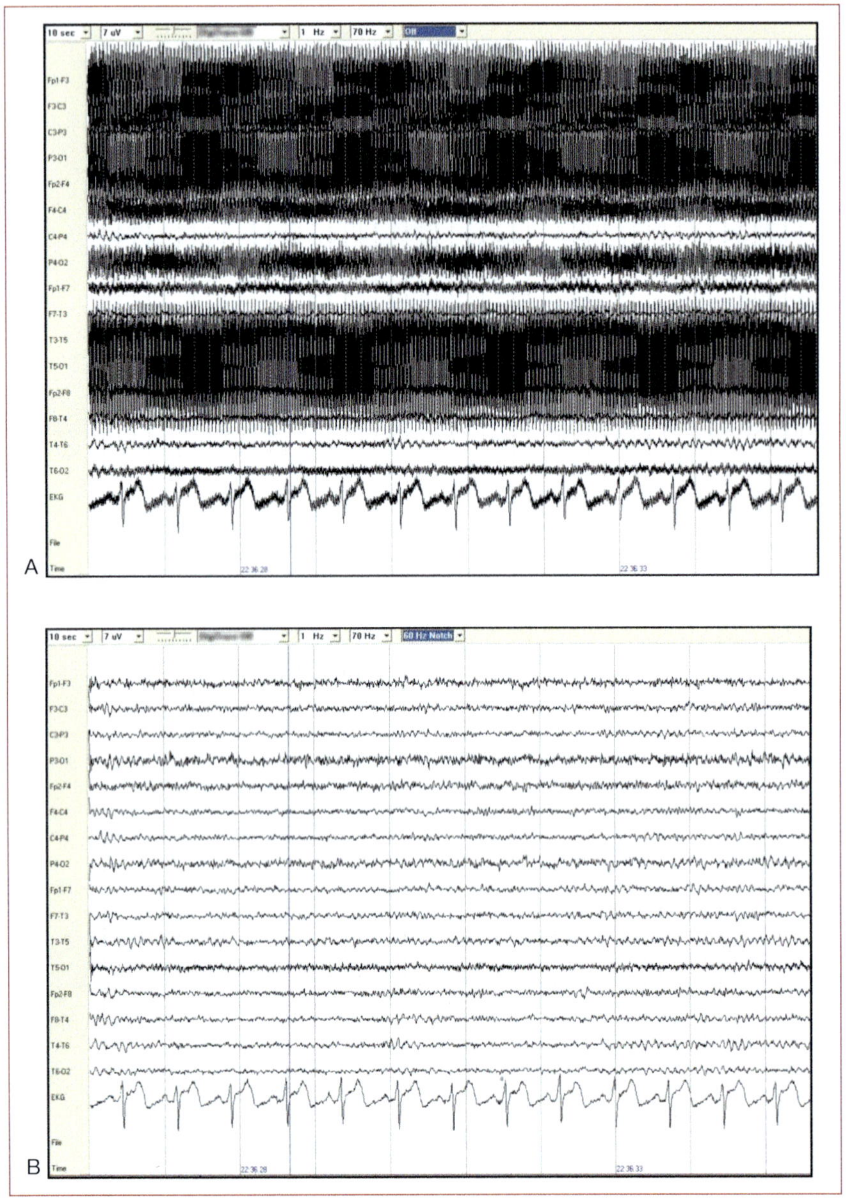

FIGURE 7.43: (A) 60-Hz artifact during ambulatory EEG. (B) 60-Hz artifact resolved following application of the 60-Hz notch filter. Note that without the notch filter, the aEEG would be uninterpretable.

aEEG, ambulatory EEG.

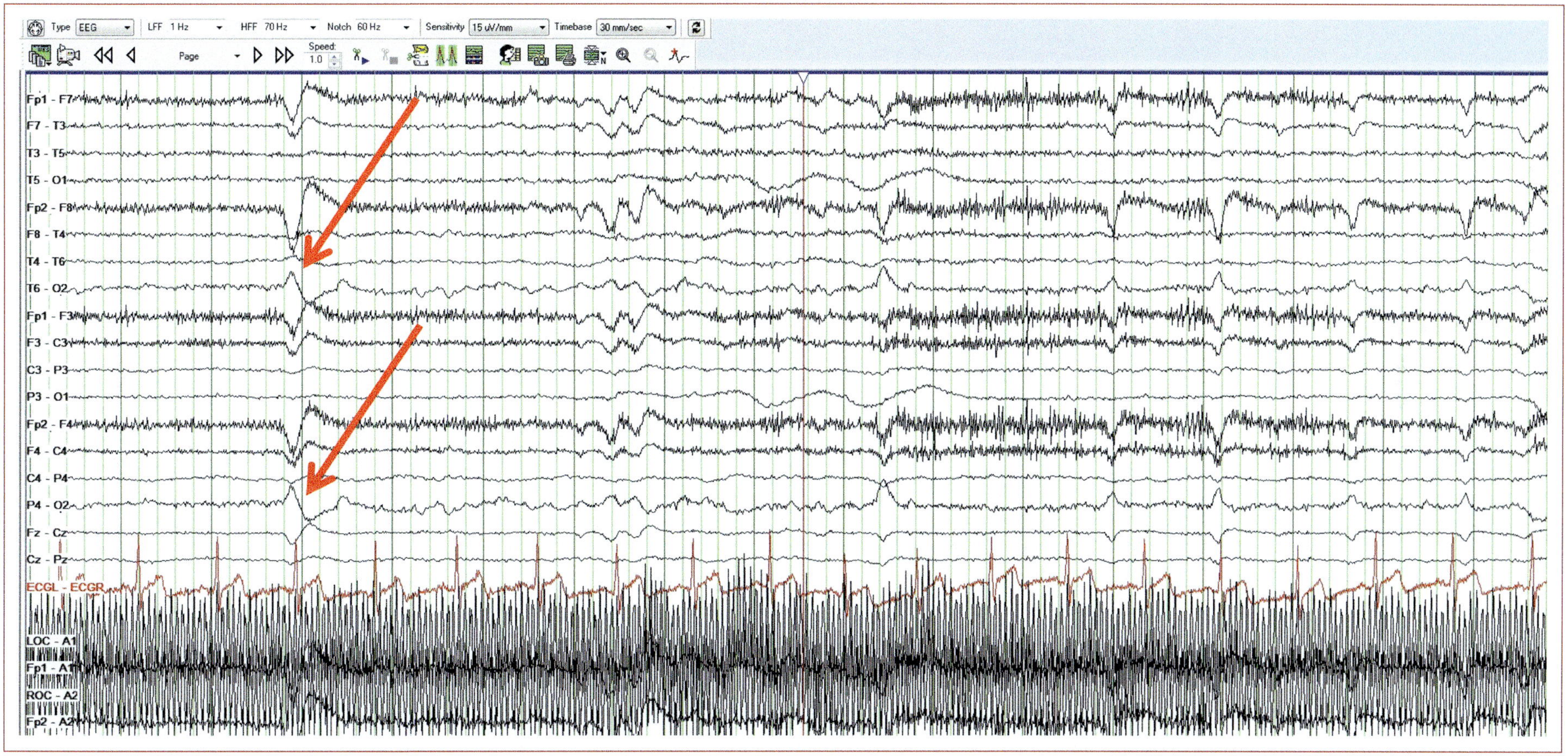

FIGURE 7.44: Ground loop recording in the right occipital electrode (O_2). Note the similar morphology but opposite polarity in a single channel (arrows) due to the amplifier "seeing" the ground instead of O_2.

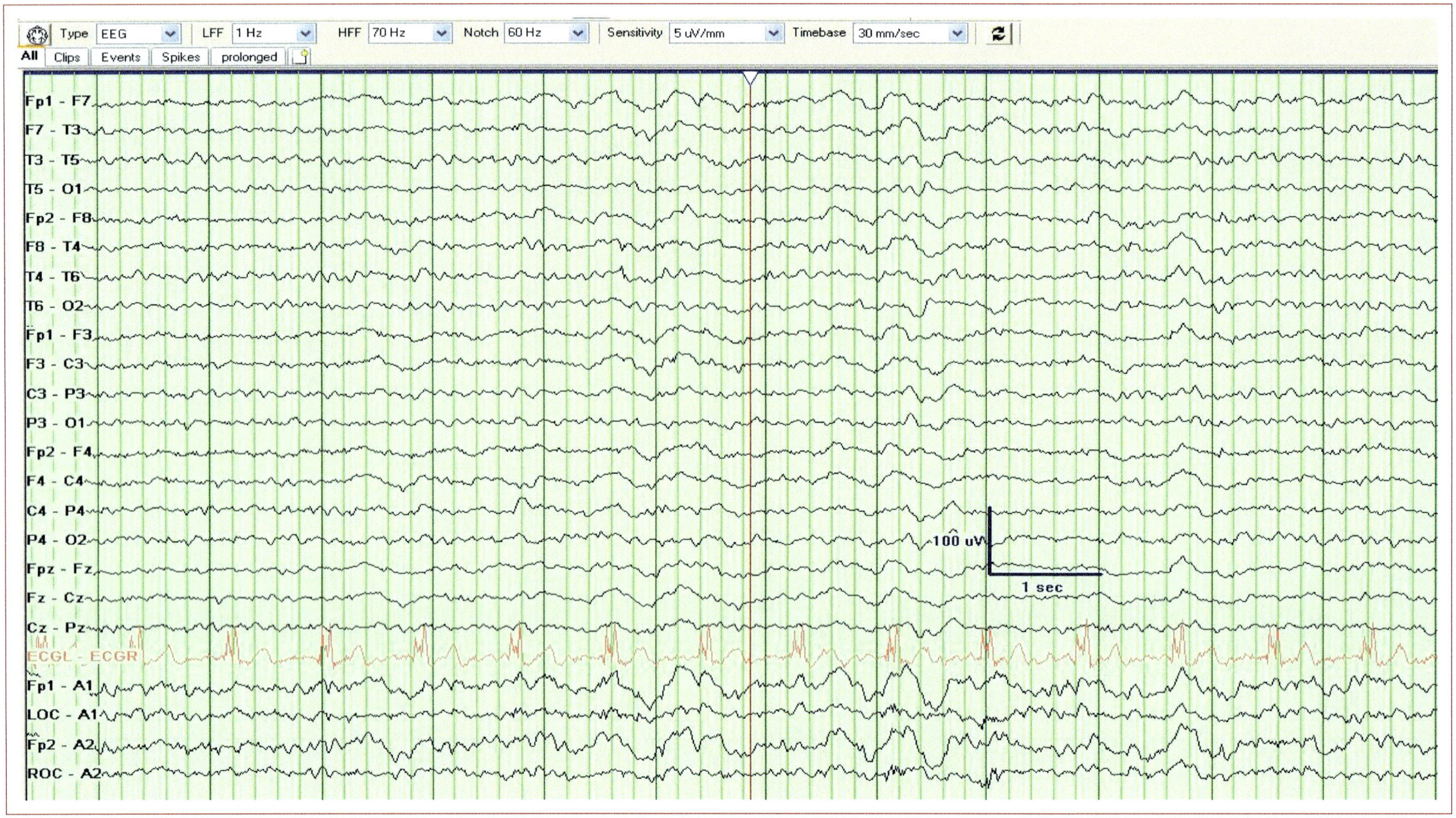

FIGURE 7.45: Pacemaker artifact present in the ECG lead. During sleep, paroxysmal atrial fibrillation led to pacemaker dependence identified during EEG.

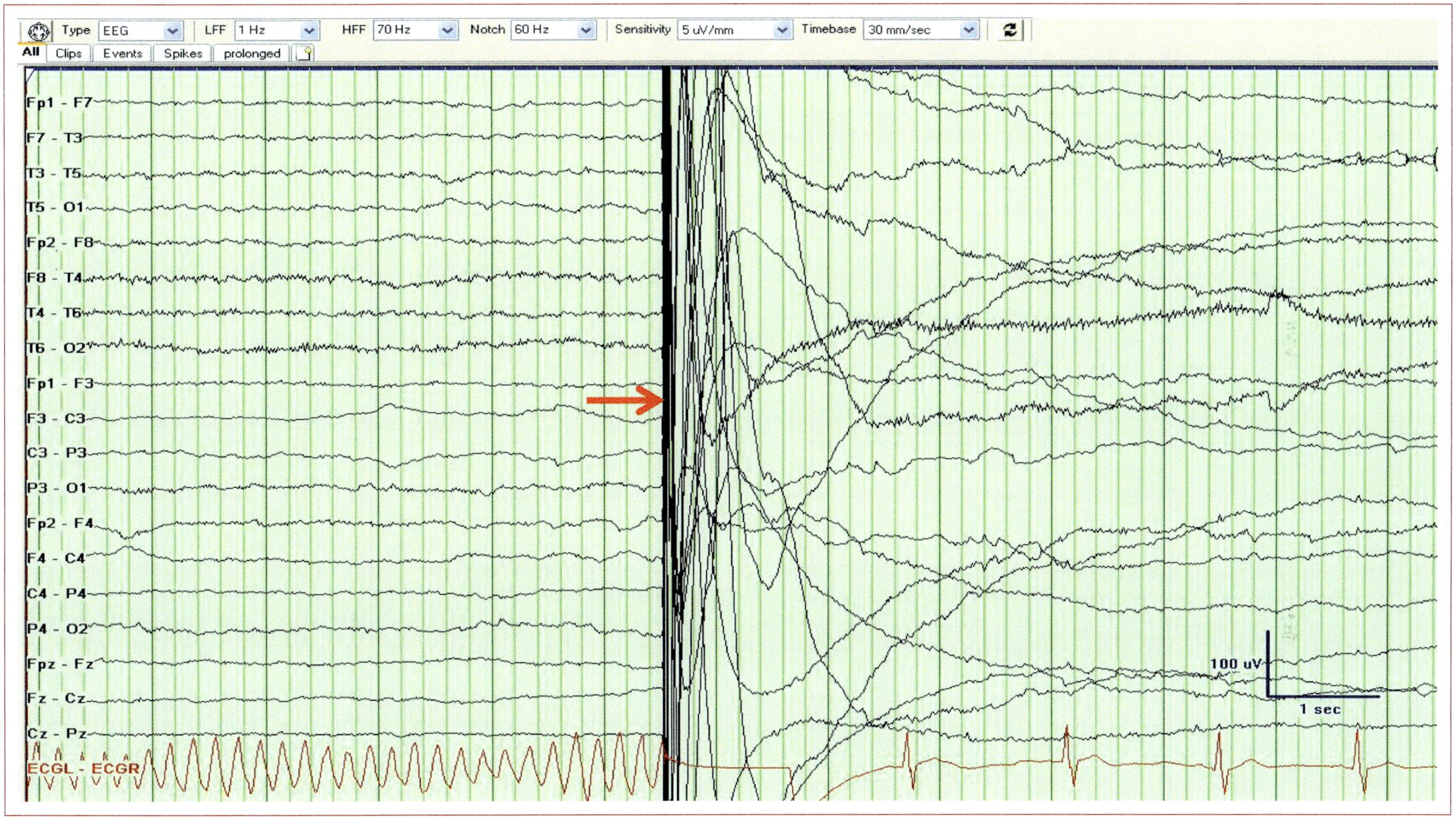

FIGURE 7.46: Generalized artifact during second 6 caused by an implantable cardiac defibrillator. Note the ventricular tachycardia on the ECG in the first half of the recording, and normal sinus rhythm after the artifact due to the "shock" (arrow).

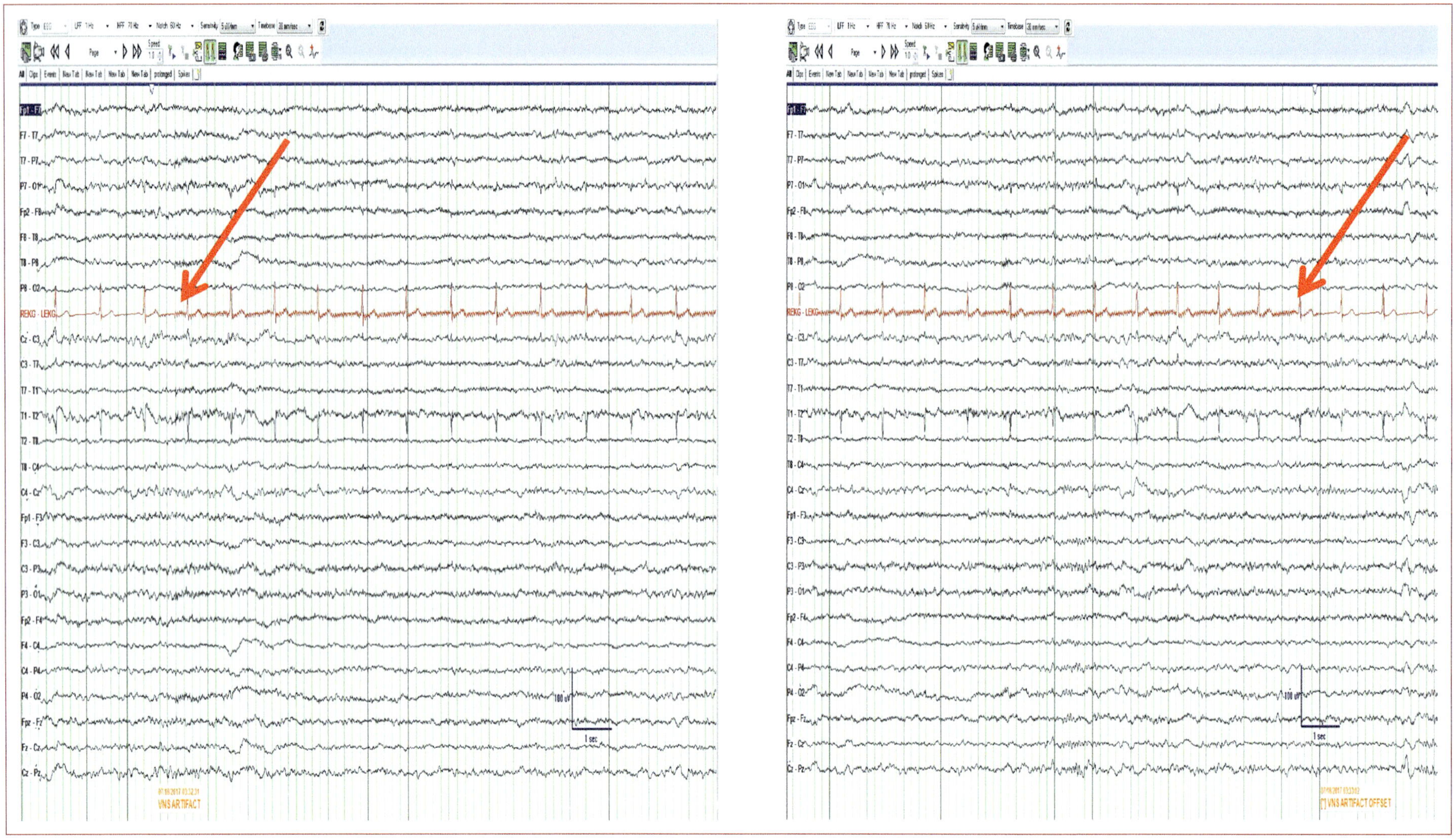

FIGURE 7.47: VNS artifact. During EEG recording, the patient complained the VNS was "not working." However, VNS artifact was present in the EEG (broken panels below) for 30 seconds. Later interrogation demonstrated intact stimulation with standard settings of 30 seconds ON and 5 minutes OFF.

VNS, vagus nerve stimulator.

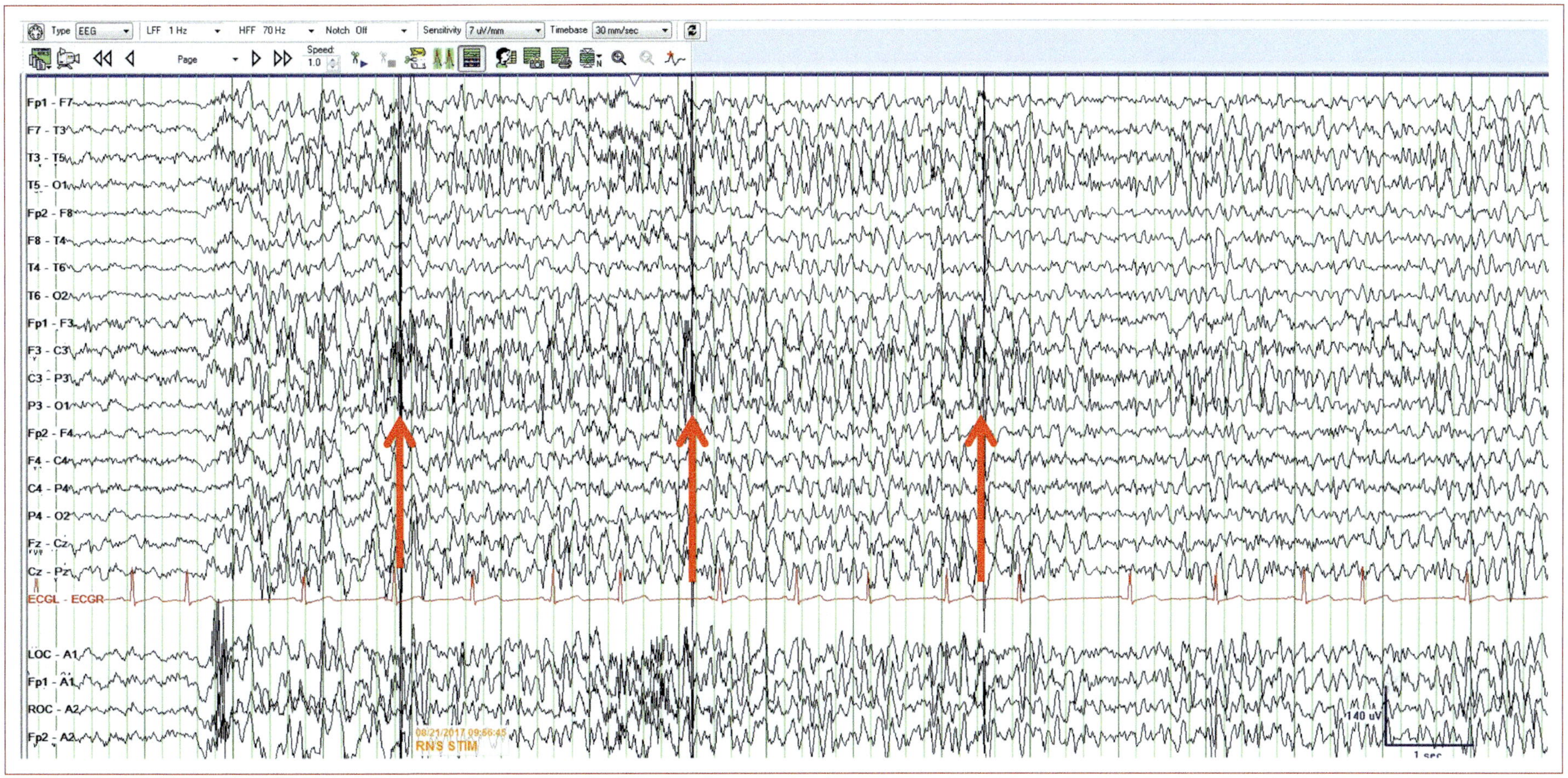

FIGURE 7.48: Electrical artifact due to discharge of the responsive neurostimulator during scalp EEG recording when a left extratemporal seizure was inadvertently captured.

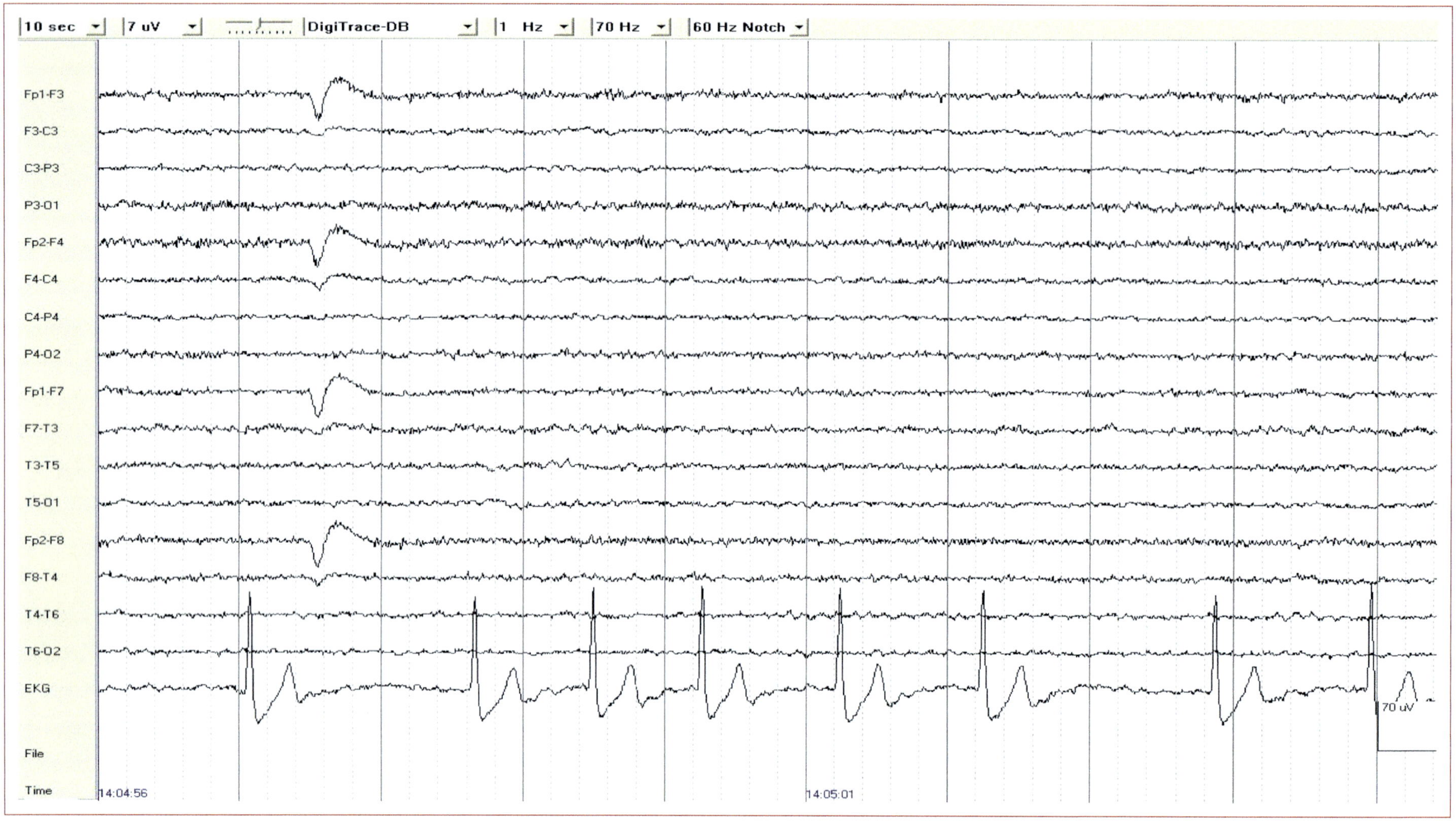

FIGURE 7.49: Ambulatory EEG performed for evaluation of "spells" unexpectedly detected paroxysmal atrial fibrillation during prolonged overnight recording, leading to cardiogenic near-syncope.

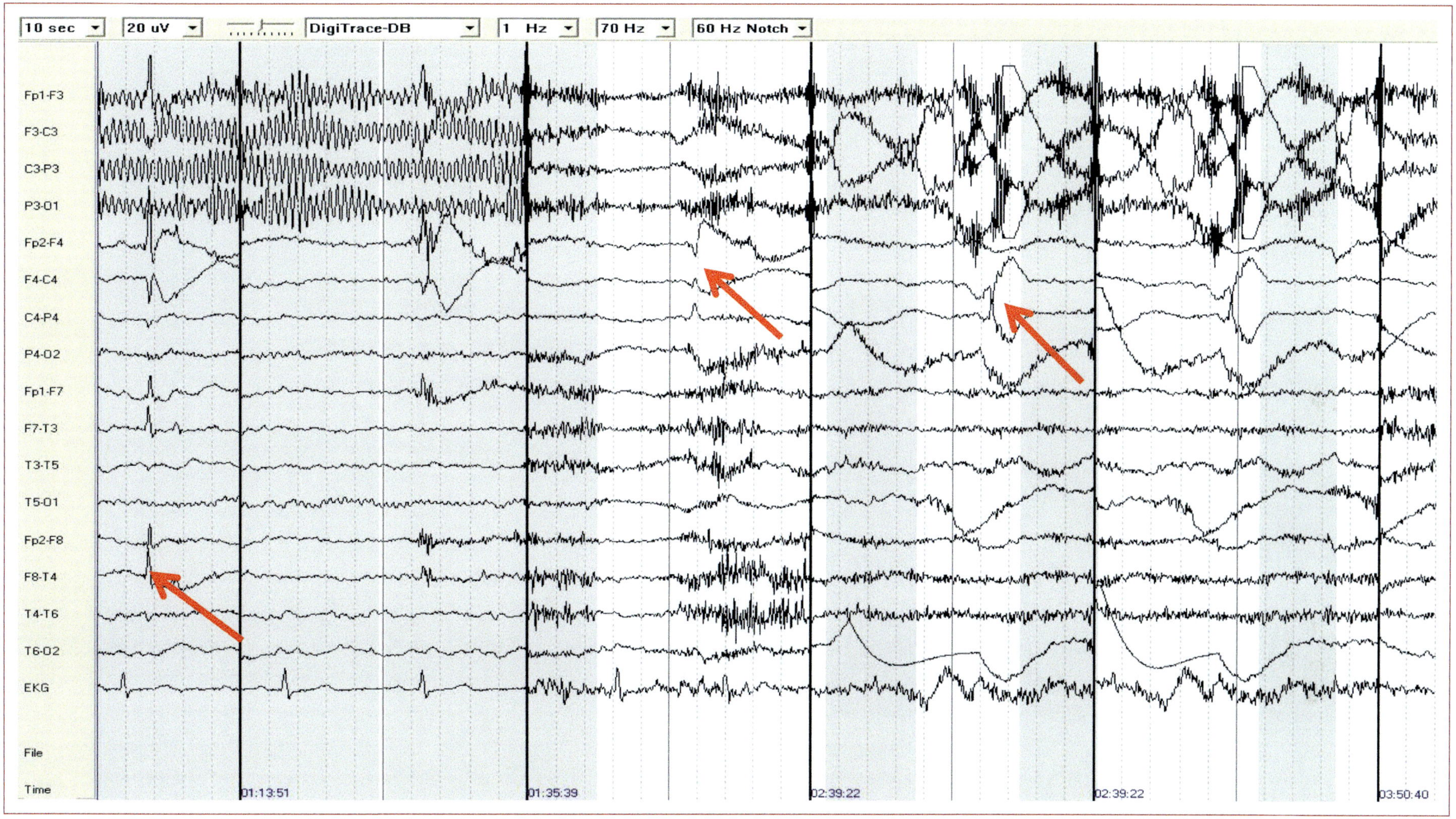

FIGURE 7.50: Spike detections (arrows) by the aEEG associated with multiple artifacts identified as spikes by the algorithm. Multiple artifacts including 60 Hz, electrode, myogenic, ECG, and movement generated.

Source: From Tatum WO. Artifact and ambulatory EEG. In: Tatum WO, ed. *Ambulatory EEG Monitoring*. New York, NY: Demos Medical Publishing; 2017:43.

aEEG, ambulatory EEG.

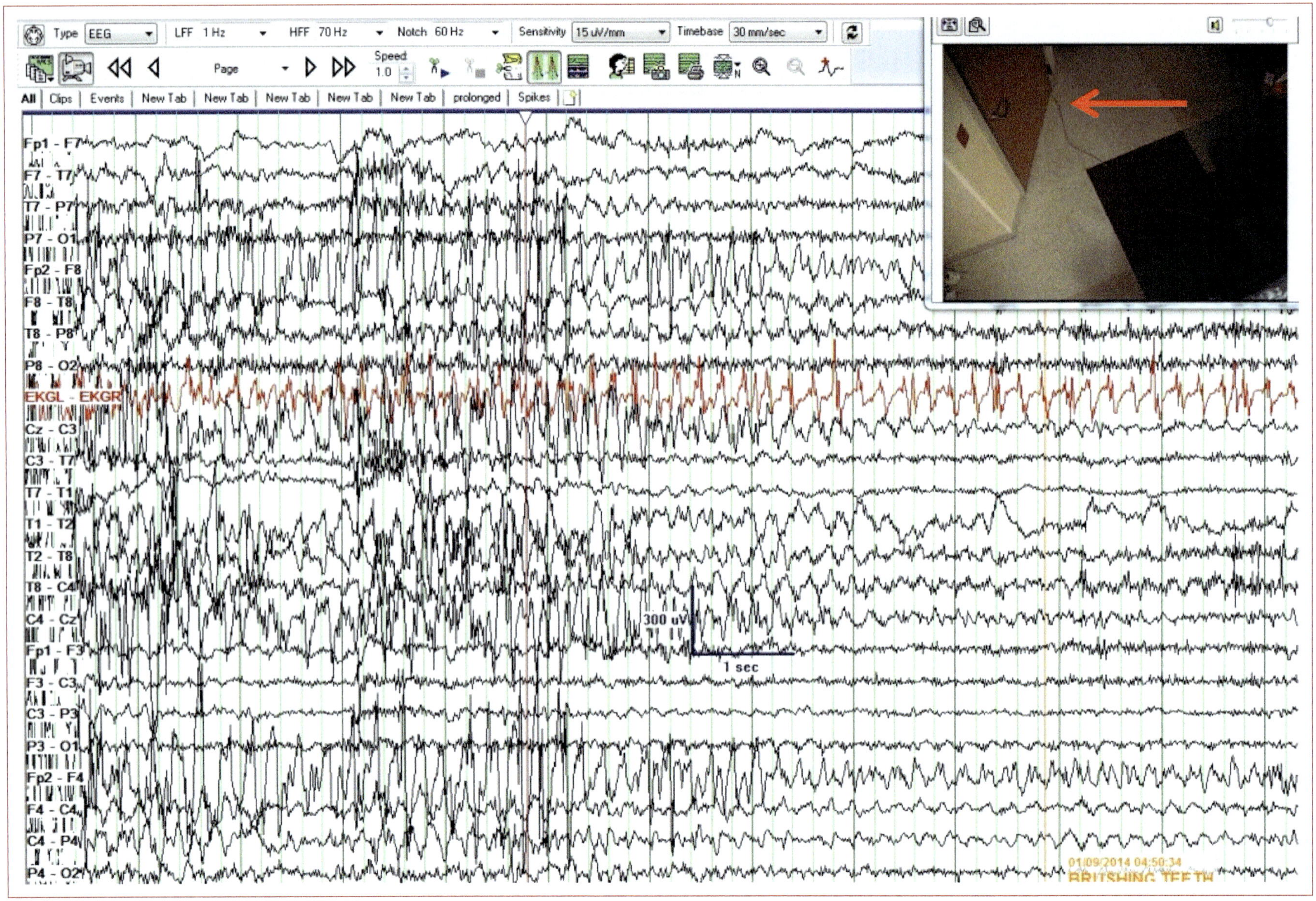

FIGURE 7.51: Toothbrushing artifact during EMU admission. Note the rhythmical 4-Hz activity mimicking a focal seizure. The video in the upper right-hand corner is unable to correlate with the EEG findings. See the cable (arrow) leading into the bathroom.

Source: From Benbadis, SR. The EEG in nonepileptic seizures. J Clin Neurophys. 2006;23(4):340-352.

EMU, epilepsy monitoring unit.

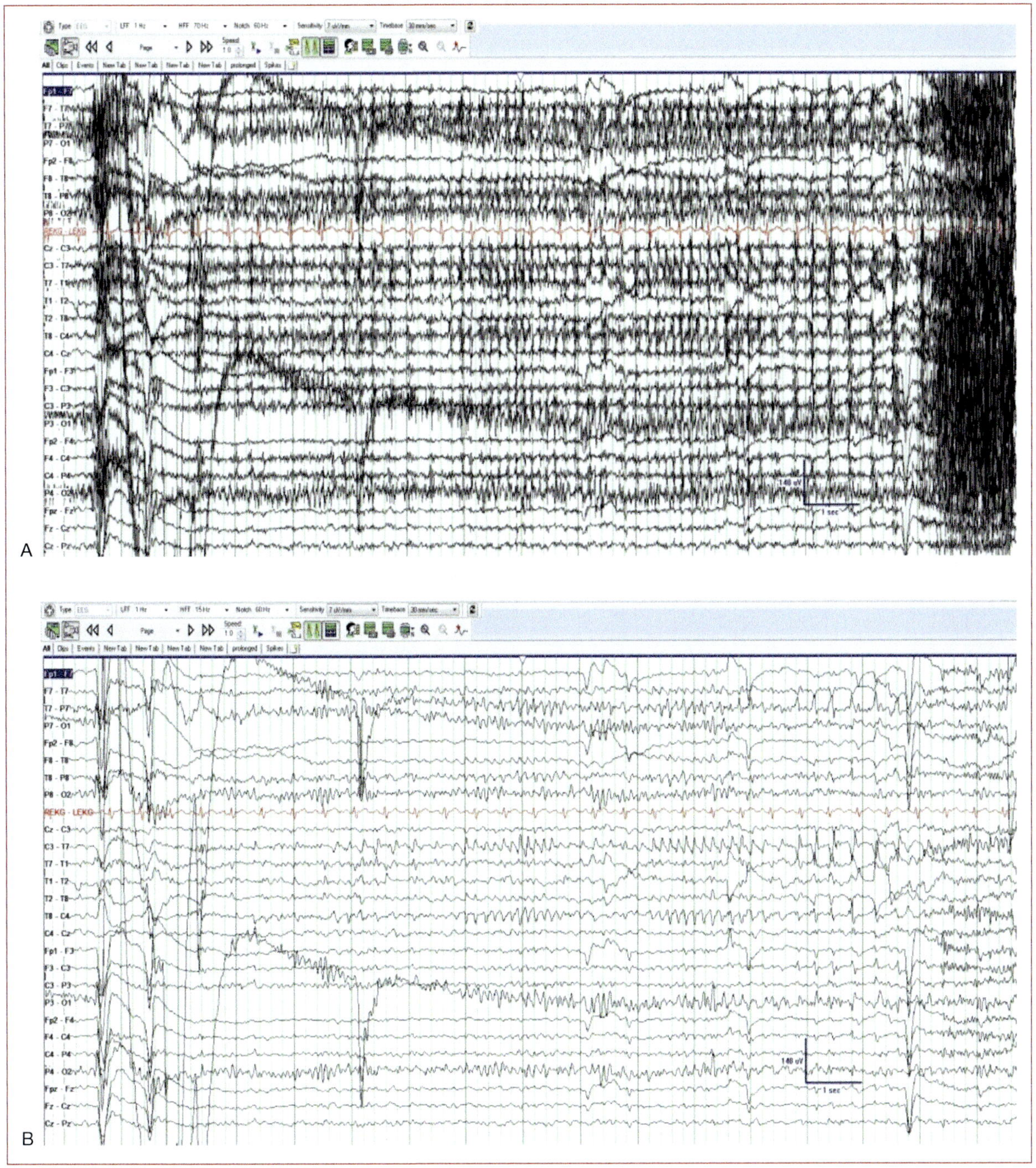

FIGURE 7.52: EEG obscured by phasic myogenic artifact during a seizure in (A) with 70-Hz HFF and (B) after a 15-Hz LFF is applied. Note the false representation of the ictal recording in (B) when overfiltering is used to "clean up" the tracing.

HFF, high-frequency filter; LFF, low-frequency filter.

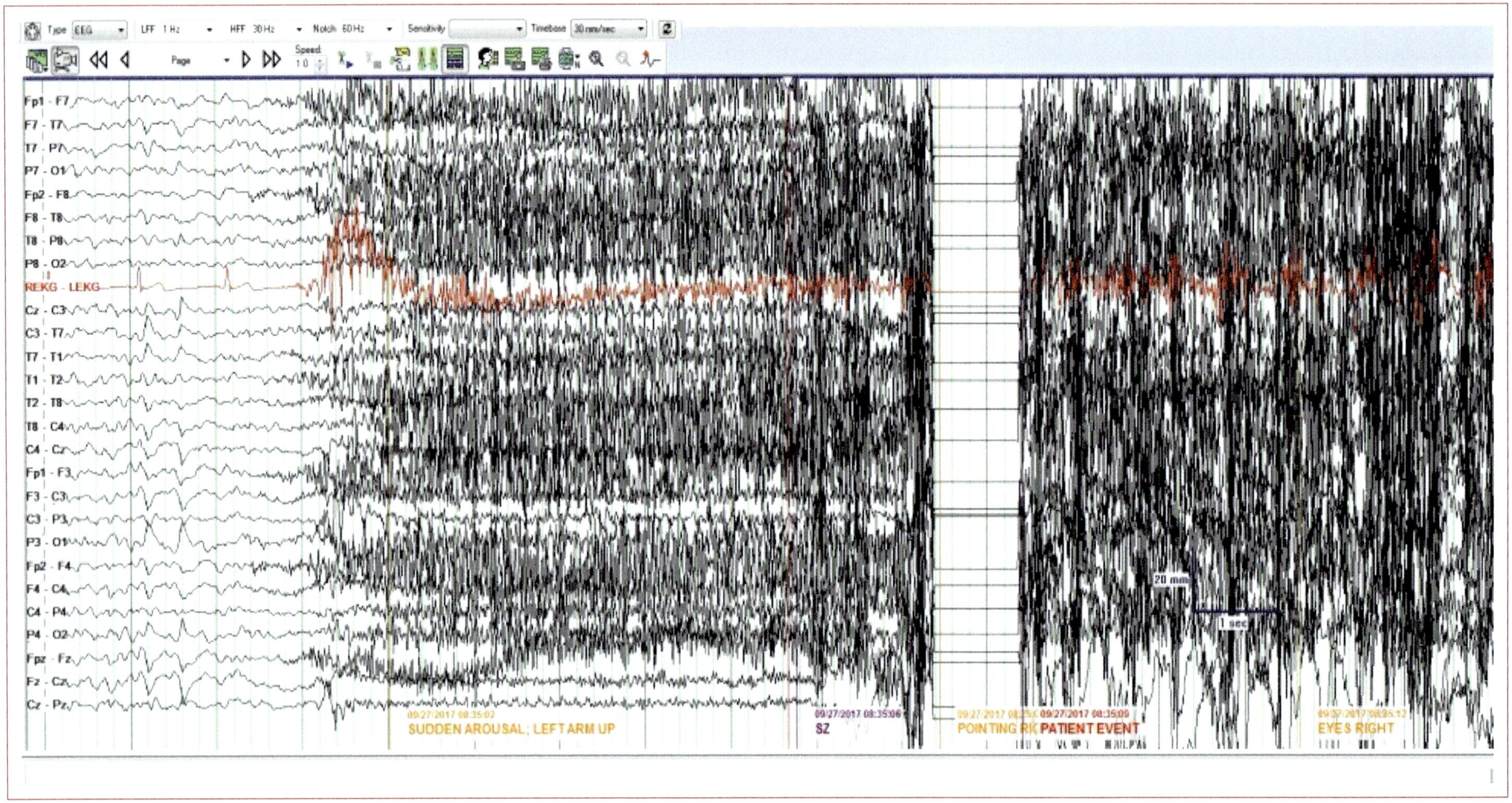

Figure 7.53: Seizure monitoring in the EMU with obscuration of seizure onset by myogenic and movement artifact. Note in addition the transient instrumental artifact during second 10 due to loss of the reference electrode.

EMU, epilepsy monitoring unit.

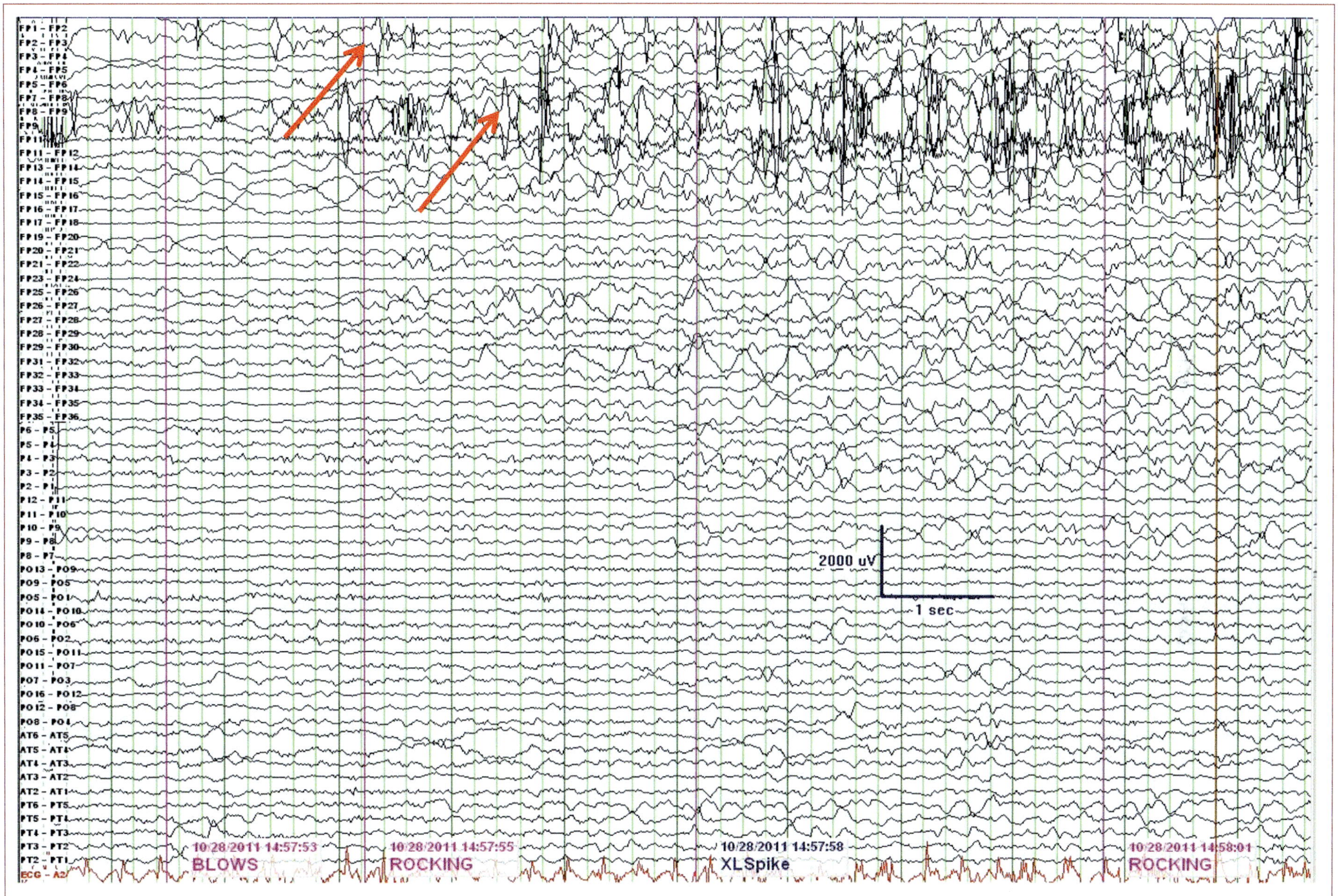

FIGURE 7.54: Intracranial ictal EEG during onset of a frontal lobe seizure emanating from the frontopolar head region. Note the superimposed grid electrode artifacts (arrows) produced by patient movement.

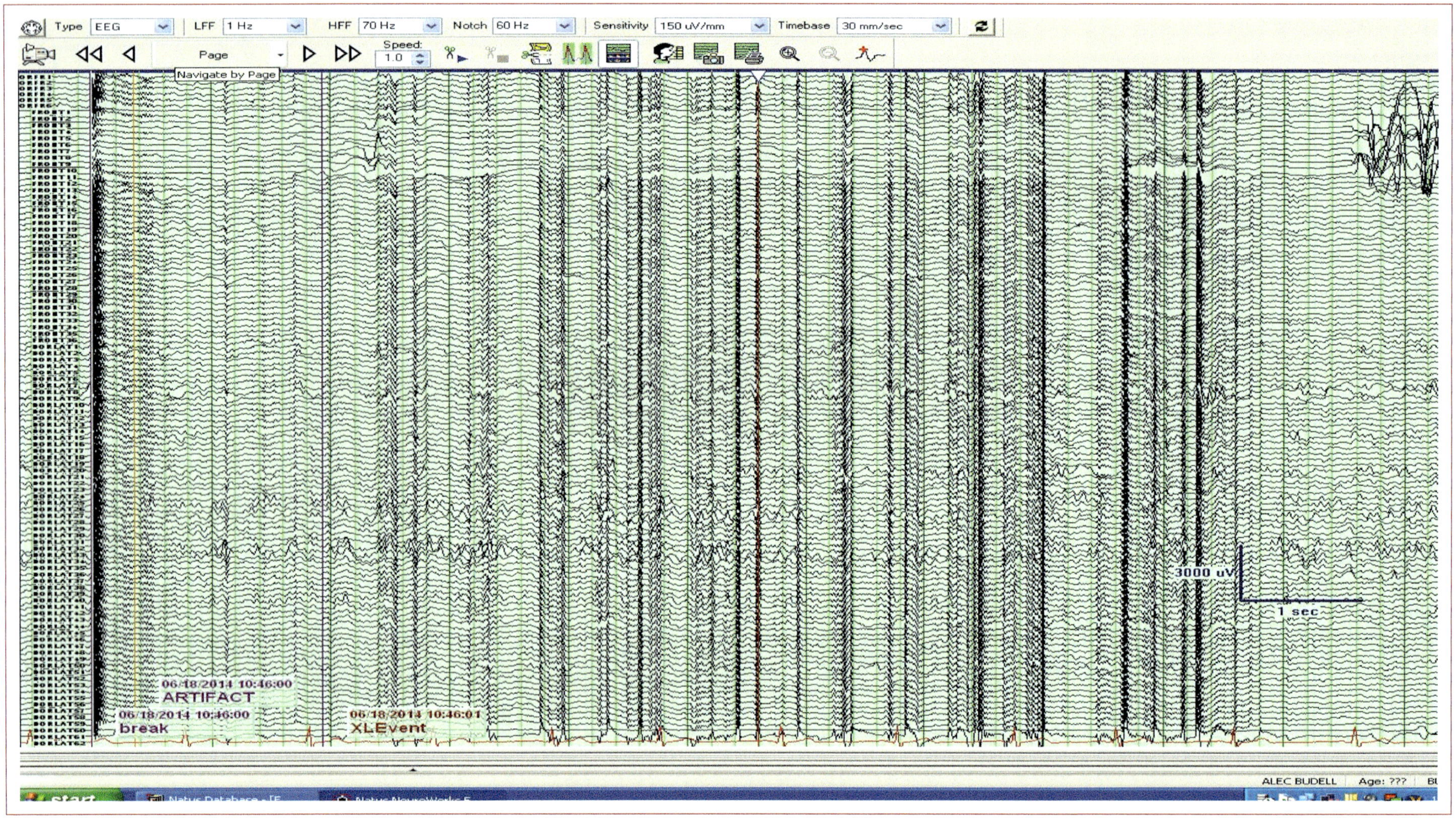

FIGURE 7.55: Generalized artifact obscuring intracranial EEG due to rolling of the "tail" prior to connecting to the cable.

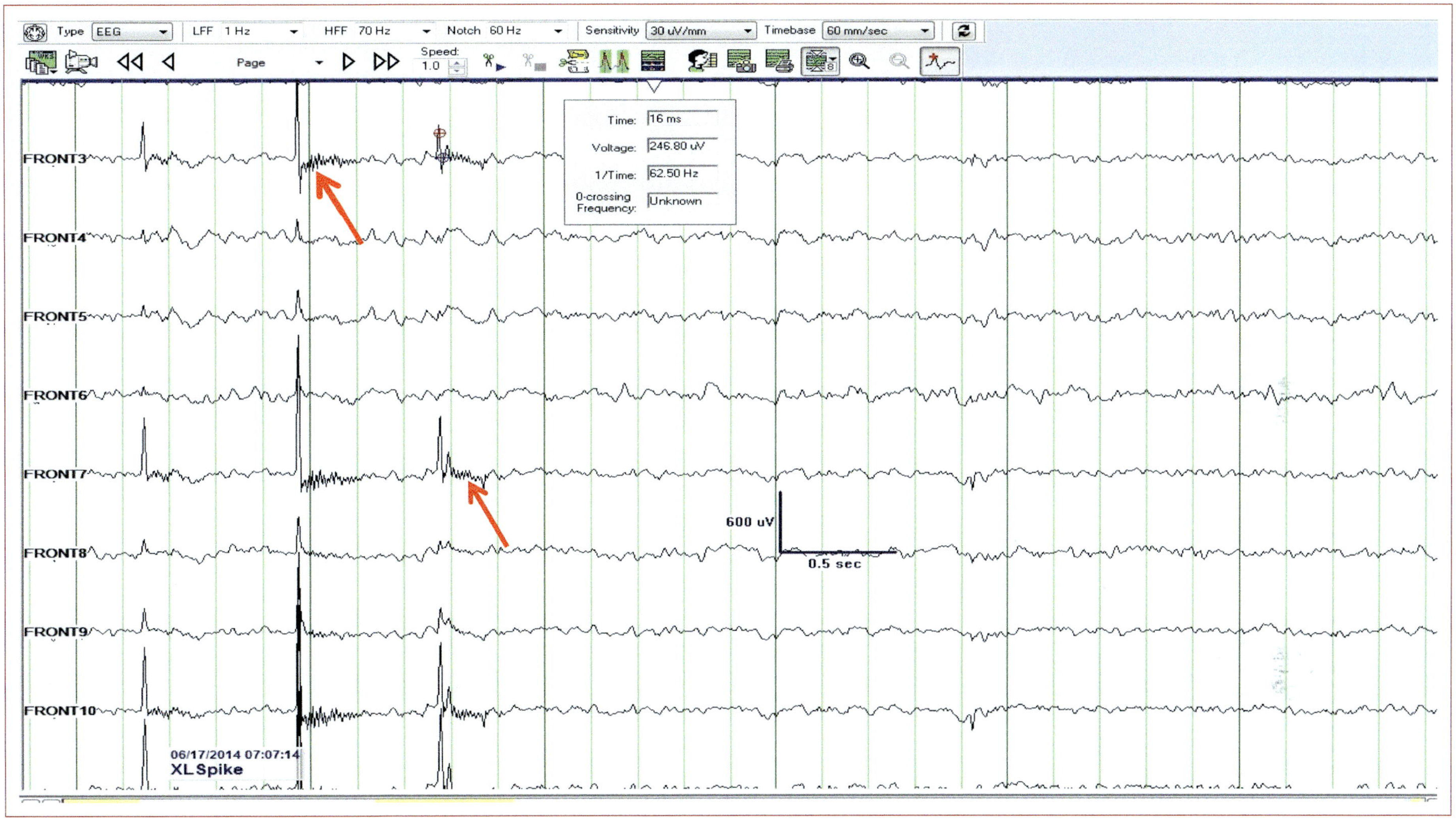

FIGURE 7.56: Artifactual spikes during iEEG recording. Note the pseudohigh-frequency oscillations (gamma frequency) associated with the spike (arrows).

iEEG, intracranial EEG.

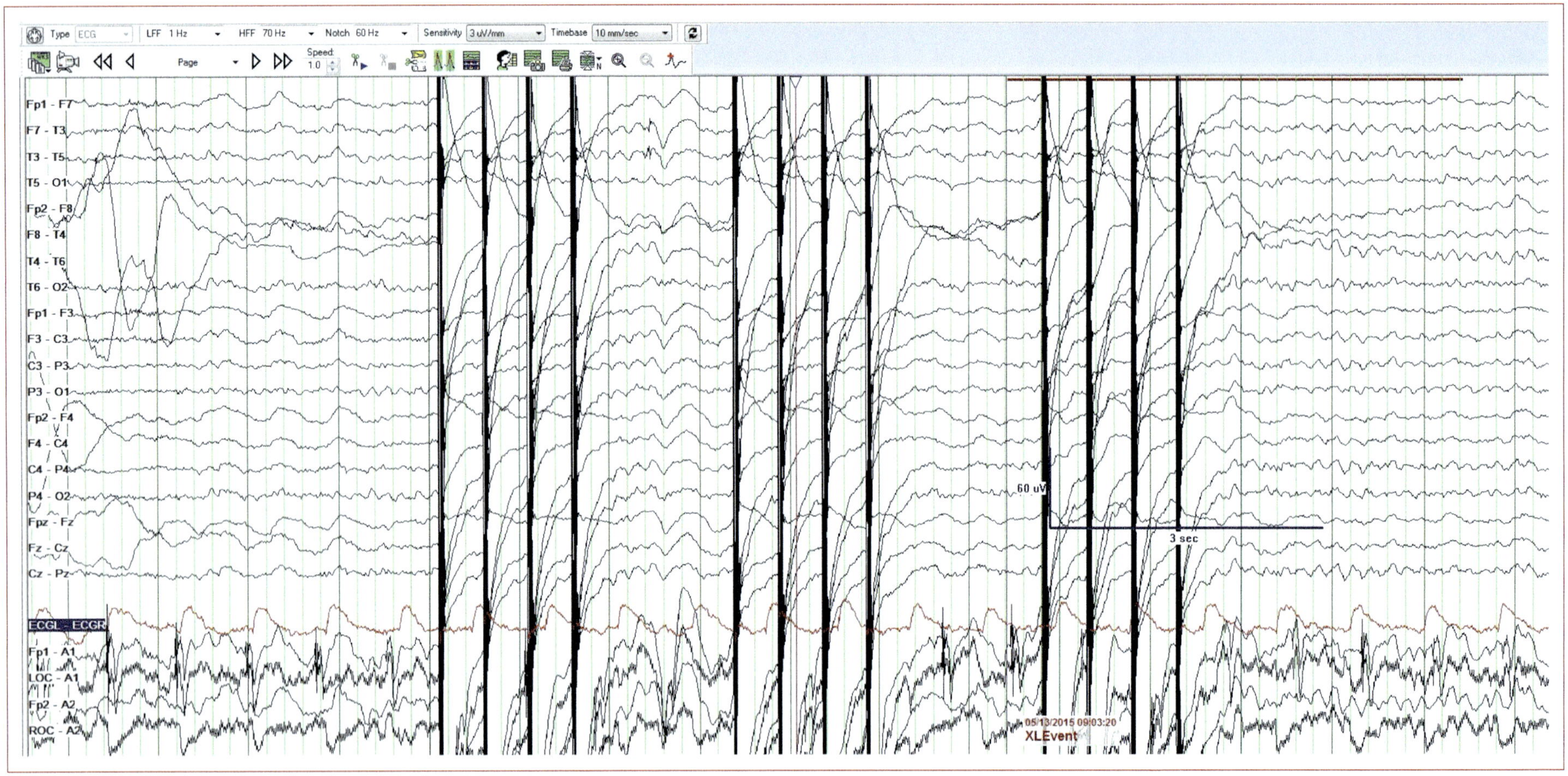

FIGURE 7.57: Characteristic train of four artifact produced in the operating room during carotid endarterectomy to ensure adequate anesthesia.

Source: From Tatum WO, Reinsberger C, Dworetzky B. Artifacts of recording. In: Schomer DL, Lopes da Silva FH, eds. *Niedermeyer's Electroencephalography: Basic Principles, Clinical Applications, and Related Fields*. 7th ed. New York, NY: Oxford University Press; 2018:307, with permission.

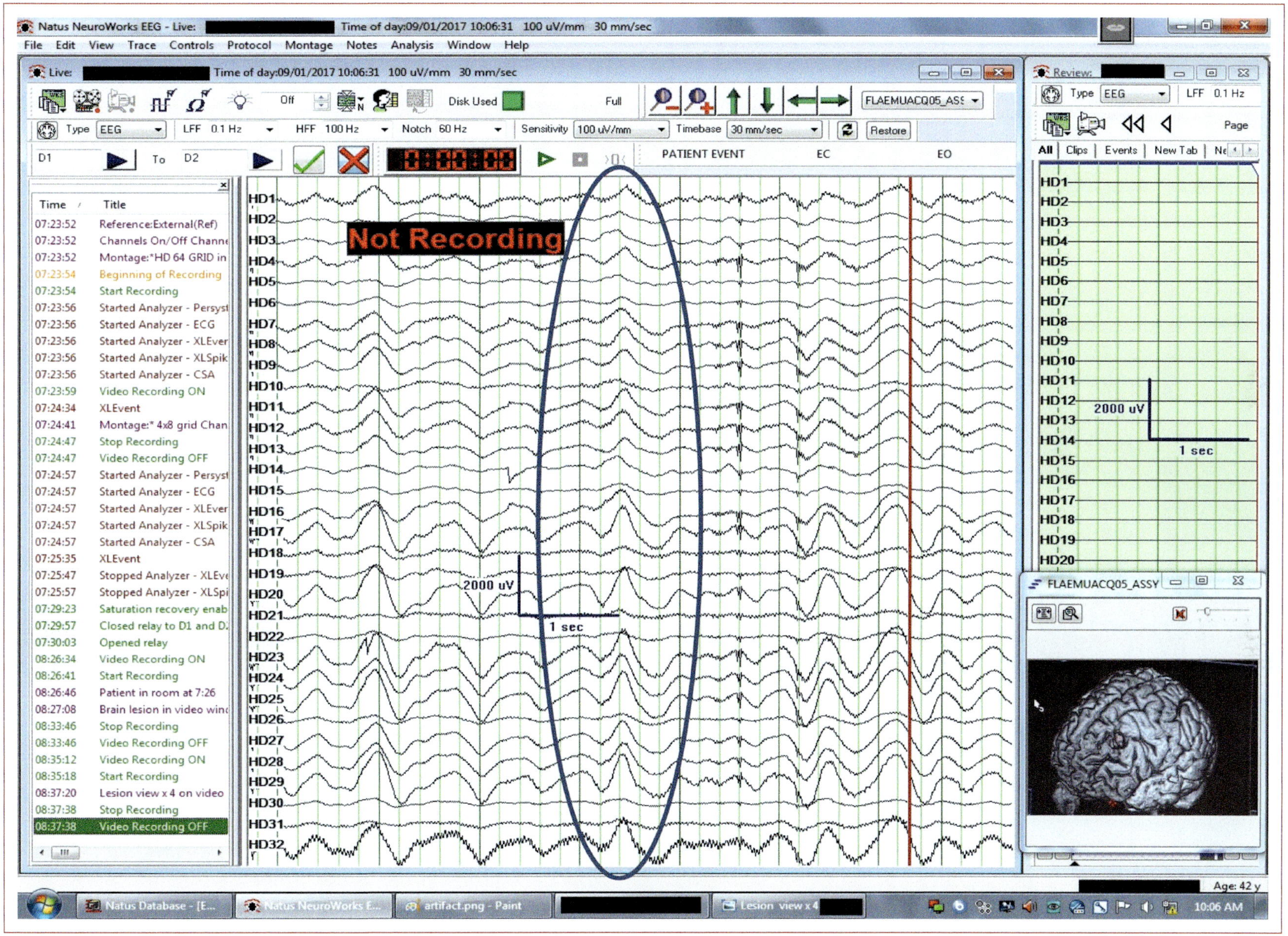

FIGURE 7.58: Electrocorticography performed in the OR with a 32-channel grid not in contact with the patient's brain. Note the waveforms (oval) despite an absence of recording noted in the reviewer box in the right upper corner.

OR, operating room.

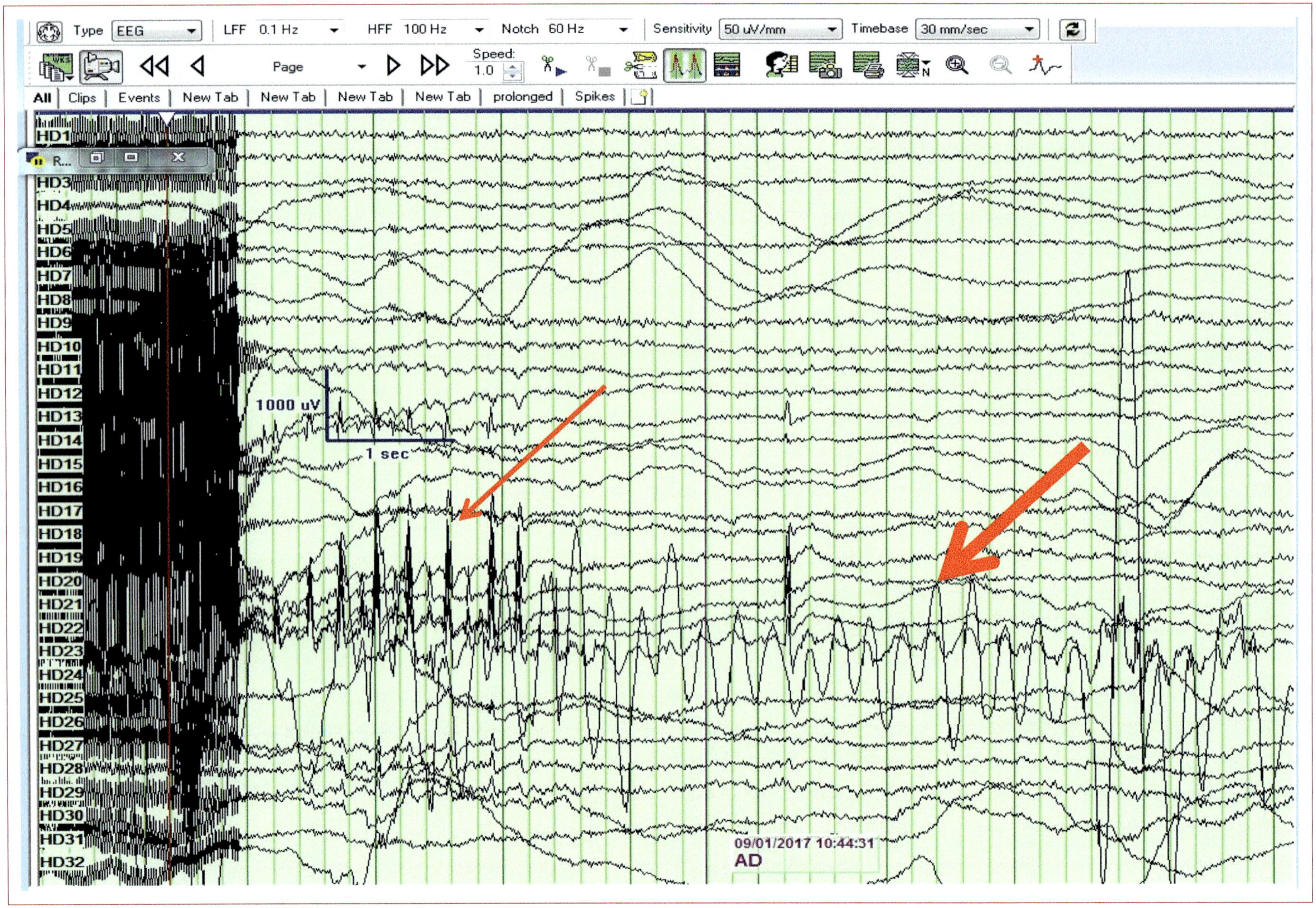

FIGURE 7.59: Intraoperative ECoG with an initial stimulation artifact during electro-cortical stimulation and the artifactual after-discharge (thick arrow) that follows a true after-discharge (thin arrow).

ECoG, electrocorticography.

REFERENCES

1. Olejniczak P. Neurophysiologic basis of EEG. *J Clin Neurophysiol*. 2006;23: 186-189. doi:10.1097/01.wnp.0000220079.61973.6c.
2. Klass DW. The continuing challenge of artifacts in the EEG. *Am J EEG Tech*. 1995;35:239-269. doi:10.1080/00029238.1995.11080524.
3. Tatum WO. EEG interpretation: common problems. *Clin Pract*. 2012;9(5): 527-538. doi:10.2217/cpr.12.51.
4. Beniczky S, Aurlien H, Brogger JC, et al. Standardized computer-based organized reporting of EEG: SCORE. *Epilepsia*. 2013;54(6):1112-1124. doi:10.1111/epi.12135.
5. Tatum WO. Normal "Suspicious" EEG. *Neurology*. 2013;80(suppl 1):S4-S11. doi:10.1212/WNL.0b013e31827974df.
6. Maulsby RL. Some guidelines for assessment of spikes and sharp waves in EEG tracings. *Am J EEG Technol*. 1971;11(1):3-16. doi:10.1080/00029238.1971 .11080808.
7. Krauss GL, Abdallah A, Lesser R, et al. Clinical and EEG features of patients with EEG wicket rhythms misdiagnosed with epilepsy. *Neurology*. 2005;64:1879-1883. doi:10.1212/01.WNL.0000163991.97456.03.
8. Tatum WO, Dworetzky BA, Schomer DL. Artifact and recording concepts in EEG. *J Clin Neurophysiol*. 2011;28:252-263. doi:10.1097/ WNP.0b013e31821c3c93.
9. Tatum WO. Artifact-related epilepsy. *Neurology*. 2013;80(1):S12-S25. doi:10.1212/WNL.0b013e3182797325.
10. Tatum WO. How not to read an EEG: introductory statements. *Neurology*. 2013; 80(1):S1-S3. doi:10.1212/WNL.0b013e318279730e.
11. Benbadis SR, Tatum WO. Over-interpretation of EEGs and misdiagnosis of epilepsy. *J Clin Neurophysiol*. 2003;20:42-44. doi:10.1097/0000469120030 2000-00005.
12. Lesser RP, Luders H, Dinner DS, et al. An introduction to the basic concepts of polarity and localization. *J Clin Neurophysiol*. 1985;2(1):45-61. PMID: 4056016.
13. American Clinical Neurophysiology Society. Guidelines and consensus statements. https://www.acns.org/practice/guidelines#electroencephalography. Accessed August 20, 2017.
14. Chadwick D. Diagnosis of epilepsy. *Lancet*. 1990;336:291-295. doi:10.1016/ 0140-6736(90)91815-R.
15. Aurlien H, Gjerde IO, Aarseth JH, et al. EEG background activity described by a large computerized database. *Clin Neurophysiol*. 2004;115(3):665-673. doi:10.1016/j.clinph.2003.10.019.
16. Ebersole JS. Cortical generators and EEG voltage fields. In: Ebersole JS, Pedley TA, eds. *Current Practice of Clinical Electroencephalography*. 3rd ed. Philadelphia, PA: Lippincott Williams & Wilkins; 2003:12-31.
17. Sullivan L. Introduction. EEG Artifacts. In: *American Society of Electroneurodiagnostic Technologists*. Kansas City, MO: American Society of Electroneurodiagnostic Technologists; 2008:5.
18. Ebersole JS, Hawes-Ebersole S. Clinical application of dipole modeling in the localization of epileptiform activity. *J Clin Neurophysiol*. 2007;24(2): 120-129. doi:10.1097/WNP.0b013e31803ece13.
19. Bonnet M, Carley D, Carskadon M, et al. EEG arousals: scoring rules and examples. *Sleep*. 1992;15:173-184. doi:10.1016/S1087-0792(97)90011-3.
20. Tatum WO, Reinsberger C, Dworetzky B. Artifacts of recording. In: Schomer DL, Lopes da Silva FH, eds. *Niedermeyer's Electroencephalography: Basic Principles, Clinical Applications, and Related Fields*. 7th ed. Philadelphia, PA: Wolters Kluwer Health/Lippincott Williams & Wilkins; 2017.
21. Mayor LC, Burneo J, Ochoa JG. *Handbook of Electroencephalography*. Bogotá, Columbia: Universidad de los Andes; 2013:221-255.
22. Klem GH. Artifacts. In: Ebersole JS, Pedley TA, eds. *Current Practice of Clinical Electroencephalography*. 3rd ed. Philadelphia, PA: Lippincott Williams & Wilkins; 2003:271-287.
23. Reilly EL. EEG recording and operation of the apparatus. In: Niedermeyer E, Lopes Da Silva F, eds. *Electroencephalography: Basic Principles, Clinical Applications, and Related Fields*. 4th ed. Philadelphia, PA: Lippincott Williams & Wilkins; 1999:122-142.
24. Tatum WO. Normal EEG. In: Tatum WO, Husain A, Benbadis SR, et al., eds. *Handbook of EEG Interpretation*. New York, NY: Demos; 2008:1-50.
25. Lagerlund TD, Cascino GD, Cicora KM, et al. Long-term electroencephalographic monitoring for diagnosis and management of seizures. *Mayo Clin Proc*. 1996;71(10):1000-1006. doi:10.1016/S0025-6196(11)63776-2.
26. Tatum WO. Artifact and ambulatory EEG. In: Tatum WO, ed. *Ambulatory EEG Monitoring*. New York, NY: Demos Medical; 2017:41-73.
27. Tatum WO. Long-term EEG monitoring: a clinical approach to electrophysiology. *Am J EEG Technol*. 2003;43(2):74-97. doi: 10.1080/1086508X.2003.11079423.
28. Bridgers SL, Ebersole J. Ambulatory cassette EEG in clinical practice. *Neurology*. 1985;35(12):1167-1168. doi:10.1212/WNL.35.12.1767.

29. Shih JJ, Tatum WO. Computer-assisted ambulatory electroencephalography. In Daube JR, Rubin DI, eds. *Clinical Neurophysiology*. 4th ed. New York, NY: Oxford University Press; 2016:167-175.

30. Liporace J, Tatum W, Morris GL, et al. Clinical utility of sleep-deprived versus computer-assisted 16-channel ambulatory EEG in epilepsy patients: a multi-center study. *Epilepsy Res*. 1998;32:357-362. doi:10.1016/S0920-1211(98)00069-2.

31. Schomer DL. Ambulatory EEG telemetry: how good is it? *J Clin Neurophysiol*. 2006;23(4):294-305. doi:10.1097/01.wnp.0000228495.29014.82.

32. Chang BS, Ives JR, Schomer DL, et al. Outpatient EEG monitoring in the presurgical evaluation of patients with refractory temporal lobe epilepsy. *J Clin Neurophysiol*. 2002;19:152-156. doi:10.1097/00004691-200203000-00006.

33. Balogh EP, Miller BT, Ball JR, eds. *Improving Diagnosis in Health Care*. Washington, DC: National Academies Press; 2015.

34. Benbadis SR. The EEG in nonepileptic seizures. *J Clin Neurophysiol*. 2006;23(4):340-352. doi:10.1097/01.wnp.0000228863.92618.cf.

35. Serles W, Caramanos Z, Lindinger G, et al. Combining ictal surface-electroencephalography and seizure semiology improves patient lateralization in temporal lobe epilepsy. *Epilepsia*. 2000;41:1567-1573. doi:10.1111/j.1528-1167.2000.01567.x.

36. American Clinical Neurophysiology Society. Guideline twelve: guidelines for long-term monitoring for epilepsy. *J Clin Neurophys*. 2008;25:170-180. doi:10.1097/WNP.0b013e318175d472.

37. Conradsen I, Moldovan M, Jennum P, et al. Dynamics of muscle activation during tonic-clonic seizures. *Epilepsy Res*. 2013;104(1-2):84-93. doi:10.1016/j.eplepsyres.2012.09.004.

38. Vinton A, Carino J, Vogrin S, et al. Convulsive nonepileptic seizures have a characteristic pattern of rhythmic artifact distinguishing them from convulsive epileptic seizures. *Epilepsia*. 2004;45(11):1344-1350. doi:10.1111/j.0013-9580.2004.04704.x.

39. Beniczky S, Conradsen I, Moldovan M, et al. Automated differentiation between epileptic and non-epileptic convulsive seizures. *Ann Neurol*. 2015;77(2):348-351. doi:10.1002/ana.24338.

40. Jiruska P, Alvarado-Rojas C, Schevon CA, et al. Update on the mechanisms and roles of high-frequency oscillations in seizures and epileptic disorders. *Epilepsia*. 2017;58(8):1330-1339. doi:10.1111/epi.13830.

41. Zijlmans M, Worrell GA, Dumpelmann M, et al. How to record high-frequency oscillations in epilepsy: a practical guideline. *Epilepsia*. 2017;58(8):1305-1315. doi:10.1111/epi.13814.

42. Tatum WO, Dworetzky B, Freeman WD, Schomer DL. Artifact: recording EEG in special care units. *J Clin Neurophysiol*. 2011;28(3):264-277. doi:10.1097/WNP.

43. Sahota PK, Bray F, Garcia-Mendez L. Respiration-related artifact presenting as intermittent rhythmic theta activity. *Am J EEG Tech*. 1993;33(2):121-128. doi:10.1080/00029238.1993.11080440.

44. De Clercq W, Vergult A, Vanrumste B, et al. A new muscle artifact removal technique to improve the interpretation of the ictal scalp electroencephalogram. *Conf Proc IEEE Eng Med Biol Soc*. 2005;1:944-947. doi:10.1109/IEMBS.2005.1616571.

45. Hamaneh MB, Chitravas N, Kaiboriboon K, et al. Automated removal of EKG artifact from EEG data using independent component analysis and continuous wavelet transformation. *IEEE Trans Biomed Eng*. 2014;61(6):1634-1641. doi:10.1109/TBME.2013.2295173.

46. Akhtar MT, Mitsuhashi W, James CJ. Employing spatially constrained ICA and wavelet denoising for automatic removal of artifacts from multichannel EEG data. *Signal Processing*. 2012;92(2):401-416. doi:10.1016/j.sigpro.2011.08.005.

47. Jung TP, Makeig S, Humphries C, et al. Removing electroencephalographic artifacts by blind source separation. *Psychophysiology*. 2000;37:163-178. doi:10.1111/1469-8986.3720163.

48. Romero S, Mananas MA, Barbanoj MJ. A comparative study of automated techniques for ocular artifact reduction in spontaneous EEG signals based on clinical target variables: a simulation case. *Comput Biol Med*. 2008;38:348-360. doi:10.1016/j.compbiomed.2007.12.001.

49. Persyst. Persyst artifact reduction—detect and reduce artifact with the touch of a button. http://www.persyst.com/technology/artifact-reduction/. Accessed August 29, 2017.

50. Gao J, Yang Y, Sun J, et al. Automatic removal of various artifacts from EEG signals using combined methods. *J Clin Neurophysiol*. 2010;27:312-320. doi:10.1097/WNP.0b013e3181f534f4.

51. Stern JM, Engel J Jr. *Atlas of EEG Patterns*. Philadelphia, PA: Lippincott Williams & Wilkins; 2005:55-86.

52. Newman-Toker DE, Pronovost PJ. Diagnostic errors: the next frontier for patient safety. *JAMA*. 2009;301:1060-1062. doi:10.1001/jama.2009.249.

53. Nuwer MR, Comi G, Emerson R, et al. IFCN standards for digital recording of clinical EEG. *Electroencephalogr Clin Neurophysiol*. 1998;106(3):259-261. doi:10.1016/S0013-4694(97)00106-5.

CHAPTER 8

Artifacts in Pediatric and Adult Magnetoencephalography

Christos Papadelis, Michel AlHilani, and Phillip L. Pearl

INTRODUCTION

Magnetoencephalography (MEG) records the magnetic brain activity that is measurable using extracranial sensors. The measured magnetic fields created by electric currents in the brain are extremely weak and prone to multiple artifacts. Artifacts can be generated by strong ambient magnetic fields (ambient artifacts) external to the patient's body or by electromagnetic sources inside the patient's body (biological artifacts). Both ambient and biological artifacts can obscure the MEG signal, rendering the electromagnetic activity generated by the human brain uninterpretable. Moreover, artifacts can be falsely attributed to cerebral sources, significantly altering the results and clinical interpretation of the MEG recording. There are artifacts that are unique to the MEG setup and there is limited literature that provides a detailed description of artifacts in MEG (1–3). In this chapter, we give examples of ambient and biological artifacts that are encountered in the clinical performance of MEG used for children and adults.

AMBIENT ARTIFACTS

Ambient sources include interference from power lines and electrical motors or from large, moving objects made of ferromagnetic materials. The interference from power lines contains the main frequency (50 Hz in Europe, Asia, and Australia; 60 Hz in the United States and most countries in North and South America) and its harmonics. Artifacts from electrical motors also have a constant frequency that corresponds to the rotating frequency of the motor. Both power mains and electrical motors generate artifacts that are almost always present in MEG recordings and can be easily recognizable. Common sources of moving objects in urban hospital settings include cars, commuter trains, subways, elevators, metallic furniture, and hospital beds. The electromagnetic signals generated by moving objects are characterized by temporal scales similar to the movement; the frequency is predominantly below 1 Hz (2). Although most of these artifactual sources are distant, they are still difficult to identify and eliminate because (a) they are not always present in the signal, (b) the location of the source is often not static, and (c) they often resemble pathological or normal variants of brain origin. For example, magnetic fields from a car travelling at a distance of 2 km are roughly equivalent to those produced by the human brain (4). Mechanical vibrations from the buildings transmitted to the magnetically shielded room (MSR) might also be another source of artifacts in the MEG recordings. Paramagnetic and ferromagnetic materials that might be contained in exogenous or endogenous sources can give rise to large-amplitude artifacts that obscure the brain's MEG signal (1,5). Exogenous sources of artifacts include jewelry, watches, keys, glasses, dyes, spectacles, hearing aids, clothing (i.e., underwire bras and zippers), or even facial makeup (i.e., mascara and face glitter). Endogenous sources include dental work, fillings and braces, tattoos, and implanted medical devices that are either active (i.e., defibrillators, neurostimulators, cochlear implants, and drug pumps) or passive (i.e., hip/knee joint replacements, heart valves, aneurysm clips, coronary stents, and breast implants). These types of artifacts generally produce very large, but low-frequency signals in the MEG data. They increase when the patient is moving his or her torso, upper or lower extremities, or jaw and can be easily recognized by asking the patient to blink or move, thereby reproducing the artifact. Artifacts from dental work and facial makeup may be made worse if the patient was recently scanned in an MRI device because such materials may become magnetized.

BIOLOGICAL ARTIFACTS

MEG recordings are more often confronted by interference from the patient rather than from the environment. Eyeblink, cardiac, respiratory, and muscle artifacts are common biological sources that disturb MEG recordings. Each of these artifacts has distinct spatial and temporal characteristics which the reader should become familiar with and be able to recognize. The human heart is one of the most insidious sources of magnetic noise in MEG. Cardiac artifact reflects either the magnetic counterpart of the QRS complex or pulsation of the ECG (6,7). Cardiac artifact in MEG is characterized by relatively brief pulses occurring at the same time as the patient's heart rate. Normal cardiac function can also produce intermittent artifact by the ballistocardiographic effect. This can happen if the patient has any magnetic materials in his or her clothing that might fluctuate due to the mechanical rhythm of the cardiac muscular contraction causing an artifact in the MEG signal. Cardiac implantable devices (i.e., coronal stents) made of paramagnetic or ferromagnetic materials may also produce artifacts. Respiratory artifacts appear as slow, low-amplitude waves in MEG. Although they are usually not troublesome, they may be amplified by other factors. For example, magnetic lung contamination or magnetic material in clothing may cause slow shifts due to movement during respiration. Ocular artifacts (eye movements and blinks) are manifest as high-amplitude deflections less than a second in duration that appear predominately in the frontal channels. Other muscular artifacts can also contaminate the MEG signal. For example, tense neck muscles may emit continuous or bursting high-frequency noise, which becomes more prominent the closer the muscle is to the sensor array.

EXAMPLES OF ARTIFACTS

Commuter Train

Large moving objects that are located quite far from the MSR can cause enormous technical artifacts in the MEG dominating the brain activity signal and rendering the recording unreadable. Figure 8.1 presents an example of ambient artifact in the MEG from a commuter train. The artifact has an amplitude composed of a few thousands pico tesla (pT) compared to the brain activity magnitude of femto tesla (fT) (~100 fT for a cerebral evoked response and ~1,000 fT for cerebral alpha rhythm) and dominates the brain MEG activity. Such large amplitude corresponds to thousands of microvolts (mV) in EEG.

Cardiac Pulse Artifact

MEG is more sensitive to cardiac artifacts than standard scalp EEG. The most common biological artifact in MEG is caused by the heartbeat. It appears as relatively brief pulses occurring at the same frequency as the heart rate. It may transiently overlap with interictal epileptiform discharges, or rarely the ictal onset during MEG, distorting the source localization of the epileptiform activity. It appears more prominent on magnetometers than gradiometers (Figure 8.2). It has a specific spatial distribution in the topographic plot of the MEG signal that is perpendicular to the topography of EEG. Simultaneous ECG recordings are essential to recognize the cardiac pulse artifact in the MEG signal.

Ocular Artifacts

Moving eyeballs act as two large magnets and generate relatively prominent artifacts. Ocular artifact can either be due to eye blinks contaminating particularly the lower frequencies or due to saccadic eye movements that interfere with the MEG signal at higher frequency ranges. Certain saccadic movements may produce spiky artifacts that reflect high-frequency myogenic artifact (i.e., lateral rectus spikes). The myogenic spikes generated by eye movement are an important artifactual signal because they can mimic abnormality. It is observed at the onset of even tiny saccadic eye movements and is characterized by strong electrical transients that are believed to reflect contraction of the extraocular muscles in the orbit (8). Figure 8.3 shows an example of a typical eyeblink artifact as it looks in MEG traces. It appears as a short (between ~100 and ~400 ms), large deflection with highest amplitude in the sensors of the frontal head regions. Simultaneously, recording electrooculography (EOG) is useful to recognize vertical eyeblink artifacts in the MEG signal. Figure 8.4 shows an example of artifact due to saccades, which are visible mostly in horizontal EOG. The deflection has the maximum amplitude at the frontal and occipitoparietal areas, and its topography is 90 degrees out of phase compared with the vertical eyeblink artifact.

Myogenic Artifacts

Myogenic artifact is the main barrier against obtaining high-quality MEG recordings. This artifact can be identified as high-frequency activity that is usually present bilaterally and is seen most prominently in temporal and frontal head regions. Muscular activity produces artifact that appears within the bandwidth of frequencies between 20 and 300 Hz with most of its power at the lower end of the frequency range (9). Some facial muscles with intricate function are smaller in size and have higher nerve–muscle innervation density capable of generating myogenic activity that are high frequency, reaching up to 600 Hz (9). Most relevant to the MEG are the myogenic artifacts involved in chewing (50–60 Hz) that is generated by the masseter muscle in addition to the frontalis muscle, which controls wrinkling of the brow (30–40 Hz). Muscular activity may overlap entirely with the spectral bandwidth of high-frequency oscillations generated by neural activity (gamma, ripples, and fast ripples), making their distinction from artifact almost impossible (3,10). Figure 8.5 shows an example of myogenic activity in the MEG signal due to contraction of the right frontalis muscles. The topography across different times helps to indicate the exact location of the muscle that is contracting. Figure 8.6 illustrates an example of chewing artifact contained within the MEG signal. Note the topography of the signal indicates a bilateral frontotemporal source for the artifact. Figure 8.7 is an example of myogenic artifact due to slight head movement that results from elbow flexion from arm movement. Myogenic artifacts can cause significant distortion in the topographic maps masking the spatial origin of pathological activity and affecting the reliability of the magnetic source imaging (MSI). Figures 8.8 and 8.9 show the distortion of EEG and MEG topographic maps due to myogenic artifact, which are concordant to an interictal epileptiform discharge (green arrows) in a pediatric patient with focal epilepsy. Figure 8.10 demonstrates the dislocation of an equivalent current dipole (ECD) at the peak of a spike due to the presence of a myogenic artifact in the MEG signal.

Movement Artifact

Patient movement artifacts are more likely to impact MEG than EEG due to the MEG sensors that are in fixed locations relative to the head compared to EEG sensors that move with the head.

Large movements of the patient's extremities may cause a mixture of low- and high-frequency artifact to occur in the MEG signal (see Figure 8.7). Sometimes, the rhythmicity, polarity, and location of an artifact can look suspiciously like an electrographic seizure. This is especially true for neonates who are prone to focal seizures that may be seen in only one to two electrodes. Figure 8.11 (11) shows a patting artifact as seen on a MEG tracing that resembles an electrographic seizure. Use of concomitant video to identify movement patterns that parallel artifactual patterns is critical in these situations to differentiate extracerebral activity. Similarly, close observation of the MEG is important to assess patterns of evolution and propagation present in electrographic seizures, which are less likely to be seen in a purely artifactual pattern.

Medical Devices

On many occasions, technical artifacts from exogenous and endogenous medical devices, such as activated implantable medical devices, can generate nonphysiologic artifact rendering the MEG signal uninterpretable. Figure 8.12 demonstrates an artifact generated in the MEG due to transcranial electric stimulation. Figure 8.13 illustrates artifact during an MEG recording in an adult patient with a cochlear implant. Note that most magnetometers are saturated by the cochlear implant disturbance, becoming unable to record any brain activity from the patient. Figure 8.14 represents artifact present in the MEG signals in an adult person with epilepsy implanted with a vagus nerve stimulator (VNS). Note the precisely periodic deflections that overlap the background activity in the MEG. Figure 8.15 reflects device-related artifact during MEG acquired from an adult during electrocochleography.

ARTIFACT REDUCTION IN MEG

Artifact reduction is an important issue, not only for securing interpretable MEG recordings, but also for performing accurate source localization (12). This is particularly important during the presurgical evaluation of patients with epilepsy where the presence of artifacts in the MEG signal can alter the reliability of the MSI, providing inaccurate information about the exact location of the seizure onset zone (see Figure 8.10) and the eloquent cortex (Figure 8.16) (13). Countermeasures that are used to minimize artifacts consist of (a) precautions that are taken during the setup and connection of the MEG system, (b) precautions and intervention during the recording, and (c) usage of artifact reduction software for post hoc signal analysis of the recorded MEG signals. Some MEG devices use gradiometers that are less sensitive to interference from ambient artifact sources far away. Other MEG devices also incorporate an array of reference sensors situated at a greater distance from the head, which are used to subtract external artifacts. To prevent the occurrence of artifacts from mechanical vibrations from the building, the MSR should be isolated as much as possible. However, despite these precautions, most recordings are still subject to numerous artifacts. To improve the efficiency of recording, all magnetic materials should be avoided in the clothing of the patient. In case of dental implants, fillings, bridges, or braces, demagnetization using special equipment may prove helpful to reduce the high-amplitude magnetic signals produced by metals. A simple but effective way to minimize ocular and myogenic artifacts is to ask the patient to fixate on a single point to restrict eye movement or relax the muscles involved in producing artifact (e.g., jaw). Obviously, this approach may be impractical for some younger pediatric patients and patients with neurodevelopmental disabilities. Therefore, in these situations simultaneous recording of video, ECG, EOG, and electromyographic (EMG) signals are essential to recognize artifacts.

At the preprocessing stage of data analysis, filtering the data in the frequency range of interest (usually between 1 and 70 Hz) is fundamental for minimizing artifacts. This is particularly true for artifacts that lie outside the brain's traditional frequency range. The main power line and video artifacts are typically reduced using notch or comb filters (at 50 or 60 Hz). **Figure 8.17** shows MEG signals before and after filtering with a 60-Hz notch filter. These digital notch filters cannot be overly narrow because the main power line frequency is not absolutely constant at a single frequency. Narrow filtering may also introduce "ringing" in the time domain and may filter out MEG components at the notch filter frequency. Furthermore, filtering is not a solution when the frequency range of artifacts overlaps with the spectrum of cerebral activity (i.e., myogenic artifact). Elimination techniques to exclude selected sensors that contain continuous artifact are helpful to avoid undesired effects on source analysis though they may also exclude underlying MEG signals. More advanced signal-processing techniques may also be helpful to remove artifact composed of common sources as well as techniques that compensate for motion. For example, regression-based or blind source separation-based techniques (such as independent component analysis) may be useful for removing specific patterns of artifacts (e.g., heartbeat and ocular artifacts) (14–16). Some of these methods require the simultaneous recording of ECG, EOG, and EMG signals that are essential not only for the recognition of artifacts but also for their elimination. More recently, the signal source separation (SSS) method has been proposed (17), which decomposes the MEG signals into two components which are generated from sources inside and outside of the sensor space, and removes the latter component. The temporally extended SSS also considers temporal signal correlation (18,19) and is widely used in clinical practice. Finally, to deal with motion artifacts that distort the geographic information of the head and sensors, special compensatory methods have been developed that continuously track the head position during acquisition of the MEG signal. This technique is particularly useful for analyzing ictal data where head deviation sometimes occurs during seizures, introducing artifact (20,21).

CONCLUSIONS

Both ambient and biological artifacts can obscure the MEG signal, rendering the electromagnetic activity generated by the human brain uninterpretable. Moreover, artifacts may be falsely attributed to cerebral sources significantly affecting the clinical interpretation of MEG recordings. Accurate discrimination of artifact from cerebral sources is a critical skill for the MEG interpreter. The use of time-locked video together with the simultaneous recording of ECG, EOG, and EMG signals is indispensable for determining the source of some artifacts and differentiating them from interictal epileptiform discharges and electrographic seizures. Special precautions before and during the recording may help minimize interference from a variety of artifacts. Finally, the use of more advanced signal-processing tools can successfully address a plethora of persistent artifacts that occur during MEG recordings obtained in adult and pediatric patients.

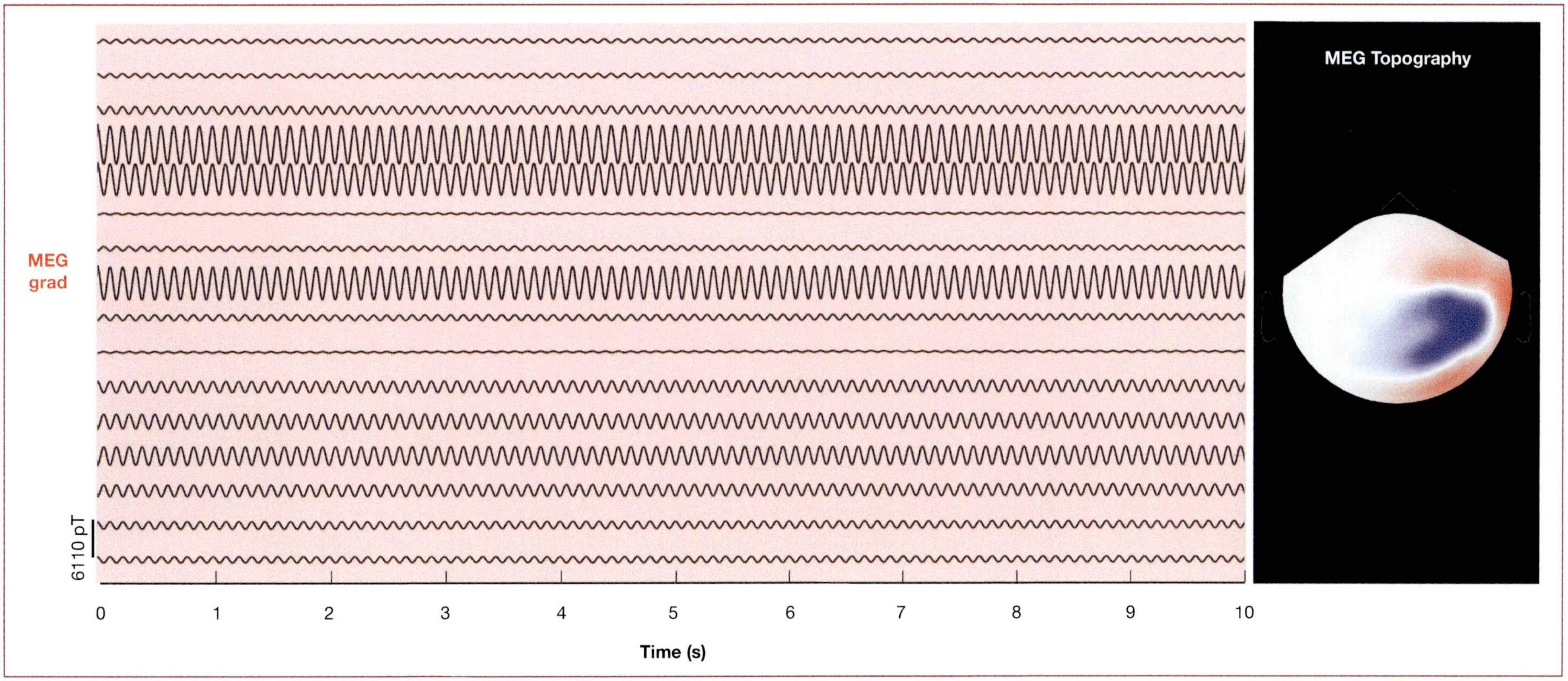

FIGURE 8.1: Continuous sinusoidal artifact from a commuter train recorded with Neuromag Triux (Elekta Instrument AB Stockholm, Sweden) system in the MEG unit at the Centre for Cognitive Neuroscience of the University of Salzburg, Austria (Courtesy of Gianpaolo Demarchi). Please note the enormous signal amplitude (units are in the magnitude of pT).

MEG, magnetoencephalography.

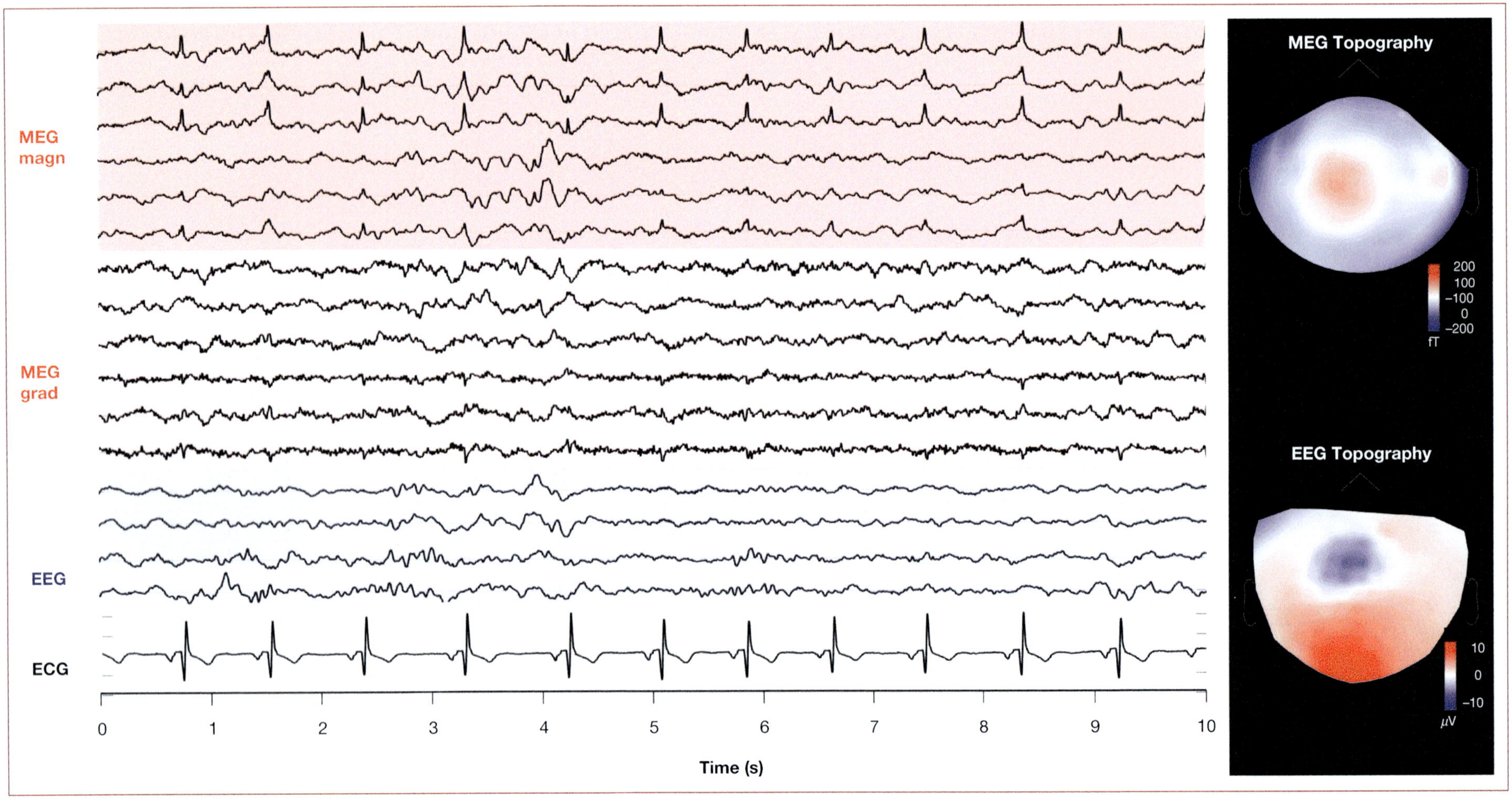

FIGURE 8.2: Pulse artifact seen in simultaneous MEG and EEG recordings obtained in a 13-year-old boy with drug-resistant epilepsy. MEG recordings are performed with the Neuromag Vectorview (Elekta Instrument AB Stockholm, Sweden) system, comprising 306 MEG channels (two planar gradiometers and a magnetometer at each of 102 sites). Recordings from both magnetometers (MEG magn.) and gradiometers (MEG grad.) are shown. Recordings from EEG are displayed in a bipolar montage (F7-T7, T7-P7, F4-C4, and C4-P4 electrodes). The ECG was recorded simultaneously with MEG and EEG. Right panels: topographic mapping of MEG and EEG at the peak of the cardiac pulse artifact in the MEG signal.

MEG, magnetoencephalography.

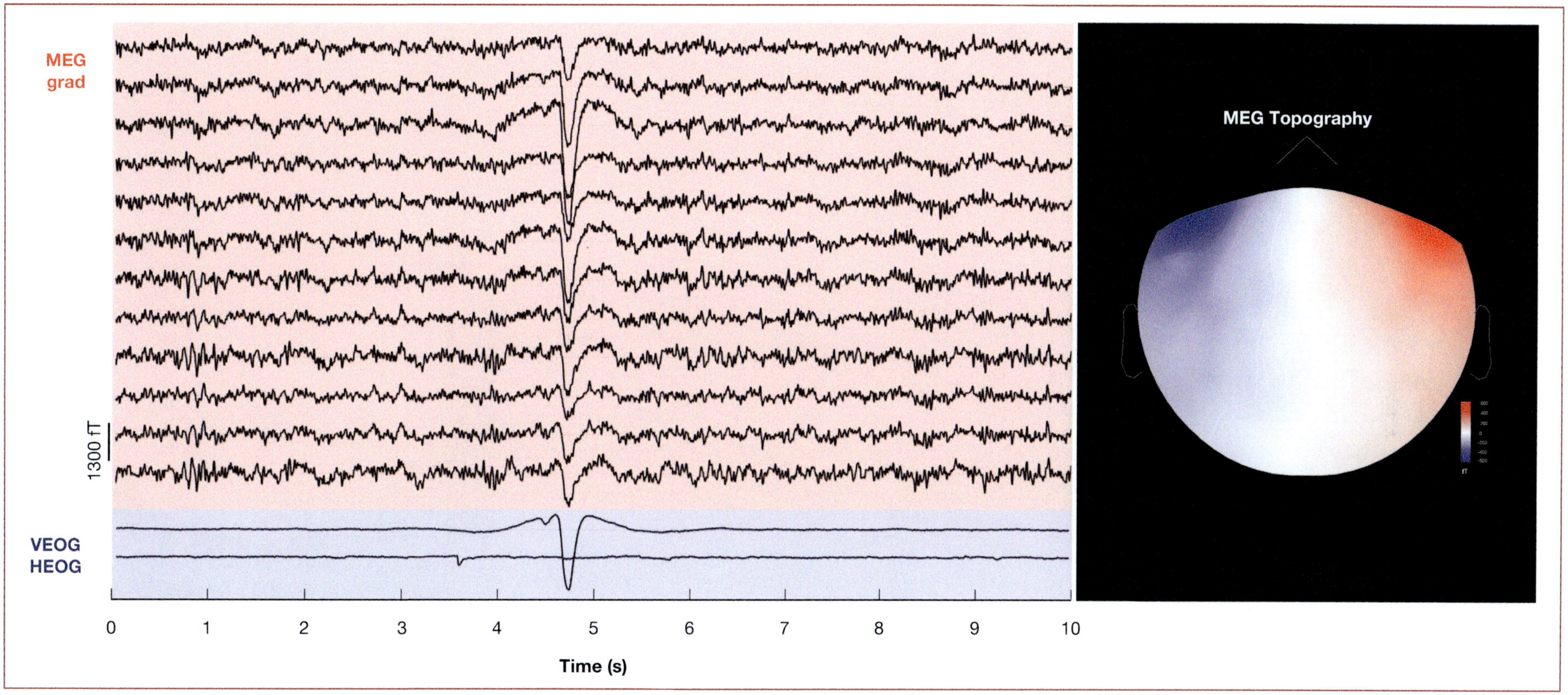

FIGURE 8.3: Vertical eyeblink artifact recorded with simultaneous MEG (red panel) and vertical (VEOG) and horizontal EOG (HEOG) recordings (blue panel). MEG recordings from a 24-year-old healthy man performed with the CTF system (CTF MEG International Services LP, British Columbia, Canada), composed of 151 MEG axial gradiometers. Right panel: corresponding MEG topography at the peak of the eyeblink deflection; red and blue areas indicate maximum influx and efflux of magnetic activity.

MEG, magnetoencephalography.

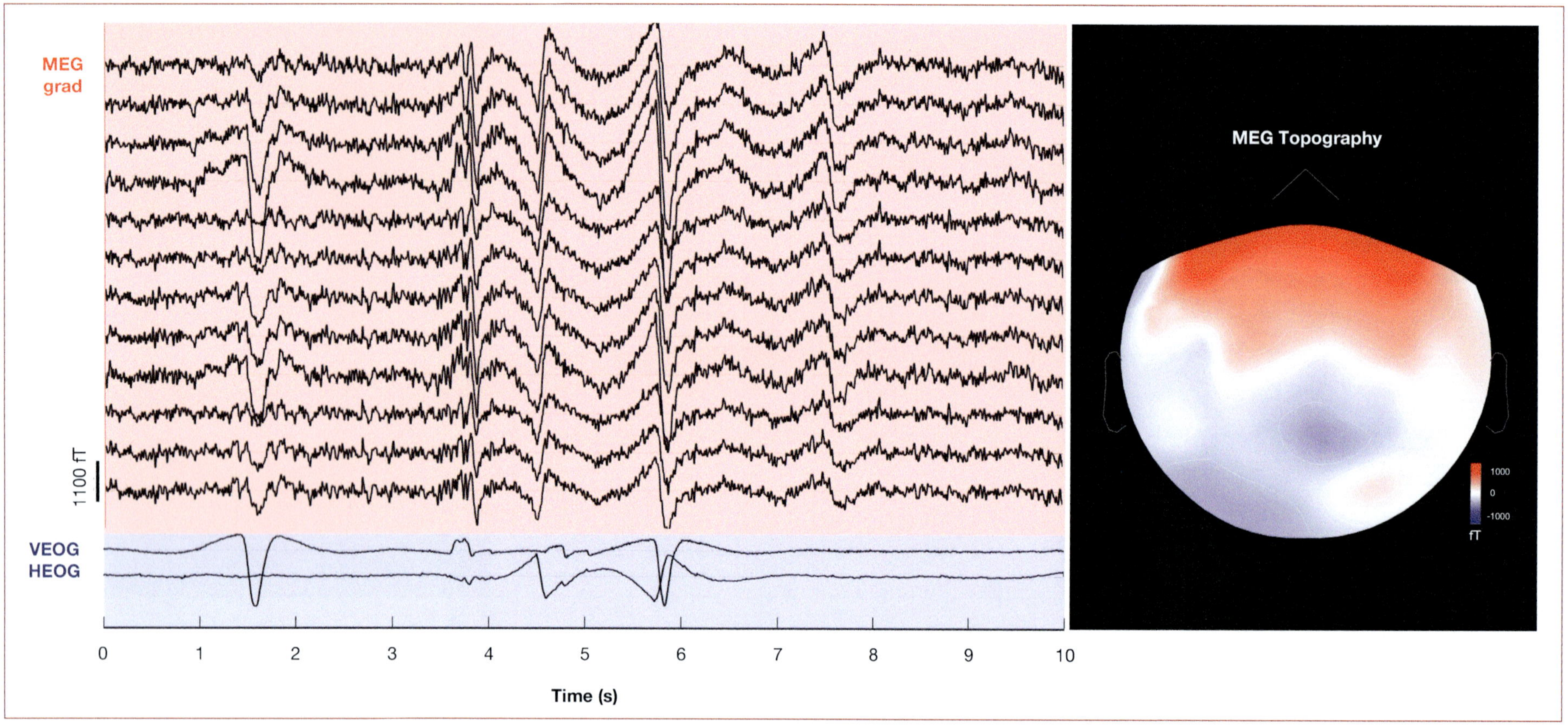

FIGURE 8.4: Saccadic eye movement artifact recorded with simultaneous MEG (red panel), VEOG, and HEOG recording (blue panel). MEG is recorded from the same subject as in **Figure 8.3** performed using the CTF system (CTF MEG International Services LP, British Columbia, Canada) composed of 151 MEG axial gradiometers. Right panel: corresponding MEG topography at the peak of saccadic deflection. The red and blue areas indicate maximum influx and efflux of magnetic activity.

HEOG, horizontal electrooculography; MEG, magnetoencephalography; VEOG, vertical electrooculography.

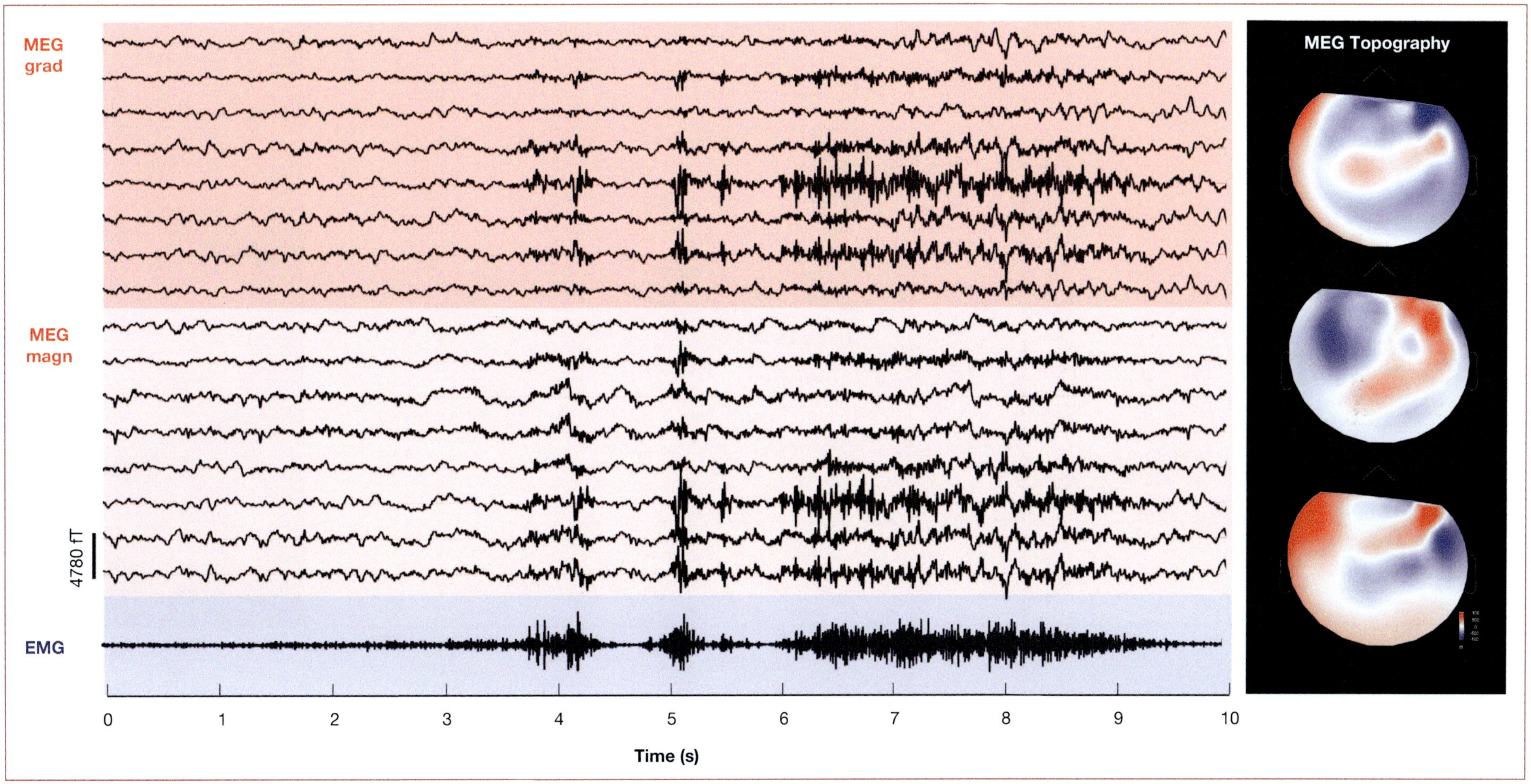

FIGURE 8.5: Myogenic artifact recorded with simultaneous MEG (red panel) and EMG recording (blue panel). MEG recording from a 9-year-old boy with drug-resistant epilepsy performed with the Neuromag system (Elekta Instrument AB Stockholm, Sweden). Right panel: corresponding MEG topographies at different times during the myogenic artifact. The red and blue areas indicate maximum influx and efflux of magnetic activity.

EMG, electromyography; MEG, magnetoencephalography.

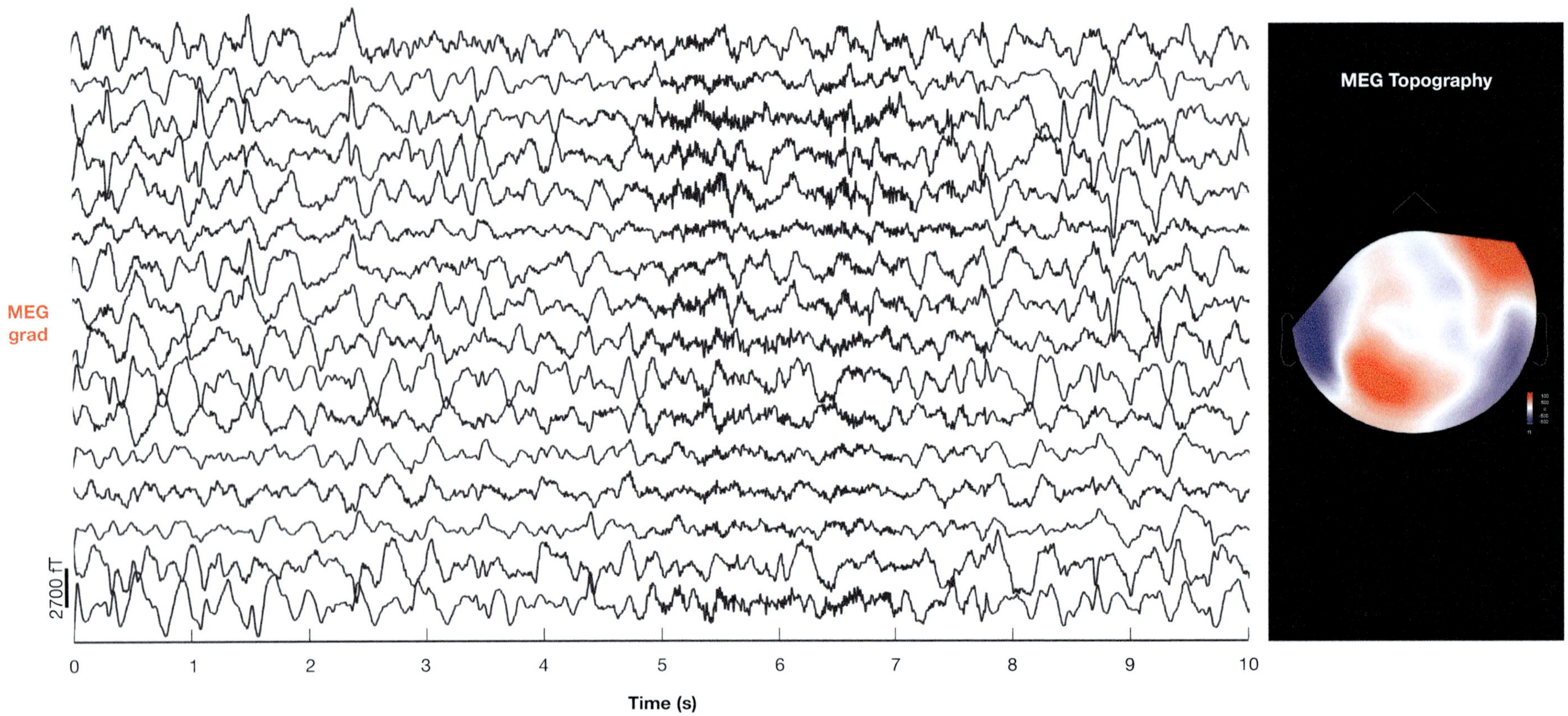

FIGURE 8.6: Chewing artifact recorded with MEG from a 10-year-old child with epilepsy performed with Neuromag (Elekta Instrument AB Stockholm, Sweden). Right panel: corresponding MEG topography during the artifact. The red and blue areas indicate maximum influx and efflux of magnetic activity.

MEG, magnetoencephalography.

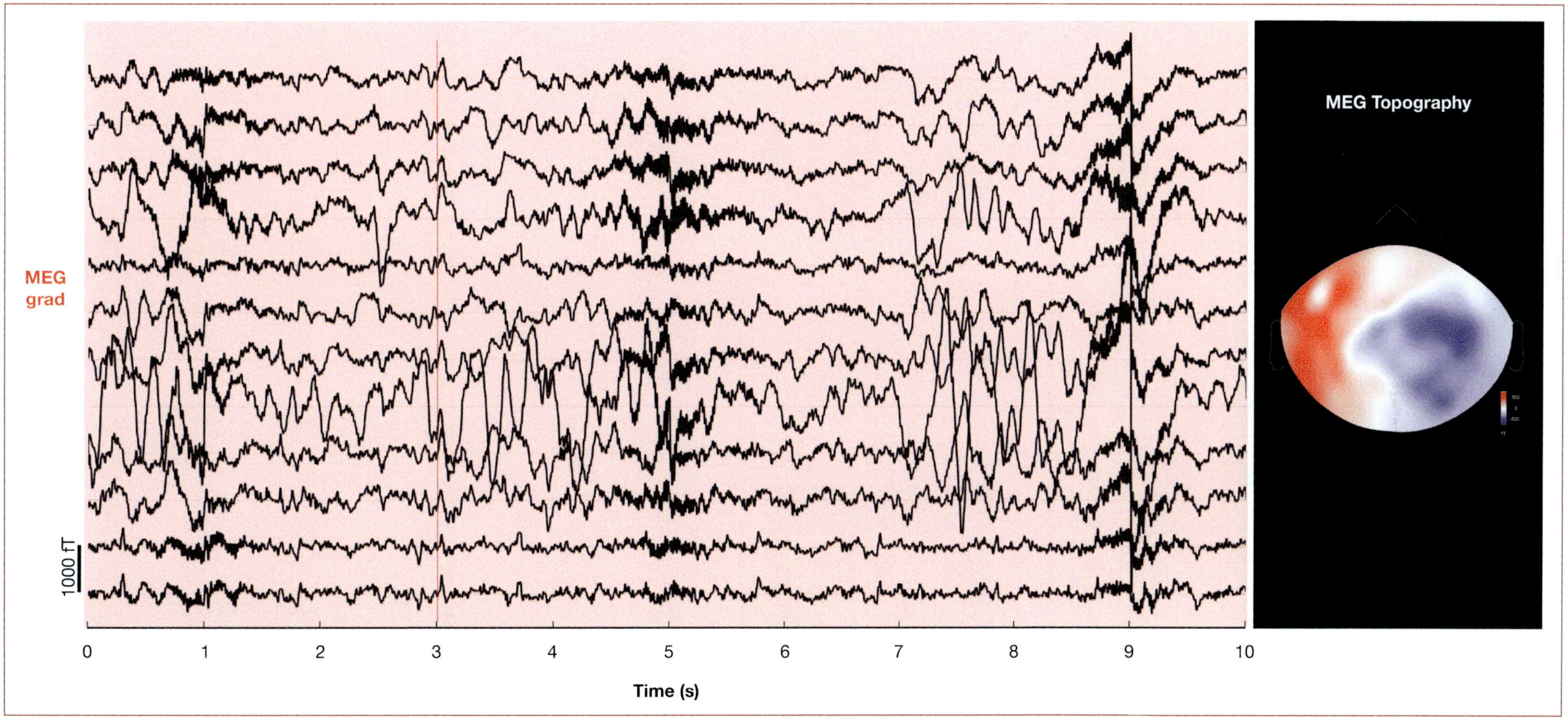

FIGURE 8.7: Myogenic artifact in the MEG signal due to head movement after elbow flexion once every ~4 seconds. Recording from a 45-year-old man with a CTF (CTF MEG International Services LP, British Columbia, Canada) system in the MEG laboratory at the Children's Hospital of Philadelphia (Courtesy of William C. Gaetz). Right panel: topography at the peak of MEG activity during elbow flexion.

MEG, magnetoencephalography.

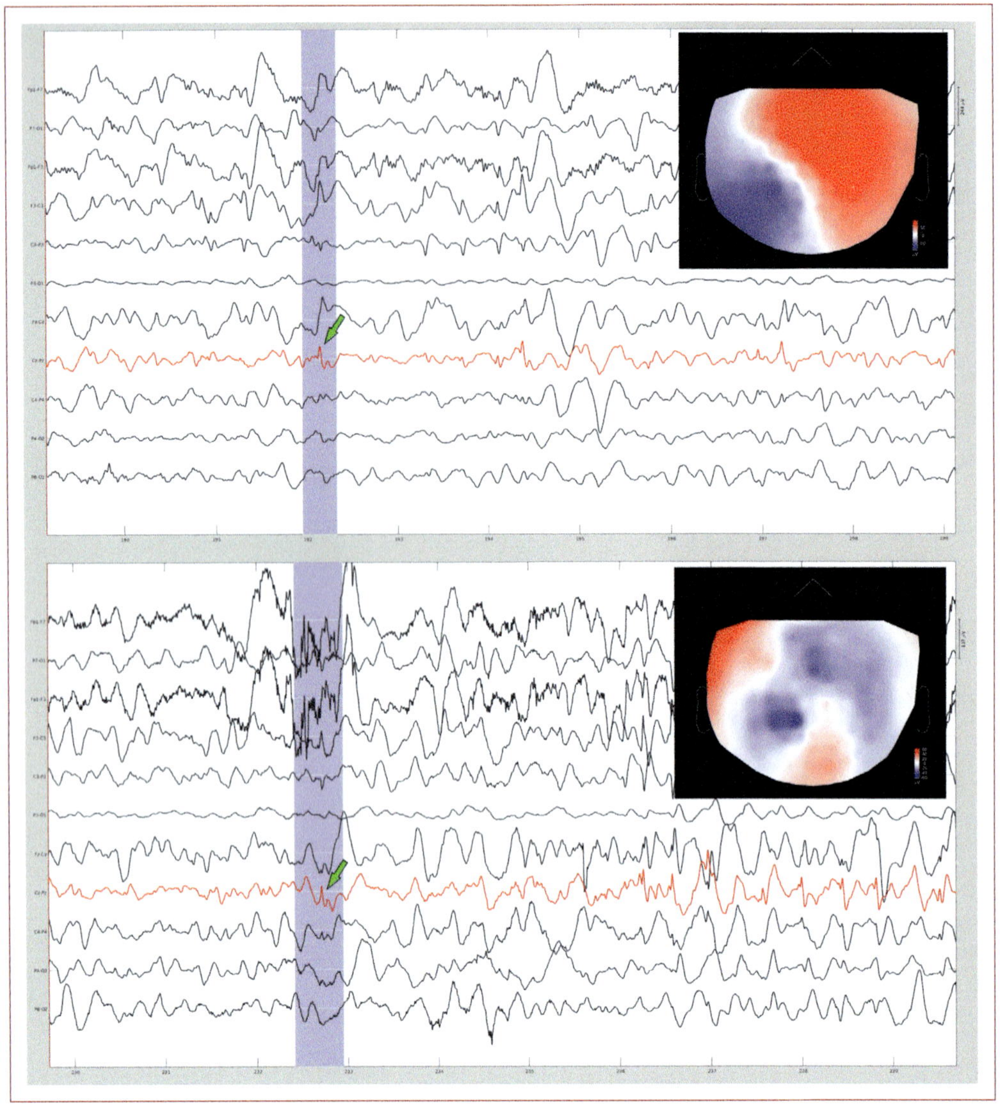

FIGURE 8.8: Interictal epileptiform discharges on EEG signal (green arrows pointing to spikes on Cz-Pz) and topoplot maps of spike discharges at the peak. Upper panel: 10 seconds of EEG (bipolar longitudinal montage) with no artifacts. Lower panel: 10 seconds of EEG signal (bipolar longitudinal montage) where spikes (green arrow) are concurrent with myogenic artifact. MEG recording from a 10-year-old girl with drug-resistant focal epilepsy due to cortical dysplasia. Note that topography in the upper panel indicates a focal source on vertex. Topographic map in the lower panel is distorted due to the presence of myogenic artifact.

MEG, magnetoencephalography.

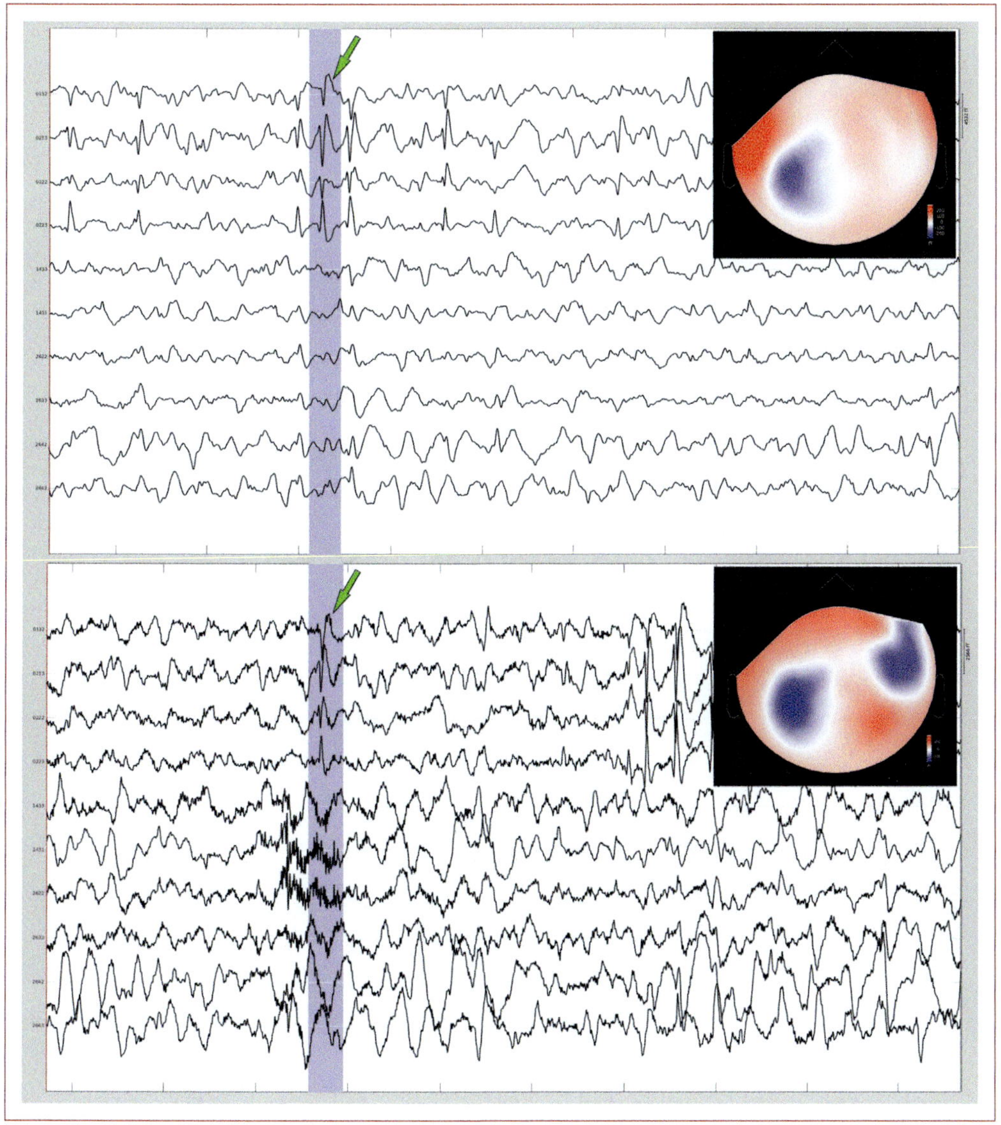

FIGURE 8.9: Interictal epileptiform discharges on MEG signal (green arrows) and topoplot maps at the peak of the spikes. Upper panel: 10 seconds of MEG (gradiometers covering the left temporal lobe) with no artifacts. Lower panel: 10 seconds of MEG signal (gradiometers covering the left temporal lobe) where spikes (green arrow) are concurrent with myogenic artifacts. MEG recording from a 12-year-old boy with drug-resistant focal epilepsy. Note that topography in the upper panel indicates a focal source in the left temporal lobe. Topographic map in the lower panel is distorted due to the presence of myogenic artifact.

MEG, magnetoencephalography.

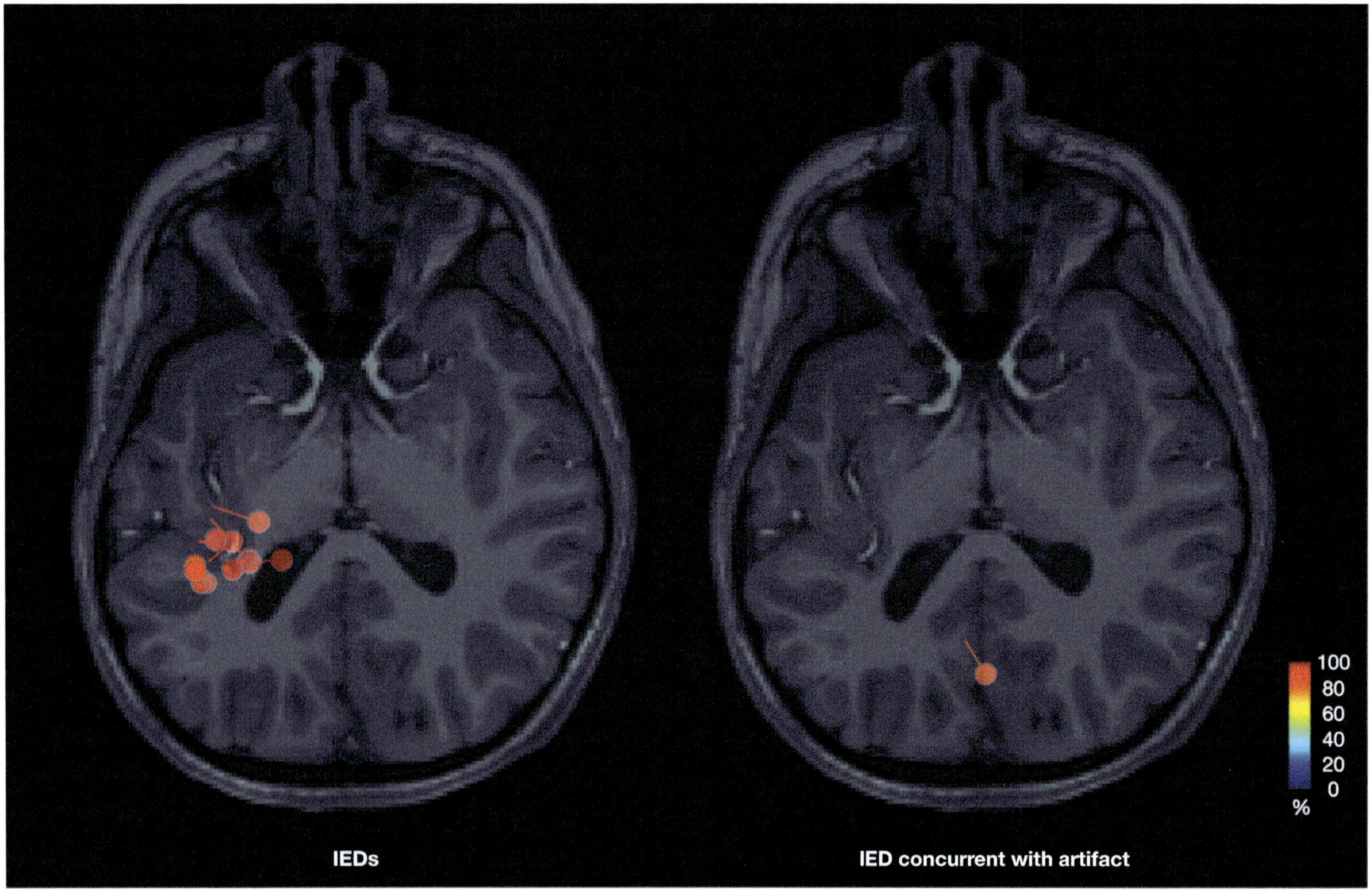

FIGURE 8.10: ECDs at the peak of IEDs overlaid on the patient's brain MRI. Left panel: All ECDs taken from 10-minute recordings (goodness of fit: >85%). Right panel: ECD from a spike that was concurrent with myogenic artifact. Note the formed cluster of ECDs at the left temporal lobe and the distant location of the ECD that was concordant with the artifact. MEG recordings from a 12-year-old boy with drug-resistant epilepsy.

ECD, equivalent current dipole; IED, interictal epileptiform discharge; MEG, magnetoencephalography.

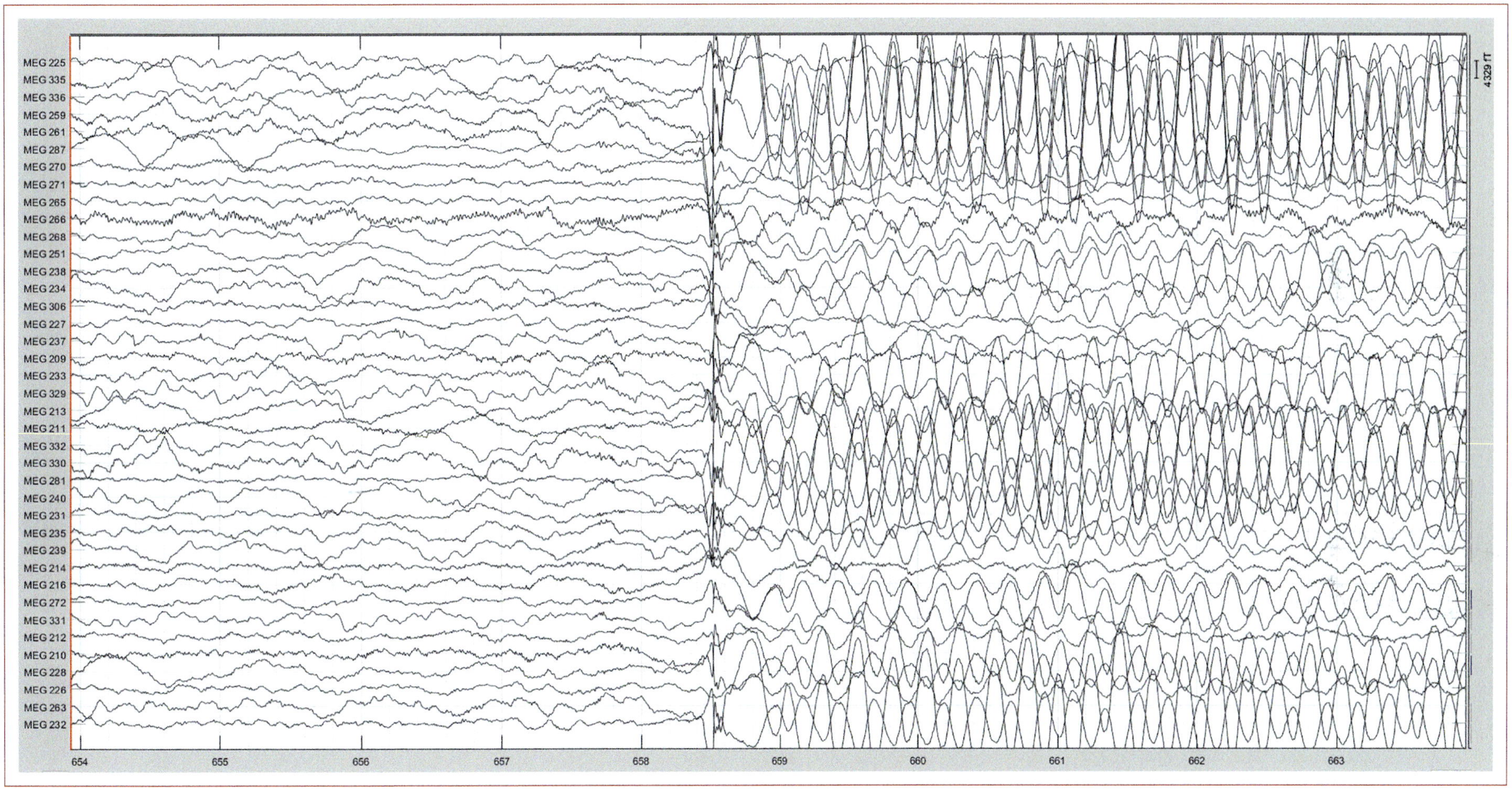

FIGURE 8.11: Patting artifact recorded from a 13-month-old boy with epilepsy using the BabyMEG system (MagView™; Tristan Technologies Inc., San Diego, California) that is specifically designed for pediatric use and equipped with 375 magnetometers (11).

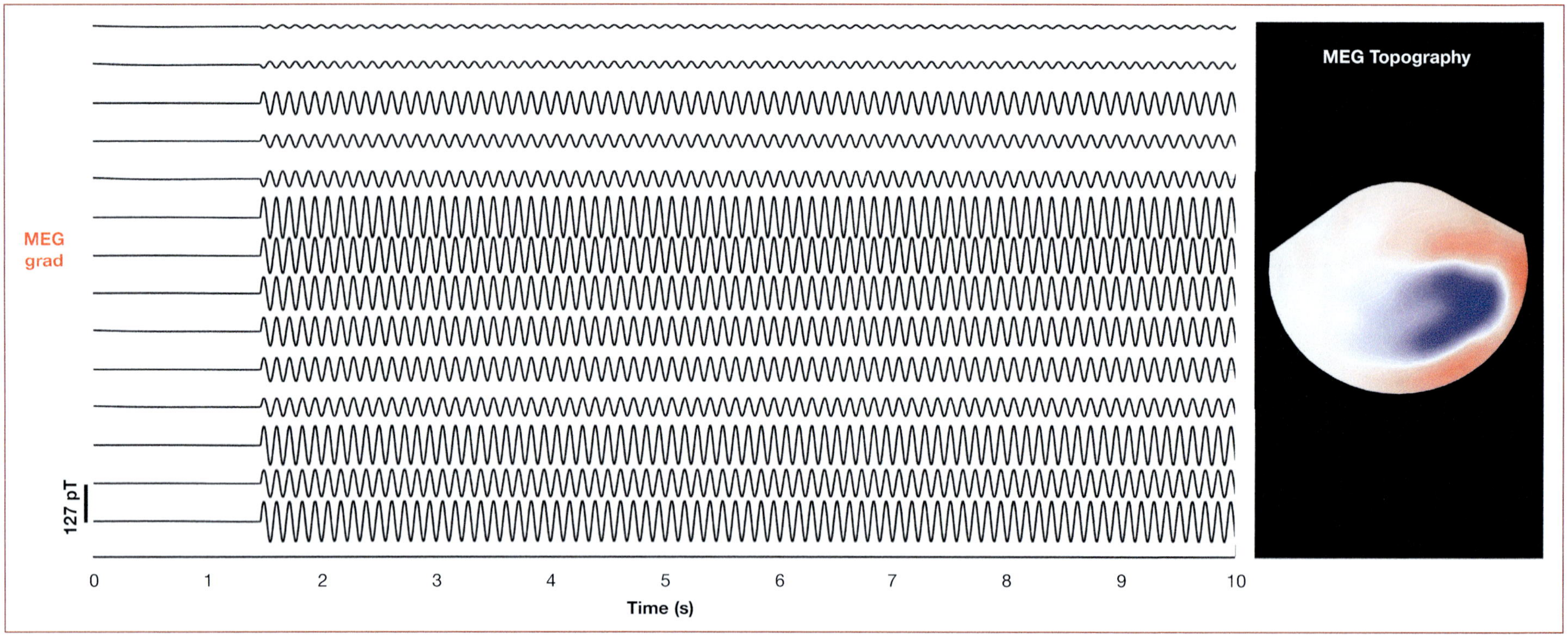

FIGURE 8.12: MEG nonphysiologic artifact due to transcranial alternating current electric stimulation recorded from a 38-year-old healthy man with the Neuromag Triux system (Elekta Instrument AB Stockholm, Sweden) at the MEG unit of Centre for Cognitive Neuroscience at the University of Salzburg, Austria (Courtesy of Gianpaolo Demarchi).

MEG, magnetoencephalography.

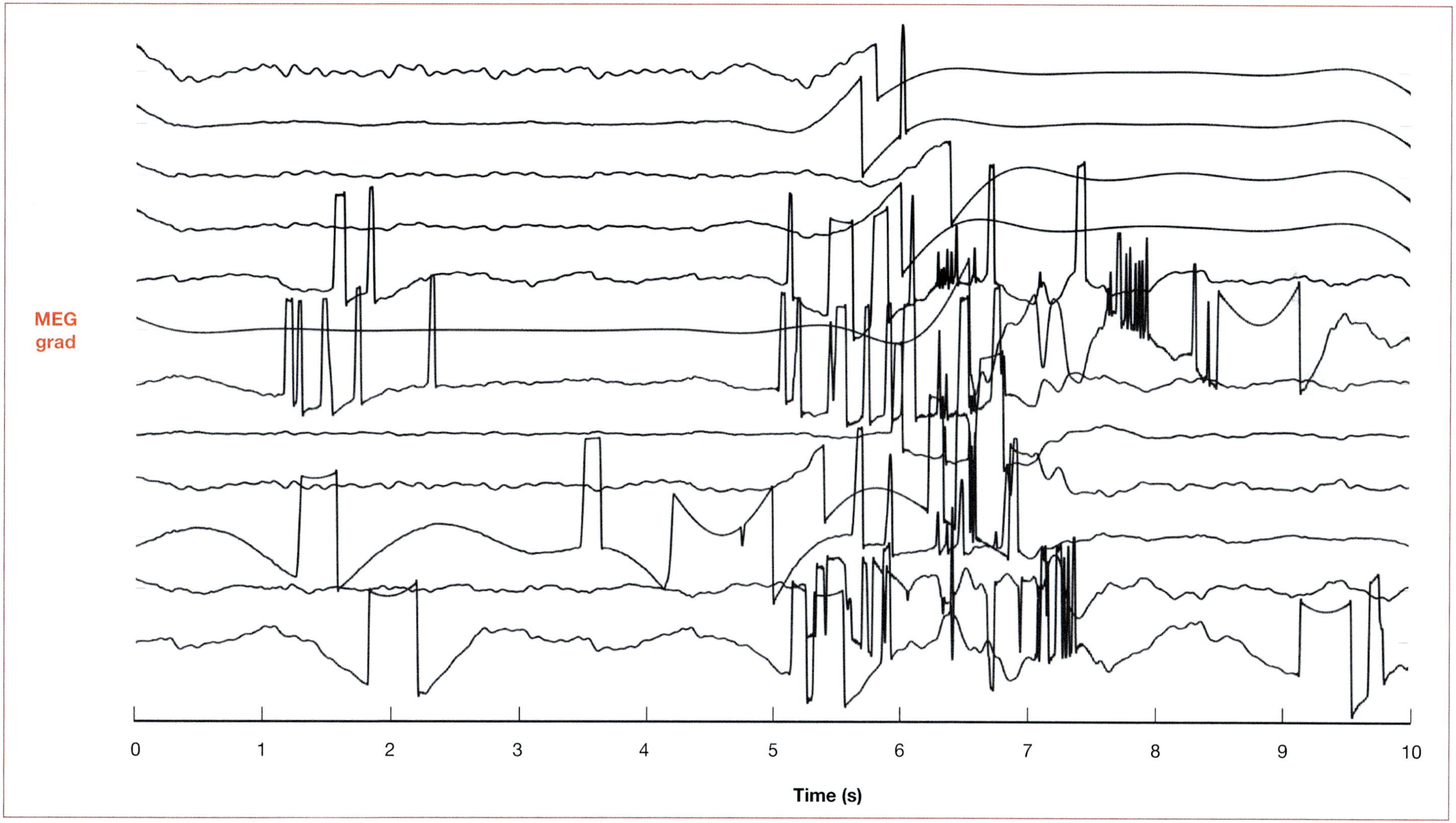

FIGURE 8.13: Nonphysiologic artifact due to a cochlear implant in a 42-year-old man recorded with the Neuromag Triux system (Elekta Instrument AB Stockholm, Sweden) at the MEG unit in the Centre for Cognitive Neuroscience at the University of Salzburg, Austria (Courtesy of Gianpaolo Demarchi). Note the enormous amplitude (units in the magnitude of nano tesla) of the MEG signal causing saturation of most magnetometers.

MEG, magnetoencephalography.

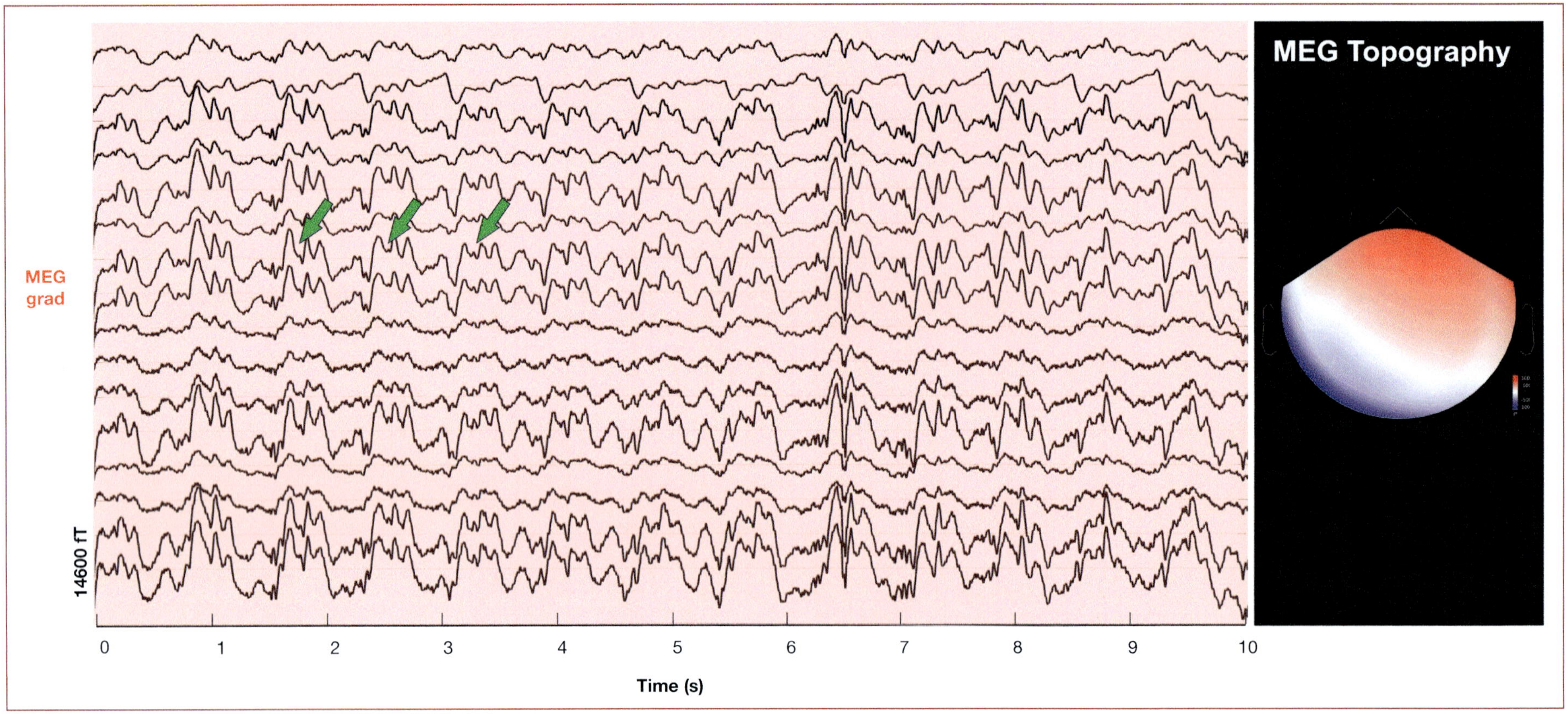

FIGURE 8.14: Nonphysiologic artifact generated by the VNS in a 32-year-old man with drug-resistant epilepsy recorded with the Neuromag Triux (Elekta Instrument AB Stockholm, Sweden) system at the MEG unit in the Centre for Cognitive Neuroscience at the University of Salzburg, Austria (Courtesy of Gianpaolo Demarchi).

MEG, magnetoencephalography; VNS, vagus nerve stimulator.

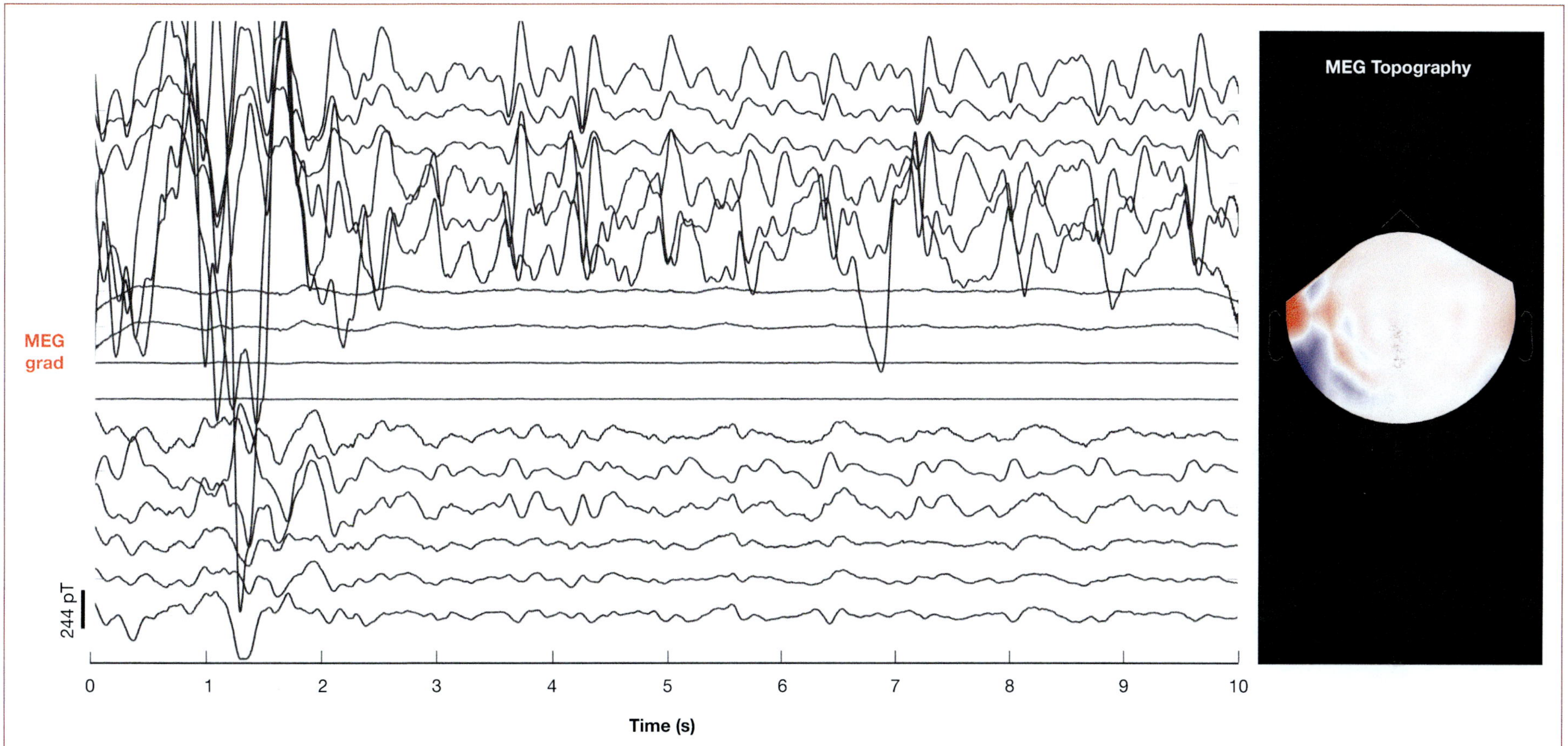

FIGURE 8.15: Nonphysiologic artifact seen in the MEG signal during electrocochleography (ECochG) performed in a 32-year-old man with tinnitus recorded with the Neuromag Triux (Elekta Instrument AB Stockholm, Sweden) system at the MEG unit in the Centre for Cognitive Neuroscience at the University of Salzburg, Austria (Courtesy of Gianpaolo Demarchi).

MEG, magnetoencephalography.

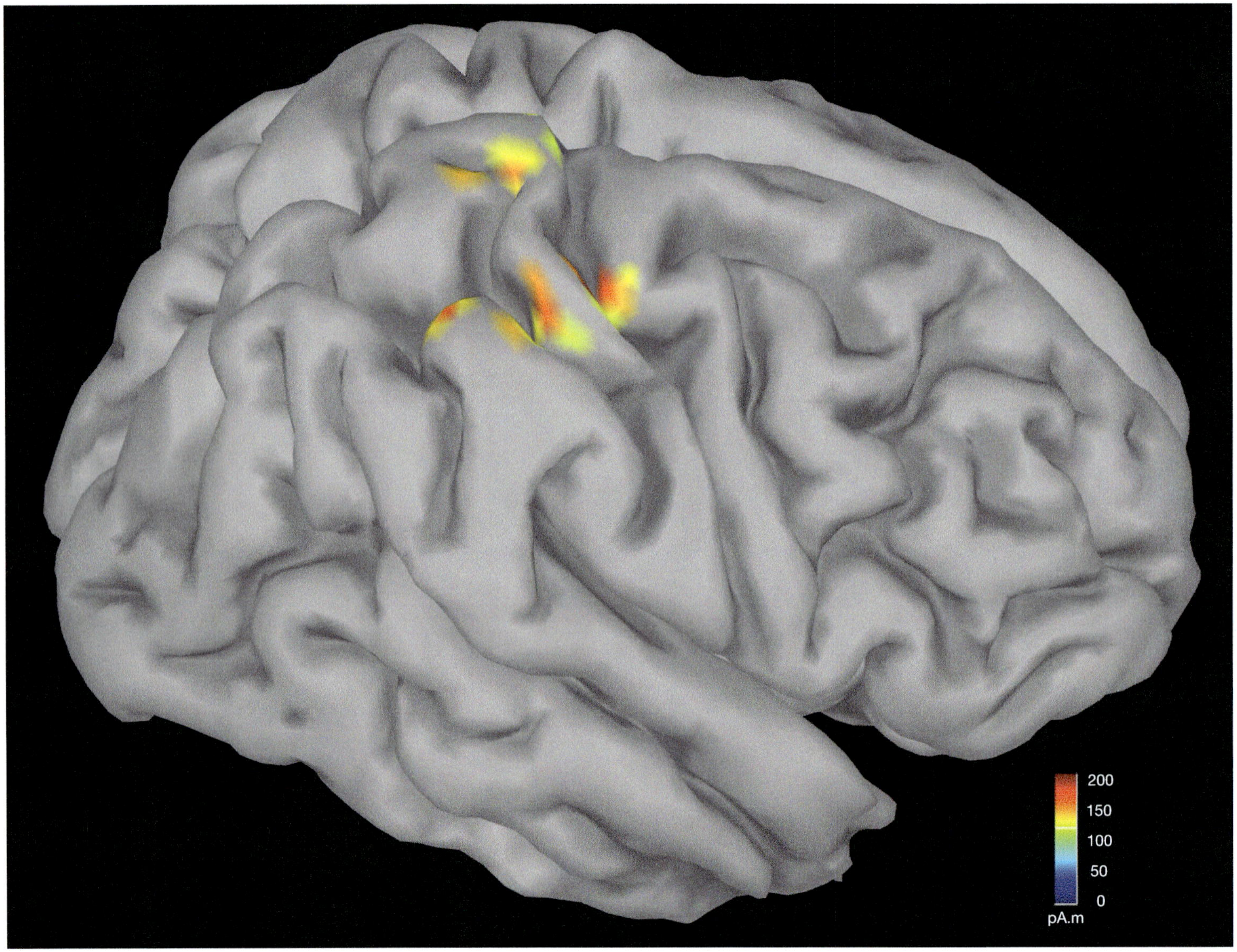

FIGURE 8.16: Mapping of the somatosensory cortex in a 4-year-old child with epilepsy and spastic diplegia. Recordings were performed using the BabySQUID system (Tristan Technologies Inc., San Diego, California) during tactile stimulation of the left thumb with a pneumatic stimulator (13). MSI was performed using the minimum norm estimates (activity thresholded at 90%).

MSI, magnetic source imaging.

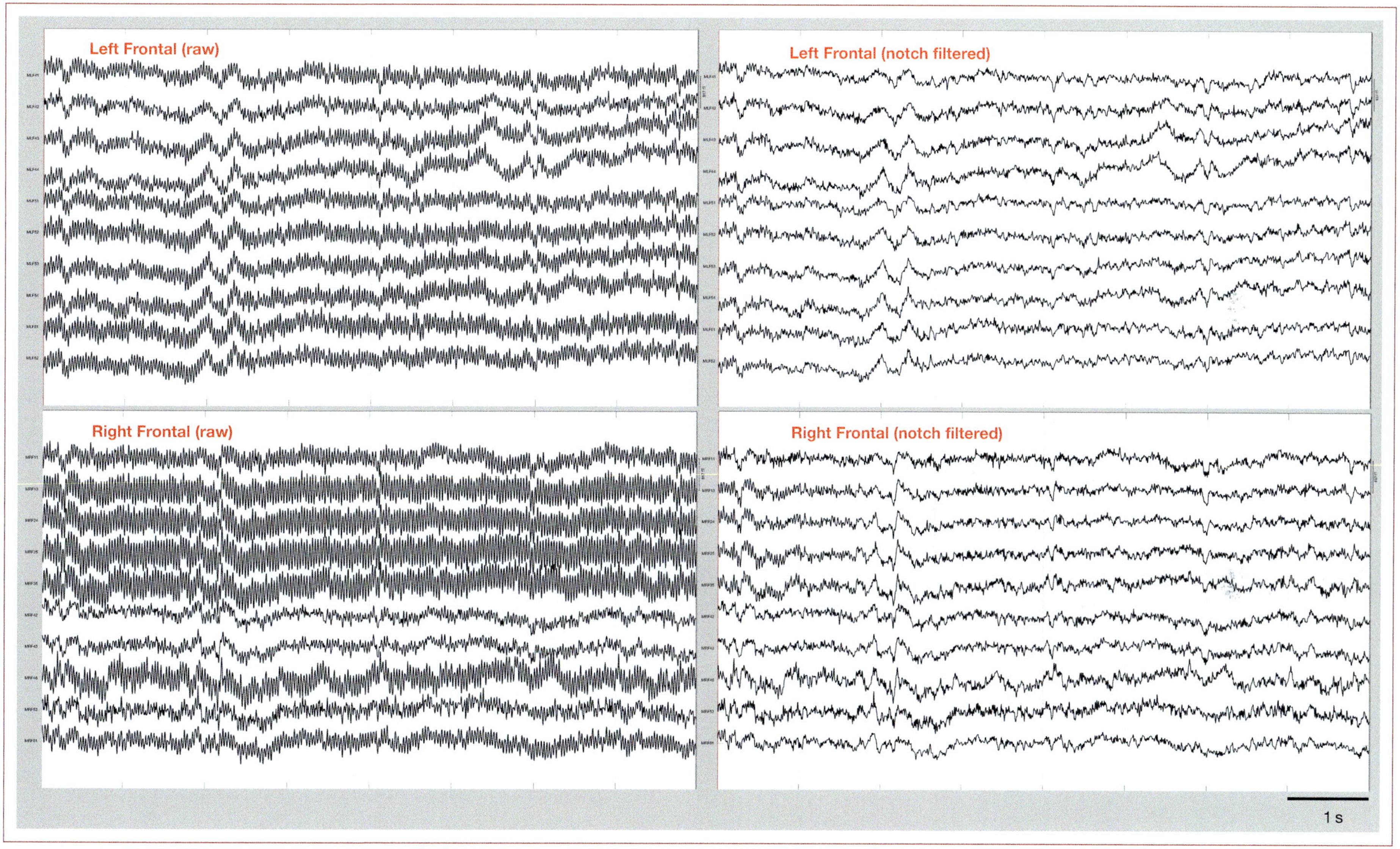

FIGURE 8.17: MEG from left and right frontal sensors before and after applying a 60-Hz notch filter. Recording from a 45-year-old man with a CTF (CTF MEG International Services LP, British Columbia, Canada) system at the MEG laboratory at the Children's Hospital of Philadelphia.

Source: Courtesy of William C. Gaetz.

REFERENCES

1. Hari R. Magnetoencephalography as a tool of clinical neurophysiology. In: Schomer DL, Lopes da Silva FH, eds. *Niedermeyer's Electroencephalography*. 4th ed. Philadelphia, PA: Wolters Kluwer/Lippincott Williams and Wilkins; 1999:1107-1134.

2. Parkkonen L, Salmelin R. Measurements. In: Hansen PC, Kringelbach ML, Salmelin R, eds. *MEG: An Introduction to Methods*. New York, NY: Oxford University Press; 2010:71-80.

3. Muthukumaraswamy SD. High-frequency brain activity and muscle artifacts in MEG/EEG: a review and recommendations. *Front Hum Neurosci*. 2013;7:138. doi:10.3389/fnhum.2013.00138.

4. Gaetz W, Otsubo H, Pang EW. Magnetoencephalography for clinical pediatrics: the effect of head positioning on measurement of somatosensory-evoked fields. *Clin Neurophysiol*. 2008;119(8):1923-1933. doi:10.1016/j.clinph.2008.04.291.

5. Velmurugan J, Sinha S, Satishchandra P. Magnetoencephalography recording and analysis. *Ann Indian Acad Neurol*. 2014;17(5):113-119. doi:10.4103/0972-2327.128678.

6. Jousmäki V, Hari R. Cardiac artifacts in magnetoencephalogram. *J Clin Neurophysiol*. 1996;13(2):172-176. doi:10.1097/00004691-199603000-00008.

7. Samonas M, Petrou M, Ioannides A. Identification and elimination of cardiac contribution in single-trial magnetoencephalographic signals. *IEEE Trans Biomed Eng*. 1997;44:386-393. doi:10.1109/10.568914.

8. Carl C, Açık A, König P, et al. The saccadic spike artifact in MEG. *Neuroimage*. 2012;59(2):1657-1667. doi:10.1016/j.neuroimage.2011.09.020.

9. Criswell E. *Cram's Introduction to Surface Electromyography*. London, UK: Jones & Bartlett; 2011.

10. Tamilia E, Madsen JR, Grant PE, et al. Current and emerging potential of magnetoencephalography in the detection and localization of high-frequency oscillations in epilepsy. *Front Neurol*. 2017;8(1):14. doi:10.3389/fneur.2017.00014.

11. Okada Y, Hamalainen M, Pratt K, et al. BabyMEG: A whole-head pediatric magnetoencephalography system for human brain development research. *Rev Sci Instrum*. 2016;87:094301. doi:10.1063/1.4962020.

12. Tanaka N, Stufflebeam SM. Clinical application of spatiotemporal distributed source analysis in presurgical evaluation of epilepsy. *Front Hum Neurosci*. 2014;8:62. doi:10.3389/fnhum.2014.00062.

13. Papadelis C, Butler EE, Rubenstein M, et al. Reorganization of the somatosensory cortex in hemiplegic cerebral palsy associated with impaired sensory tracts. *Neuroimage Clin*. 2017;17:198-212. doi:10.1016/j.nicl.2017.10.021.

14. Vigario RN. Extraction of ocular artifacts from EEG using independent component analysis. *Electroencephalogr Clin Neurophysiol*. 1997;103:395-404. doi:10.1016/s0013-4694(97)00042-8.

15. Kobayashi K, Merlet I, Gotman J. Separation of spikes from background by independent component analysis with dipole modeling and comparison to intracranial recording. *Clin Neurophysiol*. 2001;112:405-413. doi:10.1016/s1388-2457(01)00457-6.

16. Klados MA, Papadelis C, Braun C, et al. REG-ICA: a hybrid methodology combining Blind Source Separation and regression techniques for the rejection of ocular artifacts. *Biomed Signal Process Control*. 2011;6(3):291-300. doi:10.1016/j.bspc.2011.02.001.

17. Taulu S, Kajola M, Simola J. Suppression of interference and artifacts by the signal space separation method. *Brain Topogr*. 2004;16(4):269-275. doi:10.1023/b:brat.0000032864.93890.f9.

18. Taulu S, Simola J. Spatiotemporal signal space separation method for rejecting nearby interference in MEG measurements. *Phys Med Biol*. 2006;51(7): 1759-1768. doi:10.1088/0031-9155/51/7/008.

19. Taulu S, Hari R. Removal of magnetoencephalographic artifacts with temporal signal-space separation: demonstration with single-trial auditory-evoked responses. *Hum Brain Mapp*. 2009;30(5):1524-1534. doi:10.1002/hbm.20627.

20. Medvedovsky M, Taulu S, Bikmullina R, Paetau R. Artifact and head movement compensation in MEG. *Neurol Neurophysiol Neurosci*. 2007;29:4.

21. Kakisaka Y, Wang ZI, Mosher JC, et al. Clinical evidence for the utility of movement compensation algorithm in magnetoencephalography: successful localization during focal seizure. *Epilepsy Res*. 2012;101(1-2): 191-196. doi:10.1016/j.eplepsyres.2012.03.014.

CHAPTER 9

Nerve Conduction Studies and Needle Electromyography

Devon I. Rubin and Ruple S. Laughlin

INTRODUCTION

In clinical electromyography (EMG), electrical signals from muscle fibers or nerves are recorded and analyzed to determine the function of nerves, neuromuscular junctions, and muscle fibers. In disease states, alterations in the signals on nerve conduction studies (NCSs) and/or needle EMG indicate the presence and type of disorder. In contrast to EEG where the physiologic electrical signals originating in the central nervous system are of extremely low voltage, the signals generated from peripheral nerve axons and muscle fibers are somewhat larger. As a result, external electrical artifacts less commonly interfere with the physiologic signals during NCS and needle EMG. Furthermore, advances in modern equipment, the use of common mode rejection differential amplifiers, and appropriate grounding of equipment have significantly reduced nonphysiologic artifacts. Nonetheless, artifacts such as 50- or 60-Hz signals from nearby external sources or artifacts from sources such as pacemakers or nerve stimulators still do occur and may be recorded during needle EMG. Since some of the artifacts can impede reliable interpretation of true physiologic responses or may mimic physiologic waveforms, recognition of artifacts is critical to prevent misinterpretation of a study. This chapter will review a variety of external artifacts as well as artifactual responses due to technical errors during NCS and needle EMG.

NCS ARTIFACTS

NCSs are a component of an electrodiagnostic examination during which a nerve is stimulated with an electrical stimulator and the action potentials propagating along the nerve or a muscle innervated by that nerve are recorded, usually with surface recording electrodes. Although nonphysiologic artifacts are uncommon during the performance of NCS with modern-day equipment, "artifactual" responses are frequent. Artifactual responses refer to recorded waveforms that do not accurately represent the true or optimal physiologic response, and are frequently due to technical problems in the performance of an NCS. Artifactual responses can occur due to many factors, including problems with nerve stimulation, errors in nerve or muscle recording, physiologic conditions such as low surface temperature, or the presence of anomalous variant nerve anatomy. These artifactual responses may be more difficult to identify than external nonphysiologic artifacts, as the responses obtained may look "real" but still not be the optimal responses. As a result, the presence of these artifactual responses may result in false-positive (misdiagnosis of a disease) or false-negative interpretations of a study. This section will discuss and demonstrate artifactual responses due to technical problems as well as external, nonphysiologic artifacts in NCS.

ARTIFACTS DURING MOTOR NCS

The goal of a motor NCS is to test the integrity of an individual nerve, the neuromuscular junctions, and the muscle fibers innervated by that nerve. A motor NCS is performed by electrically stimulating (and depolarizing) all of the axons within a nerve and recording the summation of all of the muscle fiber action potentials generated in the innervated muscle. This study requires appropriate placement of the recording electrodes over the muscle and appropriate stimulation of the nerve. Technical problems with recording and stimulating can produce artifactual and inaccurate responses (1).

Artifactual Low Amplitude–G1 Electrode Placement

This median motor NCS was recorded from a 49-year-old man with hand pain and demonstrates low compound muscle action potential (CMAP) amplitude (Figure 9.1A). In our laboratory, the normal amplitude from the elbow stimulation site is greater than 4.0 mV and in this study it is 3.2 mV. Low CMAP amplitude would be suggestive of a process anywhere along the motor unit, including loss of anterior horn cells or motor axons, a severe neuromuscular junction defect, or severe loss of muscle fibers in a myopathy. However, technical problems such as incorrect placement of the G1 (active) recording electrode can also result in low CMAP amplitude.

The ideal placement of the G1 recording electrode during a motor NCS is directly over the endplate zone. At this site, the action potentials are initiated along the muscle fibers and propagate away from the electrode along the course of the muscle fibers. Since the extracellular electrical field generated from the inward sodium ion flow during the action potential generation is negative at the site of sodium channel opening and positive on the preceding and trailing "tails" of the moving potential, a CMAP waveform recorded directly over the endplate will have an upward deflection from the baseline and appear as a biphasic, negative (upward)–positive (downward) wave. When the G1 electrode is placed along the muscle at a site away from the endplate zone, the preceding positive electrical field from the action potential moving toward the electrode will produce an initial "positive dip" in the CMAP morphology and result in a triphasic, positive–negative–positive waveform. Additionally, since the electrical field density is lower, the further the electrode is from the endplate zone, the more gradual the negative slope and the lower the amplitude of the CMAP (1).

In most cases in which the G1 electrode is not placed directly over the endplate zone, the CMAP amplitude will be lower than it should be and an initial positive deflection will be present. However, a low CMAP can occur without the "positive dip." Therefore, a problem with G1 electrode placement should always be considered first when an unexpectedly low CMAP amplitude is recorded. In this case, the G1 electrode was moved and the amplitudes significantly increased. After the G1 electrode was moved along the muscle belly, much higher amplitude (11.6 mV) was recorded in this patient (Figure 9.1B).

Artifactual Low Amplitude–Stimulator Off Nerve

The tibial motor response was recorded from a 57-year-old woman with foot burning and a normal neurologic examination and demonstrates a much lower CMAP amplitude at the knee (8.8 mV) than at the ankle (18.3 mV) (Figure 9.2A). During a motor NCS, when all of the axons within the nerve being tested are depolarized by electrical stimulation, all of the muscle fibers innervated by that nerve will elicit action potentials. The summation of each of the muscle fiber action potentials produces the CMAP response, and the amplitude of the CMAP directly reflects the number of muscle fibers depolarized and indirectly reflects the number of axons present within the nerve. Therefore, accurate CMAP amplitude requires depolarization of all of the axons within the nerve. When the electrical current administered through the stimulator is not sufficient to depolarize some of the axons, the recorded CMAP amplitude may be lower than the actual amplitude and does not reflect the true integrity of the nerve or muscle. Artifactual low amplitudes from inadequate nerve stimulation can result from placement of the stimulator at a distance from the nerve or may occur when certain anatomic factors are present, such as limb edema, prior nerve transposition, and in limbs with a larger amount of subcutaneous tissue (1). In the most severe situation when the stimulator is located far away from the nerve being tested, no response will be recorded. In other cases, artifactual low amplitude is obtained since only a portion of the axons are depolarized. If submaximal stimulation occurs at a proximal stimulation site but not the distal site, the artifactual low proximal CMAP amplitude may mimic a conduction block.

Techniques to ensure maximum stimulation of a nerve include sliding the stimulator parallel to the expected course of the nerve to determine the highest amplitude response at low stimulus intensity (1). A higher amplitude response at a different site (without a change in the stimulus intensity) indicates closer proximity to the nerve. The stimulator is moved several times in both directions until the site of the maximum amplitude waveform is identified. At that site, the stimulus intensity is then increased until a supramaximal response is obtained. Ensuring that the stimulus intensity is increased by 5% to 10% after the waveform appears to be maximal is important to ensure that all axons have been depolarized. In this case, after sliding the stimulator and ensuring supramaximal stimulation, the CMAP amplitude increased to 13.8 mV (Figure 9.2B).

Artifactual High Amplitude–Overstimulation

The peroneal motor NCS was performed in a 60-year-old patient with leg pain and demonstrates larger CMAP amplitude with stimulation at the knee (3.7 mV) than at the ankle (3.1 mV) (**Figure 9.3A**). Since motor axons within a nerve all have approximately the same diameter and degree of myelination, they all conduct action potentials at approximately the same rate. However, given slight variations in the conduction along the motor axons, when a nerve is stimulated at two different sites (such as at the elbow and axilla), there is a slight dispersion of the CMAP waveform and slight reduction in the amplitude from the more proximal stimulation site compared to the distal site. In every normal motor nerve, the CMAP amplitude at the distal site should be either slightly higher than or equal to the amplitude at the proximal site. A higher CMAP amplitude at a proximal site than distal site indicates either a technical problem or anomalous anatomic variation.

Overstimulation is one common technical problem that can result in an artifactual high CMAP amplitude (1). When too much current is administered to a nerve, the excess current will spread through the extracellular tissue and will not only depolarize the nerve of intent, but may also spread to another nearby nerve (or portion of the brachial plexus when stimulating at Erb's point). When another nerve is additionally depolarized and muscles supplied by that nerve are in the vicinity of the G1 recording electrode, stimulation of multiple nerves may yield artifactual large CMAP amplitude due to the summation of responses of multiple nerves and the subsequent activation of muscle fibers in the vicinity of the recording electrode. Overstimulation can also change the waveform morphology and result in inaccuracies in marking the onset latencies of the waveform, yielding inaccurate conduction velocities and latency measurements. Additionally, overstimulation may mimic anomalous innervation if the amplitude of the response is higher proximally than distally.

When performing motor NCS, careful observation of the waveform as well as the visible muscle movement elicited by stimulation is important. If the waveform changes in morphology when stimulation is increased in 5% to 10% increments, or if the muscle twitch is not one expected from stimulation of the intended nerve, it is important to reassess and reduce stimulation intensity, slide the stimulator, and begin again. In this case, overstimulation at the knee led to current spread to and depolarization of the tibial nerve, in addition to the peroneal nerve. The G1 electrode over the extensor digitorum brevis (EDB) recorded action potentials from tibial-innervated foot muscles. The waveform morphologies were different and the patient's foot was noted to change from dorsiflexion to plantar flexion as the stimulus intensity increased. When only the peroneal nerve was stimulated, the amplitudes were similar between the ankle and knee (**Figure 9.3B**).

Artifactual High Amplitude–Martin-Gruber Anastomosis

The median motor study was performed in a 60-year-old woman with arm numbness, and demonstrates higher CMAP amplitude at the elbow (13.5 mV) than at the wrist (8.4 mV) (**Figure 9.4**). When a higher CMAP amplitude at a proximal site compared to a distal site is encountered, technical factors such as submaximal stimulation at a distal site or overstimulation at a proximal site should be considered. When these technical problems have been excluded, another possible cause is anomalous anatomy. During a median motor NCS, when the CMAP amplitude at the elbow is higher than at the wrist, a Martin-Gruber anastomosis may be present. This is a common anatomic variation that consists of a communication between the median and ulnar nerve fibers in the forearm, whereby fibers that are destined to supply ulnar-innervated muscles course through the median nerve in the upper arm and proximal forearm, and "cross over" to the ulnar nerve in the forearm before innervating the destined muscles (2–5). When the crossing-over fibers supply ulnar muscles that are located in the hand adjacent to the thenar region (such as first dorsal interosseous, adductor pollicis, or abductor pollicis brevis), an artifactual high CMAP amplitude with elbow stimulation during a routine median motor NCS is recorded. This results from the summation of the volume-conducted CMAP response from the nearby ulnar-innervated muscles that are supplied through the crossing-over fibers to the "normal" median CMAP response originating from the abductor pollicis brevis and opponens pollicis. This addition of other muscle fiber action potentials results in a higher CMAP amplitude at the elbow than at the wrist (where only the true median fibers are activated).

Artifactual High Amplitude–Accessory Peroneal Nerve

The peroneal motor NCS, with recording from the EDB, was recorded from a 49-year-old man and demonstrates a higher CMAP amplitude with stimulation at the knee (4.1 mV) than at the ankle (3.8 mV) (**Figure 9.5A**). Anomalous innervation in the lower extremity can produce an artifactual appearing result and mimic a technical problem. In motor NCS, all of the axons within the nerve being studied should be depolarized through electrical stimulation and reflected in the resultant muscle CMAP amplitude with appropriate stimulation intensity. The CMAP amplitudes should be approximately the same at all sites of stimulation, with the proximal stimulation sites often being slightly lower than distal sites due to normal minor dispersion of the response. A higher proximal than distal amplitude never occurs from a physiologic basis, and only is seen with technical problems (e.g., overstimulation at the proximal site or understimulation at the distal site) or anomalous innervation. Technical factors should always be checked first, such as ensuring that the foot is dorsiflexing upon stimulation, sliding the stimulator if necessary, and excluding understimulation at the distal stimulation site.

If technical factors are excluded and the proximal peroneal motor CMAP amplitude is still higher than the distal site, the patient likely has an "accessory peroneal nerve." This is a normal anatomic variant, present in approximately 15% to 20% of individuals, in which the terminal branch of the superficial peroneal nerve that courses along the lateral leg and behind the lateral malleolus innervates a portion of the EDB (1). As a result, some of the axons innervating some fibers of the EDB muscle are not depolarized when the peroneal nerve is stimulated at the normal distal stimulation site at the anterior ankle. An accessory peroneal nerve can easily be confirmed by stimulation behind the lateral malleolus, in which a response will be recorded from the EDB due to this anomalous pathway. This was confirmed in the patient in **Figure 9.5B**.

Artifactual Slowed Conduction Velocity–Incorrect Distance Measurement

This ulnar motor NCS was performed in a 35-year-old woman with hand tingling, and demonstrates a mildly slowed conduction velocity (CV) (49 m/sec, normal >51 m/sec) across the elbow (**Figure 9.6A**). In motor NCS, CV between two or more sites of stimulation is calculated to assess the integrity of the axons and myelin in a specific nerve segment. The CV is calculated by determining the difference in onset latencies of the recorded waveforms between the different sites of stimulation divided into the distance between the stimulation sites, usually measured in millimeters. Accurate calculation of the CV requires precise and accurate measurement of the actual course of the nerve being studied. Measurement is made by holding a measuring tape along the skin surface of the limb between the stimulation points. If the tape measure is not accurately placed along the actual course of the nerve, the recorded distance will not reflect the actual length of the nerve. When a falsely short measurement is recorded, such as when the tape measure is placed in front of the medial epicondyle rather than behind the epicondyle through the ulnar groove, the CV will be artifactual slowed and may mimic disease (1). This may occur more commonly in the ulnar nerve around the elbow, where it is more difficult to know the actual course of the nerve. The effect of measurement error is proportional to the distance between the two stimulation sites, with a much greater error the shorter the distance. In this case, when the nerve measurement was accurate, the CV was normal (**Figure 9.6B**).

Artifactual Fast CV–Martin-Gruber Anastomosis

The median motor NCS was performed in a 79-year-old woman with a moderate left median neuropathy, and demonstrated a CV of 75 m/sec (**Figure 9.7**). A normal CV of motor axons in most nerves in most patients ranges from approximately 50 to 60 m/sec. This patient had an artifactual, excessively fast CV, which is outside of the normal range expected for a patient of this age. Artifactual fast CVs can occur as the result of technical errors, such as incorrect distance measurement or overstimulation and depolarization of adjacent nerves. In this case, technical problems were excluded. What is also noted in this case is that the waveform morphology between the wrist and elbow sites differs with the elbow waveform, demonstrating a "notch" in the waveform. This is indicative of a Martin-Gruber anastomosis in the context of a median neuropathy at the wrist (6,7). An earlier example demonstrated and discussed how a Martin-Gruber anastomosis can produce a higher CMAP amplitude at the elbow than wrist in a median motor NCS, due to the addition of muscle fibers from nearby ulnar innervated muscles supplied by the crossing-over fibers. When this is present in the context of a median neuropathy at the wrist, the slowing of the conduction across the wrist delays the latencies of the "true" median responses (the portion of the CMAP that originates from the ABP/opponens pollicis). However, the portion of the CMAP that courses through the crossing-over fibers (which are located in the ulnar nerve at the wrist and are not compressed at the wrist) is not delayed. This results in a separation between the "median" CMAP and the "crossover" CMAP. Therefore, the initial onset of the waveform at the elbow does not represent the true median fibers; however, the latency marker is usually automatically placed at the onset latency by the machine which includes the faster MGA fibers bypassing the carpal tunnel, resulting in a calculated CV that will be falsely fast. This often also results in a "notched" appearance of the proximal waveform. In severe cases, there may be a complete separation of the true median CMAP and the crossover CMAP.

ARTIFACTS DURING SENSORY NCS

Sensory NCSs are performed by electrically stimulating the axons within a nerve and recording the sensory nerve action potentials (SNAPs) at another site along the nerve. Since SNAPs are much smaller than muscle fiber action potentials (or CMAPs) recorded during motor NCS, careful attention to technique is critical to obtain the most accurate response. Problems with nerve identification during stimulation or placement of the recording electrodes, limb temperature, and stimulus and motor artifact can all interfere with obtaining the most accurate responses.

Artifactual Low Amplitude—G1 Placement Off Nerve

This medial antebrachial cutaneous NCS was performed in a 50-year-old man with arm paresthesia demonstrating fairly low amplitude (5 μV) (**Figure 9.8A**). Sensory NCS record the summated SNAPs traveling along the nerve past the recording electrodes. In order to record the maximum electrical field from the travelling volley of the action potentials, the recording electrodes are placed as close as possible to the nerve. The further the G1 recording electrode is from the action potential generator, the lower the amplitude in response. This is particularly important in sensory studies where the amplitudes are much lower than motor responses. Additionally, the G1 and G2 electrodes should be placed 3.5 to 4 cm apart to maximize the amplitude of the waveform displayed through a differential amplifier. If the two electrodes are less than 3 cm apart, the SNAP amplitude decreases. In this case, the G1 electrode was located too far lateral to the actual course of the medial antebrachial nerve. Once the electrode was moved a few centimeters medially, a higher amplitude (11 μV) was recorded (**Figure 9.8B**).

Artifactual Low Amplitude—Limb Edema

The sural sensory NCS was performed in a 30-year-old woman with radicular leg pain and lower limb lymphedema, and demonstrated a low-amplitude response (**Figure 9.9A**). In most laboratories, routine NCSs are performed using surface recording electrodes placed on the skin over the nerve being studied. Since SNAPs are very low amplitude, they are much more susceptible to the effect of distance between the nerve and recording electrodes. The recording electrodes record the electrical field generated by the action potential propagating along the nerve. This electrical field is strongest immediately adjacent to the nerve and decreases further away from the nerve. Therefore, conditions that increase the distance between the skin and nerve may have a significant effect on the recorded sensory (more than motor) amplitude, producing artifactual low amplitude.

In patients with lymphedema, fluid accumulation in the subcutaneous tissue and less commonly in the muscle increases the distance between the nerve and the skin surface. This may not only impact the ability to obtain supramaximal stimulation due to the increased distance between surface shock and nerve, but also affects the recorded amplitude. Low amplitudes on NCS should be interpreted with caution in patients with lymphedema as they may not accurately reflect the integrity of the nerve. It is important to be conscientious of these limitations to avoid erroneous conclusions regarding pathology. The effects of edema are difficult to mitigate; in these cases good electrode-to-skin contact is quite important. If concern is high for a falsely low-amplitude response, needle stimulation or needle recording may be considered. In this patient, the surface stimulator was pressed more deeply into the skin to ensure that it was as close as possible to the nerve, resulting in a slightly higher amplitude (**Figure 9.9B**).

Artifactual Long Distal Latency—Cool Limb Temperature

This median antidromic sensory response was recorded from a 50-year-old man with hand numbness, and demonstrates a prolonged distal latency (**Figure 9.10A**). Although this would suggest that the patient might have carpal tunnel syndrome, the amplitude of the response is very high and the waveform morphology appears somewhat broad for a SNAP, raising the suspicion that there may be low limb temperature.

Cool limb temperature prolongs the duration of opening of the sodium and potassium channels and slows the electrotonic spread of the action potential along the nerve. This results in slowing of the conduction time along the nerve and may be seen as an artifactual prolonged distal latency (by approximately 0.2 milliseconds/°C decrease) and slowed CV (by 1.8–2.0 milliseconds/°C decrease). Additionally, both the amplitude and duration of the waveform response will be increased. The artifactual prolongation of the distal latencies due to cool limb temperature can lead to the erroneous interpretation of a study as indicative of polyneuropathy or carpal tunnel syndrome. Limb surface temperatures should always be measured prior to the performance of an NCS. The ideal temperature for the NCS should be greater than 32°C on the hand and greater than 30°C on the foot. If the limb is too cool, it should be warmed prior to the study. When the limb was warmed in this patient, the distal latency normalized (**Figure 9.10B**).

Artifactual Long Distal Latency—Cathode-Anode Reversal

This median antidromic NCS was performed in a 48-year-old woman without any hand numbness, and demonstrates a prolonged distal latency (normal <3.6 milliseconds) (**Figure 9.11A**). This could be consistent with carpal tunnel syndrome. However, technical factors should always be considered when an abnormal finding is encountered. During routine NCS using a bipolar electrical stimulator, the cathode (the site under which the nerve is depolarized) is placed directly over the nerve, pointed toward the recording electrodes, with the anode approximately 2 cm distant to the cathode. If the cathode and anode are inadvertently reversed, the nerve is depolarized approximately 2 cm further away from the recording electrode. This additional 2 cm of distance that the action potentials must travel along the nerve will increase the distal latency by approximately 0.4 milliseconds. In patients being evaluated for mild carpal tunnel syndrome, where prolongation of the sensory distal latency may be the only finding, inadvertent cathode–anode reversal may produce an artifactual long distal latency (a false-positive study). An additional effect of cathode–anode reversal is that a theoretical block of conduction of some of the fibers may occur as a result of hyperpolarization of axons at the anode. Anode block can consequently require a higher stimulus intensity to depolarize the axons. In this patient, when the cathode and anode were appropriately placed, the distal latency was normal (**Figure 9.11B**).

Artifactual Long Distal Latency–Wrong Distal Measurement

The median sensory antidromic NCS was performed in a 50-year-old man with arm pain and demonstrated a prolonged distal latency of 3.9 milliseconds(normal <3.6 milliseconds) (**Figure 9.12A**). One parameter assessed in each NCS is the distal latency, or time from the stimulus to the onset or peak of the recorded waveform with stimulation at a distal site. Normative reverence data for NCS are derived using specific laboratory techniques. Distal latency reference values are derived using standard distances between the stimulator cathode and G1 recording electrode. Therefore, the distal stimulation should be performed as close as possible to the standard distance. When an incorrect and excessively long distal distance is used, the actual length of the nerve segment being tested will be longer than normal. Therefore, the time for the action potentials to reach the recording electrode will increase, producing artifactual long distal latency. This could result in a false-positive study and an incorrect diagnosis in a normal patient. Falsely long distal distances can occur with imprecise measurement technique, in situations where the stimulator was moved (sliding technique) to optimally identify the nerve, or in patients with long limbs, such as a long hand. In cases where sliding resulted in a longer distal distance, the study should be repeated at a more accurate distance. In this example, the initial distance was 15 cm and, after stimulating at 13 cm, the distal latency was 3.4 milliseconds (**Figure 9.12B**).

Shock/Stimulus Artifact

This medial plantar NCS was recorded from a 40-year-old patient with foot pain and demonstrated prominent shock artifact, resulting in artifactual low amplitude (**Figure 9.13A**). Shock artifact, also called stimulus artifact, is the artifact that occurs from the spread of the stimulating current over the skin directly to the recording electrode. While shock artifact is present on every NCS, it is much more prominent in sensory than motor NCS due to the high signal amplification needed to display sensory waveforms. The shock artifact can alter the actual recorded waveform or run into the actual waveform, particularly if the distance between the stimulator and recording electrodes is short. The most common scenario is a distortion of the baseline by the shock artifact, hindering accurate marking of waveform onset for latency measurements. Methods to reduce shock artifact include minimizing the amount of electrical conducting paste placed on the stimulator as well as reducing impedance with good skin preparation prior to electrode application. Utilizing a smaller stimulating head may also limit current spread due to the closer relationship between anode and cathode. When the shock artifact does interfere with the SNAP baseline or waveform, rotating the stimulator anode around the cathode can reduce the impact of the shock artifact on the recorded response by finding a position in which the electrical field difference is the smallest, allowing the electrical stimulus to reach both the G1 and G2 electrodes to a similar degree and cancel out. When this was performed in the same patient, the onset baseline became more accurate and the amplitude increased to 20 μV (**Figure 9.13B**).

Motor Artifact

This ulnar sensory antidromic NCS was performed in a 50-year-old patient with hand pain, and demonstrates prominent motor artifact (arrows) (**Figure 9.14A**). Some sensory NCSs are performed by stimulating a mixed nerve (with motor and sensory fibers) and recording over a site where only sensory axons are present, such as over a digit in the hand. In these studies, although the intended response to be analyzed is the SNAP response, the electrical field from the muscle fibers that are also depolarized may be picked up by the recording electrodes through volume conduction through the extracellular tissue. Since sensory axons conduct at a slightly faster rate than motor axons, the SNAP will occur earlier than the motor response. However, the motor response is much larger than the SNAP amplitude and can distort or interfere with the identification and marking of the SNAP response. In cases where the SNAP is absent, a portion of the motor artifact may be misinterpreted as the sensory response. This is most commonly seen in ulnar antidromic studies, where the abductor digit minimi is in close proximity to the 5th digit. Motor artifact can be reduced by moving the G1 recording electrode a short distance away from the stimulator (such as over the proximal interphalangeal joint instead of the metacarpal phalangeal joint) and shielding the recording electrodes with gauze. In this case, moving the G1 electrode slightly more distal on the digit reduced the artifact (8) (Figure 9.14B).

60-Hz Artifact

This radial sensory NCS was attempted in a 70-year-old patient in the ICU and demonstrates prominent 60-Hz artifact that interfered with the recorded response (Figure 9.15A). During routine NCS, 60-Hz artifact can interfere with the recorded waveforms. This artifact is most problematic in areas where other electrical equipment is present (e.g., intravenous [IV] pumps or ventilation devices), such as a hospital room or an ICU setting. The green ground electrode applied to the patient is a common reference point that is used in differential amplifiers in EMG machines to attempt to reduce 60-Hz artifact that is common to both the G1 and G2 electrodes. However, it does not perfectly reduce the artifact. When 60-Hz artifact is prominent, high-amplitude sinusoidal waves can interfere with the identification of the true nerve response due to their inability to obtain a clear baseline, and signal distortion. Sensory NCSs are much more affected by such artifacts due to their filter settings and low amplitude, requiring greater amplification (which also amplifies the 60-Hz artifact). Methods used to reduce the artifact include the use of a larger ground electrode and reducing the possible sources as much as possible (e.g., turning off lights, unplugging a hospital bed). When a larger ground was used and equipment was turned off, a radial response was able to be recorded (Figure 9.15B).

ARTIFACTS DURING REPETITIVE NERVE STIMULATION

Repetitive nerve stimulation (RNS) is an NCS technique that consists of administering several electrical stimuli at various rates (2–50 Hz) to assess the adequacy of neuromuscular transmission. In normal persons without impaired neuromuscular transmission, supramaximal stimulation at low rates of a nerve results in depolarization of all of the innervated muscle fibers; therefore, the CMAP amplitude and area remain the same with each stimulus. In some neuromuscular junction diseases, such as myasthenia gravis, the amplitude and area of the CMAP decrease with each stimulus, since there is a reduction in the endplate potential at some of the postsynaptic junctions, resulting in an insufficient depolarization to produce action potentials in some of the muscle fibers. The presence and degree of "decrement" in the CMAP amplitude and area helps to diagnose neuromuscular junction diseases. RNS studies are difficult and frought with technical factors that can produce artifactual false decrement (false-positive studies) or, rarely, artifactual normal (false-negative) studies. Technical problems that produce artifactual responses include submaximal stimulation, unstable baselines due to muscle contraction or recording electrode movement, and cool limb temperature (which improves decrement).

Artifactual False Decrement–Stimulator Movement

The spinal accessory RNS study was performed in a 60-year-old man with weakness and appears to demonstrate a maximum amplitude decrement of 52% between the first and fourth stimuli (Figure 9.16A). During RNS, the stimulator must remain in a completely fixed position over the nerve to ensure reliable and reproducible responses. Movement or sliding of the stimulator off the nerve during each stimulus results in a variability and possibly a reduction in the number of axons that are depolarized, thereby resulting in lower CMAP amplitude. This drop in amplitude can mimic real decrement. The pattern of true, physiologic decrement from a neuromuscular junction disorder is a maximum decrease in amplitude (or area) between the first and second stimuli, with less of a drop with each subsequent stimulus. If the pattern of amplitude reduction is not physiologic (such as the largest drop occurring between the third and fourth stimuli), technical factors are likely. The stimulator should be carefully held in a stable position on the skin and supramaximal nerve stimulation should be administered to reduce this artifactual response. In this case, when another set of four stimuli were given and careful attention was made to holding the stimulator still, no significant decrement (2%) was seen (Figure 9.16B).

Artifactual False Decrement–Muscle Contraction

This ulnar RNS study was performed in a 50-year-old man with weakness and appears to demonstrate a maximum amplitude decrement of 11% between the first and fourth stimuli (Figure 9.17A). During RNS, the recording electrodes must remain in a completely fixed position over the muscle to ensure reliable and reproducible responses. Even slight movement of the G1 electrode along the muscle may change the position of the electrode relative to the endplate zone, affecting the morphology and amplitude of the CMAP. This may result in CMAP variability with each stimulus and may mimic decrement. Movement of the electrode can occur when the patient tenses up or contracts the muscle during stimulation. If the morphology of the CMAP waveforms with each stimulus varies, or the pattern of apparent decrement is not physiologic, technical factors are likely. In this case, when the study was repeated and the patient remained relaxed, no decrement was seen (Figure 9.17B).

Artifactual Normal Study–Cool Limb Temperature

This ulnar RNS study was performed in a 42-year-old woman with weakness and positive acetylcholine receptor antibodies, and demonstrated no decrement (Figure 9.18A). The patient was noted to have a cool hand temperature of 27.8°C. Cool limb temperature improves neuromuscular transmission by prolonging the open time of the acetylcholine receptors as well as lowering the activity of acetylcholinesterase at the neuromuscular junction, thereby increasing the safety margin of neuromuscular transmission (9–11). Therefore, RNS performed on a cool limb in a patient with myasthenia gravis may improve the actual decremental response and result in an artifactual normal (false-negative) study. Warming the limb has been shown to increase the degree of decrement and the sensitivity of repetitive NCS in myasthenia gravis. In this patient, when the limb was warmed to 32.2°C, a reproducible 8% decrement was recorded (Figure 9.18B).

ARTIFACTS DURING NEEDLE EMG

During needle EMG, a recording needle electrode is inserted into a muscle and the electrical signals generated from muscle fibers are recorded and amplified. The presence of various abnormal signals from fibers and alterations in the motor unit potential (MUP) morphologies help to determine whether there is an underlying neuromuscular disorder. The electrical signals generated from muscle fibers are very small in amplitude, in the range of 10 µV to 1 to 2 mV, and therefore must be amplified for interpretation. Due to the small amplitude of the signals, various external artifacts and other factors can interfere with the recordings. To reduce the contribution of external artifactual signals, all electrical activity recorded from an "active" wire at the tip of the needle electrode is compared to the activity recorded at a reference site at the same point in time. Through the use of a differential amplifier in the EMG machines, the difference in the voltages between the active and reference sites is amplified and displayed. Therefore, artifactual signals that are recorded equally at the active and reference sites will essentially be cancelled out and minimized. This cancellation effect is higher when needle EMG is performed with a concentric needle electrode (in which the reference electrode is the needle shaft) compared to a monopolar needle electrode (in which the reference electrode is a separate needle or surface electrode placed at some other site on the limb). However, because the signals are recorded to a slightly different degree at the active and reference sites, artifactual signals are not completely eliminated and artifacts can be recorded with both types of electrodes. The use of a ground electrode can help to minimize, but not completely eliminate, external artifacts, by serving as a common reference for the active and reference recording sites. When the ground electrode is not well attached to the patient, external artifacts are more likely to be recorded.

In contrast to external artifacts, artifactual responses can occur from physiologic factors (such as abnormal movements or poor relaxation), which can interfere with the recordings and affect the ability to adequately assess for abnormal waveforms. Similarly, technical factors, related to equipment or technique of the needle examination can interfere with the recordings and lead to misinterpretation of the recordings. This section will provide examples of physiologic, technical, and external artifacts during needle EMG.

PHYSIOLOGIC ARTIFACTS

Tremor

This waveform was recorded from the pronator teres in a 70-year-old man with arm pain (Video 9.1). The recording demonstrated bursts of MUPs that recur repetitively in a regular firing pattern. Each burst consists of a different group of MUPs, as evident by the changing morphology of each burst, due to central activation of different anterior horn cells. This type of regular burst firing of groups of different MUPs is characteristic of a tremor discharge. In many cases, a visible tremor will be evident to the electromyographer during the study; however, sometimes subtle tremor may not be visible. Tremor bursts may appear similar to myokymic discharges or polyphasic MUPs, although the burst of a myokymic discharge consists of the same MUP firing within the group and polyphasic MUPs have spikes that are time-locked to the main spike and fire in a semi-rhythmic firing pattern. The presence of tremor discharges can interfere with the ability to assess for spontaneous discharges, such as fibrillation or fasciculation potentials.

Poor Relaxation

The recording was made from the thoracic paraspinal muscles in a 28-year-old man who was referred for a possible myopathy (Video 9.2). The recording was made with the patient in the lateral decubitus position with attempted relaxation of the paraspinals. During assessment for spontaneous activity, continuous activity from voluntary MUPs was recorded, despite attempts to relax the muscle. The presence of the MUPs makes it difficult to assess for fibrillation potentials. Poor relaxation can occur when patients are in discomfort or tense, have certain neurologic disorders such as spasticity or movement disorders, or in certain muscles that are difficult to relax (such as paraspinals, diaphragm, or genioglossus).

TECHNICAL ARTIFACTS

Decreased Insertion Activity

This recording was made from the anterior tibialis in a 76-year-old man with complete foot drop from an old, severe peroneal neuropathy (Video 9.3). During needle examination of each muscle, examination of a resting muscle is performed to assess for any abnormal spontaneous discharges, such as fibrillation potentials. Needle movements within a muscle typically induce a brief burst of electrical activity as the needle irritation of the fibers initiates action potentials along the fibers (insertional activity). Normal insertional activity consists of a burst of spikes that lasts only as long as the needle electrode is moved, and ceases immediately after needle movement is halted. In cases where muscle tissue has been replaced by fat or connective tissue, no action potentials can be elicited and needle movement will initiate little or no electrical activity, known as decreased insertional activity (12). Decreased insertional activity is an abnormal finding that can produce an artifactual appearing response during assessment of a resting muscle. While it is often seen in severe disease processes, it can also occur from technical factors, such as poor needle connection to the cable or when the preamplifier has not been turned on.

Low-Frequency Filter–Too High

This recording was made from the deltoid of a 35-year-old man with fatigue, and demonstrates a short duration, low appearing MUP (Video 9.4). Every EMG waveform is composed of signals of a wide range of frequencies, typically ranging from 2 Hz to 30 kHz. Various frequency signals compose different parts of the waveform, with the higher amplitude spike component composed of higher frequency waves and the lower amplitude "tails" composed of lower frequency waves. In order to minimize the effect of extraneous electrical noise that may distort the physiologic signals, amplifier filters are applied to all signals prior to signal amplification in EMG machines. During routine EMG studies, the low-frequency filter (LFF) is usually set to 20 to 30 Hz. Increasing the LFF has the effect of reducing the amplitude and contribution of the lower frequency components of the MUP, which mainly compose the preceding and trailing "tails." Filtering these components results in artifactual short duration and lower amplitude MUPs which can mimic a myopathy. When the LFF was decreased to 20 Hz from 2,000 Hz, the MUP duration normalized (Video 9.5).

LFF–Too Low

This recording was made from the first dorsal interosseous at rest in a 52-year-old woman with hand numbness (Video 9.6). The recording demonstrates prominent instability or "swaying" of the baseline during assessment of insertion activity. During routine needle EMG recording, the default LFF is typically set at 20 to 30 Hz. Decreasing the LFF has the effect of allowing more of the lower frequency components of the potentials to contribute to the waveform and results in an increase in slow movement artifact and instability of the baseline. During MUP assessment, a lower LFF allows for incorporation of more of the distant muscle fiber action potentials in the motor unit to be recorded, resulting in an increase in the baseline–baseline duration of the MUP. When normative MUP duration data were collected in the past, the LFF was set at 2 Hz. Therefore, when quantitative EMG is performed and the results are compared to normative data, the LFF should be reduced to 2 Hz for accurate comparison. However, lowering the LFF also introduces additional low-frequency waveforms, such as sweat artifact or artifact from slight movement of the needle, which reduce the stability of the baseline. In this patient, increasing the LFF from 2 to 20 Hz resulted in a more stable baseline (Video 9.7).

Too Rapid Needle Movements

This recording was made from the biceps of a 42-year-old woman with hand numbness (Video 9.8). The recording was made during assessment of insertion and spontaneous activity in the muscle at rest, particularly to assess for fibrillation potentials. Each burst of insertion activity was elicited during brief needle movement. In this example, the needle was constantly being moved with very minimal pauses between needle movements. Although this technique does not produce true artifactual recordings, it may result in artifactual false interpretations since slowly firing spontaneous waveforms (e.g., fibrillation potentials or fasciculation potentials) may be missed. This can be corrected by ensuring pauses of at least 1 to 2 seconds after each needle movement during assessment of a resting muscle (12).

EXTERNAL ARTIFACTS

60-Hz

This artifact was recorded from the anterior tibialis in a 65-year-old man with generalized weakness in the ICU (**Video 9.9**). 60-Hz artifact is the most common type of artifact recorded during needle EMG. Although this artifact does not resemble any physiologic artifact, when it is prominent it may interfere with the baseline recordings and make it more difficult to assess for other spontaneous discharges or MUP abnormalities. 60-Hz artifact is more prominent in environments with a large amount of electrical equipment (e.g., ICU), but can occur in any environment. Sometimes, just a cellphone or tablet plugged into an outlet in the EMG examination room can produce prominent 60-Hz artifact. It can be minimized by using a larger ground electrode, unplugging as much of the nearby equipment as possible, and ideally using a dedicated earth ground for the EMG equipment.

Pacemaker

This waveform was recorded from the thoracic paraspinal muscles in a 75-year-old patient with back pain (**Video 9.10**). This waveform is a single-spike waveform that fires repetitively in a regular pattern and has the sound of a ticking clock. This waveform is a cardiac pacemaker artifact. A pacemaker artifact typically appears as a single spike, usually firing in a regular pattern at a rate of approximately 1 Hz. The regular firing pattern of a single spike may mimic a fibrillation potential. Although a pacemaker artifact is most often recorded in muscles close to the pacemaker, such as thoracic paraspinals, it can be recorded from more distant limb muscles as well. In contrast to a true fibrillation potential, a pacemaker artifact does not change or disappear with needle movement and the same spike firing at the same rate is often found in more than one muscle. Additionally, the square wave morphology of the pacemaker artifact produces an artificial sound that is subtly different from a fibrillation potential.

Pacemaker (With Fibrillation Potentials)

This example was recorded from the thoracic paraspinals in a 69-year-old man with weakness (**Video 9.11**). This recording demonstrates a run of positive waveform fibrillation potentials. However, the larger amplitude single spike is a pacemaker artifact and fires at a regular rate at just under 1 Hz. This pacemaker artifact could easily be confused with a single-spike form fibrillation potential.

Transcutaneous Electrical Nerve Stimulator

This discharge was recorded from the tensor fascia lata muscle in a 50-year-old patient with leg pain (**Video 9.12**). The discharge is a recurrent single spike that fires at a rate of approximately 60-Hz. The interspike intervals between the spikes are completely fixed and do not vary, although occasionally a spike will drop out. This artifact was generated from a transcutaneous electrical nerve stimulator (TENS) unit. The fast, unchanging rate gives the discharge an artifactual sound. This discharge would not likely be misinterpreted as a physiologic waveform, although the fast, unchanging rate could appear somewhat similar to a complex repetitive discharge.

Radiofrequency Artifact

This artifact was recorded from the tensor fascia lata of a 30-year-old patient with leg pain (**Video 9.13**). Although the needle electrode was in the subcutaneous tissue, radiofrequency artifact was recorded. Visually, the artifact is very low amplitude and high frequency, and appears similar to subcutaneous tissue. However, the sound of the radio broadcast (discussing the stock market!) can be easily heard. There is also low-amplitude 60-Hz artifact as well.

Gastric Stimulator

This artifact was recorded from the iliopsoas of a 55-year-old woman with a gastric stimulator (**Video 9.14**). A single positive waveform fires repetitively at a rate of about 15 Hz with a very regular, unchanging pattern. The waveform then pauses briefly before firing again. This could potentially be misinterpreted as a myokymic discharge, but the unchanging rate and morphology of the single spike indicates that this is an artifact.

Deep Brain Stimulator

This artifact was recorded from the deltoid in a 68-year-old patient with Parkinson's disease (**Video 9.15**). This high-frequency artifact is composed of two spikes firing at rates of approximately 200 Hz, with one spike firing slightly slower (which appears to be moving to the right) than the other. This artifact was generated from a deep brain stimulator (DBS) device. Although this artifact does not mimic any physiologic EMG waveform, its prominence can interfere with recording of smaller waveforms (such as fibrillation potentials) or MUP assessment.

Printer Artifact

This artifact was recorded during needle examination of the medial gastrocnemius (**Video 9.16**). The discharge begins with a low-amplitude spike firing at about 12 Hz followed by the addition of a very high-pitched, high-frequency background artifact firing at over 500 Hz. This artifact was recorded during the printing of a waveform from the EMG machine in the exam room.

Text Artifact

This waveform was recorded while assessing spontaneous activity in a resting muscle (the first dorsal interosseous) in a 40-year-old patient with hand numbness (**Video 9.17**). After a brief period of normal spontaneous activity, a repetitive spike is initiated, firing first at 60 Hz, and then suddenly shifting to a slower rate 25 Hz. The interspike intervals between the spikes remain completely fixed and stable. This could have the appearance and sound of a complex repetitive discharge. The discharge occurred at the same moment that the electromyographer received a text message on a smartphone.

CONCLUSIONS

External artifacts and artifactual responses due to technical factors are common in clinical EMG. Recognition of these artifactual responses is critical to ensuring accurate interpretation of the NCSs and needle EMG findings. When identified, the electromyographer must take the appropriate steps to reduce or resolve the artifactual response and ensure technically reliable studies.

VIDEOS

Video 9.1: Tremor producing an electrophysiologic discharge in a resting muscle.

Video 9.2: Artifactual "active" baseline in a resting muscle due to poor muscle relaxation.

Video 9.3: Decreased insertion activity due to severe muscle atrophy.

Video 9.4: Artifactual short duration, low-amplitude motor unit potentials due to low frequency filter set too high (2000 Hz).

Video 9.5: Same motor unit potentials as Video 9.4, now with normal duration and amplitude when low frequency filter set at 20 Hz.

Video 9.6: Unstable baseline sway due to low frequency filter set too low (2 Hz).

Video 9.7: Normal baseline when low frequency filter set to 20 Hz.

Video 9.8: Rapid needle movements in a resting muscle obscure the baseline, making it difficult to assess for slow spontaneous discharges.

Video 9.9: 60-Hz artifact present during needle EMG.

Video 9.10: Pacemaker artifact recorded during needle examination of the thoracic paraspinal muscles.

Video 9.11: Fibrillation potentials present with a pacemaker artifact.

Video 9.12: TENS unit artifact recorded during needle EMG.

Video 9.13: Radiofrequency artifact recorded during needle EMG.

Video 9.14: Gastric stimulator artifact recorded during needle EMG.

Video 9.15: Deep brain stimulator artifact recorded during needle EMG.

Video 9.16: Printer artifact recorded during needle EMG.

Video 9.17: Smartphone text artifact recorded during needle EMG.

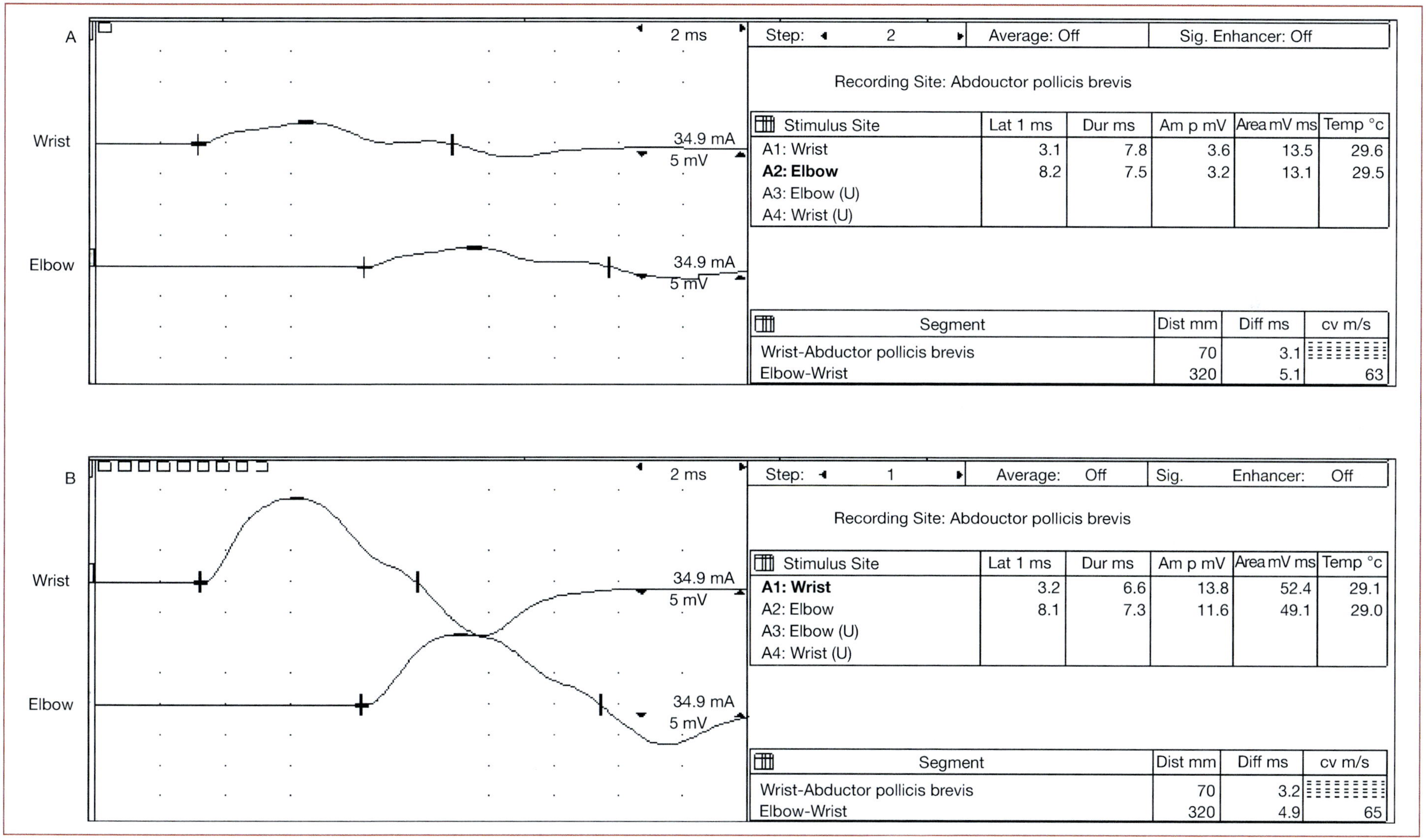

FIGURE 9.1: (A) Artifactual low-amplitude median motor CMAP due to G1 electrode placement away from the end plate zone. (B) Normal amplitude is noted after moving the G1 electrode over the end plate zone.

CMAP, compound muscle action potential.

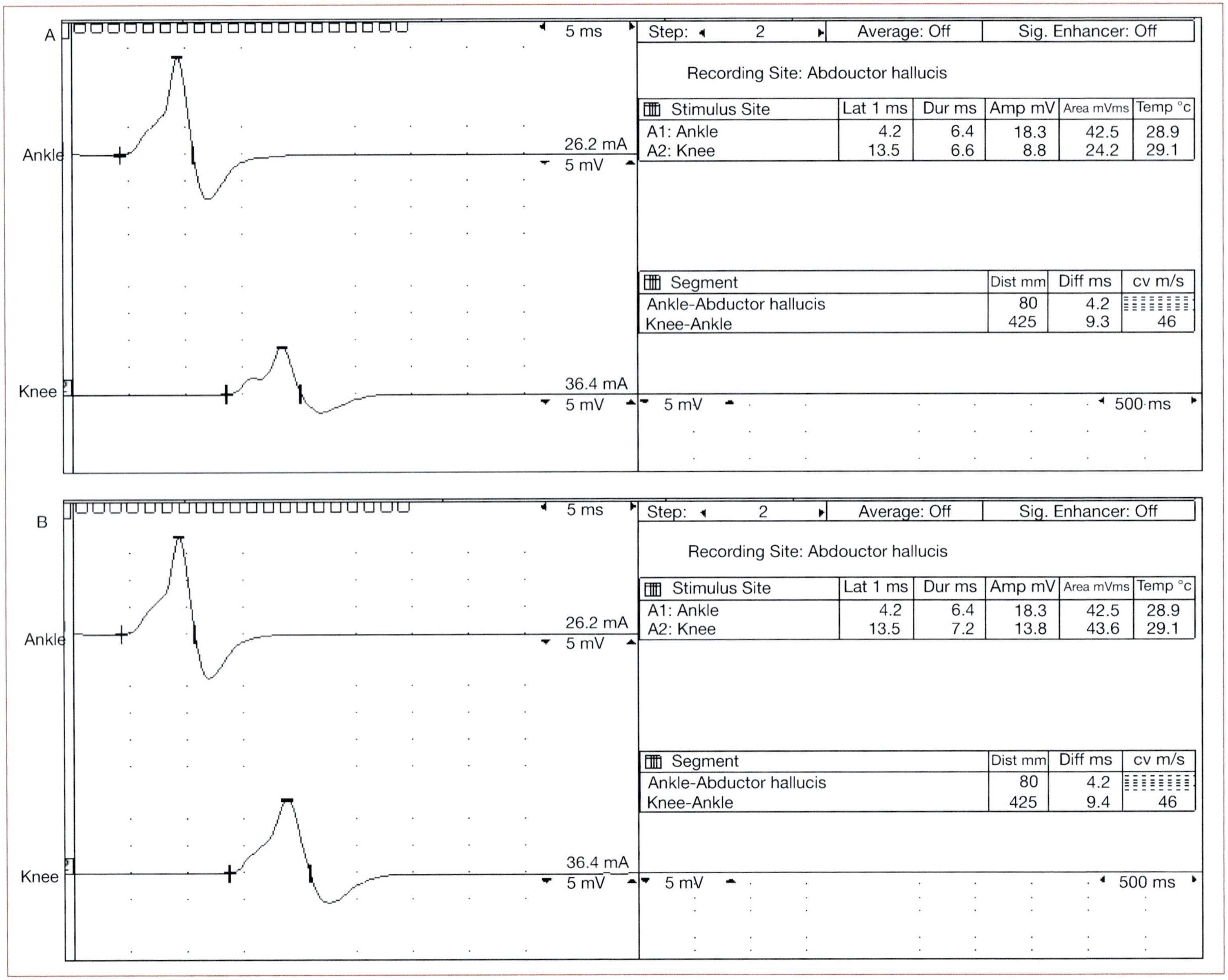

FIGURE 9.2: (A) Tibial motor nerve conduction study demonstrating a greater than 50% amplitude decrease at the knee compared to the ankle, mimicking a conduction block, due to submaximal nerve stimulation. (B) After moving the stimulator closer to the nerve, the amplitude at the knee increased.

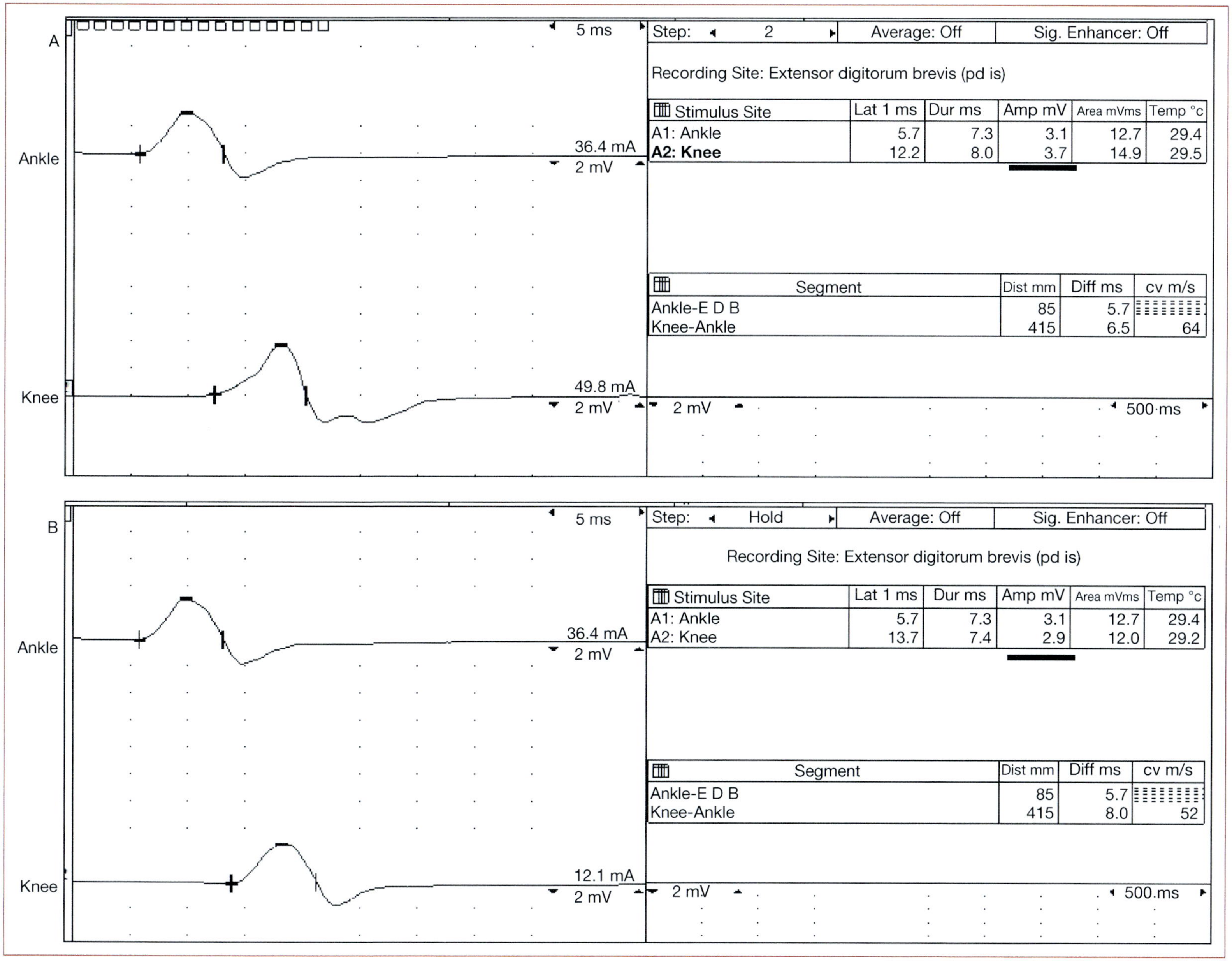

FIGURE 9.3: (A) Artifactual high CMAP amplitude at the knee due to overstimulation of the peroneal nerve at the knee. (B) Normal response with appropriate stimulation.

CMAP, compound muscle action potential.

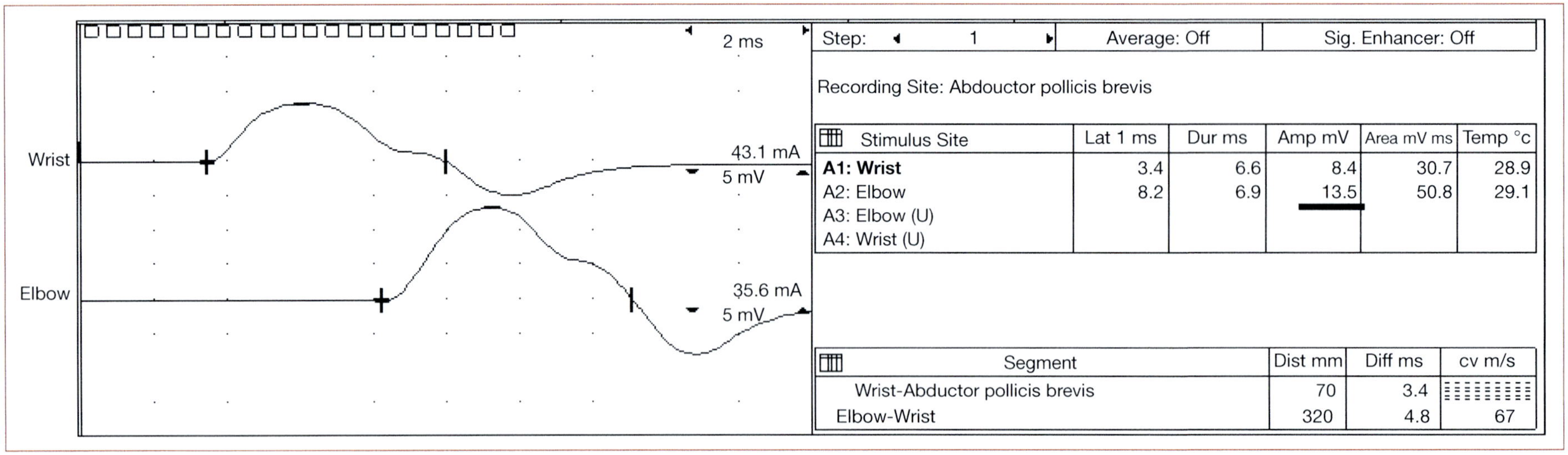

FIGURE 9.4: Median motor nerve conduction study demonstrating higher amplitude at the elbow than wrist, due to a normal anatomic variant (Martin-Gruber anastomosis).

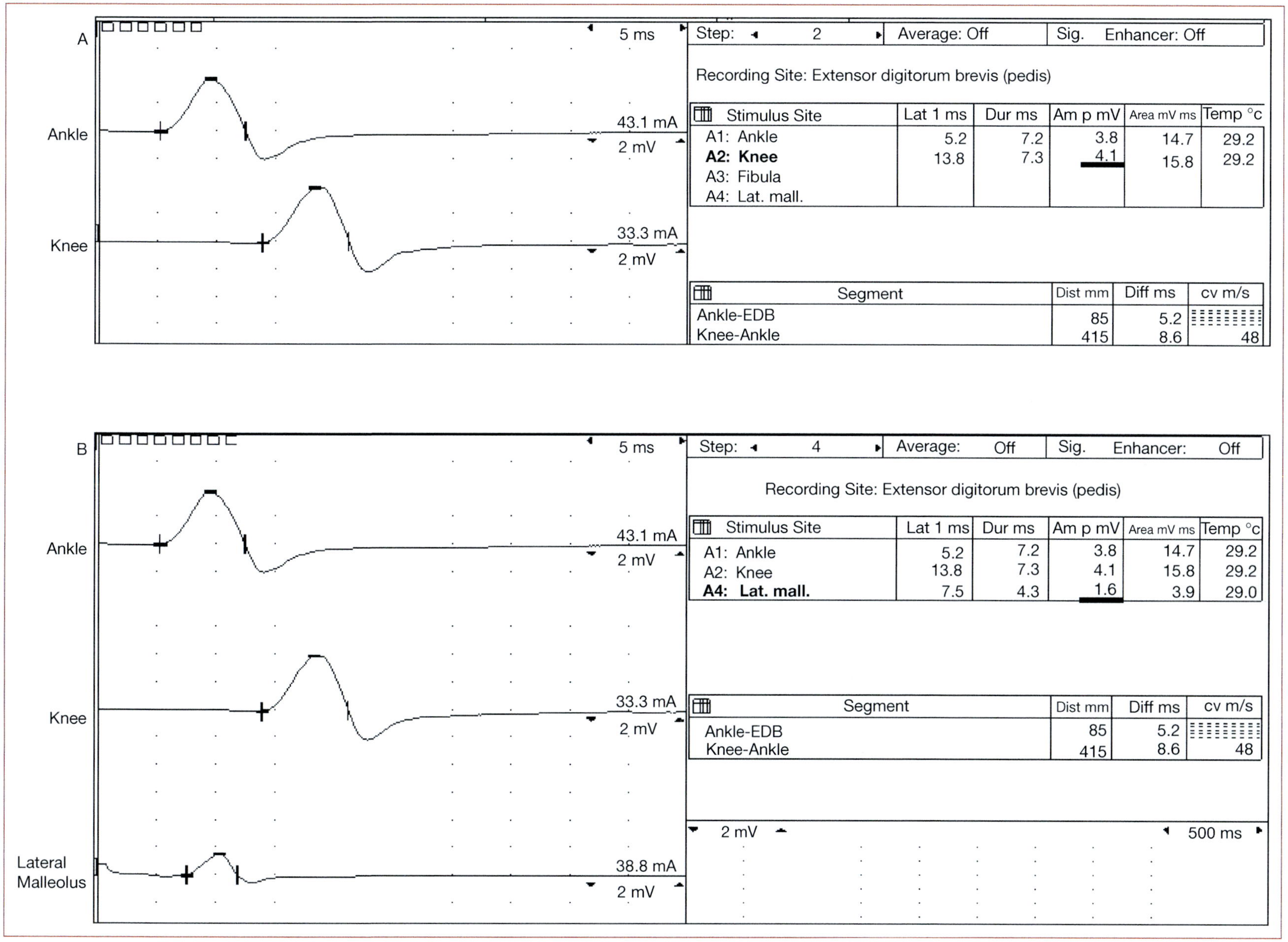

FIGURE 9.5: (A) Artifactual high CMAP amplitude at the knee in the peroneal motor nerve conduction study due to a normal anatomic variant (accessory peroneal nerve). (B) Confirmation of the variant with stimulation behind the lateral malleolus.

CMAP, compound muscle action potential.

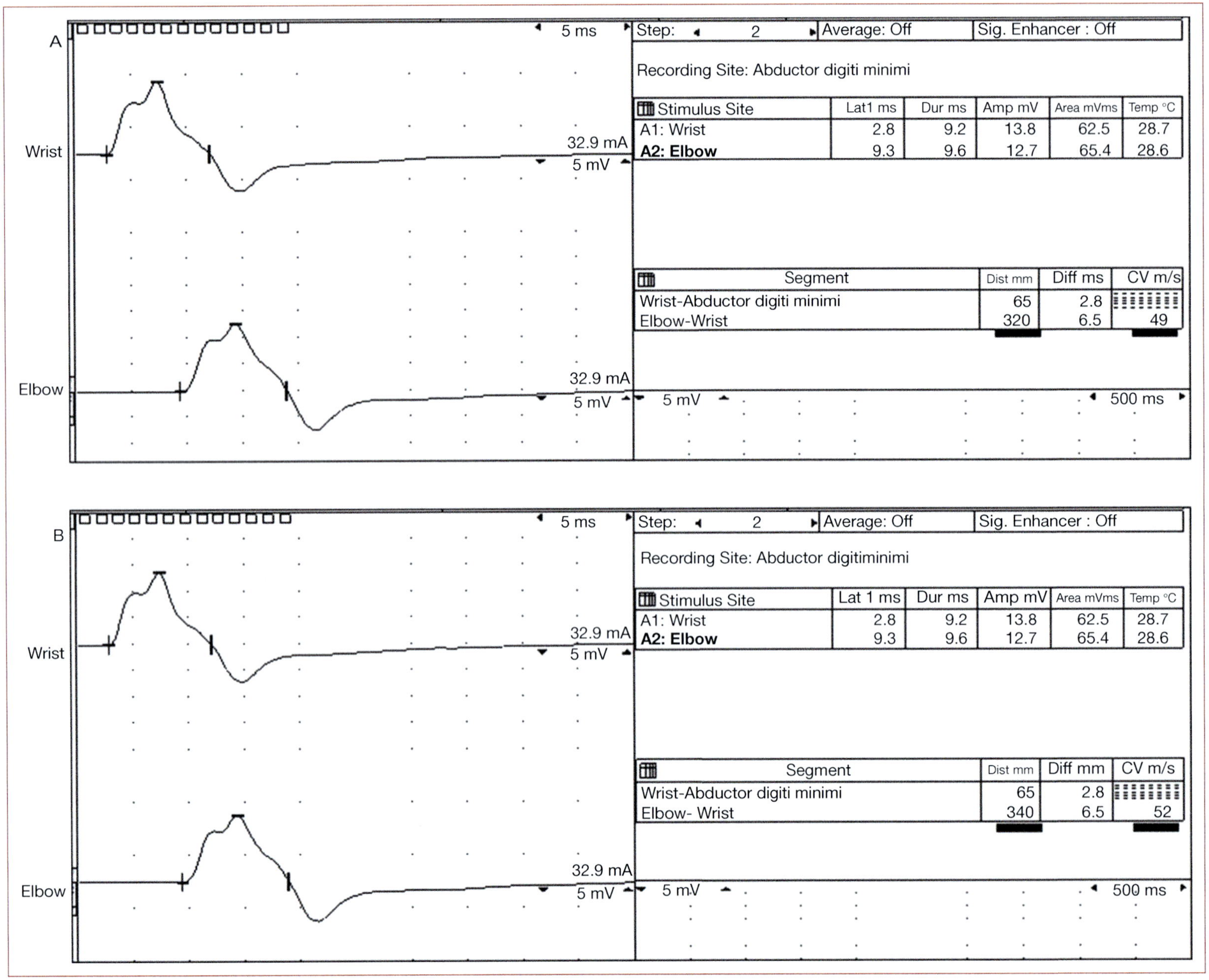

FIGURE 9.6: (A) Artifactual slowed conduction velocity in the ulnar motor nerve conduction study due to incorrect (too short) distance measurement. (B) Normal distance measurement results in a normal conduction velocity.

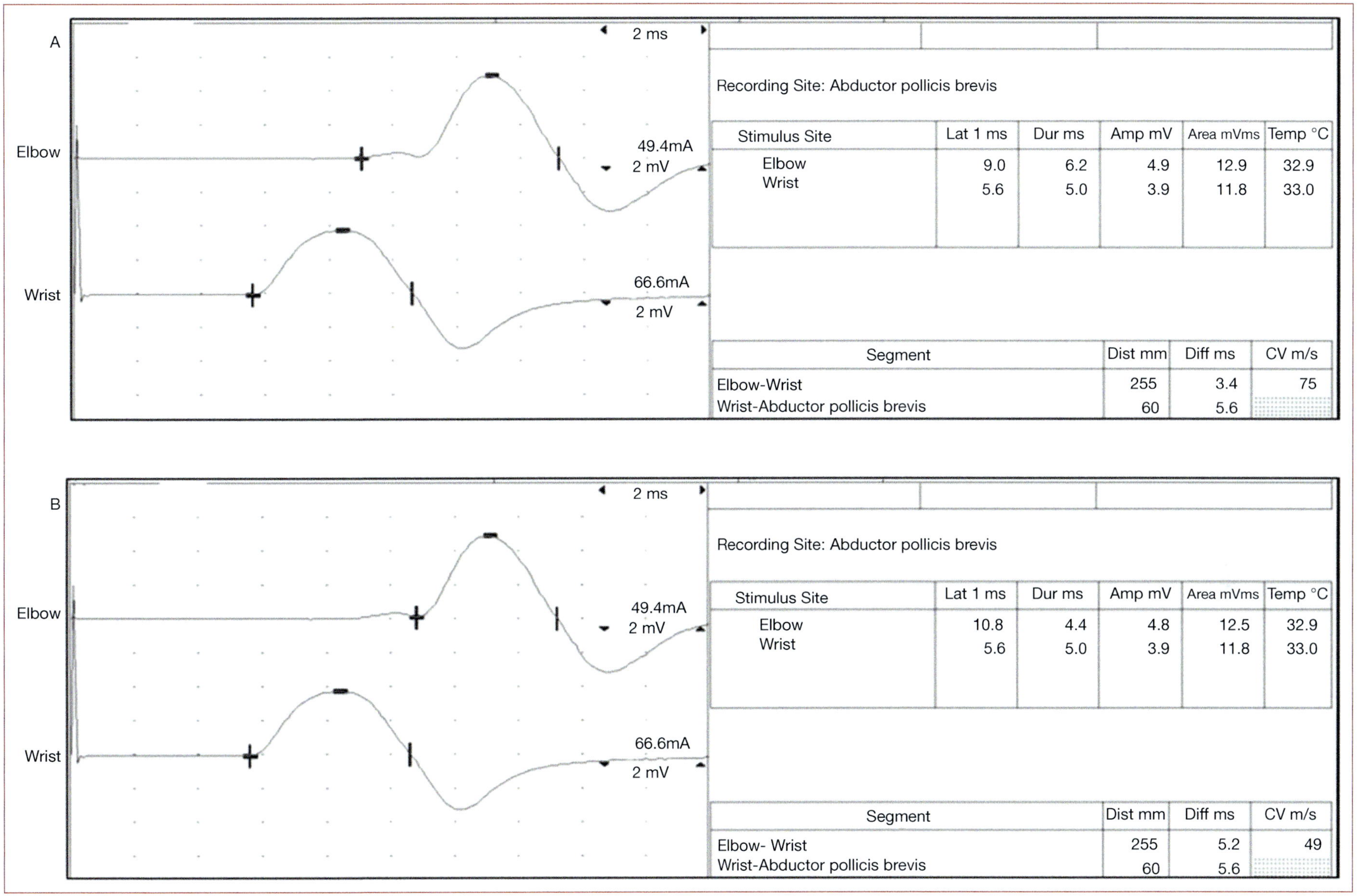

Stimulus Site	Lat 1 ms	Dur ms	Amp mV	Area mVms	Temp °C
Elbow	9.0	6.2	4.9	12.9	32.9
Wrist	5.6	5.0	3.9	11.8	33.0

Segment	Dist mm	Diff ms	CV m/s
Elbow-Wrist	255	3.4	75
Wrist-Abductor pollicis brevis	60	5.6	

Stimulus Site	Lat 1 ms	Dur ms	Amp mV	Area mVms	Temp °C
Elbow	10.8	4.4	4.8	12.5	32.9
Wrist	5.6	5.0	3.9	11.8	33.0

Segment	Dist mm	Diff ms	CV m/s
Elbow- Wrist	255	5.2	49
Wrist-Abductor pollicis brevis	60	5.6	

FIGURE 9.7: Artifactual fast conduction velocity in a median motor nerve conduction study due to the presence of a Martin-Gruber anastomosis and a median neuropathy at the wrist.

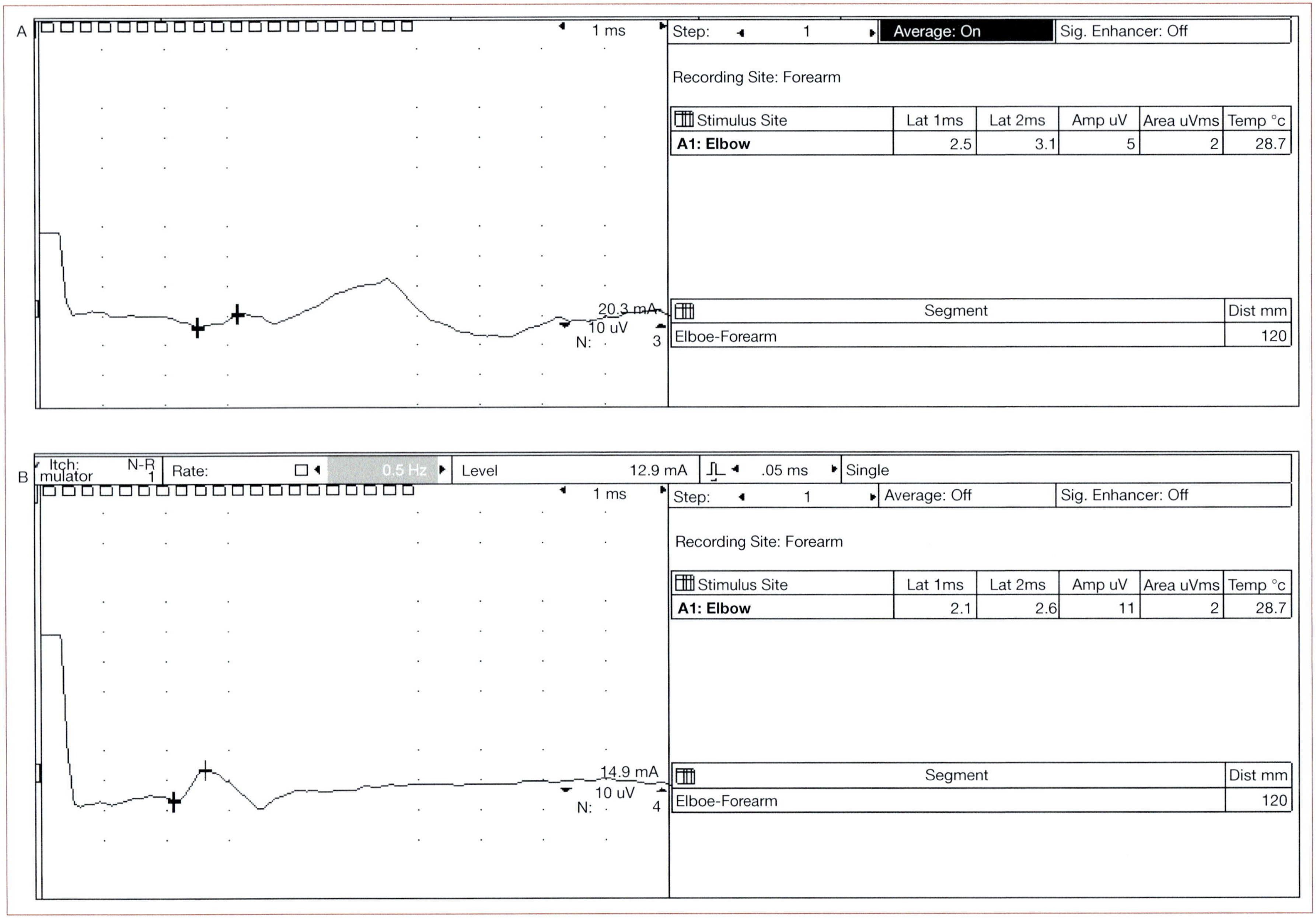

FIGURE 9.8: (A) Artifactual low medial antebrachial sensory amplitude due to inappropriate G1 placement a distance from the nerve. (B) Higher amplitude after G1 is moved closer to the nerve.

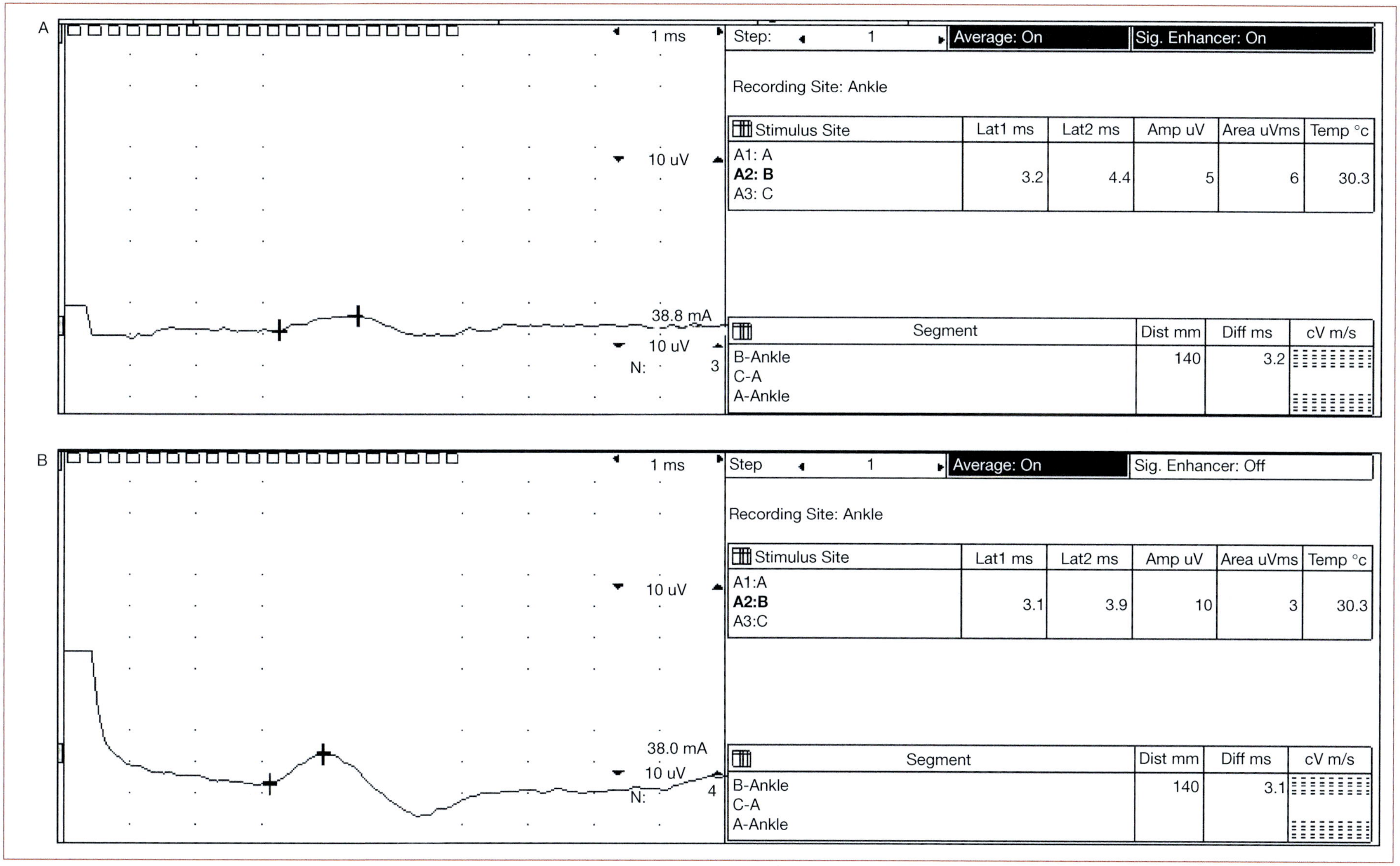

FIGURE 9.9: (A) Artifactual low sural sensory amplitude due to limb edema. (B) Improved amplitude after pressing the stimulator deeper in the skin.

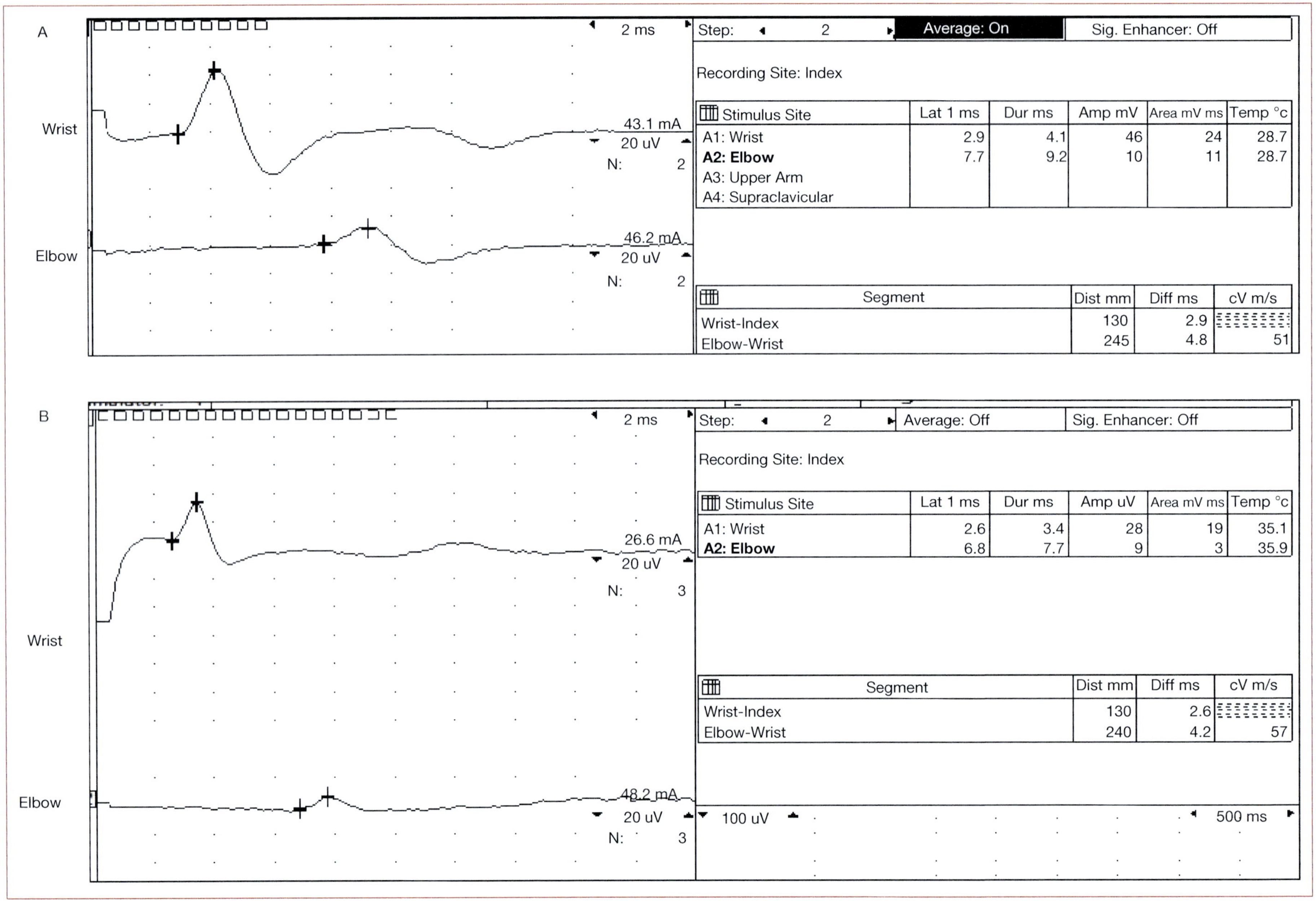

FIGURE 9.10: (A) Artifactual prolonged median sensory distal latency due to cool limb temperature and (B) normal distal latency after warming the limb.

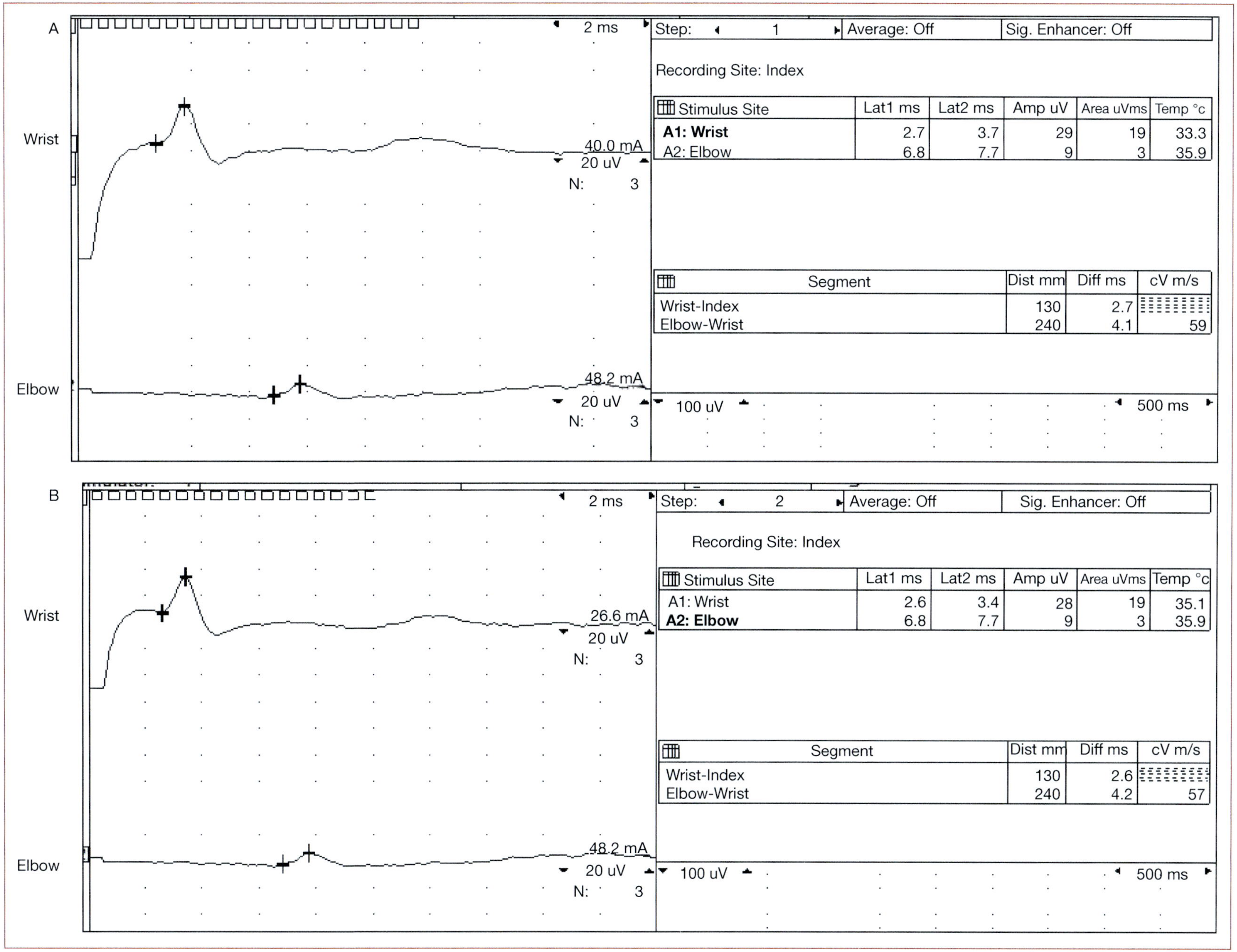

FIGURE 9.11: (A) Artifactual prolonged median sensory distal latency due to cathode-anode reversal and (B) normal latency with correction of cathode-anode reversal.

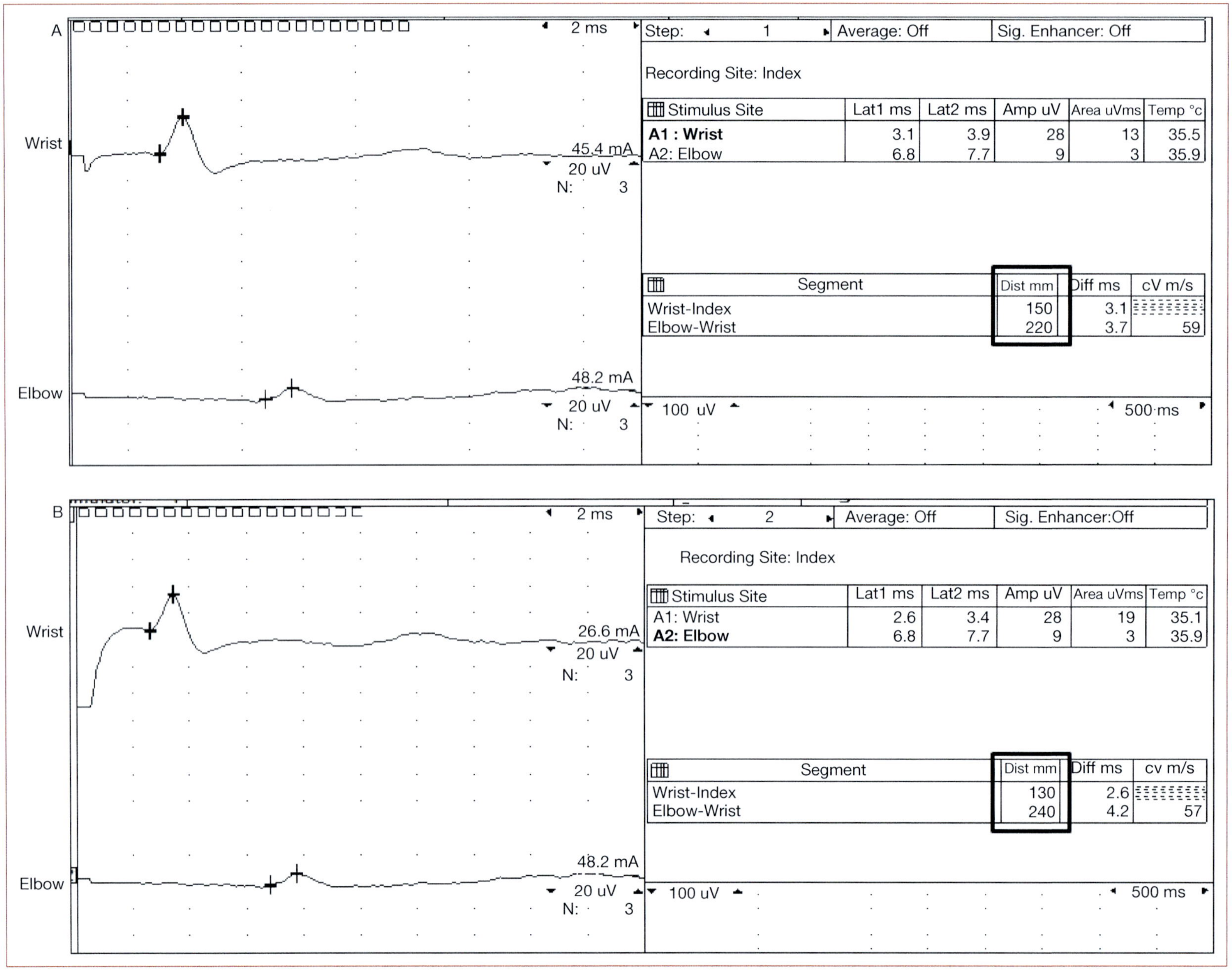

FIGURE 9.12: (A) Artifactual prolonged median sensory distal latency due to incorrect distal distance between cathode and G1 electrode and (B) normal latency with appropriate distal distance.

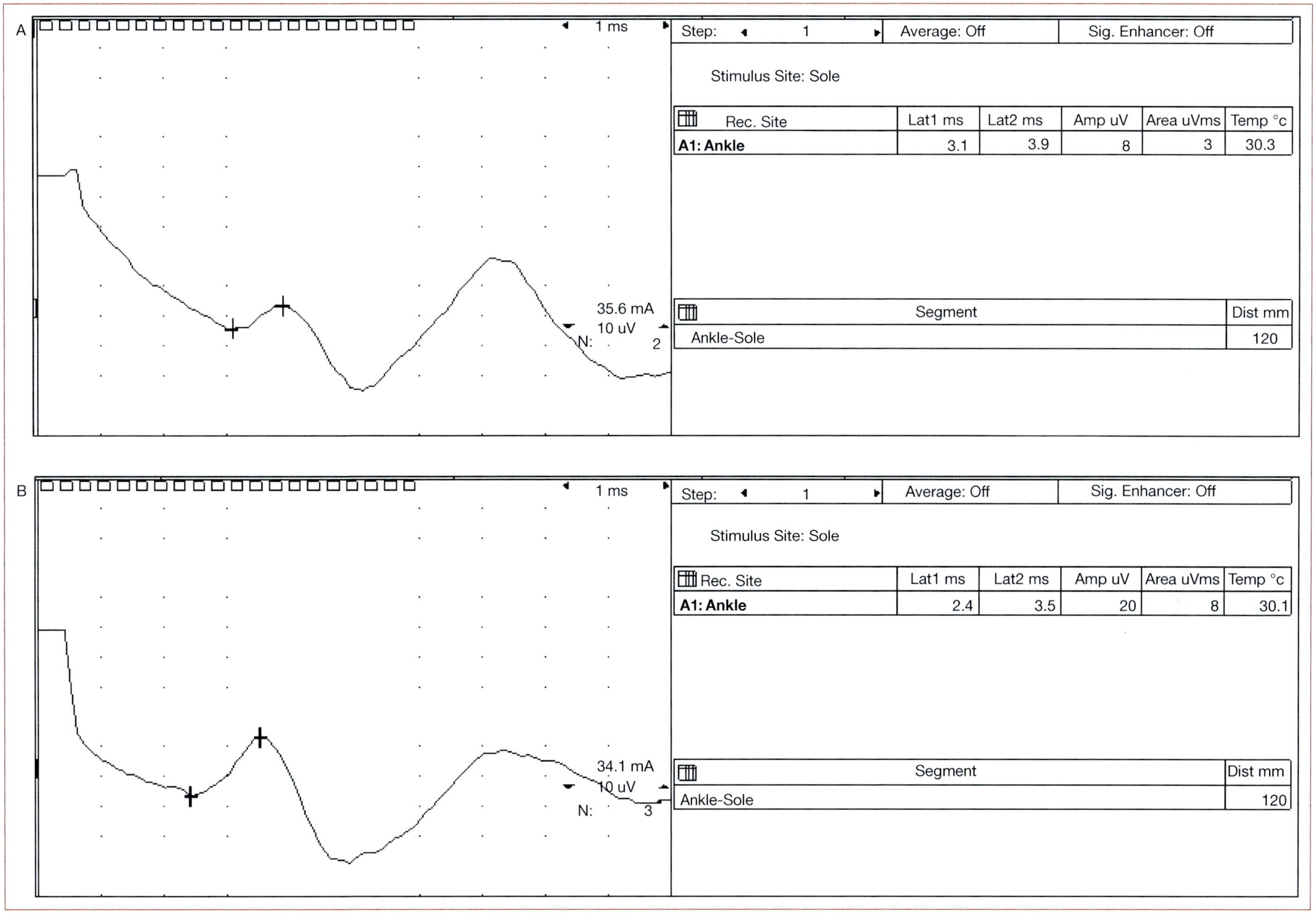

FIGURE 9.13: (A) Prominent stimulus artifact interfering with the baseline in the medial plantar sensory study. (B) Improvement in the baseline with stimulator rotation.

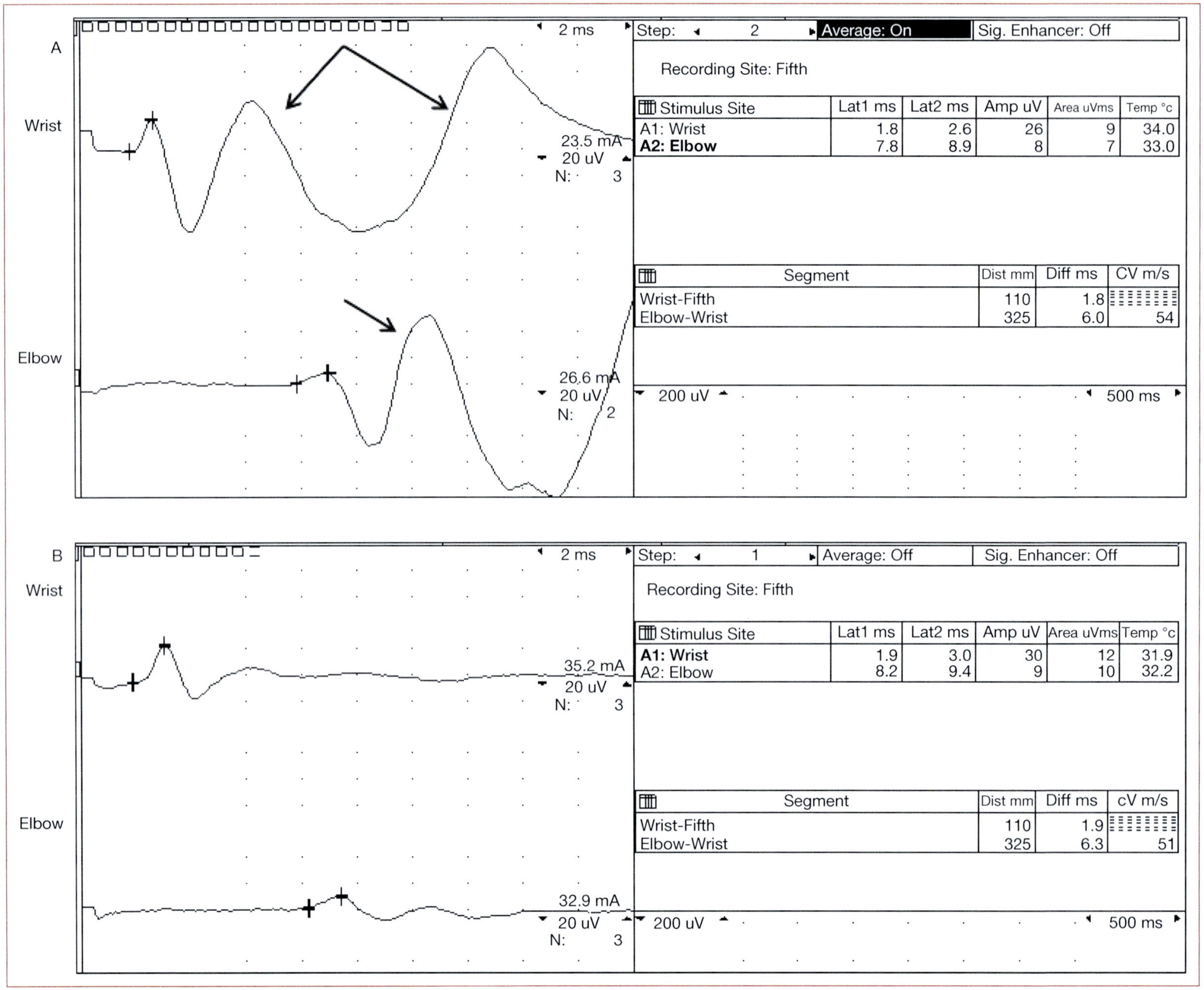

FIGURE 9.14: (A) Ulnar sensory antidromic study demonstrating prominent motor artifact. (B) Improvement in the artifact occurred with G1 electrode repositioning.

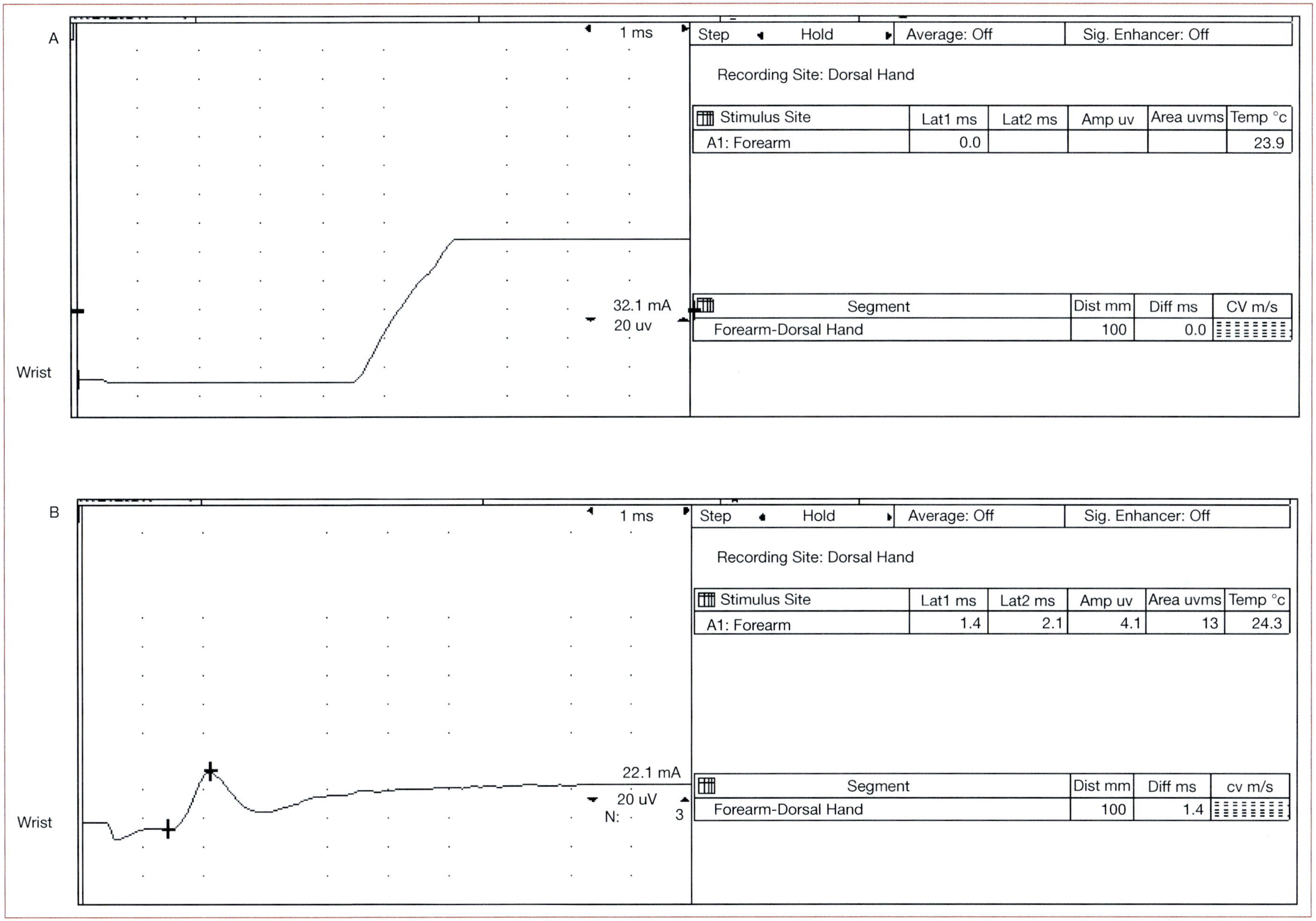

FIGURE 9.15: (A) Radial sensory study with interference by prominent 60-Hz artifact. (B) There was improvement in the baseline and response with reduction in 60-Hz interference.

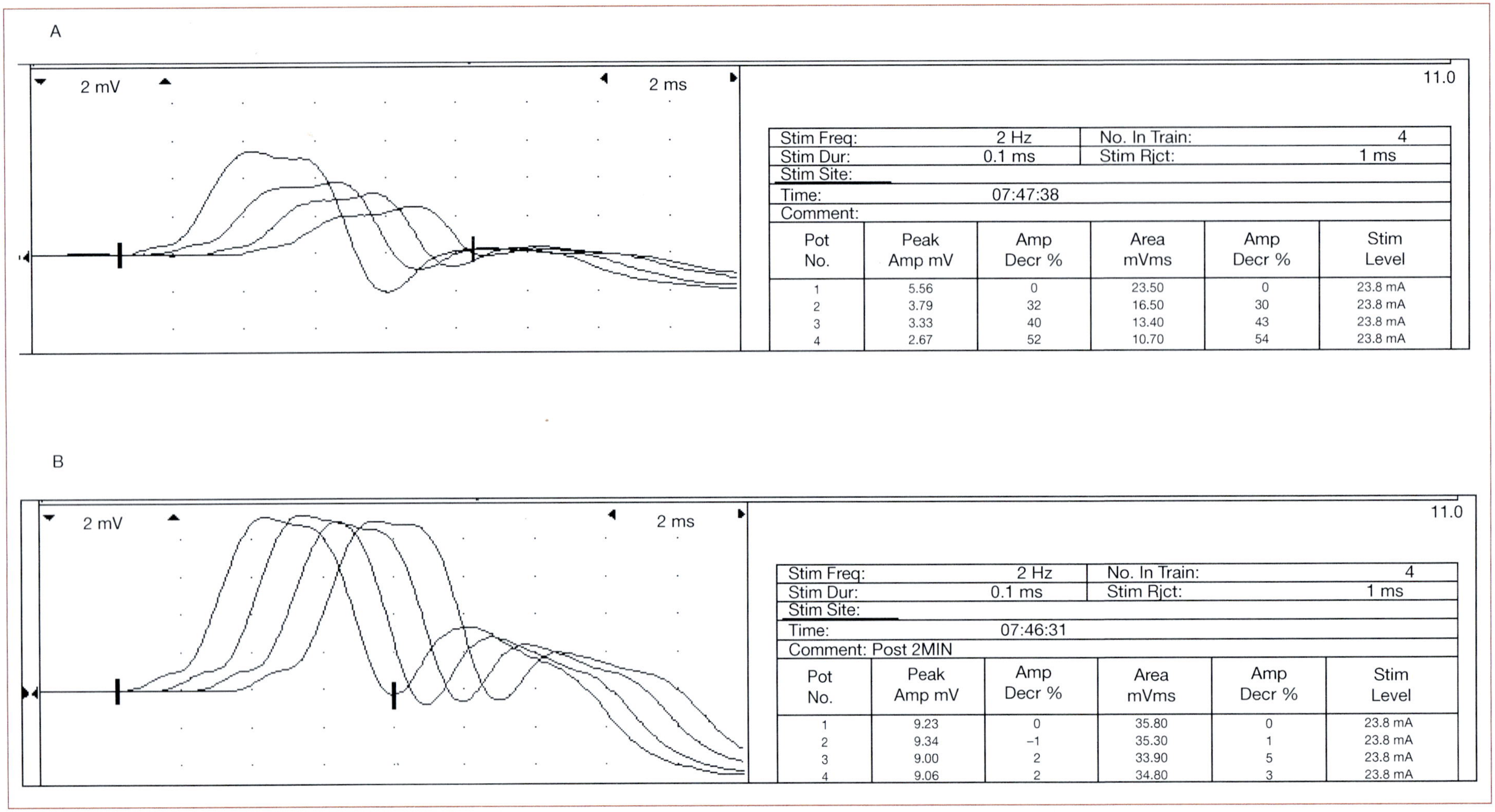

FIGURE 9.16: (A) Artifactual decrement during spinal accessory repetitive nerve stimulation caused by stimulator movement. (B) No decrement with minimization of stimulator movement.

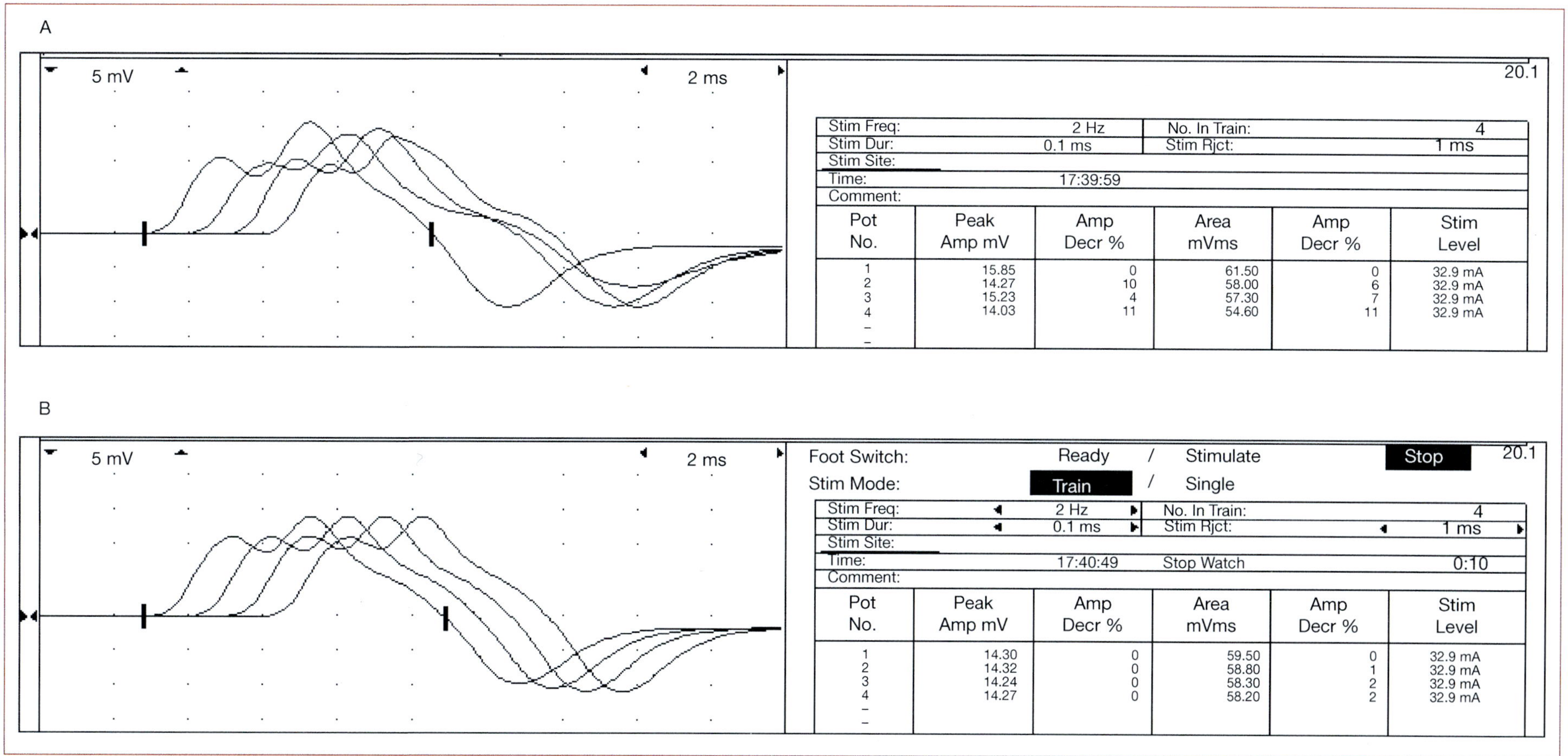

FIGURE 9.17: (A) Artifactual decrement during ulnar repetitive nerve stimulation from muscle contraction during stimulation. (B) No decrement with minimization of muscle contraction.

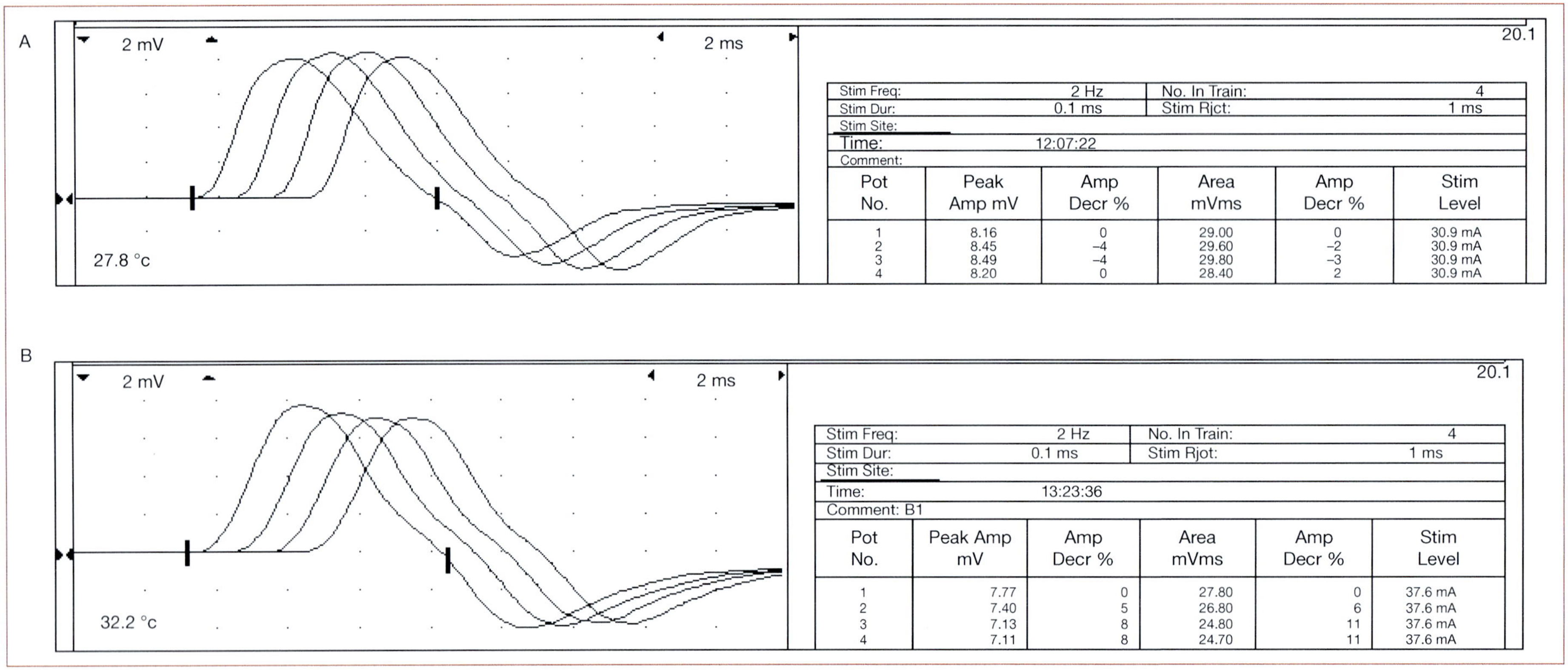

A

Stim Freq:	2 Hz	No. In Train:	4
Stim Dur:	0.1 ms	Stim Rjct:	1 ms
Stim Site:			
Time:	12:07:22		
Comment:			

Pot No.	Peak Amp mV	Amp Decr %	Area mVms	Amp Decr %	Stim Level
1	8.16	0	29.00	0	30.9 mA
2	8.45	−4	29.60	−2	30.9 mA
3	8.49	−4	29.80	−3	30.9 mA
4	8.20	0	28.40	2	30.9 mA

B

Stim Freq:	2 Hz	No. In Train:	4
Stim Dur:	0.1 ms	Stim Rjct:	1 ms
Stim Site:			
Time:	13:23:36		
Comment: B1			

Pot No.	Peak Amp mV	Amp Decr %	Area mVms	Amp Decr %	Stim Level
1	7.77	0	27.80	0	37.6 mA
2	7.40	5	26.80	6	37.6 mA
3	7.13	8	24.80	11	37.6 mA
4	7.11	8	24.70	11	37.6 mA

FIGURE 9.18: (A) Artifactual normal ulnar repetitive nerve stimulation in a patient with myasthenia gravis due to cool limb temperature. (B) After warming the limb, a mild degree of reproducible decrement was recorded.

REFERENCES

1. Rubin DI. Technical issues and potential complications of nerve conduction studies and needle electromyography. *Neurol Clin*. 2012;30:685-711. doi:10.1016/j.ncl.2011.12.008.
2. Gutmann L. AAEM minimonograph #2: important anomalous innervations of the extremities. *Muscle Nerve*. 1993;16:339-347. doi:10.1002/mus.880160402.
3. Wilbourn AJ, Lambert EH. The forearm median-to-ulnar nerve communication: electrodiagnostic aspects. *Neurology*. 1976;26:368.
4. Sun SF, Streib EW. Martin-Gruber anastomosis: electromyographic studies. Part II. *Electromyogr Clin Neurophysiol*. 1983;23:271-285. PMID:6872927.
5. Kimura J, Murphy MJ, Varda DJ. Electrophysiological study of anomalous innervation of intrinsic hand muscles. *Arch Neurol*. 1976;33:842-844. doi:10.1001/archneur.1976.00500120046007.
6. Gutmann L. Median-ulnar nerve communications and carpal tunnel syndrome. *J Neurol Neurosurg Psychiatry*. 1977;40:982-986. doi:10.1136/jnnp.40.10.982.
7. Rubin DI, Dimberg EL. Martin-Gruber anastomosis and carpal tunnel syndrome: morphologic clues to identification. *Muscle Nerve*. 2010;42:457-458. doi:10.1002/mus.21751.
8. Rutkove SB. Reduction of motor artifact in antidromic ulnar sensory studies. *Muscle Nerve*. 1999;22:520-522. PMID:10204789.
9. Rutkove SB, Kothari MJ, Shefner JM. Nerve, muscle, and neuromuscular junction electrophysiology at high temperature. *Muscle Nerve*. 1997;20:431-436. PMID:9121500.
10. Hubbard JI, Jones SF, Landau EM. The effect of temperature change upon transmitter release, facilitation, and post-tetanic potentiation. *J Physiol*. 1971;216:591-609. doi:10.1113/jphysiol.1971.sp009542
11. Rutkove SB, Shefner JM, Wang AK, et al. High-temperature repetitive nerve stimulation in myasthenia gravis. *Muscle Nerve*. 1998;21:1414-1418. doi:10.1002/(SICI)1097-4598(199811)21:11<1414::AID-MUS8>3.0.CO;2-C.
12. Daube JR, Rubin DI. Needle electromyography. *Muscle Nerve*. 2009;39(2):244-270. doi:10.1002/mus.21180.

CHAPTER 10

Artifact in Autonomic Neurophysiology Studies

William P. Cheshire, Jr.

INTRODUCTION

The past few decades have witnessed major advances in increasingly sophisticated, noninvasive neurophysiological tests to probe one of the most developmentally ancient of human body systems. The autonomic nervous system is a vast network of neurons that coordinate visceral activity throughout the body to ensure internal homeostasis and respond to external stress. Most autonomic responses are involuntary and occur below the level of conscious awareness. As autonomic dysfunction can be a hallmark or epiphenomenon of many diseases, as well as an important cause of distress and debility for patients, diagnostic testing of autonomic responses is a valuable aspect of clinical neurophysiology.

THE AUTONOMIC NERVOUS SYSTEM

Structurally the autonomic nervous system comprises central and peripheral interconnected components. The central autonomic network includes neurons located in the hypothalamus; insular, anterior cingulate, and ventromedial prefrontal cortices; stria terminalis, amygdala; periaqueductal gray matter; parabrachial nucleus, nucleus of the solitary tract; ventrolateral medulla; medullary lateral tegmental field; and intermediolateral cell column of the spinal cord.

The peripheral autonomic nervous system is organized into sympathetic, parasympathetic, and enteric divisions. The sympathetic nervous system, which is often characterized as coordinating "fight-or-flight" responses, flows from thoracolumbar segments of the spinal cord and contrasts with the parasympathetic nervous system, which has more of a role in "rest-and-digest" functions and flows from cranial nerves III, VII, IX, and X, and sacral spinal segments. Although sympathetic and parasympathetic behaviors are often antagonistic, some are functionally distinct and unopposed, whereas others are interdependent. Additionally, the enteric nervous system consists of ganglionic plexuses intrinsic to the wall of the gut.

Autonomic responses entail a sequential, two-neuron efferent pathway in which a preganglionic neuron synapses onto a postganglionic neuron that innervates the target organ. Sympathetic synapses are found in the paravertebral sympathetic chain ganglia, whereas parasympathetic synapses are found in ganglia near their target organs.

AUTONOMIC REFLEX TESTING

This chapter focuses on the components of autonomic testing of greatest importance to neurologic practice (1). In clinical neurophysiology laboratories, three categories of autonomic testing are well established. Sudomotor testing (CPT code 95923) evaluates sympathetic cholinergic function in the secretion of sweat from eccrine glands. Cardiovagal testing (CPT code 95921) evaluates parasympathetic function in the control of heart rate. Vasomotor adrenergic testing (CPT code 95922) evaluates sympathetic noradrenergic function in the regulation of blood pressure. The methodology and proper performance of these tests have been reviewed elsewhere (2).

Many other tests of autonomic function are available in other specialties. These include tests of circulating catecholamine levels and renin for the endocrinologist, pharmacologic tests of pupillary dilation and constriction for the ophthalmologist, electrocardiography or electrophysiologic testing of the heart for the cardiologist, urodynamic testing for the urologist, and gastric and bowel motility testing for the gastroenterologist. As these are not typically part of the neurologist's repertoire of clinical tests, they are not addressed here.

In routine clinical practice, autonomic neural activity cannot be measured directly. Rather, the autonomic end-organ response is measured. Clinically meaningful information may be present at rest or, more typically, is obtained by measuring the evoked response to a standardized stimulus under controlled conditions.

SOURCES OF ARTIFACTS

Six categories of potential artifacts may occur during autonomic testing (Table 10.1). For tests that require the patient's participation, inadequate cooperation can decrease autonomic responses. Also, the patient may have concurrent medical conditions that influence autonomic responses or impair his or her ability to participate in the test. Importantly, a wide variety of medications can potentially increase or decrease autonomic responses. Additionally, ambient conditions in the testing room may influence the patient's autonomic responses. Further, testing equipment malfunctions can occur. Finally, the physician who lacks sufficient training or experience in autonomic disorders may misinterpret the test results. Examples of these will be pointed out under each type of testing.

ARTIFACTS AT THE BEDSIDE

Although the focus of a textbook on artifacts in clinical neurophysiologic testing is necessarily on the ways in which technology is used and its data are interpreted in the course of patient care, the experienced physician is mindful that the history and physical examination are typically the most important elements of the diagnostic process. In regard to autonomic disorders, a careful history is the most important diagnostic test (3). Here too artifact can intervene.

An artifact can be defined as something crafted by art or as information generated by an artificial device. Insofar as taking a good history is an

TABLE 10.1: Types of Artifact Encountered in Autonomic Testing

Source of Artifact	Examples
Patient's behavior	Limb movement Inadequate effort Talking Coughing Sneezing Laughing
Concurrent medical condition	Anxiety Respiratory muscle weakness Dehydration with intravascular hypovolemia Cold limb causing vasoconstriction Vestibular dysfunction activated by tilt table motion
Medication	Anticholinergics Carbonic anhydrase inhibitors Vasopressors Vasodilators Stimulants
Room conditions	Uncomfortable heat or chill Bright overhead light Loud or sudden noise Intravenous catheter causing vasovagal response
Equipment malfunction	Electrical power failure Loose electrical connections Improperly sized blood pressure cuff Pressure or fluid leakage from cables
Misinterpretation of data	Being unfamiliar with the range of normal Noticing peaks or troughs rather than means

essential aspect of the art of medicine, artifact can occur if communication between the patient and the physician is incomplete, if pertinent questions are not asked, or if questioning follows too rigidly an algorithm or predetermined care process instead of being open-ended and inquisitive about the patient's perspective. Artifacts in the medical history take the form of gaps in information or misinterpretations based on flawed assumptions. Technology also can introduce artifacts into the medical history. Computer software that constructs a medical document by transcribing, without understanding, text from the digital patterns of spoken audio input frequently introduces errors of language that can alter the intended meaning of a clinical note, sometimes in surprising ways. The autonomic term lacrimation, for example, might be typed "like cremation." Treatment with a course of steroids might be mutated into "coarse old stories" (4).

When evaluating the patient who presents with episodic collapse, an invaluable element of the art of the physical examination is the ability to measure very quickly the pulse and blood pressure at the moment that symptoms occur. Some healthy patients will experience a transient fall in blood pressure upon standing that recovers to normal values within 20 seconds. The patient whose systolic blood pressure falls below about 70 mmHg or in whom recovery is prolonged may, after 7 seconds of cerebral hypoperfusion, lose consciousness. One of the diagnostic challenges in evaluating such spells is distinguishing orthostatic syncope, which is caused by hypotension, from psychogenic pseudosyncope, in which blood pressure remains normal during apparent loss of consciousness (5). If one knows the blood pressure at baseline, with practice one can develop the skill of ascertaining a significant change in blood pressure very rapidly using a sphygmomanometer and stethoscope. Anticipating that a spell may occur, the neurologist has the blood pressure cuff already in place when asking the patient to stand up. At the moment the patient starts to collapse, and while preventing the patient from falling, the neurologist inflates the cuff to just above the baseline value and, while auscultating the brachial artery, deflates the cuff rapidly. In this way, accurate blood pressure measurements can usually be obtained within a few seconds. In many clinical settings, however, physicians and nurses increasingly are relying on automated blood pressure devices that take about 35 seconds to obtain a blood pressure reading. That time may be too long to correlate with symptoms if the blood pressure has already recovered by the time the machine registers a value. If the blood pressure is below the range of pressures the machine is designed to measure, it may return an error message (**Figure 10.1**), an artifact that is of little value compared to personally obtained blood pressure measurements.

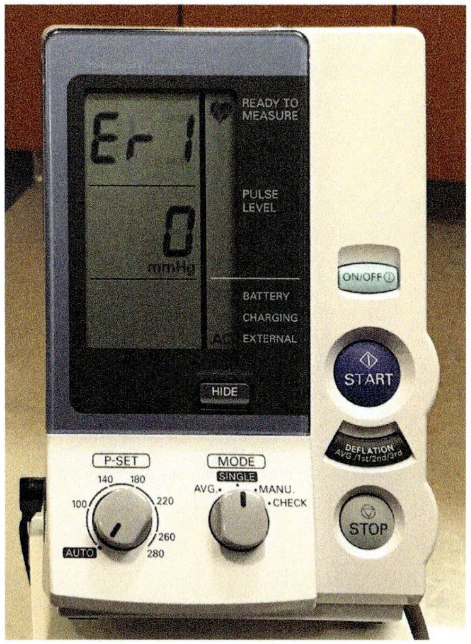

FIGURE 10.1: Automated blood pressure measurement device displaying an artifactual error message because the patient's low blood pressure was out of range for the device to quantify.

ARTIFACTS DURING SUDOMOTOR TESTING

Tests of sudomotor function are commonly utilized in assessing small fiber neuropathy and disorders of thermoregulation. A number of methodologies are in common use (6). The thermoregulatory sweat test subjects the patient to a controlled, gradual heat stimulus to produce a generalized sweating response, the anatomical distribution of which is visualized by the aid of a colorimetric indicator powder, recorded, and quantified. The quantitative sudomotor axon reflex test utilizes acetylcholine, which is applied at four standardized limb sites by transcutaneous iontophoresis to reach subepidermal peripheral postganglionic sympathetic cholinergic sudomotor neurons, which then activate innervated eccrine glands. The latency and volume over time of the resulting secretion of sweat outflow is recorded. Another method is the silastic imprint technique, which evaluates the number and size of evoked sweat droplets per measured area of skin.

All sudomotor tests are subject to the potentially confounding effects of medication. If the patient is taking an anticholinergic agent or a drug that blocks carbonic anhydrase, it may not be possible to distinguish hypohidrosis or anhidrosis on testing from a small fiber peripheral neuropathy affecting sudomotor nerves. For this reason, it is preferred that patients hold all anticholinergic agents (including tricyclics, bladder and gut antispasmodics, and antihistamines) and carbonic anhydrase inhibitors (topiramate and acetazolamide) for five half-lives prior to testing. These medications do not always interfere with sudomotor responses, but in some patients they can exert a potent effect, and it is not possible to predict in advance which patients are susceptible. The many drugs that can affect sudomotor responses have been extensively reviewed elsewhere (6,7).

It is sometimes assumed that, whereas a distal small fiber neuropathy might impair the sudomotor response only at the foot, a drug effect would be seen uniformly across sites; this does not always hold true. Distally predominant drug effects sometimes occur (Figure 10.2).

Other medications, particularly opioids, selective serotonin and norepinephrine reuptake inhibitors, and stimulants can enhance sudomotor responses. Opioid-induced hyperhidrosis is not uncommon. As drug-induced stimulation of sweating is typically mediated centrally, assessment of peripheral sudomotor nerve function is generally not impaired. Pyridostigmine is another example of a pharmaceutical agent that can enhance the sweating response (Figure 10.3).

ARTIFACTS OF HEART RATE DURING CARDIOVAGAL TESTING

Assessment of parasympathetic cardiovagal function is accomplished by quantifying the variation in heart rate (or change in the RR interval). A number of clinical techniques exist. The most sensitive, and the least specific, measures the difference between the increase in heart rate during inspiration and the decrease in heart rate during expiration (respiratory sinus arrhythmia) under conditions that maximize this difference (Figure 10.4). The Valsalva ratio is an index of baroreflex–cardiovagal function and is obtained by having the patient exhale against resistance and calculating the ratio of the increase in heart rate to the decrease in heart rate that occurs when straining ceases. Another test is the 30:15 ratio, in which the longest RR interval at the 30th beat after standing is divided by the shortest RR interval at the 15th beat. Cardiovagal function can be assessed also by fast Fourier transformation of ECG spectra in the time or frequency domain.

When testing heart rate variability to deep breathing, if the patient does not take slow, complete, deep breaths in timing with the visual sinusoidal stimulus that, like the conductor of an orchestra, directs the patient's breathing, the magnitude of the response will be decreased (Figure 10.5). Thus, it is advisable to monitor simultaneously chest wall movement, and for the Valsalva maneuver, exhaled respiratory pressure to ensure that they are adequate in volume and force to induce the desired autonomic response.

The timing of chest wall movement in relation to changes in heart rate should also be heeded in order not to mistake a cardiac dysrhythmia for a normal autonomic response. The patient with atrial bigeminy, for example, will exhibit a heart rate that oscillates rhythmically between a high value and a low value, but the rate of change varies with the heartbeat, not with the slower respiratory rate (Figure 10.6).

In other patients, atrial bigeminy may be continuous, in which case it may be unclear how the maximum and minimum heart rates should be defined for purposes of evaluating neurally mediated heart rate variability. In such cases, it may be reasonable, when calculating the Valsalva ratio, to draw measurements from every other beat (Figure 10.7).

Valid assessment of cardiovagal function requires accurate assessment of beat-to-beat heart rate, which is typically accomplished by measuring the RR interval on a single-lead ECG. It is sometimes necessary to reposition the precordial or limb leads or select among electrode pairs in order to obtain distinct R waves that are sufficiently high in amplitude and consistently higher than the T waves. Occasionally, the ECG waveform will change during testing, and if the R waves decrease in amplitude or the T waves increase in amplitude, the software may erroneously count some of the T waves as R waves and falsely report a doubling of heart rate (Figure 10.8).

Atrial fibrillation or flutter is recognized by the characteristically erratic pattern on the beat-to-beat heart rate tracing (Figure 10.9). Sometimes, but not always, the slower, regular oscillation of neurally mediated heart rate variability can be discerned in the background.

Premature ventricular contractions are another source of artifact arising from the cardiac conduction system that may be mistaken for neurally mediated autonomic responses arising from baroreflex–cardiovagal pathways. An occasional premature ventricular contraction may appear on the beat-to-beat heart rate tracing as a sudden blip or series of blips of high amplitude in which an apparent single-beat increase in heart rate is immediately followed by an apparent single-beat decrease in heart rate to below baseline (Figure 10.10). When a series of premature ventricular contractions (PVCs) occurs during testing of heart rate variability, the peak and trough values associated with the PVCs should not be counted. Rather, the slower, smoother, sinusoidal profile of heart rate variability may be appreciated in the background (Figure 10.11).

Muscle artifact is another potential source of electrical interference with the ECG signal. As autonomic studies do not typically include electromyography, this artifact may appear only on the ECG tracing, typically as a single or clustered, arrhythmic group of heart rate peaks that are much higher than the baseline recording (Figure 10.12).

The recent introduction of personal biosensor technologies that allow patients and healthy individuals to detect heart rate changes during daily life has created a new source of artifact. Whereas, until now, detailed heart rate information had been available only to the autonomic nervous system or to medical professionals, now these devices have made heart rate information accessible to patients' conscious awareness and amateur scrutiny. It should be recognized that data acquired from personal health monitoring devices are subject to selection bias, as patients may be more likely to look at the device's display when they are experiencing palpitations or other symptoms. Patients without medical or sports physiology background may not know the normal range of heart rate and may misinterpret a normal transient increase in heart rate as a dysautonomia (8).

ARTIFACTS OF BLOOD PRESSURE DURING THE VALSALVA MANEUVER

The assessment of both baroreflex–cardiovagal and baroreflex–sympathoneural function require the rapid assessment of blood pressure on a beat-to-beat basis. This is accomplished by technologies such as photoplethysmography, which quantifies blood pressure indirectly by measuring the absorption of infrared light transmitted through the finger as an indicator of changes in the volume of blood flowing through. This method is insensitive as a measure of absolute blood pressure, for which reason autonomic testing utilizes simultaneous sphygmomanometer recordings, but it is an exquisitely sensitive test of what is most important for autonomic testing: moment-to-moment changes in blood pressure.

Beat-to-beat devices will display not only information about blood pressure, but also artifact. A sudden increase in apparent blood pressure in response to the patient's emotional state, for example, could reflect a withdrawal of parasympathetic influence on heart rate, a surge of circulating catecholamines causing vasoconstriction in the fingers, or a subtle limb movement causing the device to lose track of its signal (Figure 10.13).

Additionally, coughing, sneezing, or laughing will momentarily alter the beat-to-beat blood pressure tracing. Merely speaking can, in some patients, elevate the heart rate by 5 to 10 beats/min and the blood pressure by 5 to 10 mmHg. The hemodynamic response to coughing or sneezing parallels that of the Valsalva maneuver (Figure 10.14). Profiles seen during laughing are brief and more variable, as the increased respiratory force is typically of shorter duration (Figure 10.15).

When performing the Valsalva maneuver, if the patient does not maintain a sufficient expiratory force (usually 30–40 mmHg), the magnitude of the elicited reflexes will be decreased. In these cases the physician might mistakenly conclude that the patient who has respiratory muscle weakness or who is uncooperative has autonomic failure.

ARTIFACTS OF BLOOD PRESSURE DURING TILT TABLE TESTING

Orthostatic hypotension, as defined by an international consensus committee representing the American Autonomic Society and the American Academy of Neurology, is a sustained reduction of systolic blood pressure of at least 20 mmHg or diastolic blood pressure of 10 mmHg within 3 minutes of standing or heat-up tilt to at least 60° on a tilt table (9). A number of variations on this broad definition are encountered in clinical practice and can be discerned by autonomic testing (10). Among them is an artifactual pattern that only appears to be orthostatic hypotension because initial supine blood pressure values are not verified to be a true baseline. In order to establish a valid baseline, the patient should be recumbent at rest for at least 10 minutes, if not longer. A blood pressure that decreases from an elevated baseline, barely meets the threshold for orthostatic hypotension when the table is upright, and does not increase when the table is returned to the horizontal position usually does not indicate a neurogenic form of orthostatic hypotension (Figure 10.16).

Another important distinction is between artifactual drops in blood pressure and the transient fall that occurs during neurally mediated syncope. In neurally mediated syncope, a gradual increase in heart rate typically precedes a gradual, smoothly contoured fall in the blood pressure tracing that occurs over about 30 to 60 seconds (Figure 10.17). Artefactual drops, by contrast, exhibit a different temporal profile. Artefactual deviations in blood pressure may abruptly decrease or increase during slight changes in finger cuff position, they may exhibit a stuttering pattern of inconsistent pulse detection, or they may taper off very slowly as pulse detection diminishes in the patient with peripheral vasoconstriction (Figure 10.16). Monitoring of beat-to-beat blood pressure during tilt table testing represents a special challenge, as the movement of the table may cause the patient's arm position to shift, and even a slight shift of position can interrupt the delicate positioning of the photoplethysmographic finger cuff in relation to the patient's pulse. For valid determinations, the finger cuff should be maintained at the level of the heart, and the blood pressure should always be confirmed by sphygmomanometry in the opposite arm.

Not only decreases, but also increases in blood pressure require interpretation of factors beyond the autonomic responses of primary interest. Among the situational factors that can cause an increase in blood pressure during autonomic testing are pressor drugs, anxiety, and pain (Figure 10.18). The differential diagnosis of paroxysmal hypertension also encompasses the common phenomenon of "white coat" hypertension and the very rare condition of pheochromocytoma.

Oscillations in blood pressure are frequently observed during tilt table testing and can be a sign of orthostatic intolerance in the patient whose autonomic nervous system is less capable of responding to the upright posture with the physiologic changes necessary to adapt to the force that gravity exerts on the cardiovascular system. As limb muscle tensing also can produce oscillations in blood pressure, it is important to observe the patient throughout testing and ensure that the arms and legs remain relaxed. Tremors in patients with movement disorders are much faster (3–5 Hz for Parkinsonism, 4–11 Hz for essential tremor) than sympathoneural blood pressure oscillations (Figure 10.19) and generally do not interfere with the assessment of beat-to-beat blood pressure unless they are of sufficiently high amplitude to interrupt detection of the finger pulse.

For blood pressure oscillations at frequencies of 5 to 20 Hz, correlation with respiratory rate may demonstrate a corresponding profile. In such cases the oscillations are a manifestation of respiratory sinus arrhythmia, which consists of time-locked oscillations in both beat-to-beat heart rate and blood pressure (Figure 10.20).

ARTIFACTS OF HEART RATE DURING TILT TABLE TESTING

Spontaneous variations in heart rate during tilt table testing, both supine and upright, that correspond in frequency to chest wall movement very often reflect respiratory sinus arrhythmia and are thus normal and physiologic (Figure 10.21). It is important to bear in mind this physiological pattern when assessing the overall change in heart rate accompanying the upright posture.

The postural tachycardia syndrome, which is a form of orthostatic intolerance, is defined as a sustained heart rate increment of more than 30 beats/min within 10 minutes of standing or head-up tilt in the absence of orthostatic hypotension (9). On occasion, this diagnosis is made incorrectly on the basis of a transient peak in heart rate exceeding 30 beats/min above baseline rather than a sustained increment. When analyzing tilt table hemodynamic profiles, one's eye can be drawn to the peak heart rates, which stand out from the other values. The published consensus definition, however, was based on normative values of *mean* heart rates during tilt table testing, for which reason the mean values, and not just the peaks, must be considered when distinguishing abnormal from normal heart rates (Figure 10.22).

The potential influence of medications on heart rate must also be taken into account when deciding whether a heart rate change is normal or abnormal. Among the common medications that can cause tachycardia, and hence the appearance of postural tachycardia syndrome on autonomic testing, are caffeine, pseudoephedrine, amphetamine, methylphenidate, phentermine (Figure 10.23), norepinephrine reuptake inhibitors, and anticholinergic agents (11).

CONCLUSION

This chapter has described and explained some of the most common artifacts encountered when performing autonomic testing. Many other types of artifacts can also occur, so varied are patients' disorders and the conditions of testing among neurophysiology laboratories. In all of these cases, there can be no substitute for knowledge about autonomic physiology and pharmacology, astute clinical observation, and boundless curiosity about the complexities of the human nervous system.

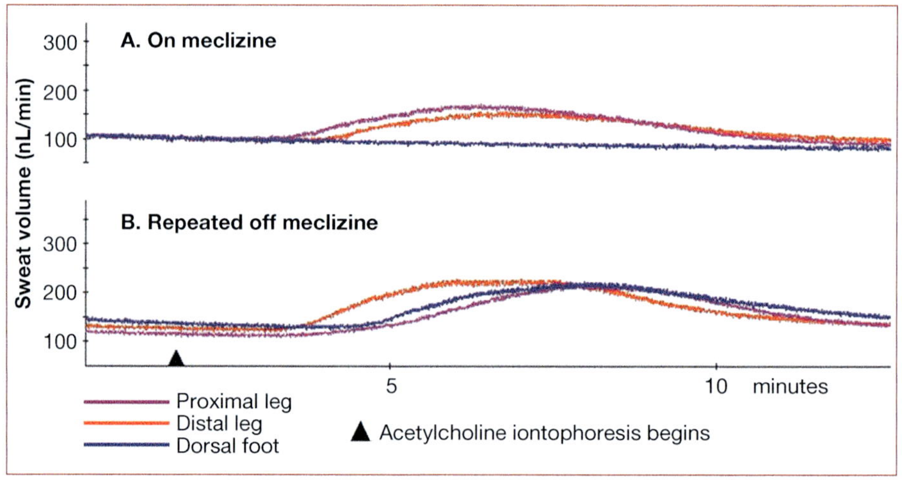

FIGURE 10.2: Quantitative sudomotor axon reflex recording in a single patient (A) while taking meclizine 25 mg TID, which has an anticholinergic effect and (B) 3 weeks after discontinuing meclizine. Sweat output is recorded from three standard sites: Purple line = proximal leg, Red line = distal leg, Blue line = dorsal foot. Sudomotor volume is determined by measuring the area under each curve. The undetectable response in recording A is an artifact of medication and might have been interpreted as evidence of a distal small fiber neuropathy if not for the normal recording B off of medication.

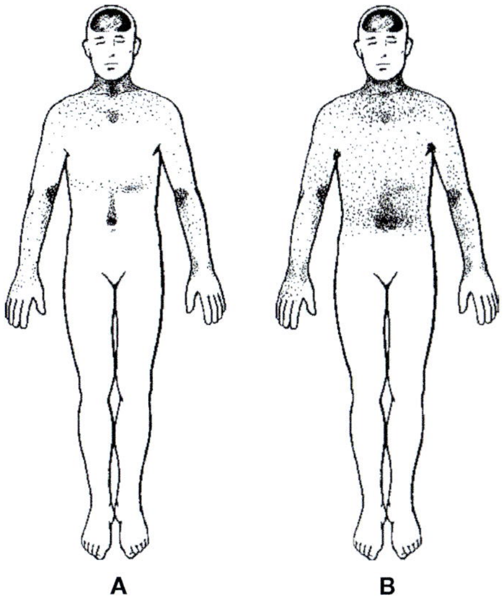

FIGURE 10.3: Thermoregulatory sweating test in a single patient with anhidrosis associated with small fiber neuropathy (A) at baseline, and (B) one hour after taking pyridostigmine 60 mg orally. Pyridostigmine, which augments sympathetic ganglionic transmission, doubled the volume of sweat the patient was able to generate in nonanhidrotic skin areas but did not recruit sweating in anhidrotic areas.

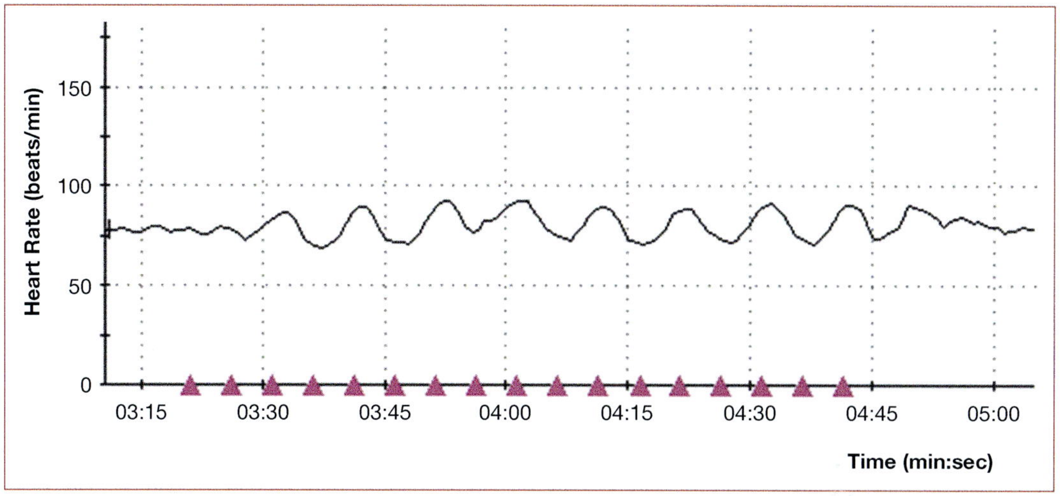

FIGURE 10.4: Example of a normal tracing of heart rate variability is shown during sinusoidal deep breathing. Each triangle indicates inspiration or expiration.

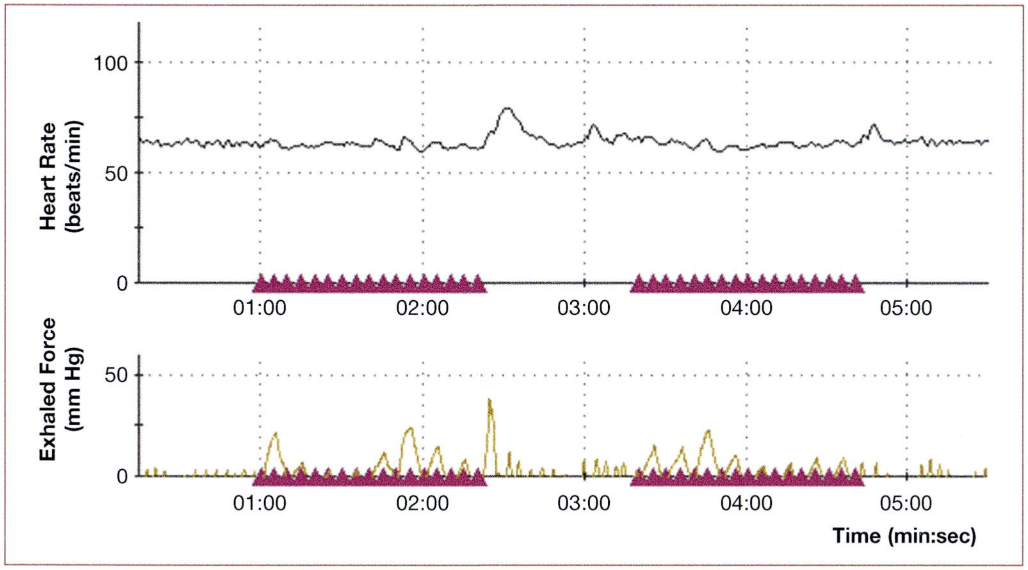

FIGURE 10.5: Heart rate variability to deep breathing in this recording is decreased in amplitude. The chest wall motion tracing (brown line in the bottom) demonstrates that this is not due to impaired cardiovagal function, but rather to the patient's inadequately deep breaths. This might reflect the patient's poor effort, poor understanding of instructions, anxiety, or respiratory muscle weakness. Several normal breaths are achieved and serve as comparison. Notably, the largest breath (at 2 minutes 20 seconds) is associated with a normal magnitude (18) of heart rate change for this 40-year-old patient, whereas the average of five consecutive cycles, which is the method typically used to calculate heart rate variability, gives a decreased value (5.9).

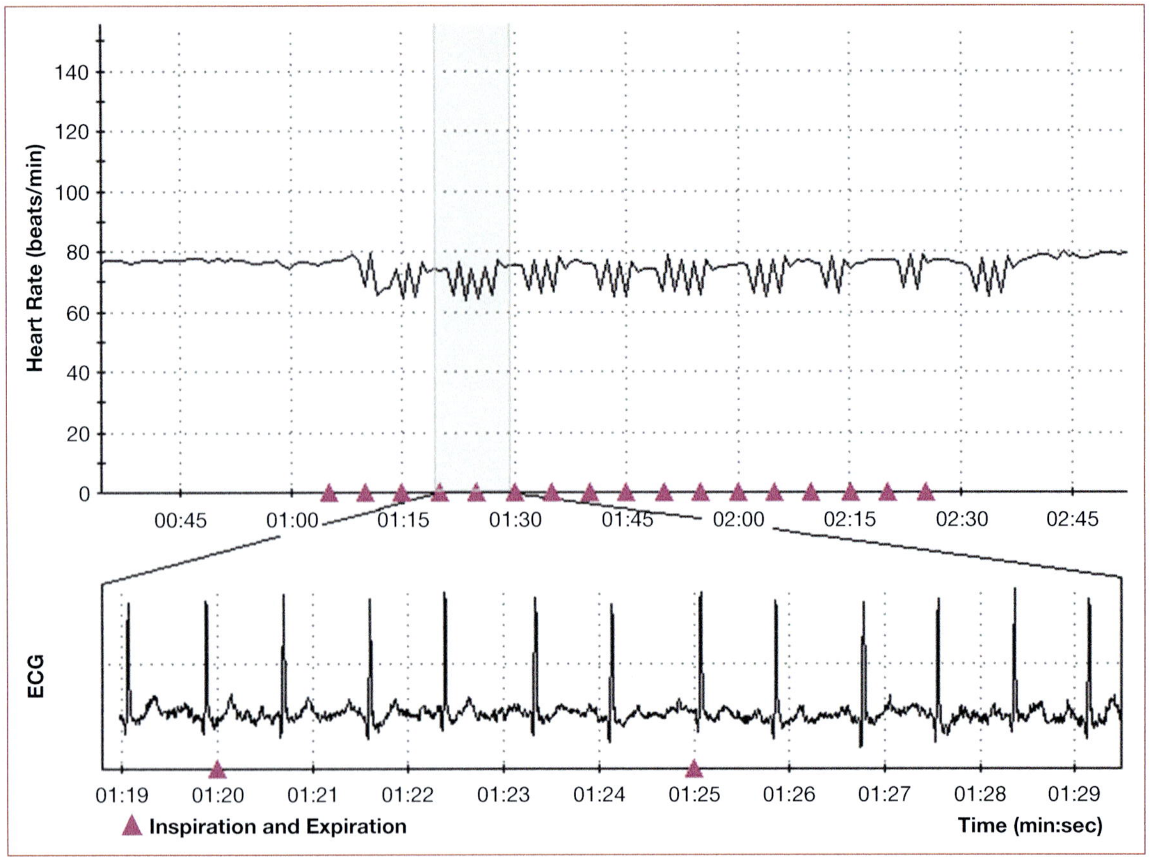

FIGURE 10.6: Heart rate recorded during sinusoidal deep breathing with inspiration and expiration marked by triangles. Two waveforms are evident. The true waveform of respiratory sinus arrhythmia, which is synchronous with the respiratory cycle, appears as a low amplitude sinusoidal wave. The more prominent sawtooth-shaped waveform should not be mistaken for neurally mediated heart rate variability. The expanded view (bottom) is the associated electrocardiogram tracing, which shows atrial bigeminy. The heart rate waveform in the upper tracing, which is derived from sequential RR intervals, thus shows an alternating beat-to-beat pattern.

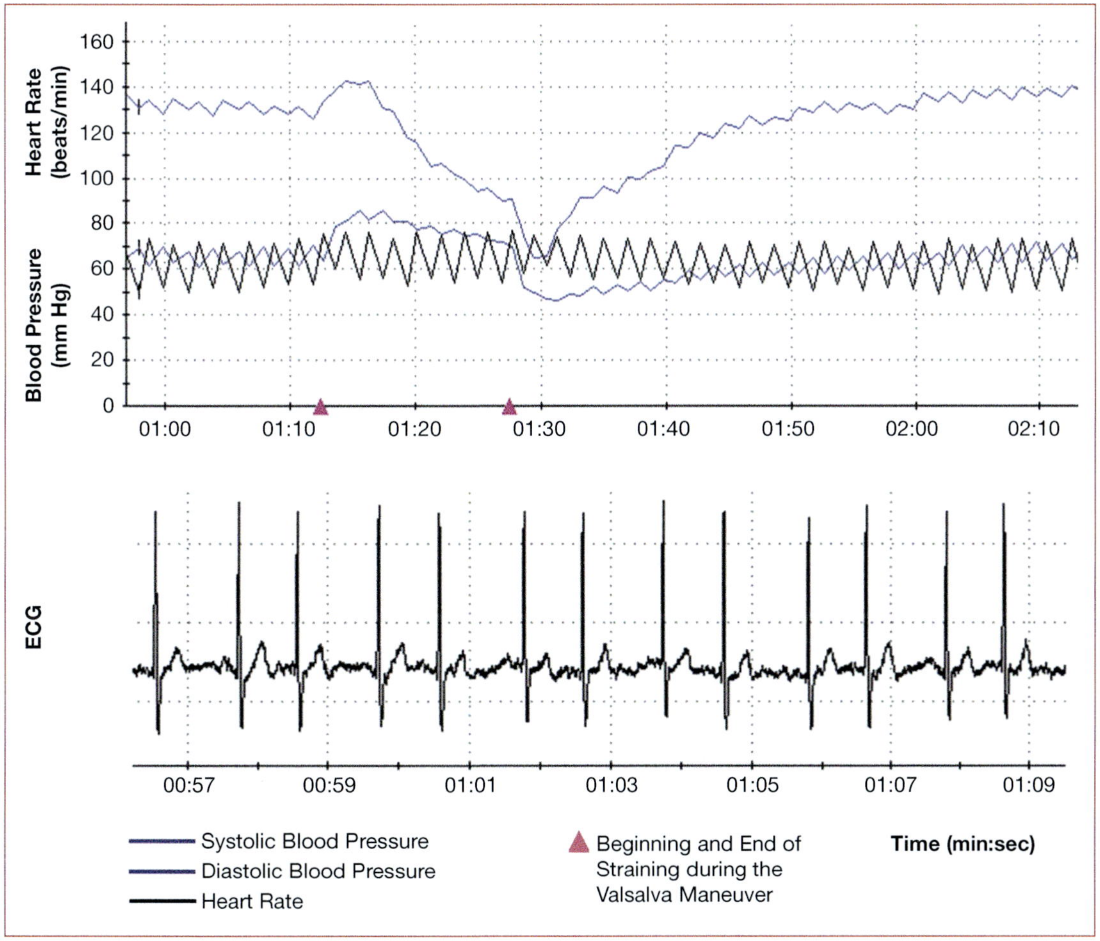

FIGURE 10.7: Beat-to-beat trace during systolic and diastolic blood pressure measurement (blue lines) and heart rate (black line) during Valsalva maneuver. The beginning and end of straining at 40 mmHg respiratory force are marked by triangles. Here, as in the previous figure, atrial bigeminy, seen in the expanded ECG view (bottom) produces a sawtooth pattern on the heart rate tracing which, to a lesser degree, is reflected also in the blood pressure curves. This artifact, if not recognized as being of cardiac atrial origin, could lead to incorrect calculation of the Valsalva ratio, which is the ratio of the maximum heart rate during phase II (at about time 1:28) to the minimum heart rate during phase IV (at about 1:55). Rather than take a peak value at time 1:28 and a trough value at time 1:55, which would give a falsely high number, an accurate Valsalva ratio requires taking peak values from both timepoints.

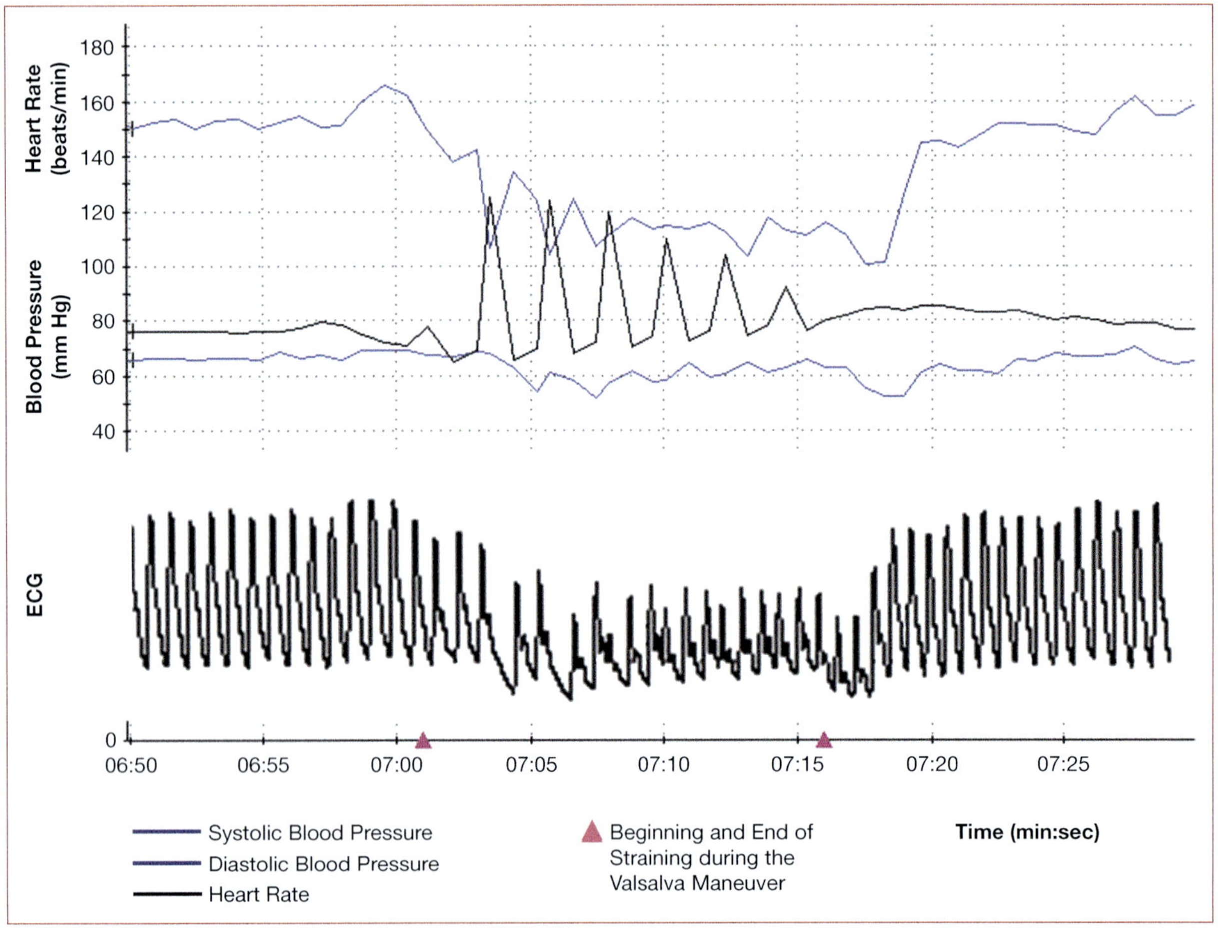

FIGURE 10.8: Beat-to-beat trace during systolic and diastolic blood pressure measurement (blue lines) and heart rate (black line) during Valsalva maneuver in which the heart rate trace shows a series of artifactual peaks. These peaks represent a doubling of the true heart rate caused by the RR wave detection software erroneously counting T waves as separate heart beats. The associated ECG tracing shown (bottom), demonstrates how, from time 7:03 to time 7:15, the magnitude of the recorded R waves decreases nearly to the amplitude of the T waves.

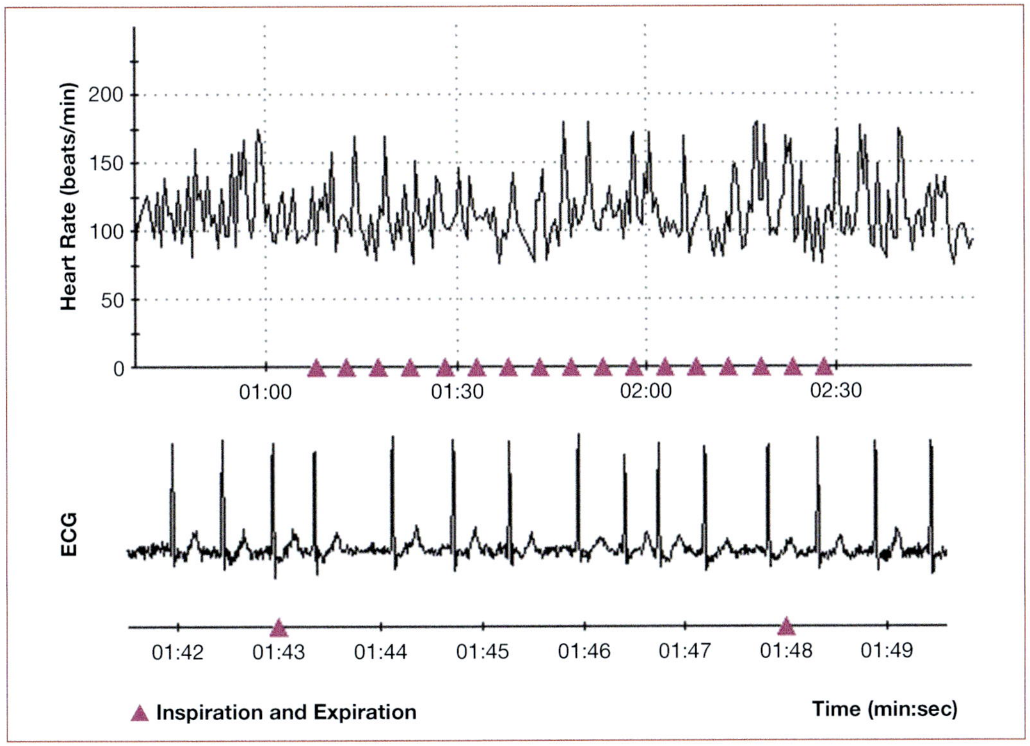

FIGURE 10.9: Tracing demonstrating beat-to-beat variability of heart rate during sinusoidal deep breathing that was present in a patient with atrial fibrillation. The irregularly irregular heart beats, as shown in the expanded ECG tracing (bottom), dominate the tracing and can prevent the identification or quantification of respiratory sinus arrhythmia in the background. If the highest peaks and lowest troughs were used to calculate heart rate variability, the result would be incorrect as it would not reflect neurally mediated heart rate variability.

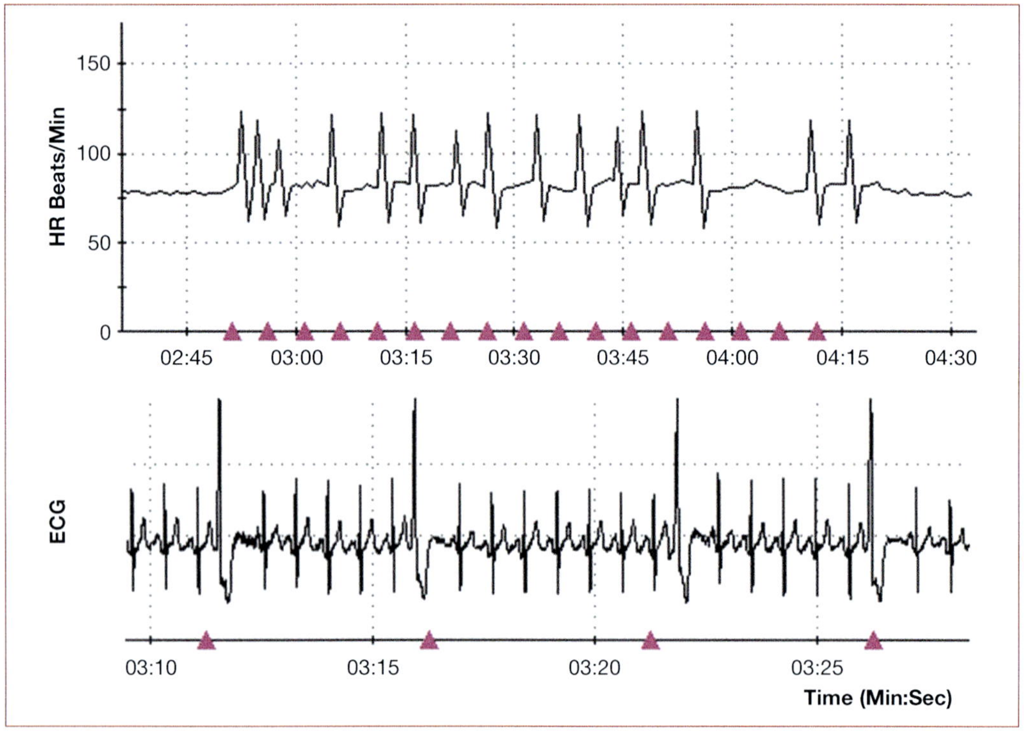

FIGURE 10.10: Tracing demonstrating beat-to-beat variability of heart rate during sinusoidal deep breathing in a patient with frequent PVCs, as shown in the expanded ECG tracing (bottom). Unlike the nearly continuous obliteration of the respiratory sinus arrhythmia signal in the patient with atrial fibrillation, the interference by PVCs is intermittent, such that the slower sinusoidal waveform may be discerned, and true peaks and troughs identified, in the background.

PVC, premature ventricular contraction.

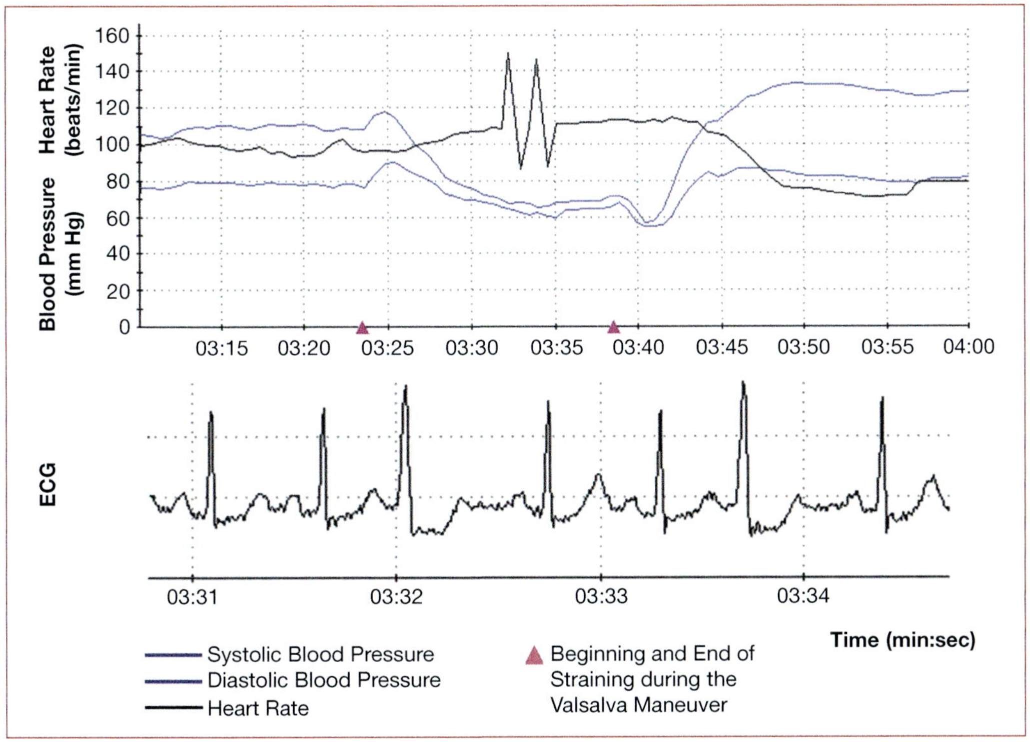

FIGURE 10.11: Tracing demonstrating beat-to-beat variability of systolic and diastolic blood pressure measurement (blue lines) and heart rate (black line) during Valsalva maneuver in a patient with occasional premature ventricular contractions. These are represented as a double blip on the heart rate tracing and in the expanded ECG tracing (bottom) as somewhat widened QRS complexes (the series of Q, R, and S waves on an ECG) lacking preceding P waves. When calculating the Valsalva ratio, the true heart rate peak is located, not at time 3:33, but at time 3:42.

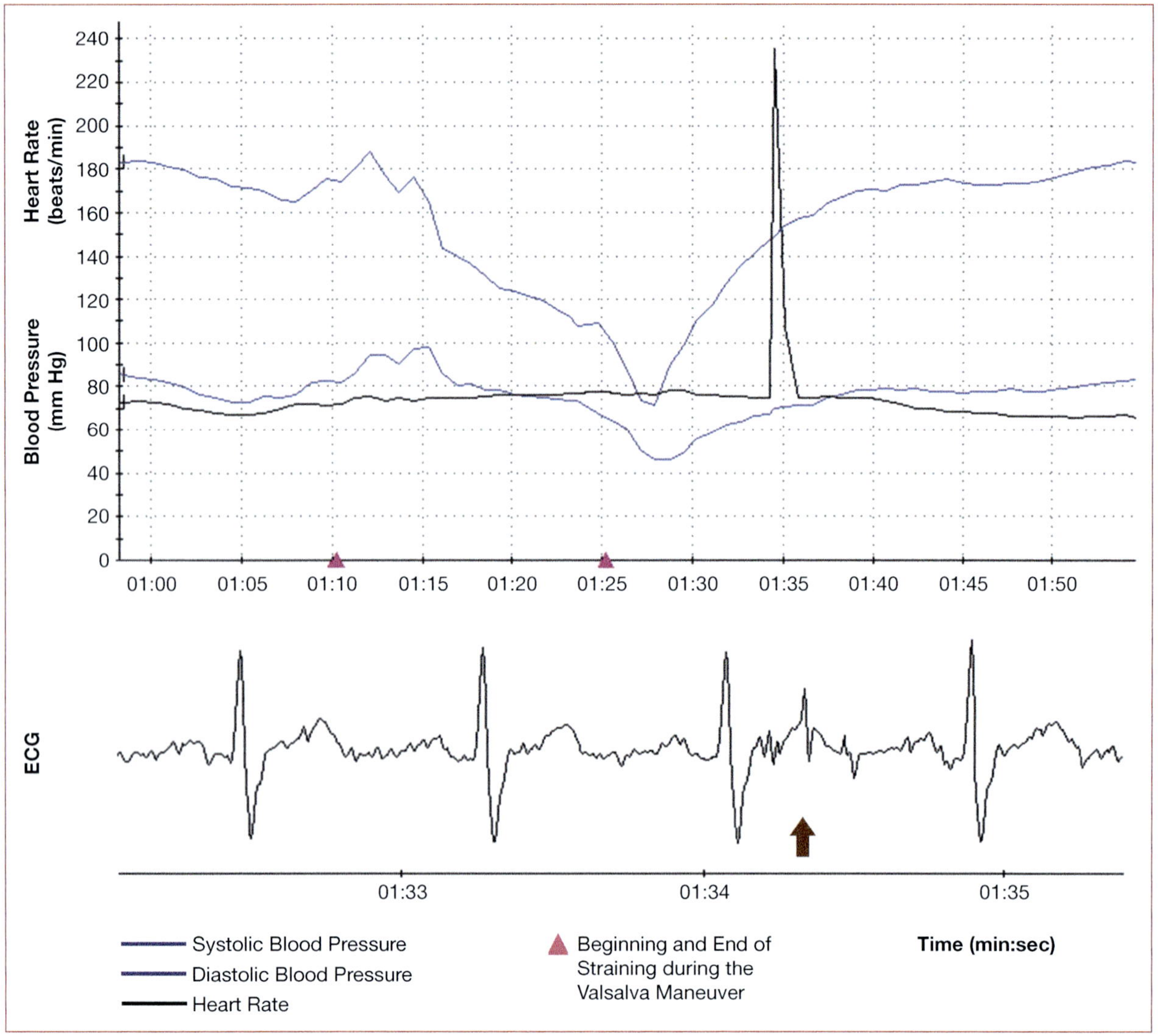

FIGURE 10.12: Tracing demonstrating beat-to-beat variability of systolic and diastolic blood pressure measurement (blue lines) and heart rate (black line) during Valsalva maneuver in a patient whose heart rate tracing shows a very large, isolated peak at time 1:35 (brown arrow). The expanded ECG tracing (bottom) shows that this is associated with a series of small amplitude, sharply contoured spikes overlying the T wave. These spikes are typical of chest wall muscle artifact, which the heart rate detection software may mistake for an R wave. This peak should be ignored when calculating the Valsalva ratio.

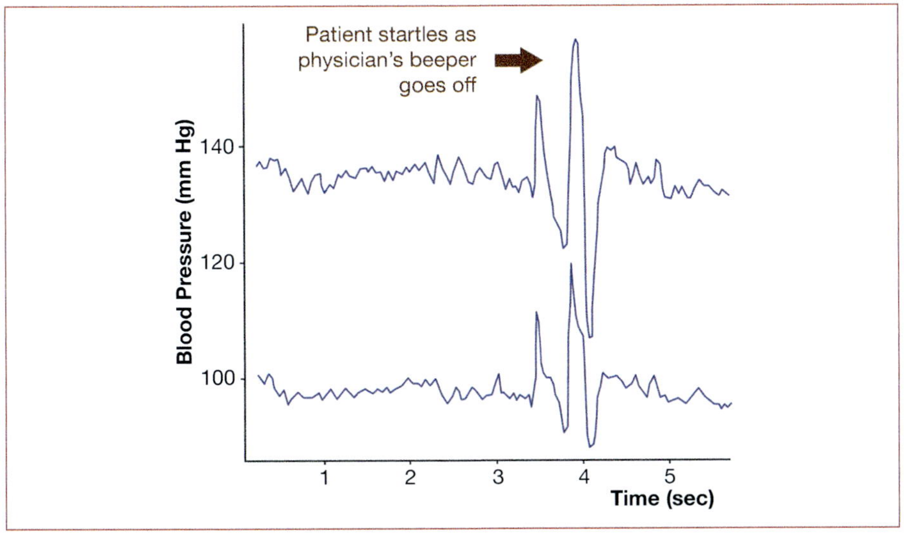

FIGURE 10.13: Tracing demonstrating beat-to-beat variability of systolic and diastolic blood pressure measurement (blue lines) in a patient tested at baseline. Just before the 4-second time mark, the physician's pager sounded a loud tone, which startled the patient and resulted in a brief rippling waveform, as if a pebble had been dropped into a quiet lake. This exemplifies how emotional states can affect sensitive autonomic recordings.

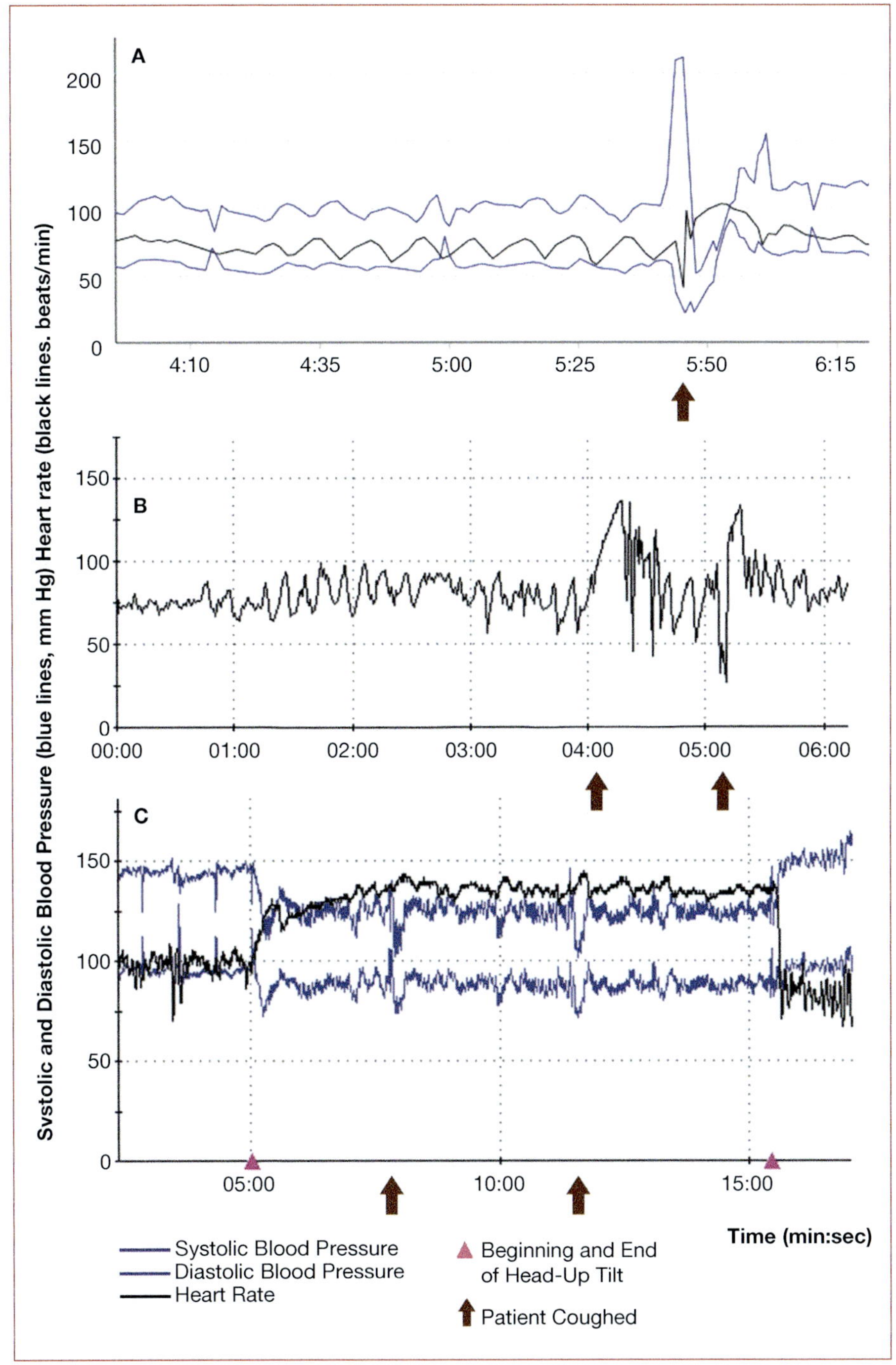

FIGURE 10.14: A composite tracing that represents three patients who coughed during autonomic testing. A and B occurred while supine at baseline, and C occurred while upright during tilt table testing. The waveform configurations are somewhat variable. One reason the appearance is variable is that the time scale is different among the recordings. In each case, the beat-to-beat blood pressure profiles demonstrate a waveform similar to, but more brief than, that of a Valsalva maneuver. An associated brief rise in heart rate also occurs. This profile should not be interpreted as autonomic instability, but rather as the physiologic effect of a transient increase in intrathoracic pressure.

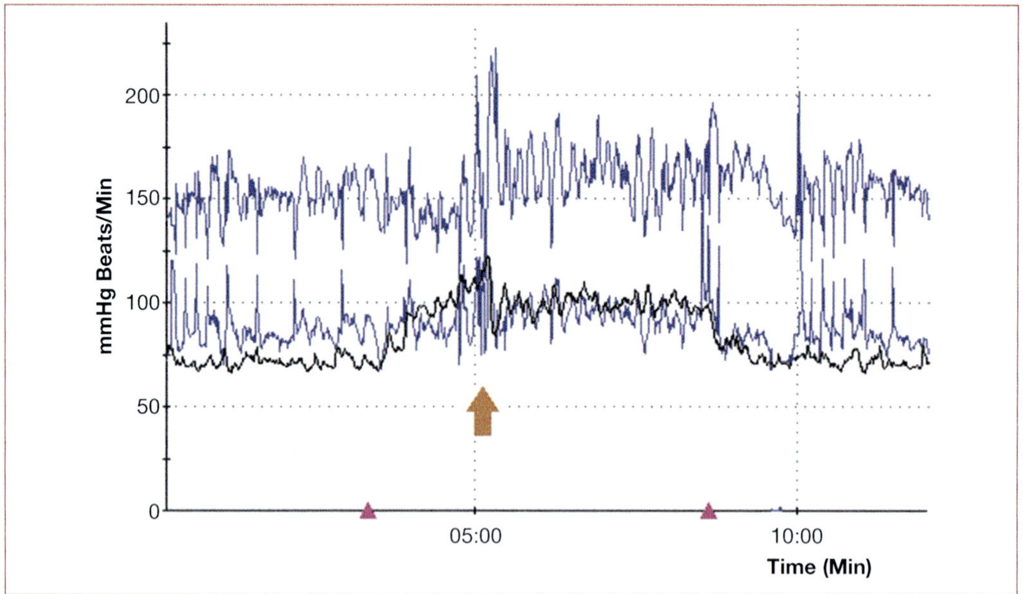

FIGURE 10.15: Beat-to-beat tracing of systolic and diastolic blood pressure (blue lines) and heart rate (black line) during a tilt table test in a patient who laughed (brown arrow at 5-minute time mark). The onset and end of head-up tilt are marked by triangles. The laughter is associated with a transient rise in blood pressure that is briefer than that caused by coughing. This profile should not be interpreted as autonomic instability, but rather as the physiologic effect of a transient increase in intrathoracic pressure.

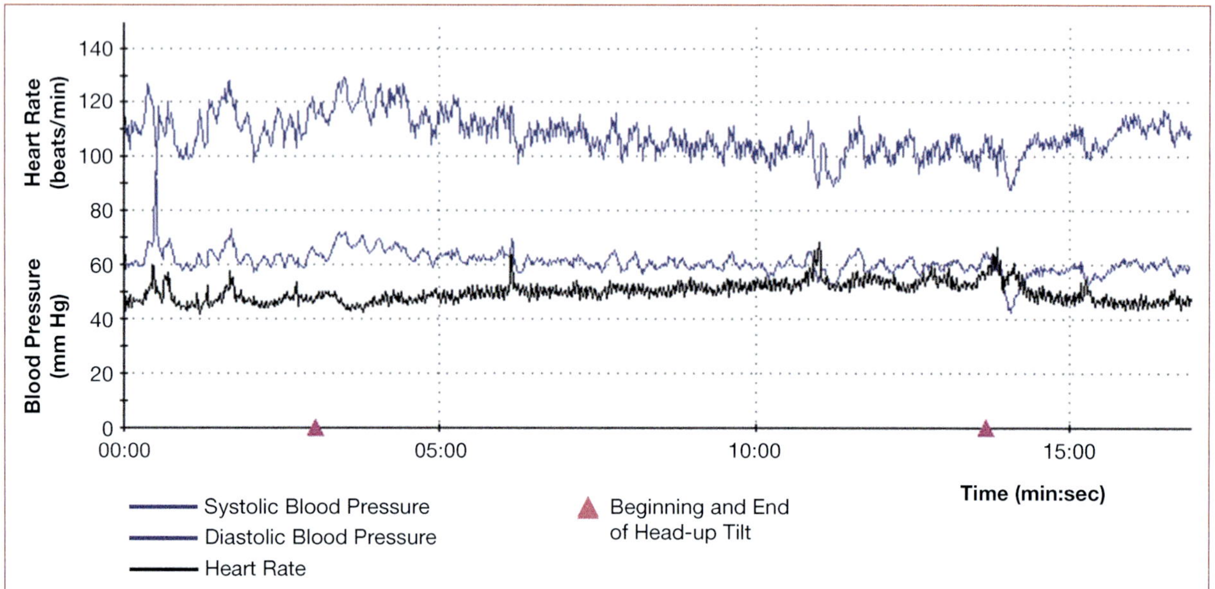

FIGURE 10.16: Beat-to-beat tracing of systolic and diastolic blood pressure (blue lines) and heart rate (black line) during a tilt table test. Although there appears to be a decline in blood pressure by 30/10 mmHg, this profile does not indicate neurogenic orthostatic hypotension. Key features are the labile supine blood pressure readings, suggesting that a true resting baseline has not been achieved, and the absence of an increase in blood pressure to the original level once the table is returned to the horizontal position.

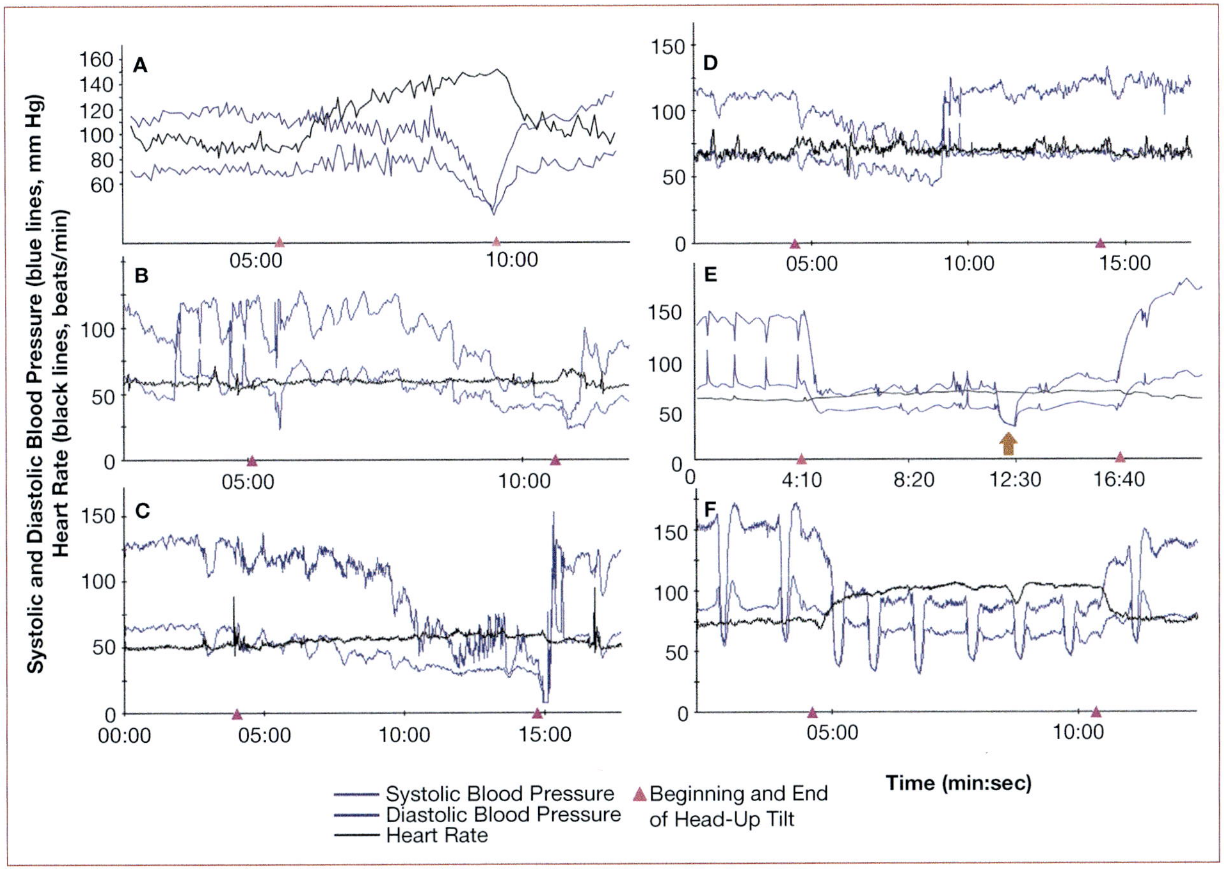

FIGURE 10.17: Composite representation of six patients who demonstrated a decrease in blood pressure during head-up tilt table testing. Beat-to-beat systolic and diastolic blood pressure (blue lines) and heart rate (black line) values are shown. (A) Neurally mediated or vasodepressor syncope. Note the preceding tachycardia and the gradual tapering of blood pressure and decrease in pulse pressure over about 1 minute. In contrast to orthostatic hypotension, which would have occurred immediately on reaching the upright posture, neurally mediated syncope is delayed in onset. This is contrasted with the temporal profiles of (B), (C), and (D), which are three separate instances of the common occurrence of the photoplethysmographic device losing detection of the patient's pulse. The loss of the pulse occurs in a stepwise manner; there is no associated tachycardia, and checking of blood pressure by ordinary sphygmomanometry in the opposite arm confirms that hypotension did not actually occur. In (D) the technologist repositioned the device and succeeded in restoring pulse detection at time 9 minutes. (E) A patient with neurogenic orthostatic hypotension happened to be wearing an ambulatory blood pressure monitor during autonomic testing. Inflation of the automated cuff is seen as a discrete notch-like dip in beat-to-beat blood pressure at the 12-minute time mark. (F) This patient also had neurogenic orthostatic hypotension but, because of previous surgery on the right arm, the left arm was used during autonomic testing both for photoplethosmography and sphygmomanometry. Several times at baseline and during head-up tilt, inflation of the automated blood pressure cuff above the elbow transiently restricted blood flow to the finger, where the appearance of an episode of hypotension was recorded.

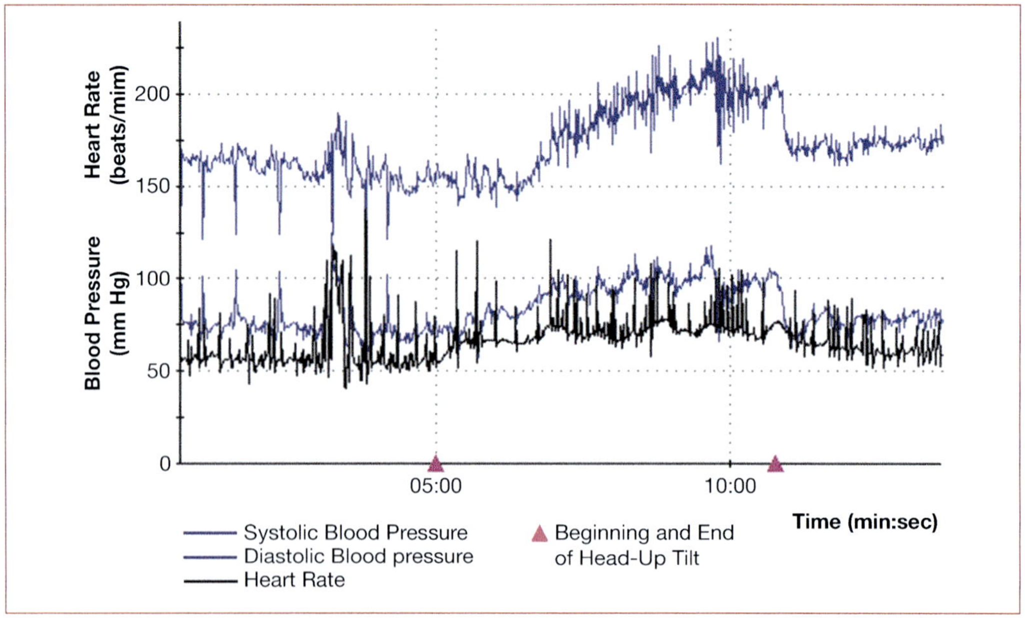

FIGURE 10.18: Beat-to-beat tracing of systolic and diastolic blood pressure (blue lines) and heart rate (black line) during a tilt table test in a patient who reported progressive urinary bladder urgency. As routine preparation for autonomic testing, patients are offered the opportunity to void the bladder, but the patient with an overactive bladder may still experience symptoms during testing. In this case, bladder discomfort caused a progressive rise in blood pressure. A similar profile can be seen in patients with autonomic dysreflexia caused by high spinal cord injuries.

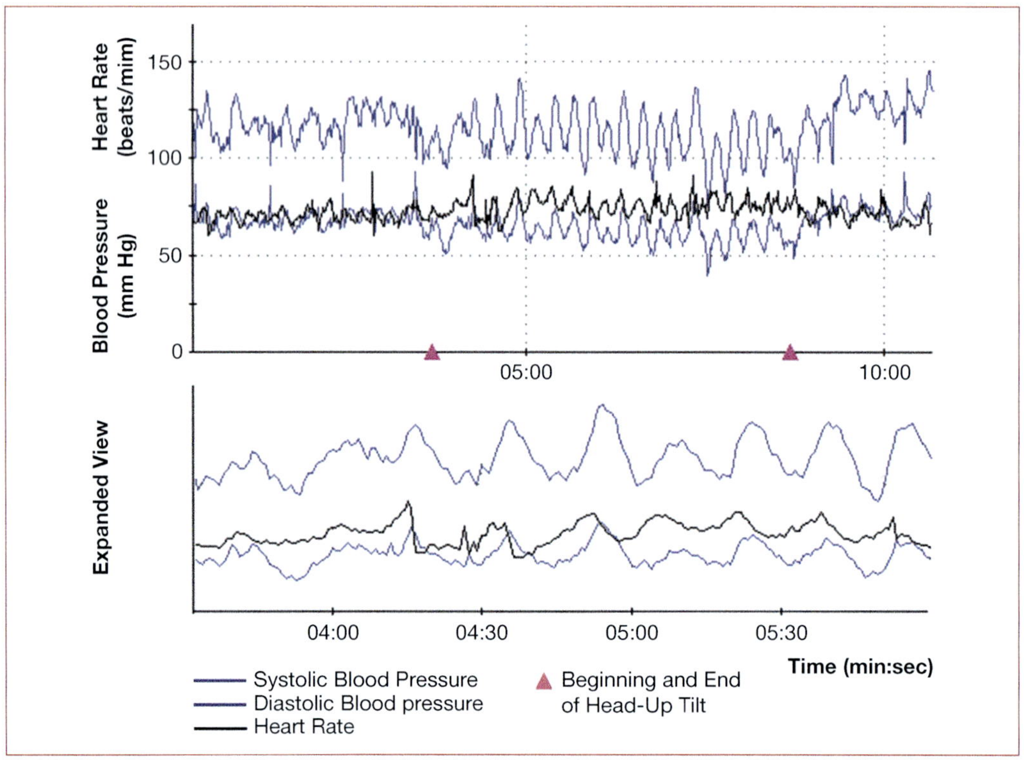

FIGURE 10.19: Beat-to-beat tracing of systolic and diastolic blood pressure (blue lines) and heart rate (black line) during a tilt table test in a patient with Parkinson's disease. The technologist commented that the tremor seemed to be causing the blood pressure oscillations while the patient was upright. The expanded blood pressure tracing (bottom) demonstrates two sets of waveforms. The oscillations in blood pressure occur at a frequency of four cycles per minute and are independent of the hand tremor. The blood pressure waveform also picks up the patient's tremor, but this is of a faster frequency of about three cycles per second and does not significantly interfere with the autonomic data.

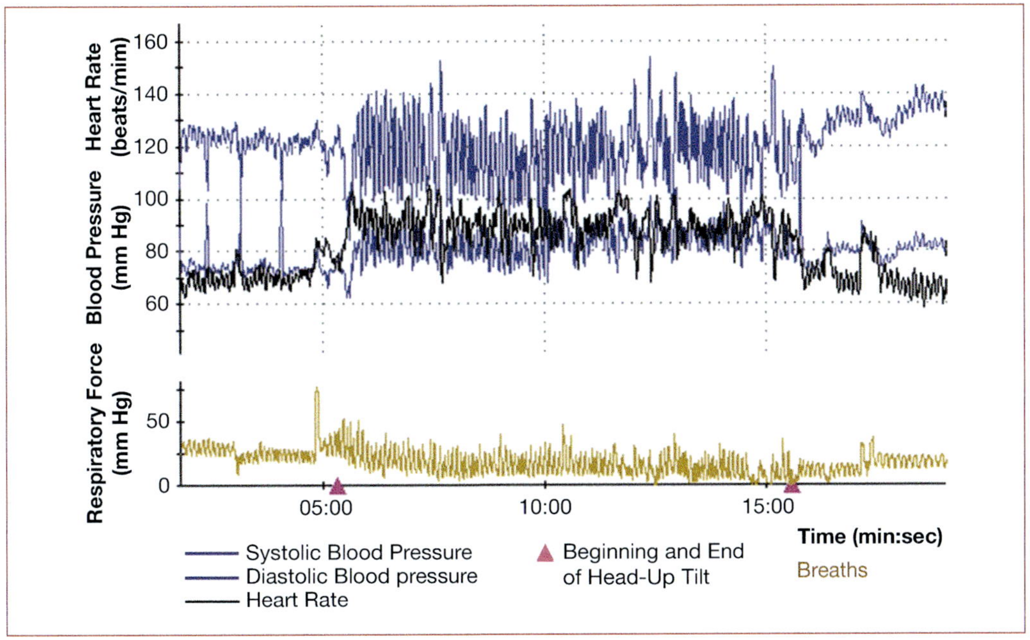

FIGURE 10.20: Beat-to-beat tracing of systolic and diastolic blood pressure (blue lines) and heart rate (black line) during a tilt table test in a patient who is hyperventilating (brown line). The variability in heart rate and blood pressure do not reflect autonomic instability but, rather, are physiologic and the consequence of respiratory sinus arrhythmia, as the respiratory frequency is time-locked with the variability in heart rate and blood pressure.

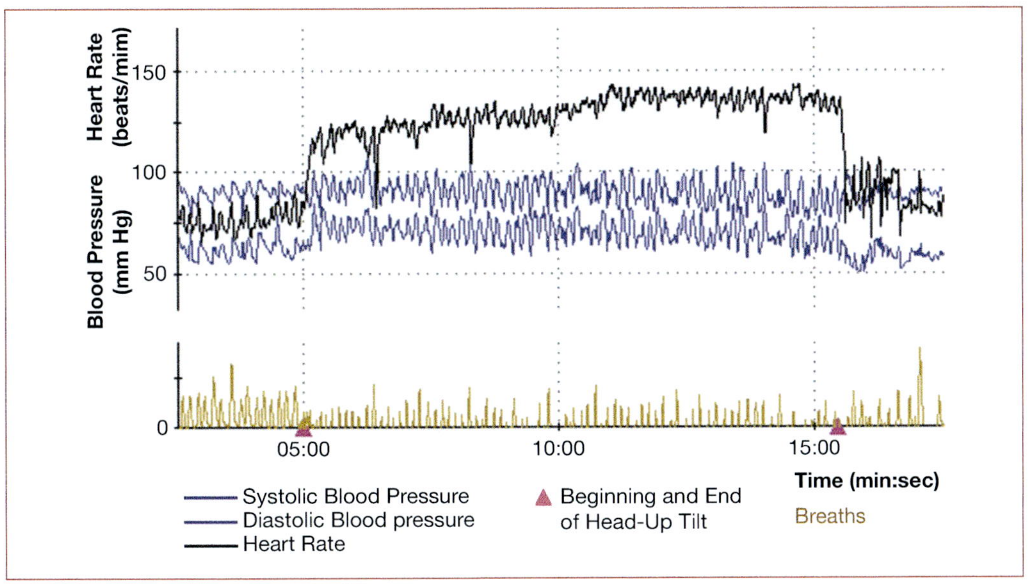

FIGURE 10.21: Beat-to-beat tracing of systolic and diastolic blood pressure (blue lines) and heart rate (black line) during a tilt table test in a patient with postural tachycardia syndrome. In the absence of orthostatic hypotension, the heart rate increases from the baseline of 76 beats/min to a sustained 125 to 135 beats/min while upright. Respiratory-associated oscillations in blood pressure and heart rate are superimposed.

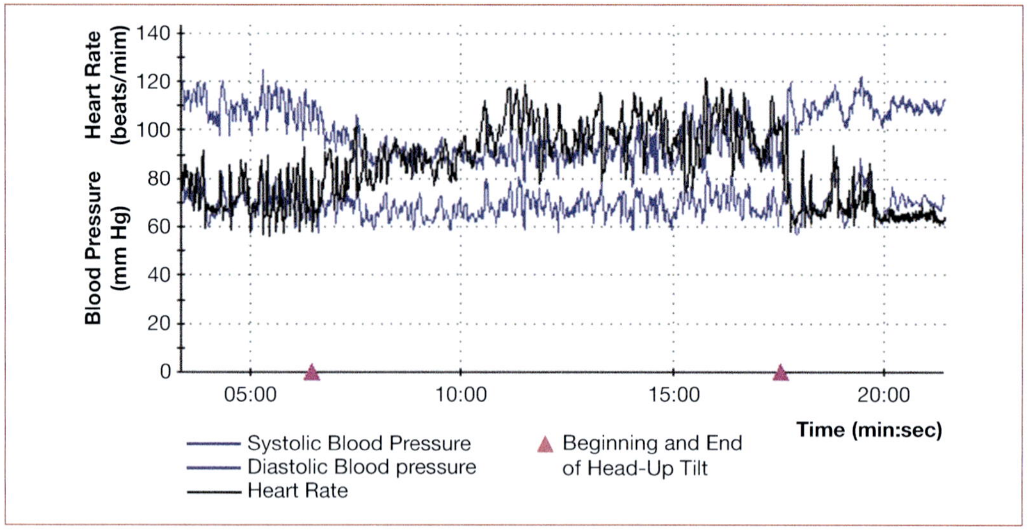

FIGURE 10.22: Beat-to-beat tracing of systolic and diastolic blood pressure (blue lines) and heart rate (black line) during a tilt table test in a patient who has a rapid heart rate upright but does not have postural tachycardia syndrome. The heart rate variations are irregular and are not synchronous with respirations (not shown). The mean heart rate supine is 68 beats/min and upright is 90 beats/min, which is within normal limits. If, instead of assessing heart rate mean values, one's eye is drawn to the heart rate peaks, isolated values of 110 to 120 stand out, which are sometimes mistaken for postural tachycardia syndrome.

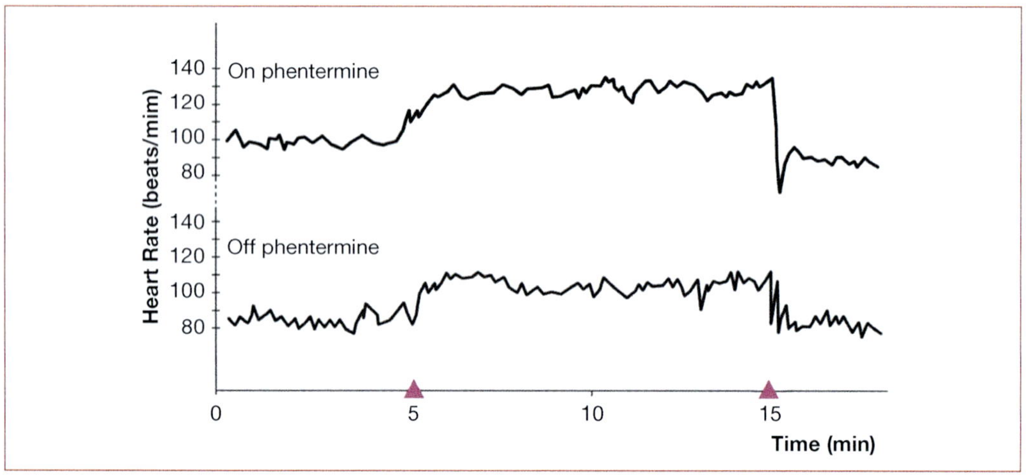

FIGURE 10.23: Beat-to-beat tracing of heart rate (black line) during a tilt table test in a patient suspected of having postural tachycardia syndrome. The heart rate increase met the criteria for this syndrome during the first recording (upper tracing) when the patient was taking the psychostimulant phentermine in an effort to lose weight, but when the test was repeated off of medication (lower tracing), the heart rate change was normal.

Source: Cheshire, WP. Stimulant medication and postural orthostatic tachycardia syndrome: a tale of two cases. *Clin Auton Res.* 2018; 26(3), 229-233. doi: 10.1007/s10286-016-0347-9.

REFERENCES

1. Gibbons CH, Cheshire WP, Fife TD. *American Academy of Neurology Autonomic Testing Model Coverage Policy*. https://www.aan.com/uploadedFiles/Website_Library_Assets/Documents/3.Practice_Management/1.Reimbursement/1.Billing_and_Coding/5.Coverage_Policies/14%20Autonomic%20Testing%20Policy%20v001.pdf. Accessed 2014.

2. Low PA, Sletten DM. Laboratory evaluation of autonomic failure. In: Low PA, Benarroch EE, eds. *Clinical Autonomic Disorders*. 3rd ed. Philadelphia, PA: Wolters Kluwer, Lippincott Williams & Wilkins; 2008:130-165.

3. Goldstein DS, Cheshire WP. The autonomic medical history. *Clin Auton Res*. 2017;27:223-233. doi:10.1007/s10286-017-0425-7.

4. Cheshire WP. Doctors' handwriting gone digital: an ethical assessment of voice recognition technology in medicine. *Ethics Med*. 2013;29:71-77.

5. Cheshire WP. Syncope. *Continuum*. 2017;23:335-358. doi:10.1212/con.0000000000000444.

6. Cheshire WP. Thermoregulatory disorders and illness related to heat and cold stress. *Auton Neurosci*. 2016;196:91-104. doi:10.1016/j.autneu.2016.01.001.

7. Cheshire WP, Fealey RD. Drug-induced hyperhidrosis and hypohidrosis: incidence, prevention and management. *Drug Safety*. 2008;31:109-126. doi:10.2165/00002018-200831020-00002.

8. Cheshire WP. Ethical assessment of personal health monitoring technologies that interface with the autonomic nervous system. *Ethics Med*. 2016;32:7-13.

9. Freeman R, Wieling W, Axelrod FB, et al. Consensus statement on the definition of orthostatic hypotension, neurally mediated syncope and the postural tachycardia syndrome. *Clin Auton Res*. 2011;21:69-72. doi:10.1007/s10286-011-0119-5.

10. Cheshire WP. Clinical classification of orthostatic hypotensions. *Clin Auton Res*. 2017;27:133-135. doi:10.1007/s10286-017-0414-x.

11. Cheshire WP. Stimulant medication and postural orthostatic tachycardia syndrome: a tale of two cases. *Clin Auton Res*. 2016;26:229-233. doi:10.1007/s10286-016-0347-9.

CHAPTER 11

Polysomnographic Artifacts

Madeleine Grigg-Damberger

INTRODUCTION

Polysomnographic artifacts are extraneous signals in a recording channel that obscure or provide false data. Because we simultaneously record multiple different biophysiological signals for long hours, artifacts in polysomnography (PSG) are ubiquitous and pervasive. Artifacts in PSG can be good, bad, or ugly. Examples may be easily identified. Artifact is good when muscle or movement artifacts herald arousals, shifts in body position, or parasomnias. Bad when false theta activity due to digital EEG aliasing is misinterpreted as EEG slowing (1). Ugly when an implanted deep brain stimulator (DBS) totally obliterates all our alternating current (AC) recorded signals (2). In this chapter, we discuss common and uncommon artifacts in PSG, their salient features, causes, clinical significance, and strategies for fixing them when needed.

UNDERSTANDING WHICH PHYSIOLOGICAL SIGNALS ARE RECORDED IN PSG

PSG is a diagnostic tool in sleep medicine during which multiple different biophysiological signals are continuously and simultaneously recorded across a sleep period to characterize sleep and identify sleep disorders. The name is derived from the Greek root πολύς (*polus* for "many, much") and the Latin root, *somnus* ("sleep"), and Greek γράφειν (*graphein*, "to write"). The resulting study is a polysomnogram (also abbreviated as PSG).

In our sleep laboratory, we typically record 11 to 16 (or more) different biophysiological variables for 6 to 8 hours when performing a comprehensive overnight in-laboratory (level 1) PSG. Given the number of different physiological signals and time duration recorded in PSG, the number and types of artifacts encountered often seem exponential.

Identifying artifacts in PSG begins by knowing which biological signals are recorded and the normal technical settings, waveforms, and patterns for each of these (3). We can score sleep/wake states using only three physiological parameters: EEG, eye movements (electrooculography [EOG]), and submentalis electromyography (chin EMG). However, far more physiological parameters are typically recorded to identify or exclude sleep pathologies and disorders.

Most comprehensive overnight in-laboratory (level 1) PSGs are recorded to identify sleep disordered breathing, most often obstructive sleep apnea (OSA). Figure 11.1 shows a 120-second epoch record in a 60-year-old man with severe OSA. Almost all of the respiratory parameters recorded in PSG provide only qualitative data. To compensate for this, multiple different respiratory signals are recorded (nasal pressure [NP] airflow, oronasal thermal sensors, thoracic and abdominal respiratory effort, electrocardiogram, and pulse oximetry); redundancy is useful when one or more fail. We additionally monitor carbon dioxide (CO_2) using end-tidal and/or transcutaneous CO_2 with capnometry when recording PSG in adults with suspected sleep-related hypoventilation and all children. Figure 11.2 shows a 120-second epoch of PSG recorded on a child with severe OSA and Down syndrome showing how we also record CO_2. When introducing and titrating positive airway pressure (PAP) to assess its effect on sleep disordered breathing, we additionally record PAP flow (Figure 11.3) and sometimes PAP pressure and leak.

Sleep laboratories are certified by the American Academy of Sleep Medicine (AASM). We record, score, and interpret PSGs using the *AASM*

Manual for the Scoring of Sleep and Associated Events (4). It provides rules for scoring sleep stages, arousals, and respiratory, cardiac, movements, and parasomnias during sleep. It also specifies standard montages, electrode placements, and digitization parameters. Table 11.1 summarizes standard low-frequency (LFF) and high-frequency filter (HFF) settings for each of the PSG signals.

Following the *AASM Scoring Manual*, we preferentially record right frontal, central, and occipital EEG referenced to left mastoid (F4-M1, C4-M1, and O2-M1) but also record F3-M2, C3-M2, and O1-M2 as backup (Figure 11.4). However, we record video-PSG with an expanded EEG montage (16–19 or more channels) when sleep-related seizures are suspected (Figure 11.5). We routinely monitor lower extremity limb EMG from the left and right anterior tibialis muscles. However, when rapid eye movement (REM) sleep behavior (REM behavior disorder [RBD]) is suspected, we also record independently left and right flexor digitorum superficialis and extensor digitorum communis muscles to detect REM sleep without atonia (RWA) because RWA and RBD events more often involve the upper extremities (Figure 11.6).

Recognizing and reducing unwanted artifacts in PSG begins and ends with biocalibration to verify proper functioning of the digital polygraph, electrodes, and sensors. The *AASM Scoring Manual* recommends systematically performing biocalibration at the start and end of the PSG recording. Biocalibration provides a wealth of information for scoring events and artifacts in the PSG. Table 11.2 summarizes the protocol and rationale for biocalibration recommended by the *AASM Scoring Manual*.

TABLE 11.1: *AASM Scoring Manual* Digital PSG Technical Specifications

	LFF (Hz)	HFF (Hz)
EEG and EOG	0.3	35
EMG	10	100
ECG	0.3	70
Oronasal thermal airflow and thoracoabdominal respiratory belts	0.1	15
Nasal pressure	DC or ≤0.03	100
PAP device flow	DC	DC
Snoring sounds	10	100

AASM, American Academy of Sleep Medicine; DC, direct current; EMG, electromyography; EOG, electrooculography; HFF, high-frequency filter; LFF, low-frequency filter; PAP, positive airway pressure.

CLASSIFYING ARTIFACTS

When forced to classify PSG artifacts into types, we favor first dividing them into two groups: *physiological* and *nonphysiological*. *Physiological* artifacts originate from the patient (e.g., cardiac, muscle, respiration, sweat, and movements of eyes, tongue, body, and limbs). Nonphysiological artifacts can be further subdivided into two types: *instrumental* (artifacts that originate from the instruments and equipment used to record the PSG) and *environmental* (artifacts that arise from nearby surrounding environment). Table 11.3 summarizes these.

ARTIFACT IDENTIFICATION STRATEGIES

Identifying artifacts in PSG begins by knowing which biological signals are recorded and the normal ranges and patterns for each of these (3). Many artifacts in PSG can be recognized by their characteristic appearance and distribution but others only identified if the technologist identifies them at the time of the recording. Identifying artifacts in PSG begins by knowing which biological signals are recorded, and the normal ranges and patterns for each (3). Observing unexpected or unusual patterns in the PSG should prompt the questions shown in Figure 11.7.

Many PSG artifacts can be reduced or eliminated by (a) proper application of recording electrodes to obtain low and nearly equal impedances, (b) electrodes and sensors placed in the proper locations and securely attached, (c) properly grounded equipment; and (d) reducing electrical and electromagnetic interference (EMI) in the surrounding recording environment. The sleep technologist identifying an artifact needs to document its presence in the comment log, determine what is needed to fix/eliminate it, and finally consider whether it affects patient safety, or prevents interpretation of the PSG. Sometimes, letting the patient sleep is the best choice.

TABLE 11.2: Biocalibration Protocol

Check, Observe, and If Needed Fix	Purpose
Check and document impedances for all the EEG, EOG, and EMG electrodes; fix if needed.	Ensure impedances for EEG, EOG, and EMG derivations are ≤5 kΩ and relatively equal
Wake EEG recorded for 30 seconds with patient lying quietly with eyes closed.	Identify presence of dominant posterior rhythm for scoring wake and sleep onset
Look up, down, left, right, and blink without moving head.	Identify presence and direction of horizontal and vertical eye movements; appreciate more subtle eyeblinking.
Grit teeth or chew.	Assess display of chin EMG; may see glossokinetic artifacts (reproduced by asking patient to say Tom Thumb or Lilt-Lilt-Lilt)
Snore or hum.	Check snoring microphone channel
Breathe in and out.	Check for sufficient sensitivity and proper polarity of airflow and respiratory effort channels
Hold breath for 10 seconds.	Ability to record an apnea
Hold breath for 10 seconds.	Ability to record an apnea
Breathe only through nose for 10 seconds, then only through mouth for 10 seconds.	Nasal pressure transducer and oronasal thermal sensors to detect air flow are functioning properly, have sufficient sensitivity and appropriate polarity
Take a deep breath and exhale slowly for 10 seconds (prolonged expiration)	Identify prolonged expiration seen with sleep-related expiratory groaning

(*continued*)

TABLE 11.2: Biocalibration Protocol (*continued*)

Check, Observe, and If Needed Fix	Purpose
Flex left foot/raise toes on left foot (×5) then flex right foot/raise toes on left foot (×5).	Optimal functioning of anterior tibialis leg EMG
Flex fingers on right hand (×5) and then left hand without bending at the two distal joints, then extend fingers on left and then right hand without moving the wrist if upper extremity EMG is recorded.	Optimal functioning and display of flexor digitorum superficialis and extensor digitorum communis when recording upper limb EMG muscles for suspected REM behavior disorder

EMG, electromyography; EOG, electrooculography; REM, rapid eye movement.

TABLE 11.3: Classifying Polysomnography Artifacts

Artifact Category	Types	Examples
Physiologic	Eye	SEMs, REMs, eye flutter, eyeblinks, nystagmus, asymmetric EOG
	Muscle and movement	Muscle; whole body movements, position shifts; sucking, chewing, eating; HT; ALMA; RMD; tremor; myokymia; hemifacial spasm; RBD events; NREM arousal parasomnias
	Sweat	Sweat; galvanic sympathetic skin response
	Oropharyngeal movements	Tongue (glossokinetic); palatal myoclonus, glottis click, inspiratory stridor, snore vibration
	Cardiac	ECG, pulse, ballistocardiographic
	Respiratory	Respiratory

(*continued*)

TABLE 11.3: Classifying Polysomnography Artifacts (*continued*)

Artifact Category	Types	Examples
Instrumental	Electrode-related	Electrode pop, high impedance, imbalanced electrode pairs, ground recording artifact
	Acquisition settings	Channel inversion, improper settings
	Recording equipment	Jack box, amplifiers
Environmental	Electrical interference	60-Hz artifact, electromagnetic, electrostatic
	Personal electronics	Smartphone, cellphone, laptop, tablets
	Oscillating devices	Oscillating beds, fans, ventilators, IV pumps, sequential compression devices
	Implanted devices	Hypoglossal nerve stimulator, deep brain stimulator, vagal nerve stimulator, cardiac pacemaker, cardiac defibrillator
	Patient care	Chest percussion, patting, rocking, feeding, CPR.

ALMA, alternating leg muscle activation; EOG, electrooculography; CPR, cardiopulmonary resuscitation; HT, hypnagogic tremor; IV, intravenous; NREM, nonrapid eye movement sleep; RBD, REM behavior disorder; REM, rapid eye movement; RMD, rhythmic movement disorder; SEM, slow eye movement.

The ability to re-reference electrodes can be invaluable for identifying and ameliorating a questionable or spurious PSG signal (3). If, after re-referencing, an artifact appears in another channel, the amplifier is not the problem. If an amplifier channel goes bad, the input can be moved to a spare channel. If the mastoid reference is bad on one side, the electrodes can be re-referenced to the ipsilateral rather than contralateral side (makes scoring the amplitude of slow wave activity in nonrapid eye movement sleep [NREM] 3 a bit off but tolerable).

Some artifacts have a stereotypical appearance, so pattern recognition of these is often helpful. When observing medium-to-high amplitude atypical waveforms in only one EEG derivation, this should warrant suspicion

TABLE 11.4: Value of Video in Comprehensive Polysomnography

- Identify the artifact, movement, or parasomnia
- Was that a snore, snort, sigh, gasp, wheeze, or stridor?
- Patient out of bed, technologist or parent in room
- Who really is snoring?
- What caused the probe to malfunction?
- Who or what caused the arousal?

that these are artifact because EEG typically distributes a maximal potential which gradually drops off with increasing distance across the scalp. Most in-laboratory PSG records have time-locked video using ultraviolet light. Video can be invaluable in confirming PSG artifacts and diagnosing sleep disorders (benefits of which are summarized in Table 11.4).

The AASM Manual specifies backup electrodes which are to be recorded and deployed if those fail (4). For example, the recommended EEG derivations are F4-M1, C4-M1, and O2-M1; but if M1 malfunctions and cannot be fixed, the backup montage is F3-M2, C3-M2, and O1-M2. Three chin EMG electrodes are mandated, such that changing pairs can eliminate the signal emanating from the bad electrode. When recording respiratory signals the preferred sensor for identifying an apnea during a diagnostic study when the oronasal thermal airflow sensor is not functioning or the signal unreliable is to use: NP sensor or respiratory inductance plethysmography (RIP) flow or sum signals. The preferred sensor for scoring hypopnea is the NP transducer sensor; if malfunctioning or unreliable, we use oronasal thermal sensors, RIP sum or flow, or dual thoracoabdominal RIP belts.

PHYSIOLOGICAL ARTIFACTS

Physiological artifacts are those which originate from the patient. Given the long duration of overnight PSG, these are diverse and pervasive. Some are welcome, helping us to recognize diagnostic sleep pathologies. Others so obscure the recording as to render parts of the recording unreadable. One of the technologist's crucial roles is to recognize artifacts and, when possible, fix or eliminate them. The most common are muscle, muscle, sweat, respiration, cardiac, and movements of the eyes, tongue, and limbs.

Muscle Artifact (Electromyography)

EMG muscle artifact is one of the most common physiological artifacts in PSG, observed when muscle groups beneath the particular electrode site contract (3). Muscle artifacts often intrude into EEG, EOG, and EMG signals. They are often of much higher amplitude (≥100 μV), two to five times higher than the EEG.

Most scalp-recorded muscle artifact in PSG emanates from frontalis, temporalis, and occipitalis muscles. Using expanded EEG montages, muscle artifact is most prominent in the frontal (F3, F4), midtemporal (T3, T4), and parietal (P3, P4) electrodes reflecting frontalis, temporalis, and masseter muscles. Occipital electrodes (O1, O2) may pick up EMG artifact from the occipitalis, trapezius, and supraspinal muscles. Like EEG tracings, muscle artifact tends to be least over the midline channels (Fz, Cz, and Pz). We use this to our advantage; when recording patients suspected of sleep-related hypermotor epilepsy, electrographic seizures may be best seen at the Cz electrode derivation (Figure 11.5).

The power spectrum of contracting striated muscle measured by surface EMG has a broad bandwidth of 20 to 300 Hz, but most of the power is between 15 and 100 Hz (5). The peak frequency of masseter muscles when chewing is 50 to 60 Hz, 30 to 40 Hz for the frontalis muscles when wrinkling the brow, and 40 to 80 Hz for the temporalis muscles when jaw clenching. The posterior head muscles have higher peak frequencies around 100 Hz although they may vary depending on the direction, force of contraction, and the patient's sex. The peak frequency can extend up to 600 Hz in some facial muscles due to their smaller size and higher innervation ratio (5).

If muscle artifact is not too prominent during wakefulness, we tolerate it, cognizant that interference will decrease with sleep onset. Skeletal EMG activity typically shows a progressive decrease with deepening NREM sleep and reaches its lowest levels in REM sleep. One of the most important biomarkers of REM sleep is a low-amplitude chin EMG. A poorly attached chin EMG can prevent optimal scoring of chin muscle atonia in REM sleep (Figure 11.8). The sudden appearance of prominent muscle artifact from NREM 3 sleep, coupled with a diffusely slowed EEG and sinus tachycardia, prompts review of the video to identify a NREM arousal parasomnia (Figure 11.9). Excessive amounts of muscle activity/movement artifact during REM sleep (accompanied by other biomarkers of REM sleep such as rapid eye movements and irregular respiration) warrants review of the video (to identify RBD events) and consideration of a diagnosis of REM sleep without atonia associated with RBD (Figure 11.10).

Movement Artifacts

Humans at sleep onset assume a posture of relative repose. The motor system reduces its level of activity and tone even before sleep onset. Subsequent movements during sleep typically occur during (a) postural shifts,

(b) arousals or awakenings, (c) sleep stage shifts, or (d) following paroxysmal events (hyperpneic phase of a respiratory event, a periodic limb movement, seizure, or parasomnia). The frequency of body movements is a fairly reliable measure of sleep and sleep stages, decreasing with increasing depth of sleep (wakefulness > NREM 1 > REM > NREM 2 and least during NREM 3 sleep) (6).

What else affects sleep-related movement? Older adults move far less in sleep than younger. One classic study found the mean hourly frequency of body position shifts (postural shifts) decreases with increasing age: from 4.7 per hour of sleep between ages 8 and 12 years to 2.1 per hour between ages 65 and 80 years (7). Progressively more intrusive stimuli lead to recruitment of progressively more extensive motor sequences. Real words or calling a sleeper's name cause a differential responsiveness. The brain appears to perform a complex set of discriminations which can lead to movement, arousal, or waking when needed. Bedpartners can influence how we move (sleeping well or poorly with each other). And last, those who are depressed and/or have suffered child abuse often exhibit increased motor activity at night (as though sleeping with one eye open).

Body movements in prolonged PSG recordings can cause electrode pops, signal blocking, and muscle artifact in EEG and ECG. Major body movements can affect every channel (**Figure 11.11**). Repetitive facial movements such as chewing, blinking, hemifacial spasm, or tremor can produce combinations of fast muscle and slow movement artifacts which resemble cerebral discharges, especially if the combinations repeat with similar shape (8). Many sleep-related movements cause stereotypical movement and muscle artifacts, which sleep specialists and technologists learn to recognize. These include chin scratching (**Figure 11.12**), mother rocking baby (**Figure 11.13**), sleep bruxism (**Figure 11.14**), rhythmic movement disorder (**Figure 11.15**), hypnagogic foot tremor (**Figure 11.16**), alternating foot tremor (**Figure 11.17**), excessive fragmentary myoclonus (**Figure 11.18**), and REM sleep with atonia (**Figure 11.10**). Observing these prototypic motor patterns when recording or reviewing a PSG should prompt video review to confirm them. It is important to understand that many sleep-related movements have no clinical consequences (do not disturb the patient's sleep nor impact upon their daytime performance) and are not considered sleep disorders. For example, rhythmic movement disorder (9), hypnagogic foot tremor, alternating leg muscle activation, and excessive fragmentary myoclonus (**Figures 11.16–11.18**, respectively) are typically asymptomatic (10).

Contrary to popular opinion and traditional teaching, motor symptoms of most diurnal movement disorders do not disappear with sleep (11). Most actually recur (and some persist) during sleep. For example, the rest tremor of Parkinson's disease (PD) tends to disappear with sleep onset and is rarely seen in deep NREM 3 sleep. Compared to wakefulness, the bursts of tremor during sleep are typically brief (<15 seconds) and most often occur after awakenings; NREM 1 sleep; and during, or in transitions to and from, REM sleep. Tremor artifact is typically rhythmic 4 to 6 Hz, begins abruptly, emanates from the nuchal muscles, and seems isolated from the rest of the EEG background, often maximal in the occipital regions (**Figure 11.19**). PD tremor is often less or even absent the first 1 to 2 hours after awakening from sleep (so-called sleep benefit). Examples of palatal myoclonus artifact (periodic, very brief, low-amplitude 100–200 millisecond bursts of pharyngeal muscle activity), frontal myogenic artifact (may appear as unilateral periodic bursts of 30–70 Hz muscle activity lasting 200–400 milliseconds, bursts recurring depending upon the individual every 1 to 5 seconds), and hemifacial spasm (prolonged high-frequency bursts lateralized to one side which last as long as the spasm).

Sweat Artifact

Sweat artifact represents long-duration, high-amplitude slow undulating shifts in the electrical potential between the skin and the recording electrodes caused by perspiration from sweat glands. Sweat contains high amounts of sodium chloride and lactic acid which react with the exposed metal of the electrode, generating action potentials which combine with skin and sweat gland potentials (12). Sweat artifact typically (a) occurs at a frequency of 0.5 Hz or slower, (b) is synchronous (but can be lateralized or asymmetric), (c) is often most prominent in frontal electrodes, and (d) can mimic slow wave activity of NREM 3 sleep (**Figure 11.20**).

To reduce/eliminate sweat artifact: (a) try cooling the patient by lowering the room temperature to less than 68°F (20°C) by either uncovering the patient or turning on air conditioning; (b) place a towel beneath the patient's head; (c) fan the patient's head using a sheet of paper but do so gently to avoid 60 Hz or movement artifact; (d) reassure the patient to reduce test anxiety; and (e) if persistent, set LFF in the affected channels to 1, 3, or 5 Hz. Realize that changing LFF to 1, 3, or 5 Hz tends to remove delta EEG frequencies important for recognizing and scoring slow wave sleep and eye movements (**Figure 11.21**). A PSG pearl: sudden onset of generalized slowing in the EEG with prominent sweat artifact in a patient with diabetes mellitus warrants consideration of nocturnal hypoglycemia (3).

Eye Movement Artifacts

To record EOG in PSG we set the LFF at 0.3 Hz and the HFF at 35 Hz, the same bandpass we use to record EEG. EOG in PSG is generated when the eyeball rotates about its axis, causing large shifts in ACs detected by electrodes placed near the eyes. The cornea is 100 mV positive compared to the retina (−100 mV). When the electropositive cornea moves toward an EOG electrode referenced to the contralateral mastoid, it results in a downward deflection. When the eyes close or blink, both eyeballs move up (Bell's phenomenon) which results in a maximum deflection in frontopolar and frontal EEG derivations. When the eyes are open, downward eye movements cause negative potentials in the frontopolar and frontal EEG derivations. Of note, when the eyeballs are in a fixed position, no change is observed in the EOG.

We use eye movements recorded in EOG and often detected in frontal EEG derivations to identify sleep/wake states. Slow eye movements appear at sleep onset (**Figure 11.22**). Slow eye movements (0.2–1 Hz) heralding the onset of NREM sleep are typically horizontal and out of phase: surface positive when positively charged cornea moves toward it, surface negative in the opposite eye. Rapid eye movements coupled with a loss of chin muscle tone and irregular respiration characterizes REM sleep (**Figure 11.4**). Of note, rapid eye movements in REM sleep are most often oblique, less often vertical, occasionally horizontal, and sometimes dysconjugate (13). When we record EOG using FPz as a common reference, the EOG also records frontopolar EEG K-complexes, and slow wave activity is typically of highest amplitude in the frontal and frontopolar derivations. K-complexes tend to cause in-phase deflections in the EOG (**Figure 11.23A**), whereas rapid eye movements cause out-of-phase deflections in recommended EOG during REM sleep (**Figure 11.23B**). EOG in PSG is typically detected in frontal and central EEG derivations (**Figure 11.23B**).

The *AASM Scoring Manual* permit recording eye movements in a PSG using either recommended or acceptable derivations (**Figure 11.24A**). Using the recommended EOG derivations, vertical or lateral conjugate eye movements result in out-of-phase deflections. EEG activity or artifacts in recommended EOG derivations typically appear as out-of-phase deflections. When the deflection in F4-M1 is downward, it means F4 is positive relative to M1. When the eyes move to the right, they cause a downward deflection in E2-M2. The acceptable derivations allow determination of the direction of eye movements. Vertical eye movements will show in-phase deflections and horizontal eye movements out-of-phase deflections. We prefer the acceptable method for recording EOG because it shows all directions of eye movements and also detects low-amplitude eye movements, such as blinking (**Figure 11.24B**).

Using *AASM Scoring Manual* recommended EOG derivations (**Figures 11.24A** and **B**), vertical or lateral conjugate eye movements result in out-of-phase deflections in both EOG derivations when one eye moves toward and the other away from one EOG electrode. EEG activity or artifacts in recommended EOG derivations typically appear as out-of-phase deflections. When the deflection in F4-M1 is downward, it means F4 is positive relative to M1. When the eyes move to the right, they cause a downward deflection in E2-M2. We prefer the alternative method for recording EOG because it shows all directions of eye movements and also detects low-amplitude eye movements, such as eyeblinking. Eyeblinks are typically brief, high-amplitude electropositive–electronegative waveforms in frontal EEG and EOG as the cornea moves upward (**Figure 11.25**).

TABLE 11.5: Causes of Asymmetric Eye Movements

- Ipsilateral eye absent or prosthetic
- Ipsilateral retinal disease
- Ipsilateral paresis of vertical gaze
- EOG electrodes asymmetrically placed
- Ipsilateral frontal skull defect
- Low-frequency filter settings set wrong

EOG, electrooculography.

Eye flutter is characterized by rhythmic 3–6 Hz activity and confined to EOG and frontal EEG derivations (**Figure 11.26**). Eye flutter more often occurs in tense or anxious patients, and can be interrupted by asking the patient to open their eyes and fixate gaze (14). A small but interesting study recorded EEG and eye movements in two healthy adults using magnetic search coil technique (15). They found that spontaneous blinks produced small eye movements directed down and inward, whereas slow or forced blinks were associated with delayed upward eye rotations (i.e., Bell's phenomenon). Both types of blinks caused positive EEG potentials with bifrontal distribution maximum at Fp1 and Fp2.

Given our dependence on EOG to score sleep, we are more concerned when encountering an asymmetric EOG in a PSG (**Figure 27**). **Table 11.5** summarizes considerations when observing decreased or absent EOG in one eye in a PSG. Two PSG eye movement artifact pearls: (a) a prosthetic eye made of glass has no electric potential but one made of metal is capable of generating a slow potential with the eye closed or open and (b) in the presence of a skull defect, the EOG will be of lower amplitude ipsilateral to the bone defect (the opposite of a breach rhythm in EEG).

Tongue and Other Oropharyngeal Artifacts

Sucking (**Figure 11.28**), swallowing, and talking (**Figure 11.29**) are common during sleep (most likely an expression of central pattern generators), involve tongue movements, and often cause artifacts which invade EEG, EOG, chin EMG, and airflow channels (16). When the tongue moves during these, it functions as a dipole (the tip relatively electronegative compared to the base). Tongue movements can produce so-called glossokinetic artifacts (Figure 11.30). When the tongue moves (particularly when touching the roof of the pharynx) the change in the electrical field spreads to involve the scalp. This results in single or brief runs of rhythmic delta activity usually maximal frontal. Glossokinetic potentials cause diffuse synchronous delta frequency slow waves that are often maximal in the frontal derivations. Glossokinetic artifacts can resemble eye movement artifacts or frontal delta activity. They can be confirmed by asking the patient when awake to say words that contain lingual consonants ("Tom Thumb" or "Lilt-lilt-lilt").

Respiratory and Vibration Artifacts

We encounter many artifacts in PSG related to respiratory effort. We preferentially record respiratory effort in PSG with LFF set to 0.1 Hz and HFF 15 Hz. Respiratory artifact often intrudes into the EEG derivations. Respiration signals are very slow and of high amplitude relative to EEG. It most often appears as a slow sway in the baseline EEG which is time-locked, occurring in-phase with phases of inspiration and expiration (Figure 11.31). Less often, respiratory effort artifact is a slow or sharp wave time-locked with inspiration and/or expiration but involves only some of the EEG electrodes (usually those on which the patient is lying) (Figure 11.32). Respiratory artifact is more often seen when the patient is lying in a manner that each breath causes a slight movement of EEG electrodes relative to the scalp. Once again, this is often most evident in electrodes which are loose or have high impedance.

To identify respiratory artifact, assess whether the artifact is time-locked to respiratory effort. Respiratory artifact is typically faster than sweat artifact and usually localized. Sweat artifact is more often generalized and involves several channels. To reduce or eliminate respiratory artifact when detecting during PSG collection: (a) check electrode impedances; if bad, regel or replace offending electrodes; (b) reposition the patient's head; and (c) reroute electrode leads so patient not lying on them. A different respiration-related artifact is snoring-related vibration, which can cause high-frequency artifacts in other channels (Figure 11.33). This artifact cannot be removed but should be recognized as snoring-related.

Cardiac Artifacts

The heart is a major source of artifacts in PSG (and EEG). It produces electrical and mechanical artifacts, both time-locked to contractions. Cardiac-related artifacts include those related to (a) ECG, (b) pulse, (c) ballistocardiographic movements, and (d) implanted cardiac pacemakers.

ECG Artifact

We record only one ECG channel (modified lead II) in PSG using a LFF of 0.3 Hz, HFF 70 Hz, and a minimum sampling rate of 200 Hz (500 Hz desirable). ECG tracings are typically recorded using a paper speed of 25 mm/sec. A 10-second time screen of PSG is roughly equivalent to a time screen of 30 mm/sec. Recording ECG in PSG using a modified level II, sinus rhythm is characterized by an upright P, R, and T waves. ECG recorded on the scalp is usually 1 to 2 µV in amplitude compared to EEG with typical amplitudes of 20 to 100 µV. ECG artifact can occur in any PSG channel, but especially in the AC-recorded EEG, EOG, and chin/limb EMG. The ECG signal has far greater amplitude (measured in mV) compared to the scalp-recorded EEG (µV).

ECG artifact in the EEG is usually diphasic (monophasic or triphasic in some). Small artifacts reflect primarily the R wave of the QRS. Larger ECG artifact may reflect other components; very large artifacts are often due to pacemakers. ECG artifact in EEG derivations is best seen in referential montages especially those to the left ear or wide interelectrode distances (all of which we typically record in PSG). The R wave is usually maximal over the left posterior head regions (Figure 11.34), lower over the right anterior head because the main cardiac vector produced a wave that is positive directed diagonally from right to left, anterior to posterior. If the head is turned, electrodes situated on left and posterior with regard to torso will still record maximum positivity. ECG artifact is enhanced in PSG when: (a) using referential montages because of their greater interelectrode distances and the field of the ECG is approximately equipotential across the head, (b) imbalanced electrode impedance between electrode pairs, (c) fatty deposits over the mastoid reference sites, and (d) individuals with short, thick necks or low-voltage scalp EEGs. ECG artifact is less noticeable in Cz or bipolar derivations.

ECG artifact usually cannot be eliminated from PSG because it is secondary to volume conduction of the ECG waveform. ECG is usually not due to a bad electrode. Given our preference for M1 and M2 as references, and that polygraphs do not easily permit linking M1 and M2, we are left with often prominent ECG artifact. Placing the ground electrode on the right side of the patient may reduce ECG artifact. Sometimes, turning the head relative to the trunk will change the field and lower the amplitude. The amplitude of the ECG artifact often changes in distribution and amplitude as the patient breathes. Breathing changes the position of the heart with respect to the head. Premature ventricular complexes are usually maximum over the posterior head regions, and are greater in amplitude and duration than the normal conducted heartbeat (Figure 11.35).

ECG artifact from cardiac arrhythmias is more challenging to recognize at first glance (Figure 11.36). Always check whether each ECG artifact is time-locked to a QRS. The heart rate tends to increase slightly with inspiration and decrease with expiration and, when prominent, this is called *sinus arrhythmia*. Heart rate cutoffs for sinus tachycardia and bradycardia are different during sleep than when awake: sinus tachycardia in adults during sleep is scored when heart rate is greater than 90 beats per minute (bpm) for greater than 30 seconds and sinus bradycardia in sleep in individuals 6 years of age or older with a heart rate less than 40 bpm greater than 30 seconds. Premature ventricular complexes are usually maximal over posterior head regions, and are greater in amplitude and duration than normal conducted heartbeats.

Pulse Artifact

Pulse artifact is caused by movement of an electrode when it rests over a pulsating artery (Figure 11.37). It appears as a smooth, periodic slow wave which follows the QRS ECG complex artifact by a slight delay (approximately 200 milliseconds); delayed by the time it takes the blood to travel from the heart to the pulsating blood vessel. Sometimes, the pulse artifact is triangular or sharply contoured. Pulse artifacts are more likely to occur in frontal, central, or temporal rather than occipital regions. To eliminate or reduce pulse artifact in PSG, first try moving the patient's head slightly off the particular electrode; if the artifact persists, reapply the electrode a small distance away from the superficial artery.

Ballistocardiographic Artifact

Ballistocardiographic artifacts are related to pulse artifacts and caused by slight recoil movements of the patient's head or body, which occur as the blood pumps from the heart. They typically occur as small "pulse waves" that correspond to cardiac contractions in the ECG tracing with a slight delay. They are cardiogenic oscillations that are most often observed in the PSG channels that record airflow or respiratory effort, but sometimes are observed in the EEG derivations. Figure 11.38 shows ballistocardiographic artifact in the abdominal respiratory effort channel and Figure 11.39 in the NP transducer and thoracic respiratory effort channel during central apneas. Some argue that this, when seen, suggests the upper airway is patent. There is considerable debate about their cause, including (a) recoil movements of the patient's head or body as the blood pumps from the heart, (b) pulsatile force on the aortic arch from abrupt redirection of blood flow, and/or (c) changes in intrathoracic pressure produced with each heartbeat, resulting in the movement of air through the patient's upper airway. There are ways to reduce or eliminate ballistocardiographic artifact. If the artifact is due to movement of the head on a pillow, try raising the head off of the bed with a roll of towels. However, this may introduce unwanted respiratory or motion artifacts. Once again, it is often seen when electrode impedances are high, so check and fix them if bad.

Cardiac Pacemaker Artifact

Pacemaker artifact appears as a high-amplitude fast spike when internal cardiac pacemaker delivers an electrical stimulus, which may be seen in the EEG and EOG channels, time-locked with ECG. The pacing spike is of much shorter duration than ECG artifact. Usually heart rate variability with respiratory events are not seen when heart rate is completely paced. This artifact cannot be eliminated. Figure 11.40 shows pacemaker artifact in a PSG tracing.

The presence of ventricular tachycardia (now called *wide complex tachycardia*) typically prompts concern when observed in overnight PSG. It needs to be distinguished from ventricular pacing in an individual with a pacemaker. Pacemakers with a single ventricular pacing lead in the right ventricle, when activated, result in a wide complex QRS, which converts to a normal sinus rhythm if the atrial rhythm falls below the set threshold or if an atrial beat is not conducted. Ventricular pacing artifact almost always occurs at a frequency less than 90 bpm, whereas ventricular tachycardia (wide complex tachycardia) is typically tachycardia.

NONPHYSIOLOGICAL ARTIFACTS

Instrumental artifacts in PSG are generated by improper calibration, application, connection, incorrect settings, and/or malfunction of instruments and other equipment used to record the PSG. These include electrode popping, reversed polarity, incorrect filter settings, high impedance, imbalanced electrode pairs, overamplification, and ground recording artifact. Environmental artifacts are those which originate from surrounding environment.

Electrical Interference Artifacts

The most common environmental artifact is electrical noise generated by power lines and nearby electrical equipment (60 Hz in North America, 50 Hz in many other countries). A 60-Hz artifact usually appears as a thick line in the channel of interest (undulations at a frequency of 60 per second can be counted if the epoch speed is changed to 1 per second per screen) and affects AC recorded PSG channels (Figure 11.41). It is caused by a problem in continuity or grounding anywhere between the patient-to-digital polygraph circuitry.

When 60-Hz artifact affects only one or a few AC-recorded channels, it often reflects high or imbalanced electrode impedance levels (Figure 11.42). When observing 60-Hz artifact, first check electrode impedances. Maximum electrode impedances for EEG and EOG in PSG need to be less than 5 kΩ and the difference between electrode pairs less than 1 kΩ. Unbalanced impedance between electrode pairs defeats the ability of the differential amplifier to cancel out the electrical noise. A 60-Hz artifact in one electrode may also be due to a broken or disconnected wire, poor electrode contact, and/or nearby electrical equipment.

If artifact involves a single electrode, press on the offending electrode, still present the regel, and if it persists, reapply. Further strategies to reduce 60-Hz artifact in AC-recorded PSG channels are as follows: (a) keep the patient's head and connections to the polygraph device as far from power cables as possible; (b) electrode wires should be as short as possible, and bound to together in a single bundled cable; and (c) identify and minimize sway of the electrode wires or movement of tubing. If 60-Hz artifact involves all AC-recorded channels, it may be a loose ground electrode (reassess and replace if needed). If not, it could be due to electrical interference: (a) first untangle and straighten cables and wires; (b) try turning off or unplugging unnecessary (briefly if necessary) equipment, systematically assessing the effect (turning back on if no effect on it); and (c) if all this fails, run the study with the 60-Hz notch filter on.

Finally, 60-Hz artifact that appears in all AC-recorded channels of all recordings made in the same recording room is likely due to unshielded electromagnetic currents flowing through nearby power cables, transformers, or electromotors (8). If so, contact your biomedical department for identification and proper shielding. Proper shielding of the room and wiring of power cables can reduce environmental EMI.

Electrode Pop Artifact

Electrode pops are single or multiple spike or sharp waveforms due to an abrupt shift in impedance, which typically occur in a single electrode at a time, do not disrupt the ongoing EEG background activity, and have no electrical field. Changes in skin temperature, movement, dry electrodes, or air bubbles in the electrode-electrolyte solution trigger transient electrode pops. When the patient moves, the electrode can pull away from the skin (Figure 11.43). When the impedance change is less abrupt, electrode pops may appear as a low-amplitude arrhythmic slow wave. Electrode popping is more often seen with (a) poor or unbalanced electrode impedances; (b) moving, jerking, or touching the lead wire; or (c) a break in skin contact. To fix electrode pops: (a) identify the electrode, (b) check electrode impedances, and (c) press and secure the electrode; if it persists, regel, and if needed reapply or replace it.

Incorrect Filter and Sensitivity Settings

Sleep specialists need to understand how to best use and display the digital PSG by reducing or eliminating channel with artifact, amplifying critical signals, or viewing the study at varying time frames for each channel and signal (3). Modern digital polysomnographic equipment is designed to permit the user to change filter and sensitivity settings for each PSG channel during and after the recording. Filter settings for different PSG parameters recommended by the AASM are summarized in **Table 11.2**. EEG and EOG are typically displayed in PSG using a bandpass of 0.3 (LFF) to 35 Hz (HFF).

Technologists sometimes adjust the filter settings of particular channel(s), and when the file is opened, we may miss these, leading to interpretative errors. When the LFF is increased from 0.3 to 1.59 or 5.3 Hz by the technologist to reduce sweat sway artifact (Figure 11.21), the amount of NREM 3 present may be underestimated. As mentioned earlier, incorrect filter setting in EOG channel may eliminate the EOG signal in that channel (Figure 11.27). REM sleep is often unscored because of falsely elevated chin EMG due to poorly attached chin EMG electrodes (Figure 11.43). Overamplification of EEG may lead to missing sleep spindles crucial for scoring NREM 2 sleep (Figure 11.44). Overamplification is most often seen in children during NREM 3 sleep when the high-amplitude slow activity (often 200–400 μV) saturates the EEG channels; correct by decreasing the channel gains from 7 μV/mm to 10 or 15 μV/mm. A tracing showing all PSG signals are flat and most often appears when the patient is disconnected from the jack box, usually to use the bathroom (Figure 11.45) or when computer shuts down (Figure 11.46). It is important for the technologist to check all the connections between the patient and amplifier.

Channel Inversion Artifacts

The polarity of each PSG channel can also be adjusted individually as per AASM recommendations. We frequently encounter inverted waveforms in one or many recording channels. If negative inputs are placed in positive ports of the headbox, the displayed signal will be inverted. This most often happens in the ECG (Figure 11.47), easily fixed by inverting the channel. Inappropriate inversions in the respiratory signals (especially in the NP), thermal sensor, and respiratory effort channels can lead to significant misinterpretations (Figure 11.48). First review the biocalibration to determine if inversion of the signal was accidental and missed.

Malfunctioning Respiratory Sensors

Most level 1 PSG recordings are to evaluate patients for sleep disordered breathing. Almost all respiratory sensors provide qualitative (not quantitative) data. Redundancy (multiple different respiratory sensors) is the name of the game when recording respiration in a PSG. Malfunctioning respiratory sensors can lead to a myriad of missing or false data. Respiratory artifacts most often appear as a low-frequency baseline sway that occurs in-phase with respiration (Figures 11.21 and 11.22); patients are often lying in a position where each breath causes a slight movement of electrode(s) relative to the scalp and a shift in the electrical potential. This is most evident in a loose or high-impedance electrode. Flattened respiratory effort channels (with or without notches), despite good respiratory effort confirmed by video, suggest the respiratory effort sensor is loose or poorly positioned.

To identify respiratory artifacts, check whether they coincide with the respiratory effort signals. Respiratory artifact is typically faster than sweat artifact and usually localized. Sweat artifact is slower and more often appears generalized. To reduce/eliminate respiratory artifact: (a) straighten electrode wires avoiding loops; (b) check electrode impedances; if the scalp contact is bad, regel or replace offending electrodes; (c) have patient change position; and/or (d) reroute electrode leads so patient is not lying on them.

NP Sensor Artifacts

NP transducer is the preferred sensor for identifying hypopneas or respiratory event-related arousals (RERAs) in PSG. However, they are particularly prone to malfunction (especially in children with profuse nasal secretions and a great dislike for the nasal cannula inserted in their nostrils) (Figure 11.49). We record NP using LFF of 0.03 Hz or direct current (DC) and the HFF set at 100 Hz. Figure 11.50 shows the NP sensor channel is inverted. The crest of the NP signal should appear sharp. If the bottom of the waveform appears sharp, flip the channels to properly identify flow limitation from obstructive hypopneas. Table 11.6 summarizes common causes for NP sensor malfunction in PSG.

Thermal Sensor Artifacts

Thermal sensors are the preferred method for identifying apneas in PSG. They measure changes in temperature induced by airflow: cooler, inspired aire causes an up signal and warmer, expired air a down signal. The signal is qualitative, not quantitative, and does not vary proportionately with airflow.

TABLE 11.6: Causes of Nasal Pressure Transducer Sensor Artifacts or Malfunction

- Patient pulled the nasal cannula out of the nose
- Obligate or intermittent mouth breather
- Profuse nasal secretions
- Supplemental oxygen during PSG dilutes NP signal
- Too small an NP prong in large nostrils may produce a small NP signal; too large an NP prong in small nostrils may cause a large signal
- Nasal prongs which partially or completely obstruct one or both nares can lead to spuriously higher apnea and arousal indexes

NP, nasal pressure; PSG, polysomnography.

Thermal sensors usually identify apneas but can overestimate ventilation and underestimate hypopneas. When the thermal sensor is dislodged or lying on the skin, it may not detect the changes in temperature between inspiration and expiration. If recognized, adjust by repositioning the thermal sensor properly. If the NP sensor is malfunctioning and forced to use the thermal sensor to assess airflow, it may fail to detect subtle changes in airway (respiratory effort-related arousals).

Pulse Oximeter Artifacts

We typically detect arterial oxyhemoglobin saturations during PSG using pulse oximeters. They calculate the oxyhemoglobin saturation (ratio of oxyhemoglobin to reduced hemoglobin in arterial blood) using spectrophotometry (the quantification of compounds by their light absorption characteristics) (17). The peak absorption frequency of reduced hemoglobin is 660 nm, and oxyhemoglobin 940 nm.

The pulse oximeter contains a photoreceptor that isolates the pulse signal from which the oxygen saturation is calculated and also generates a plethysmographic signal (the pulse waveform). Pulse waveforms are extraordinarily useful in confirming whether the pulse oximeter signal is "reliable." Observing low peripheral capillary oxygen saturation (SpO2), we confirm the pulse waveform is preserved, if blunted or absent, the SpO2 signal deemed unreliable (Figure 11.50). Pulse oximetry can be falsely peripheral for many reasons, summarized in Table 11.6. To fix poor oximeter readings: (a) reapply or select another oximeter probe; (b) remove nail polish and avoid acrylic nails; (c) try a different location (earlobe and toe). The lag time in the maximal fall in the

TABLE 11.7: Causes of Pulse Oximeter Artifact or Malfunction

- Movement artifact
- Poor perfusion in patient who is hypovolemic, hypotensive, or cold
- Inadequate light transmission detected by device because of tissue edema, nail polish, acrylic nails, dark or thick skin, improper probe placement
- Excessive ambient room light
- Venous pulsations misinterpreted as arterial
- Significantly higher SpO_2 values in heavy tobacco smokers with carboxyhemoglobin levels greater than 10%

SpO_2, peripheral capillary oxygen saturation.

oxygen desaturation related to apneas or hypopneas in a PSG varies with the location of the recording probe: 10 to 30 seconds when placed on the tip of the finger over the nail bed versus 5 to 10 seconds when attached to the earlobe. Table 11.7 summarizes causes of pulse oximeter artifact or malfunction.

PAP Tubing Artifacts

Water in the NP airflow channel causes a fast, undulating signal artifact. It appears as an M-shaped waveform with each breath as the water moves back and forth in the tubing. It occurs during diagnostic PSGs if the moisture gets into the cannula or the tubing connecting it to the NP sensor. We see it most often during continuous positive airway pressure (CPAP) titration if there is a mismatch between room temperature and the humidification in the CPAP circuit (Figure 11.51).

Computer Monitor Display Artifacts

The number of pixels on the computer monitor screen places an absolute limit on the upper range of signal frequencies which can be displayed. The AASM recommends a minimum computer monitor resolution of 1,600 × 1,200 pixels. A high-resolution, digital PSG super VGA monitor often has a horizontal screen resolution of 1,600 pixels. When sampling PSG at 10 seconds per screen, this results in a resolution of only 150 pixels per second, 72 pixels per inch. The fastest EEG frequencies seen viewing a 10-second PSG sample are less than 75 Hz, less than 20 to 25 Hz when the EEG is displayed as a 30-second time screen, and 2.7 Hz or less when viewing a 180-second epoch. To see less than 75-Hz EEG frequencies on a 30-second screen, 3,000 pixels (which are not yet commercially available) are required. Analog EEG and PSG machines recording ink on paper (of which only a few of us now recall using) had 2 to 3 times this resolution.

Frequency aliasing introduces display and potential interpretative errors in PSG and EEG. Frequency aliasing in old black and white television programs made the wagon wheels appear to be stationary or turning backward. Inadequate sampling rates can produce spurious representation of EEG activity. Epstein showed how spurious (false) theta activity in EEG channels on computer monitor display was due to aliasing EMG artifact. This was caused by undersampling of the EMG signal, resulting in errors in waveform display from exceeding Nyquist frequency on the computer screen display (1). The false theta disappeared when the HFF was turned down to 35 Hz. Such distortions can be lessened or avoided by viewing the EEG using a 10-second time screen with the HFF set at ≤40 Hz (we typically set our HFF at 35 Hz). Undersampling errors can also distort relationships between spike-and-slow waves. This is best viewed using 10-second or, even better, 5-second time screens.

Cell Phone Artifacts

Potential sources of PSG artifact change with time (environment and technology). Mobile telephones, computer tablets, and laptop computers are much more common sources of electrical interference artifact in the sleep laboratory. A cell phone ringing at the bedside can cause EMI (Figure 11.52). When the patient types on a laptop while we are recording PSG, it provokes intolerable artifact.

One case report described an EMI artifact produced by a smartphone, which was characterized by runs of 100-µV, 5- to 9-Hz sharply contoured waveforms intermixed with intermittent high-frequency (20–50 Hz) sinusoidal waves lasting for 1 to 20 seconds (18). These occurred throughout the night, and review of the audio recording revealed an intermittently rhythmic sound during the discharges. The patient had placed her mobile device 12 inches away from the recording jack box. Others have reported that the cellular telephone artifact can produce 11- to 16-Hz waveforms mimicking sleep spindles; high-amplitude short bursts of activity in chin EMG misinterpreted as REM sleep without atonia; ventricular tachycardia in the ECG channel; and unilateral saccadic eye movement artifact in EEG when repeatedly swiping to left; the ringing phone delays sleep onset, causes arousals and awakenings, and alters sleep architecture (19,20).

Cellphones are low-power radiofrequency transmitters that can cause narrowband EMI (21). They send and receive microwave frequencies from approximately 900 to 1800 Hz. Coupled with nearby electrical equipment, they can act as a radio receiver and interfere with their functioning. The fundamental principle of EMI is the level of exposure in a far field proportional to the square of the distance from the radiating source. Clinically relevant EMI at distances greater than 1 meter are negligible. The solution is to keep mobile devices greater than 3 feet (≥1 meter) from the medical device (e.g., mechanical ventilator, pacemaker, EEG, or PSG equipment). We recommend (a) electronic devices be placed at least 3 feet away from the PSG equipment, (b) preferably be turned off, (c) and the patient should not touch it when it is charging and we are recording.

Implanted Devices

Vagal Nerve Stimulation Artifacts

Artifacts due to periodic activations of implanted vagal nerve stimulators cause a periodic abrupt reduction in amplitude and a marked increase in the rate of the respiratory signals, which lasts as long as the stimulator fires (most often 30 seconds, but sometimes 17 seconds in "rapid cycling" modes) and recurs at the particular activation frequency (typically 5 minutes but sometimes 3 minutes). More often, vagus nerve stimulator (VNS) activation causes no arousal, awakening, or significant oxygen desaturation. However, case reports abound describing worsening of obstructive sleep disordered breathing (especially among those with OSA). This may be due to spasm in the upper airway muscles or laryngeal vocal cord dysfunction when the VNS activates, resulting in obstructive apneas. If symptomatic, reduce the current flow (lower VNS stimulus frequency from 30 to 20 Hz) or tape magnets across the stimulator to turn it off when the patient sleeps (22). Illustrative examples of this can be found in these references (23–25).

DBS Artifact

DBSs are used in the United States to treat PD, dystonia, neuropsychiatric disorders, and medically refractory epilepsy. DBS generates electrical artifact that affects every PSG signal recorded using AC. Bipolar DBS causes fewer artifacts than unipolar DBS. Unfortunately, turning off the DBS during the recording often results in emergence of tremor artifact in patients with PD. Bilateral monopolar DBS produces a high-frequency artifact which obscures most channels of EEG and is most pronounced in those with long interelectrode distances. Bipolar DBS causes fewer artifacts. Figure 11.53 shows an example of DBS artifact in PSG.

Artifacts Which Require Technologist or Video to Identify

It is best for the technologist recording the study to identify the artifact for the reader. Figure 11.54 shows a recurring electrographic interference artifact due to a heating pad repeatedly turning on. After the fact, we observed the heating blanket when the patient kicked off her blanket.

CONCLUSION

Because overnight PSGs are recorded for hours and many different biologic parameters recorded, artifacts are ubiquitous. Some artifacts in PSG are useful, helping us identify an arousal, body position change, respiratory event, or parasomnia. However, other artifacts may obscure significant signals in the PSG containing important diagnostic information. Some artifacts have a stereotypical appearance, so pattern recognition of these is often helpful. The ability to re-reference electrodes can be invaluable for identifying and ameliorating a questionable or spurious PSG signal. Failure to recognize artifacts may lead to false-positive reports that may contribute to errors in clinical management. The sleep technologist identifying an artifact needs to document its presence in the comment log, determine the source and perform what is needed to eliminate it from the recording, and finally consider whether it affects patient safety, or prevents interpretation of the PSG. Sometimes, letting the patient sleep even when artifact is present is the best choice.

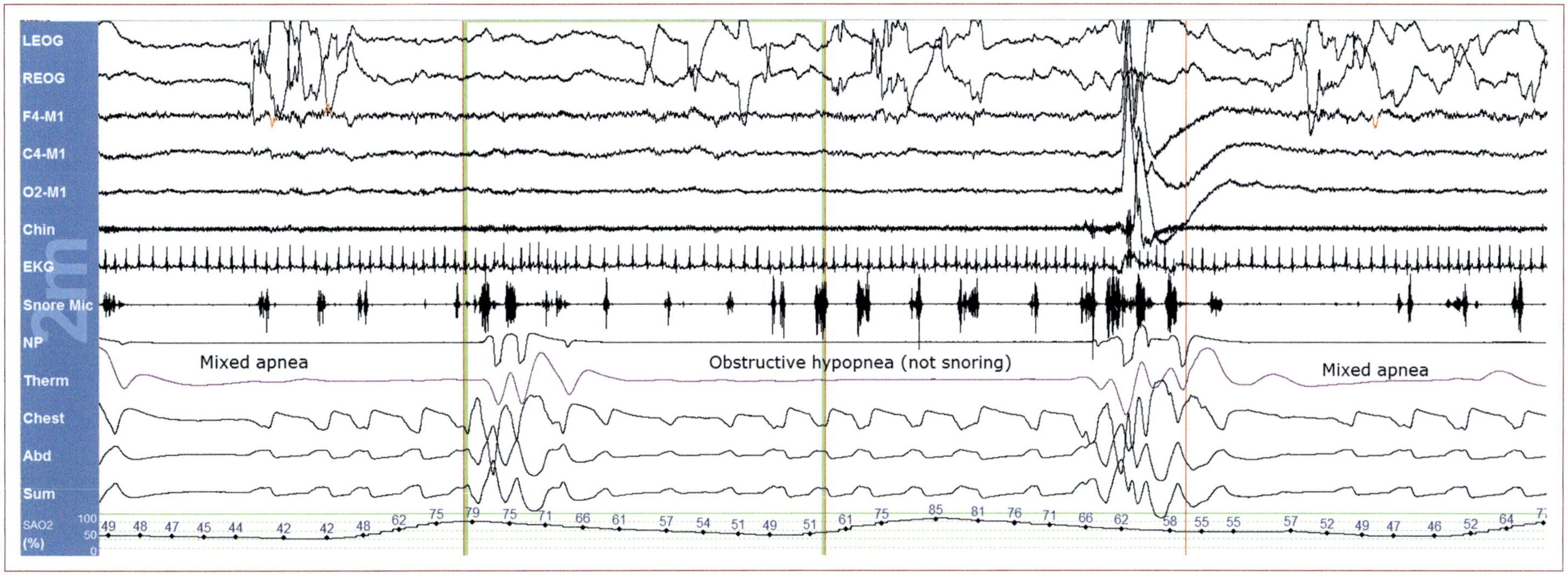

FIGURE 11.1: A 120-second polysomnographic epoch recorded in a 60-year-old man showing mixed apneas and obstructive hypopneas, which cause oxygen desaturations as low as 46% to 49% from 79% to 85%, sinus bradycardia-tachycardia response, arousals.

Abd, abdominal respiratory effort; C4-M1, right central, right central-left mastoid; Chest, thoracic respiratory effort; ECG, modified lead II; F4-M1 right frontal EEG, right frontal-left mastoid; L EOG, left extraocular muscles; NP, nasal pressure sensor; O2-M1, right occipital EEG (right occipital-left mastoid); R EOG, right extraocular muscles; SaO_2 (%), pulse oximetry signal; Snore Mic, snore microphone; Sum, summed signal of thoracic and abdominal respiratory effort signals; Therm, oronasal thermal sensor.

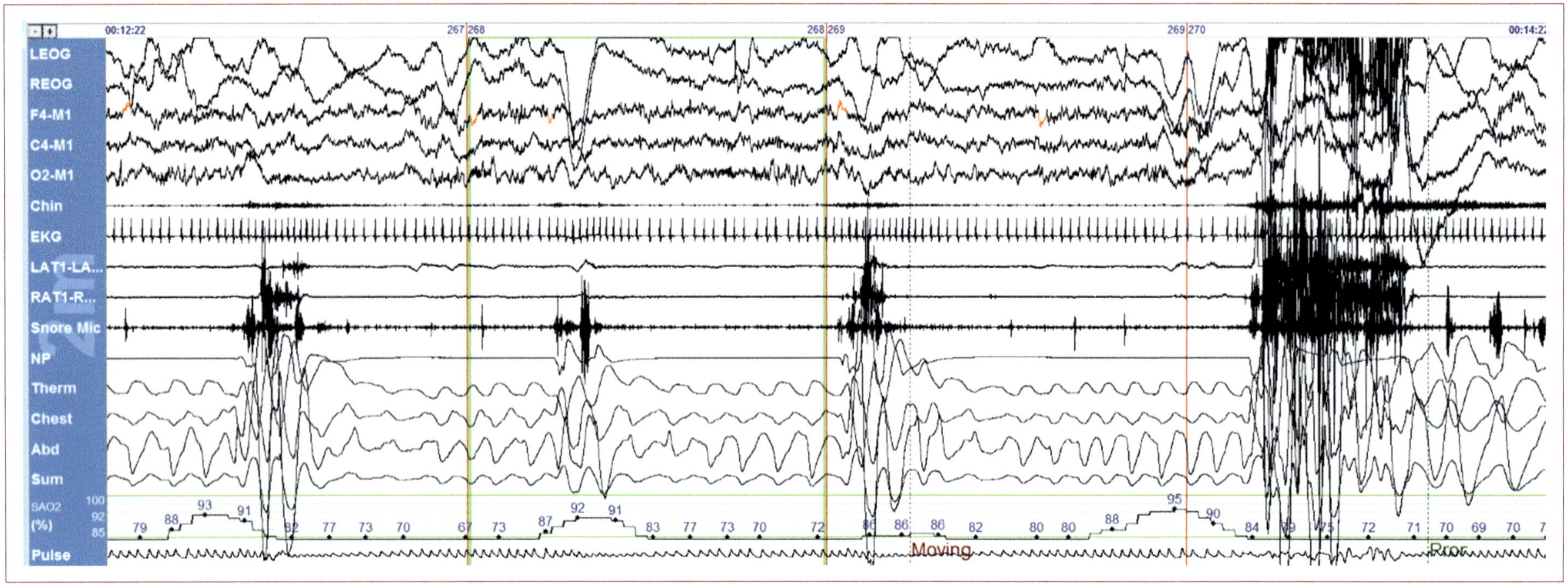

FIGURE 11.2: A 2-minute epoch of PSG during REM sleep supine recorded on a 13-year-old boy with severe obstructive sleep apnea. Five respiratory events are shown, which are obstructive and mixed apneas and obstructive hypopneas. They often last 8 to 11 seconds, cause desaturations as low as 83% obstructive hypopneas which cause desaturations as low as 67% to 69%.

Abd, abdominal respiratory effort; C4-M1 right central, right central-left mastoid; Chest, thoracic respiratory effort; ECG, modified lead II; F4-M1, right frontal EEG, right frontal-left mastoid; L EOG, left extraocular muscles; NP, nasal pressure sensor; O2-M1 right occipital EEG, right occipital-left mastoid; R EOG, right extraocular muscles; SaO_2 (%), pulse oximetry signal; Snore Mic, snore microphone; Sum, summed signal of thoracic and abdominal respiratory effort signals; $tcCO_2$, transcutaneous carbon dioxide; Therm, oronasal thermal sensor.

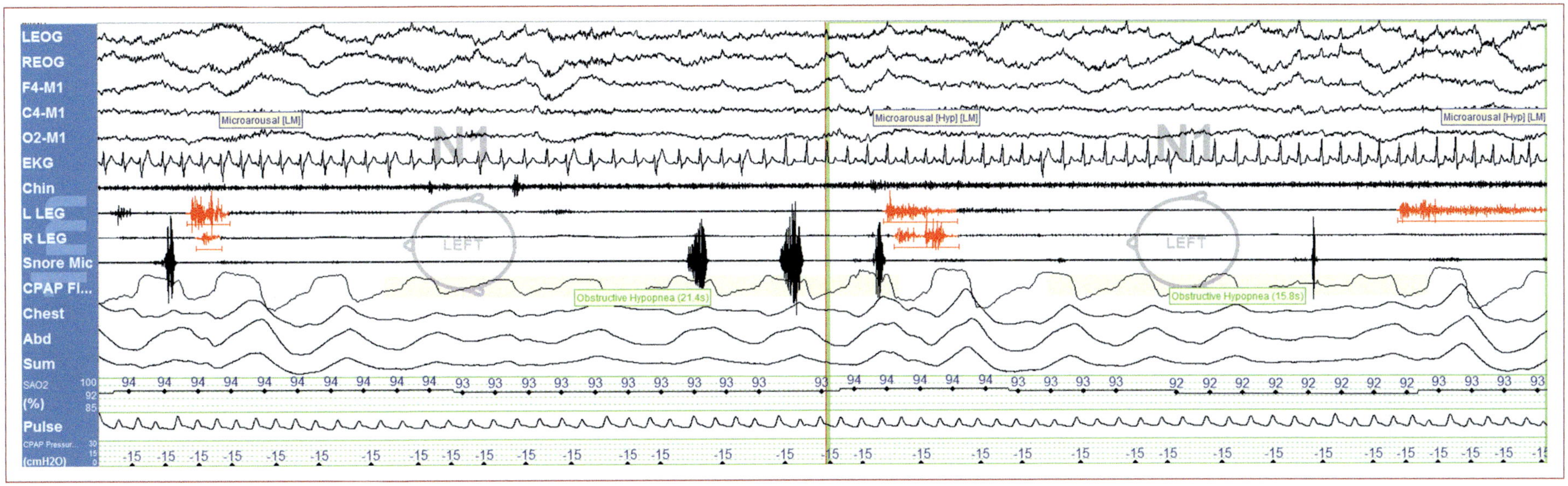

FIGURE 11.3: When titrating CPAP, we typically record CPAP flow and pressure.

Abd, abdominal respiratory effort; C4-M1 right central, right central-left mastoid; Chest, thoracic respiratory effort; Chin, chin EMG; CPAP pressure, continuous positive airway pressure; CPAP Fl, CPAP flow; ECG, modified lead II; F4-M1, right frontal EEG, right frontal-left mastoid; L EOG, left extraocular muscles; L LEG, left anterior tibialis EMG; NP, nasal pressure sensor; O2-M1, right occipital EEG, right occipital-left mastoid; Pulse, pulse waveform; R EOG, right extraocular muscles; R LEG, right anterior tibialis EMG; SaO_2 (%), pulse oximetry signal; Snore Mic, snore microphone; Sum, summed signal of thoracic and abdominal respiratory effort signals.

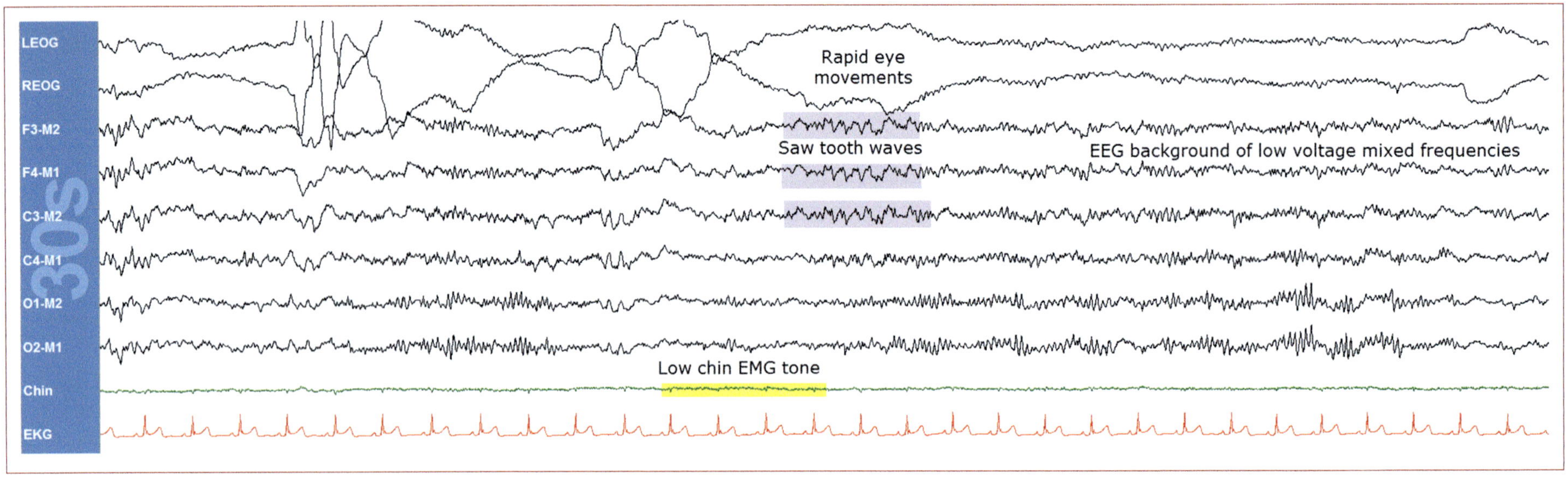

FIGURE 11.4: A 30-second PSG tracing showing standard EEG derivations recorded during REM sleep. Note the reduced muscle tone signified by low-amplitude EMG signal.

C3-M2, left central, right central-left mastoid; C4-M1, right central, right central-left mastoid; F3-M2, left frontal EEG, left frontal-right mastoid; F4-M1, right frontal EEG, right frontal-left mastoid; L EOG, left extraocular muscles; O2-M1, right occipital, right occipital-left mastoid; R EOG, right extraocular muscles.

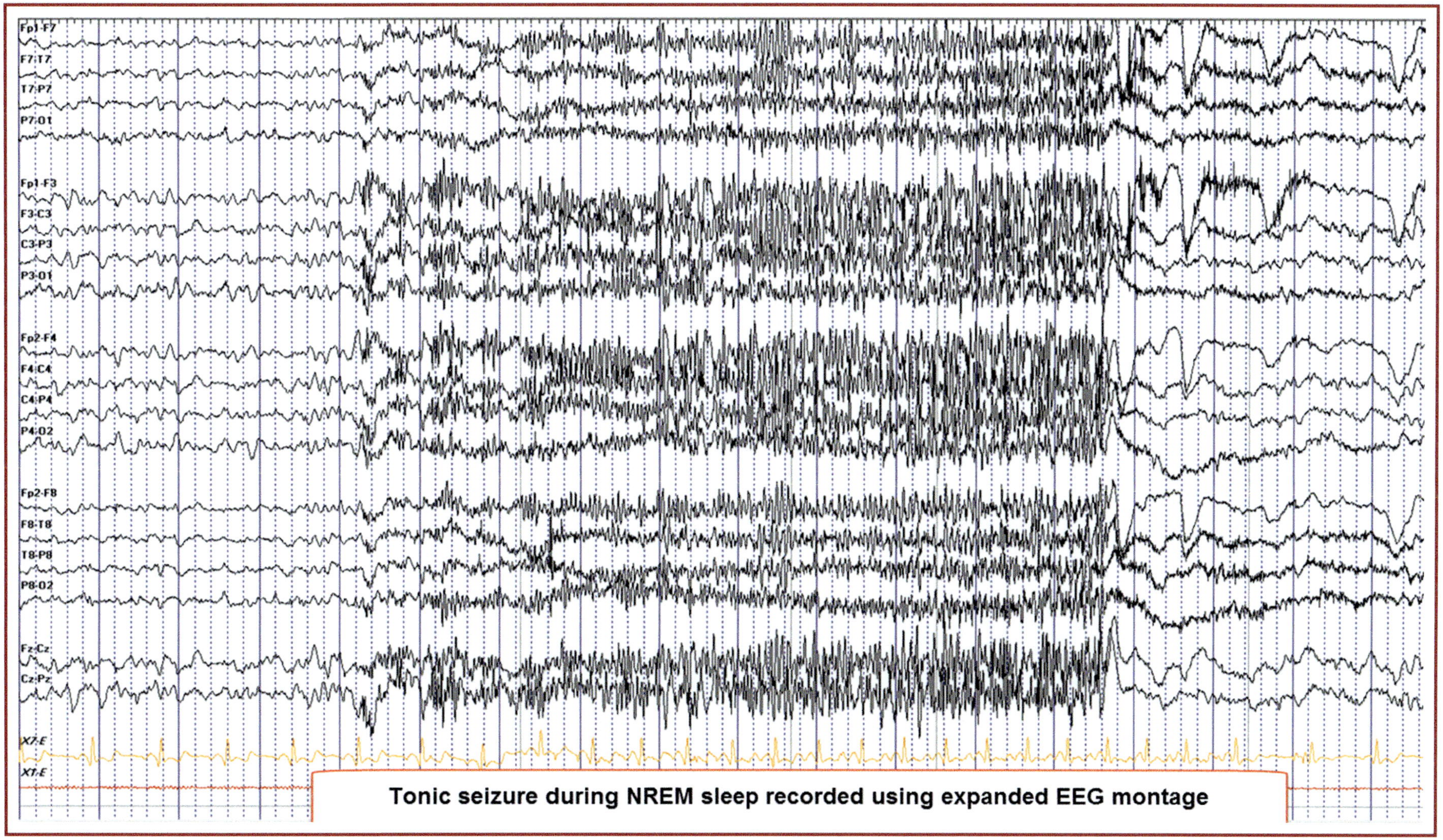

FIGURE 11.5: A 30-second PSG with expanded EEG montage used when seizures or epilepsy is suspected or known. An electroclinical tonic seizure was captured directly out of sleep.

PSG, polysomnography.

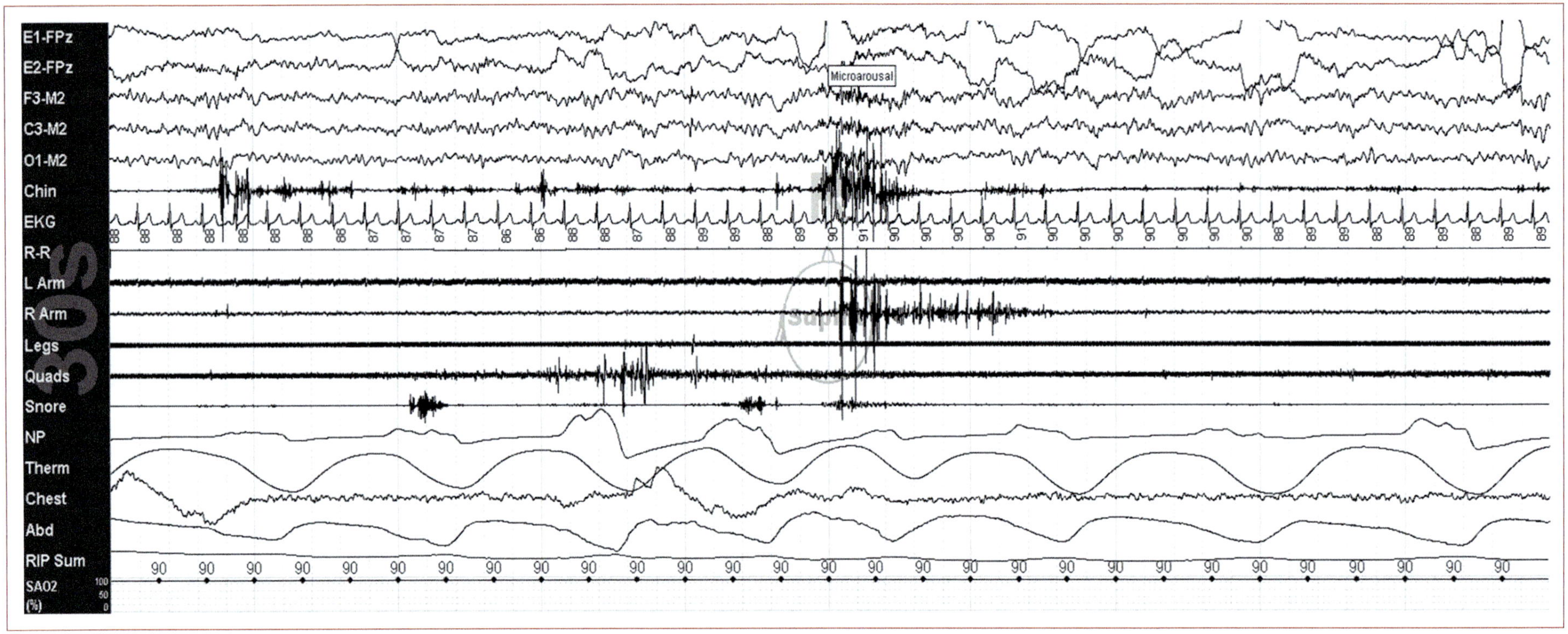

FIGURE 11.6: A 30-second epoch of polysomnogram showing additional surface EMG electrodes to the wrist extensors (L arm, R arm) and quadriceps to identify loss of REM sleep atonia (RWA). Notice inappropriate muscle activity in the right arm channel (oval).

EMG, electromyography; REM, rapid eye movement; RWA, REM sleep without atonia.

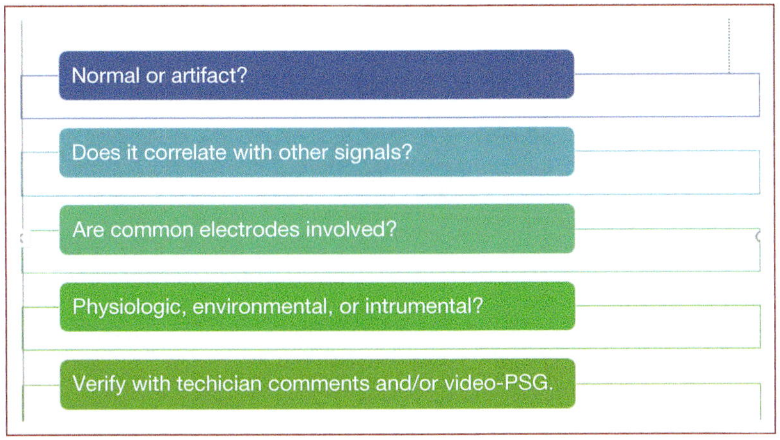

FIGURE 11.7: Observing unexpected or unusual patterns in the PSG should prompt the following questions.

PSG, polysomnography.

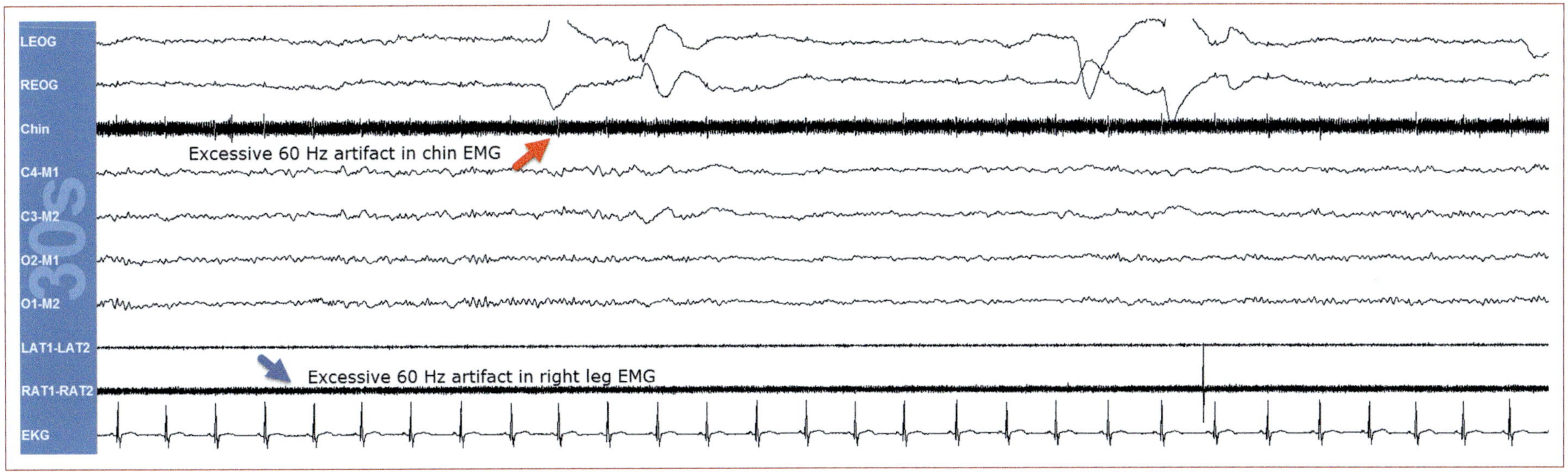

FIGURE 11.8: Poorly applied chin EMG defeats the ability to score REM sleep in a PSG (red arrow). Poorly applied right leg EMG makes it difficult to score leg movements (blue arrow). Sixty-hertz artifact in these channels is due to poorly attached surface EMG electrodes.

EMG, electromyography; PSG, polysomnography; REM, rapid eye movement.

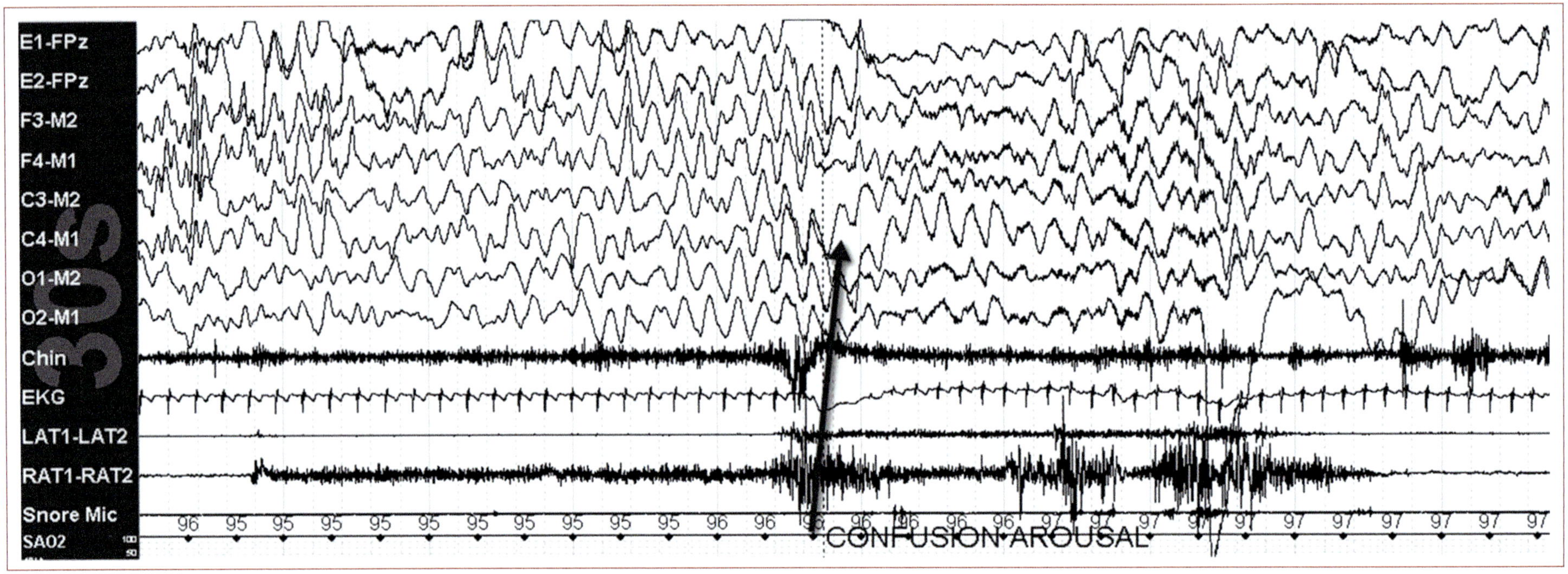

FIGURE 11.9: The sudden appearance of prominent muscle artifact from NREM 3 sleep coupled with a diffusely slowed EEG and sinus tachycardia prompts review of the video to identify a NREM arousal parasomnia.

NREM, nonrapid eye movement sleep.

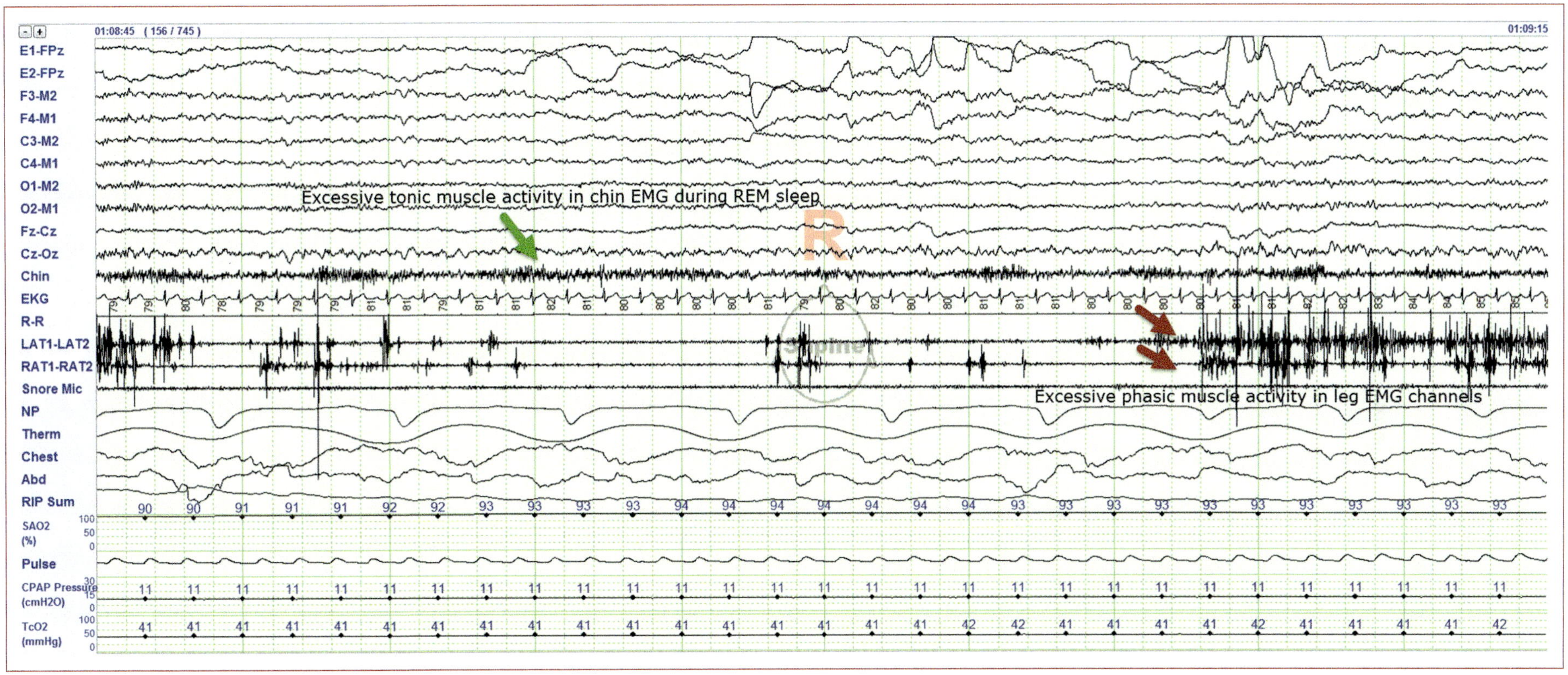

FIGURE 11.10: Excessive amounts of muscle activity/movement artifact (green arrow) during REM sleep when accompanied by other biomarkers of REM sleep such as rapid eye movements and irregular respiration warrants review of the video. This will help to identify excessive phasic muscle activity during RBD events (red arrows) to support a clinical diagnosis of REM sleep without atonia associated with RBD.

RBD, REM behavior disorder; REM, rapid eye movement;

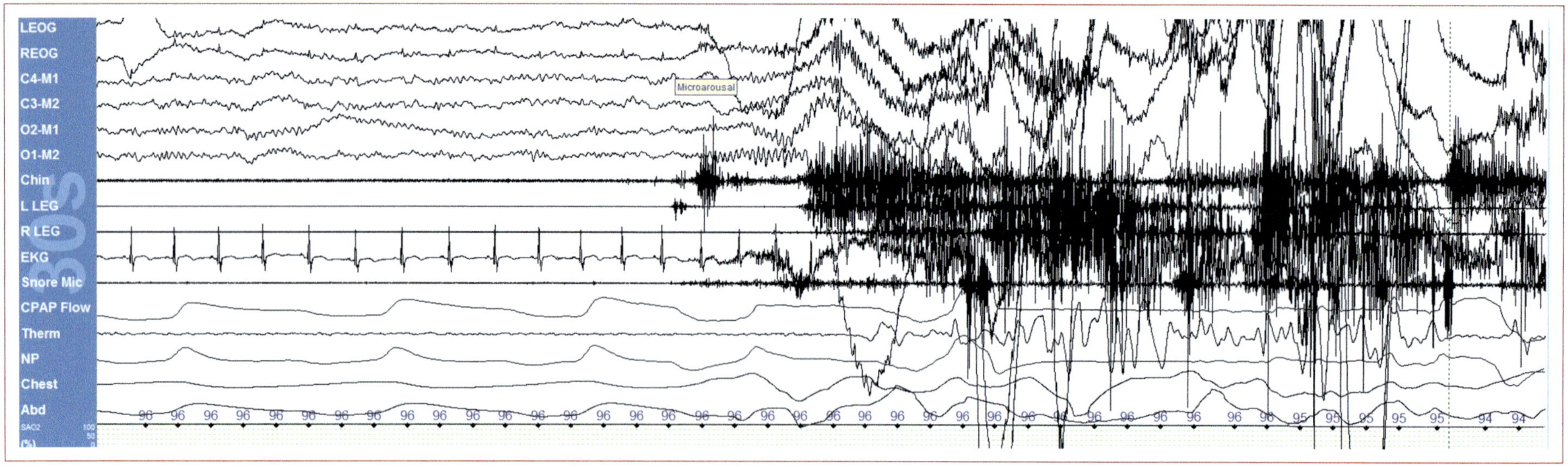

FIGURE 11.11: Whole body movements affect almost every recording channel in the PSG. Note the arousal that occurs in the middle of the epoch resulting in excessive artifact.

PSG, polysomnography.

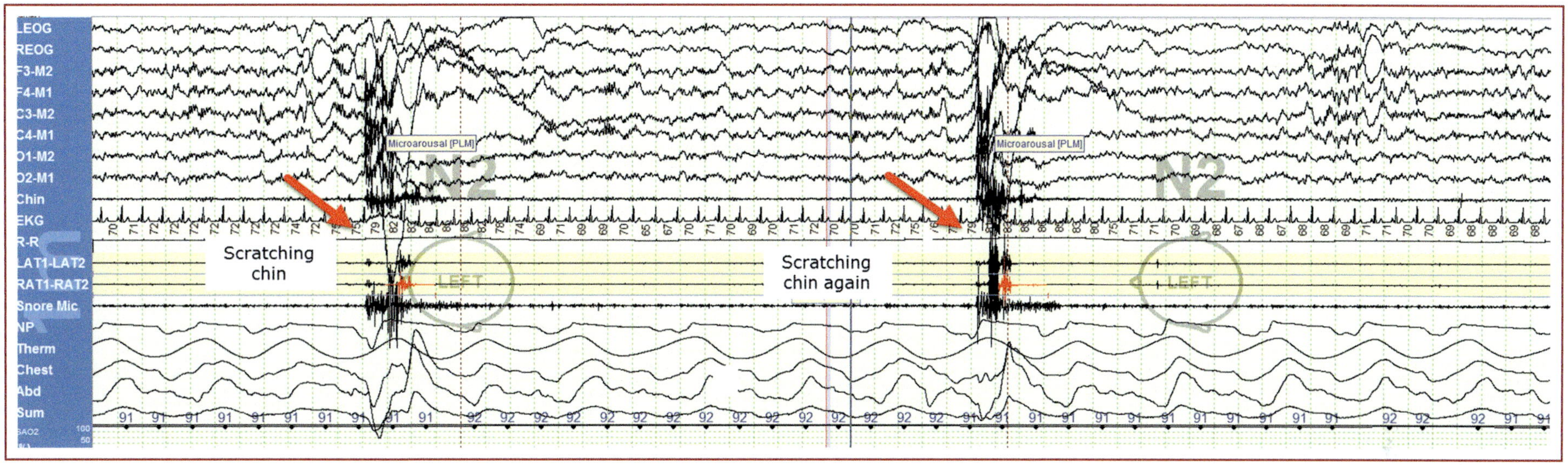

FIGURE 11.12: Artifact in the PSG due to scratching the chin. Note the involvement in chin EMG, ECG, and EEG channels (red arrows).

EMG, electromyography; PSG, polysomnography.

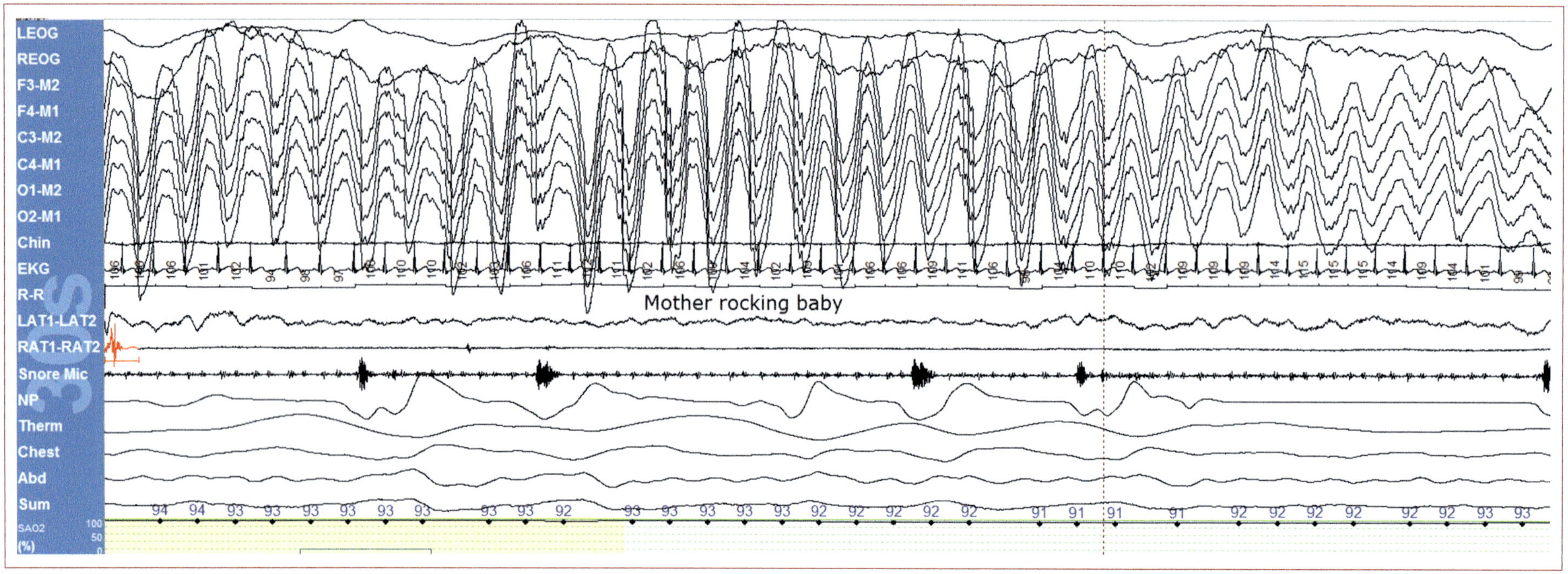

FIGURE 11.13: Mother rocking her infant. Note the prominent rhythmic high-amplitude movement artifact that appears in the EEG channels.

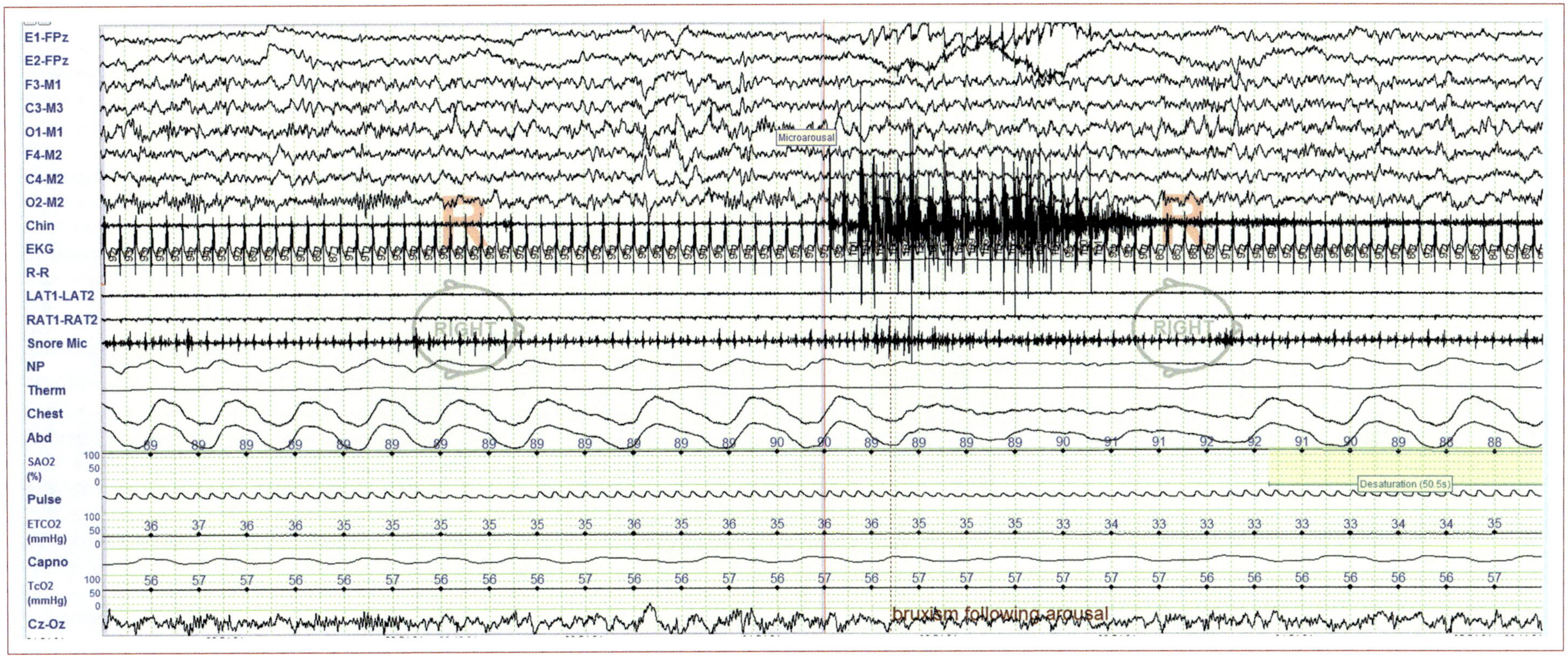

FIGURE 11.14: Sleep bruxism results in regular movement artifact present in the chin EMG channels of the PSG.

EMG, electromyography; PSG, polysomnography.

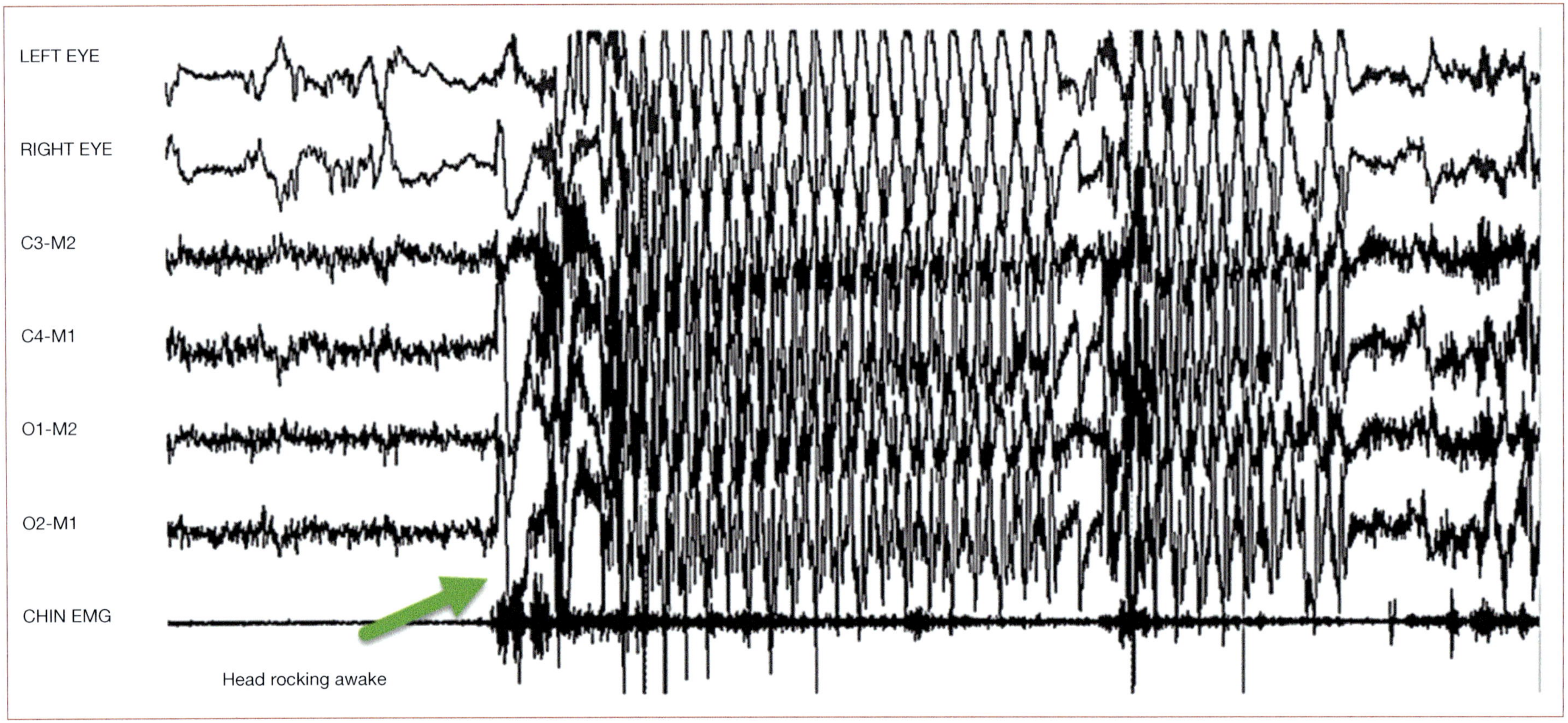

FIGURE 11.15: Rhythmic movement disorder (head rocking). This child exhibited a run of sustained movement artifact (green arrow) in the EOG and EEG due to head rocking while awake before sleep onset.

EOG, electrooculography.

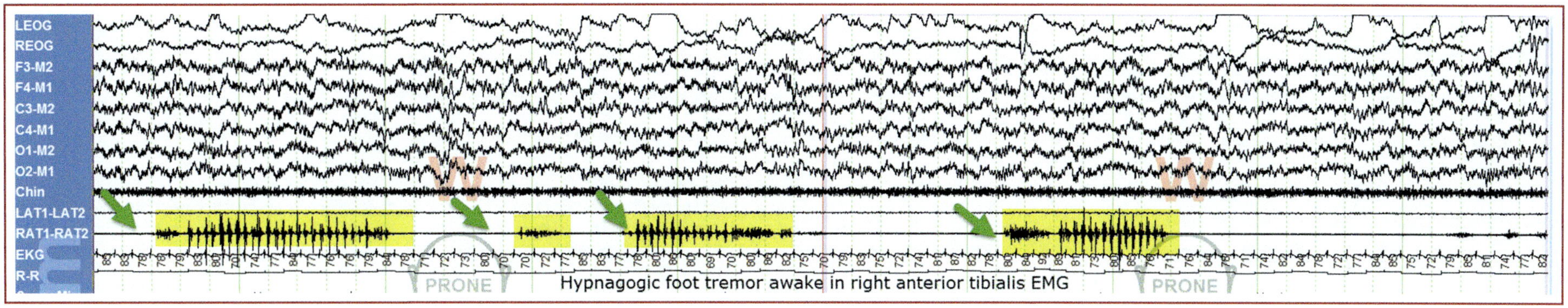

FIGURE 11.16: Hypnagogic foot tremor is present in a 60-second epoch of PSG during wakefulness in an adult. Brief runs of rhythmic, 2 to 3 per second right-leg jerking in wakefulness are shown in this epoch of PSG (green arrows). Hypnagogic foot tremor is typically asymptomatic, and is more often seen in individuals who are treated with antidepressants and/or have restless legs. It does not require treatment.

C3-M2, left central-right mastoid; C4-M1, right central, right central-left mastoid; Chin, chin EMG; ECG, modified lead II; F3-M2, left frontal-right mastoid; F4-M1, right frontal-left mastoid; L EOG, left extraocular muscles; L LEG, left anterior tibialis EMG; O1-M2, left occipital-right mastoid; O2-M1, right occipital-left mastoid; R EOG, right extraocular muscles; R LEG, right anterior tibialis EMG; R-R, R-R ECG interval.

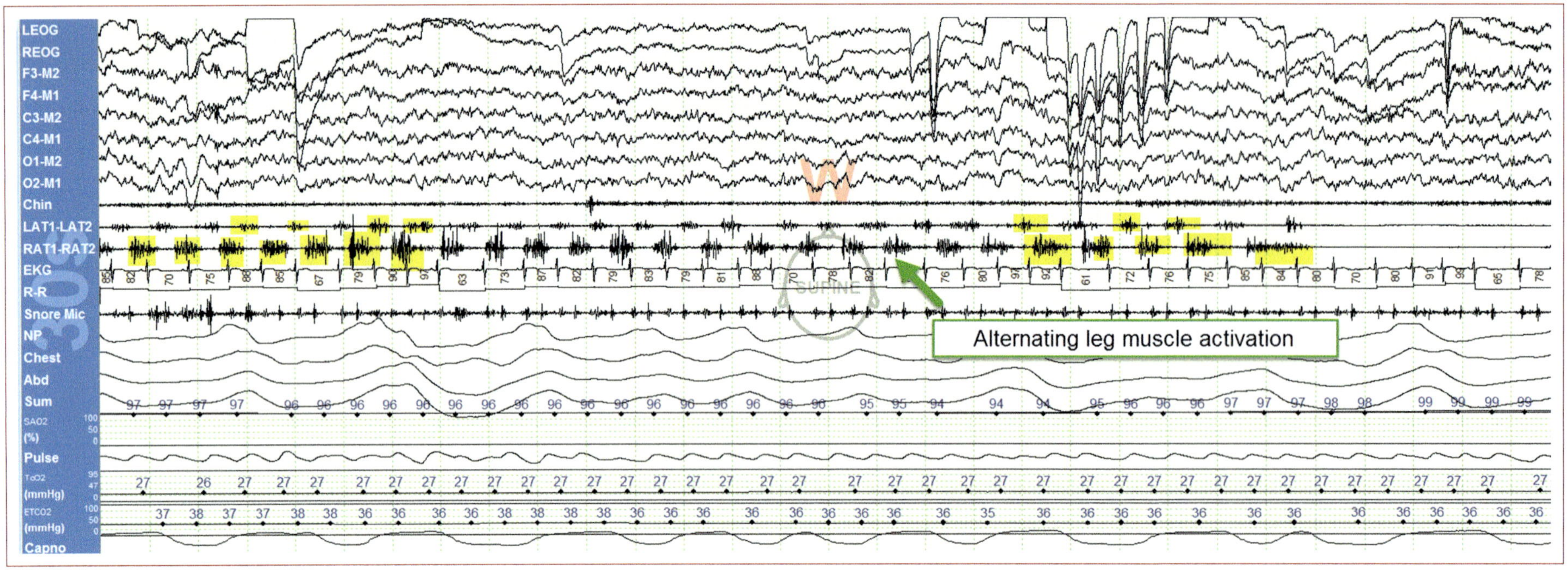

FIGURE 11.17: Alternating leg movements manifest as bursts of surface EMG "artifact" present in the electrodes applied over the anterior tibialis muscles (in yellow).

EMG, electromyography.

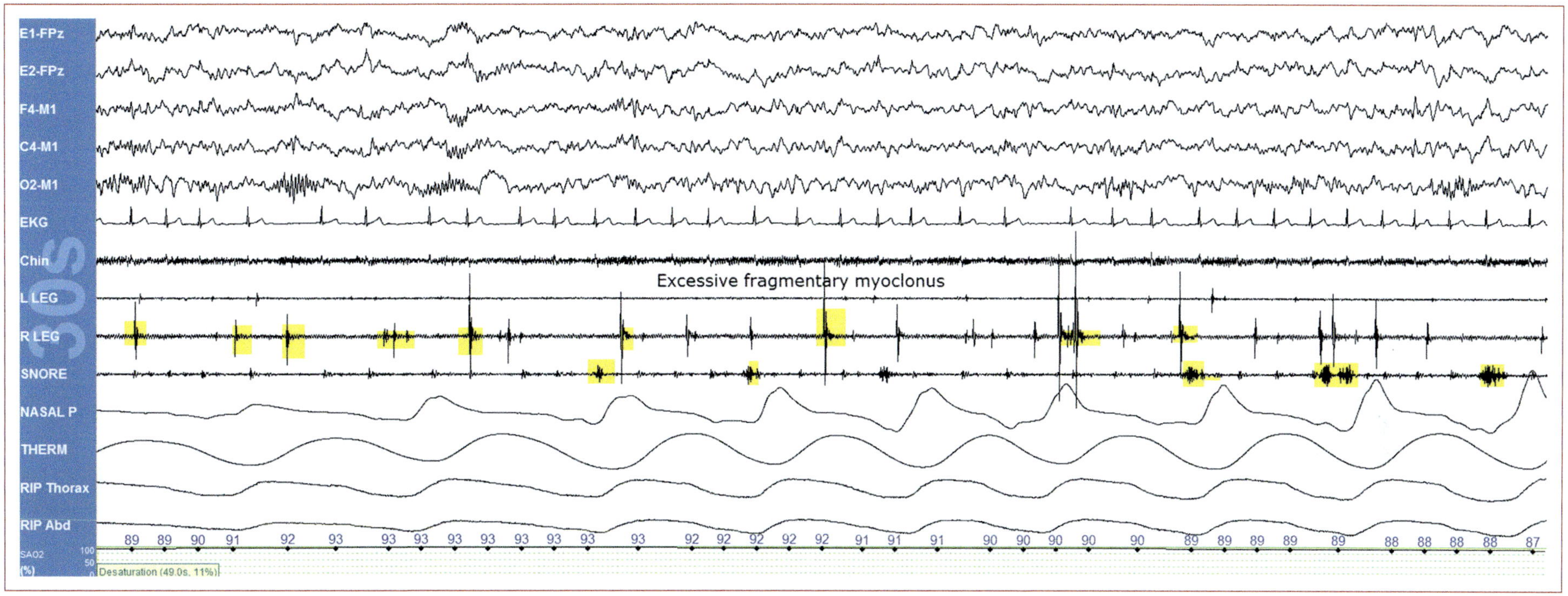

FIGURE 11.18: Excessive fragmentary myoclonus that is especially prominent in the right leg (in yellow). Note the brief paroxysmal muscular activity that is transient compared to the bursts present during RBD (**Figure 11.17**).

RBD, REM behavior disorder.

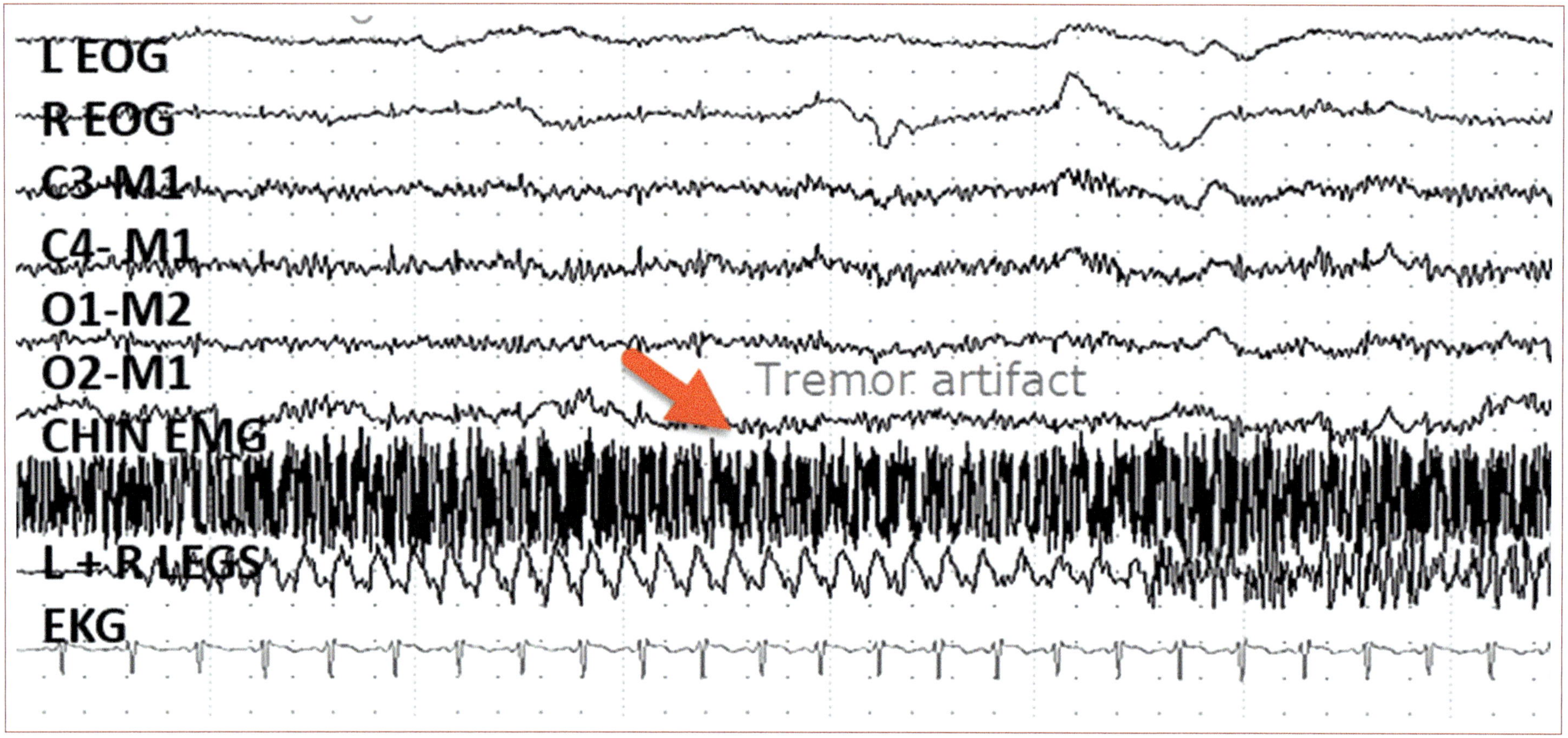

FIGURE 11.19: Tremor artifact is typically rhythmic 4 to 6 Hz which is seen in the combined leg EMG channels. Tremor involves the chin EMG but is obscured in this epoch by movement artifact.

EMG, electromyography.

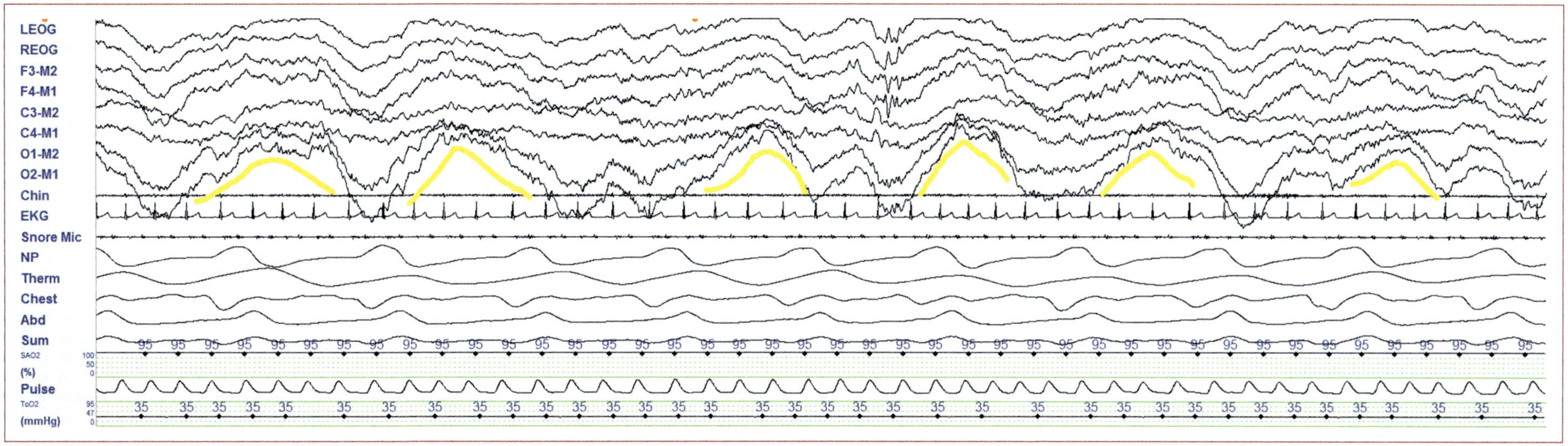

FIGURE 11.20: Sweat artifact in the EEG channels during PSG (in yellow).

PSG, polysomnography.

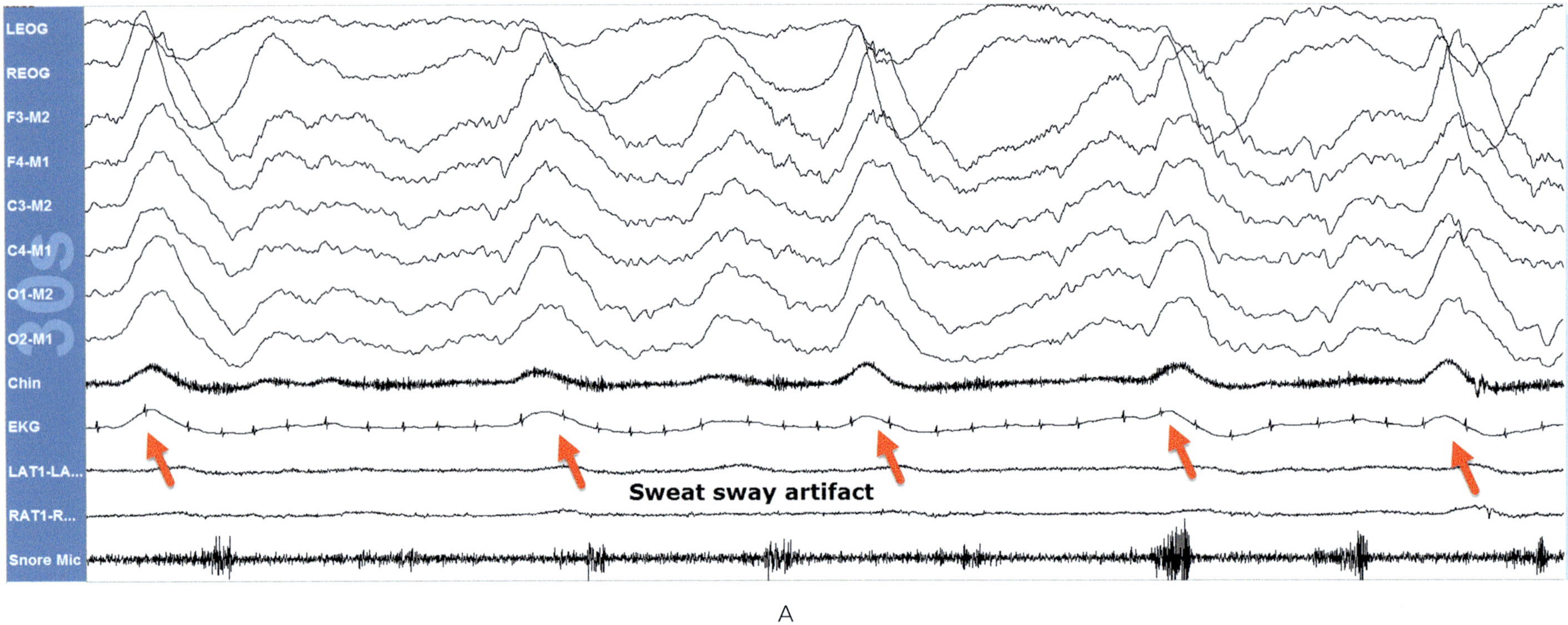

FIGURE 11.21: Effect of digital filtering noted in the PSG. (A) Low-frequency filter setting at 0.3 Hz. (*continued*)

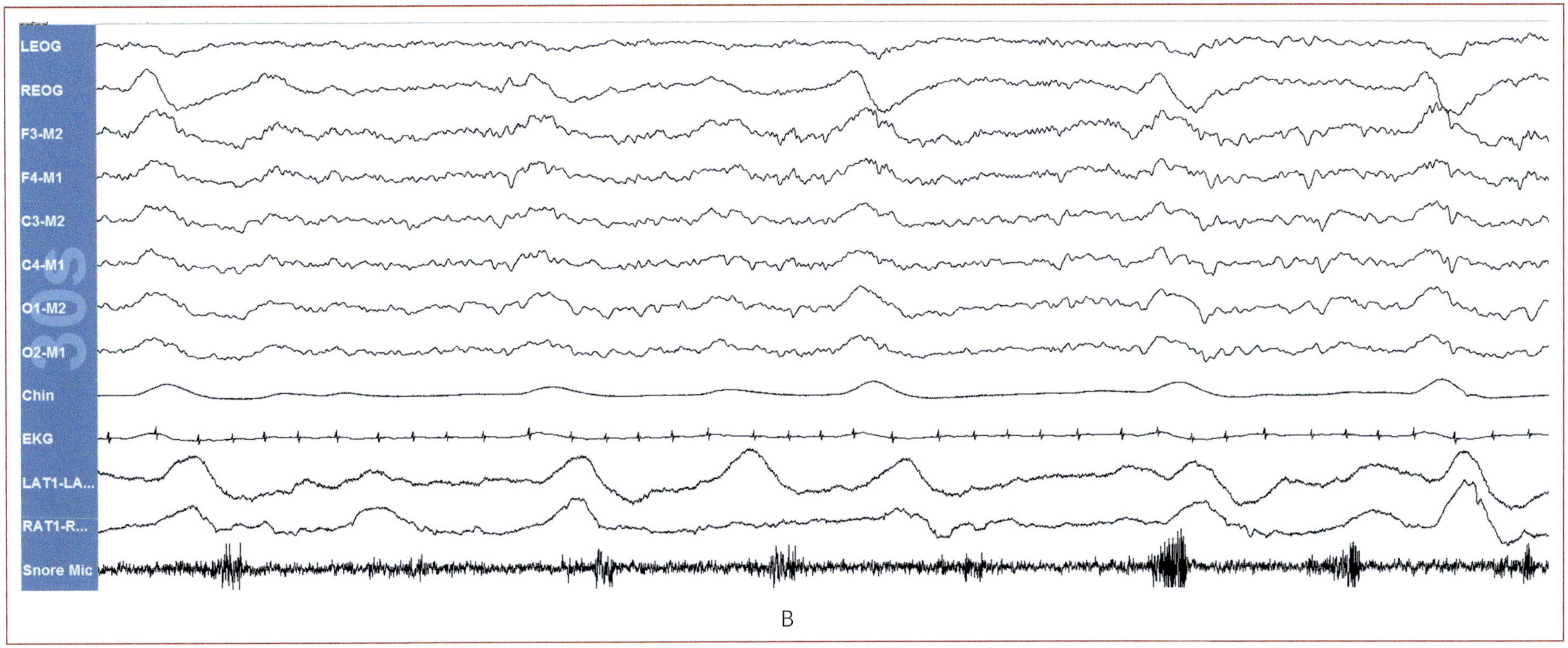

FIGURE 11.21: (*continued*) (B) Low-frequency filter setting at 1.59 Hz. (***continued***)

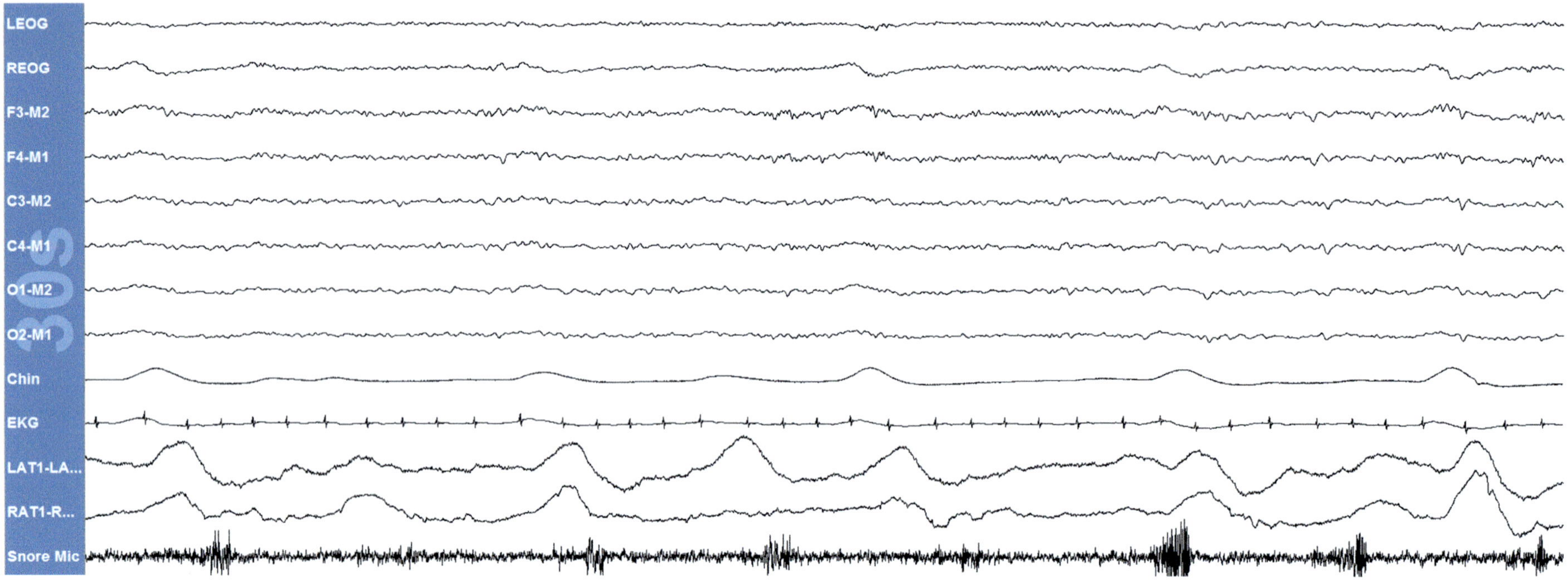

C

Figure 11.21: (*continued*) (C) Low-frequency filter setting at 5.3 Hz. In A, note the prominent slow frequencies present using a low-frequency filter setting (high pass) modified (red arrows) as the filter setting is raised (B and C).

PSG, polysomnography.

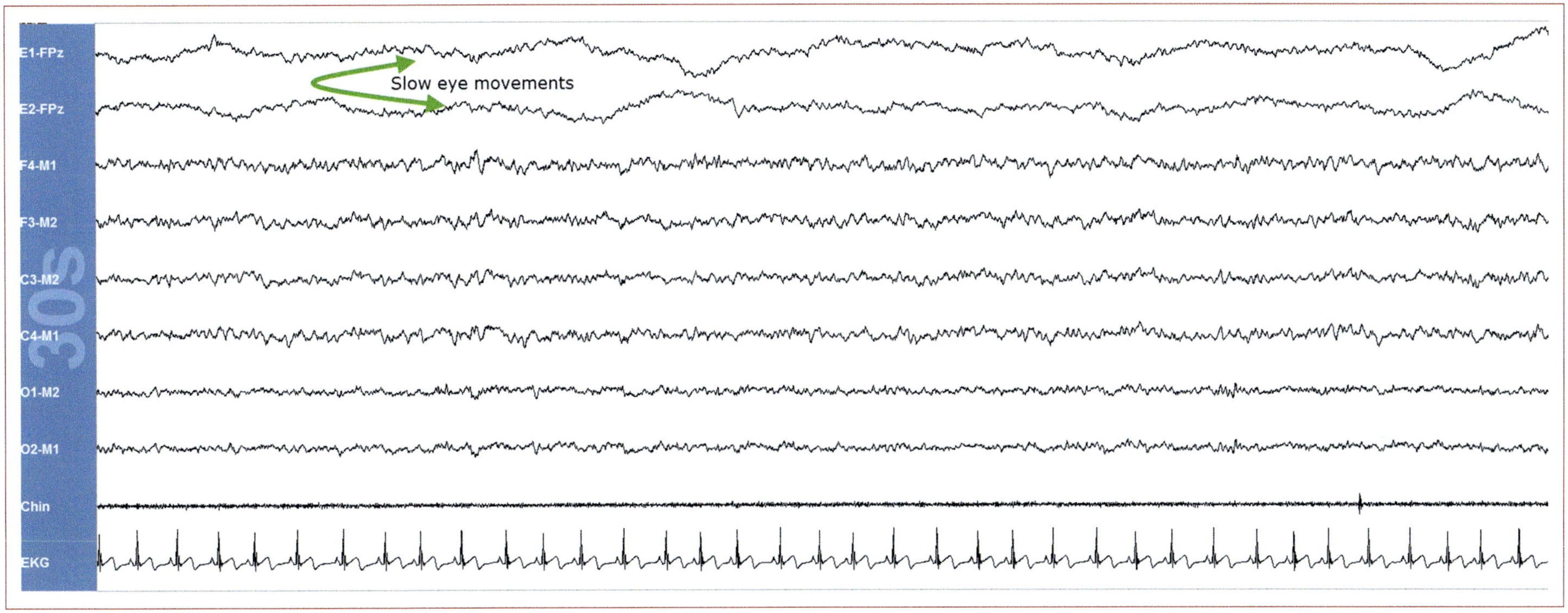

FIGURE 11.22: Slow rolling eye movements monitored by EOG herald sleep onset.

EOG, electrooculography.

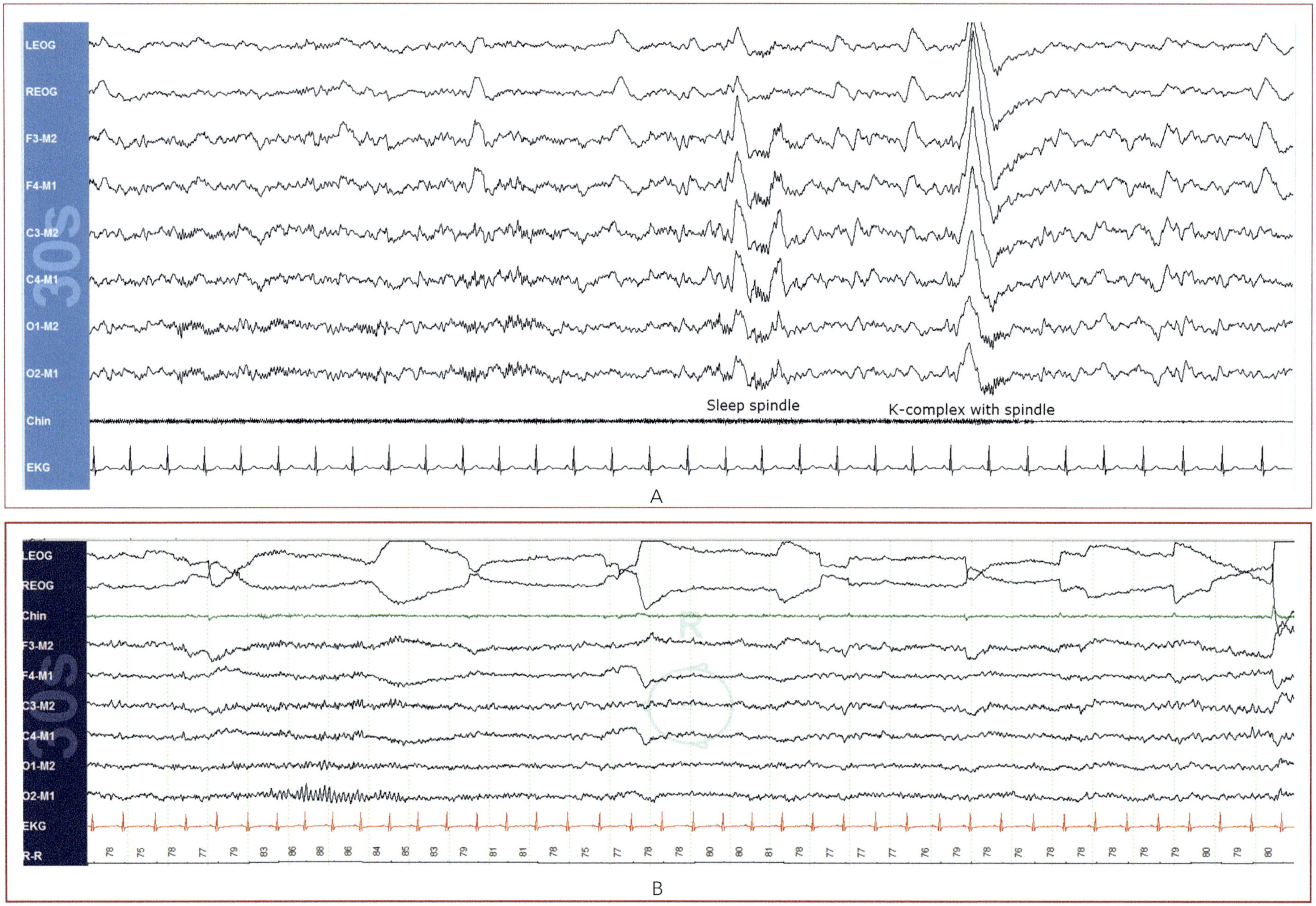

FIGURE 11.23: (A) Note how K-complex in NREM 2 is maximal frontal and in phase in EOG channels. (B) Note that REMs during REM sleep are out of phase in the left and right EOG channels. REMs are detected in the left and right frontal EEG derivations.

EOG, electrooculography; NREM, nonrapid eye movement sleep; REM, rapid eye movement.

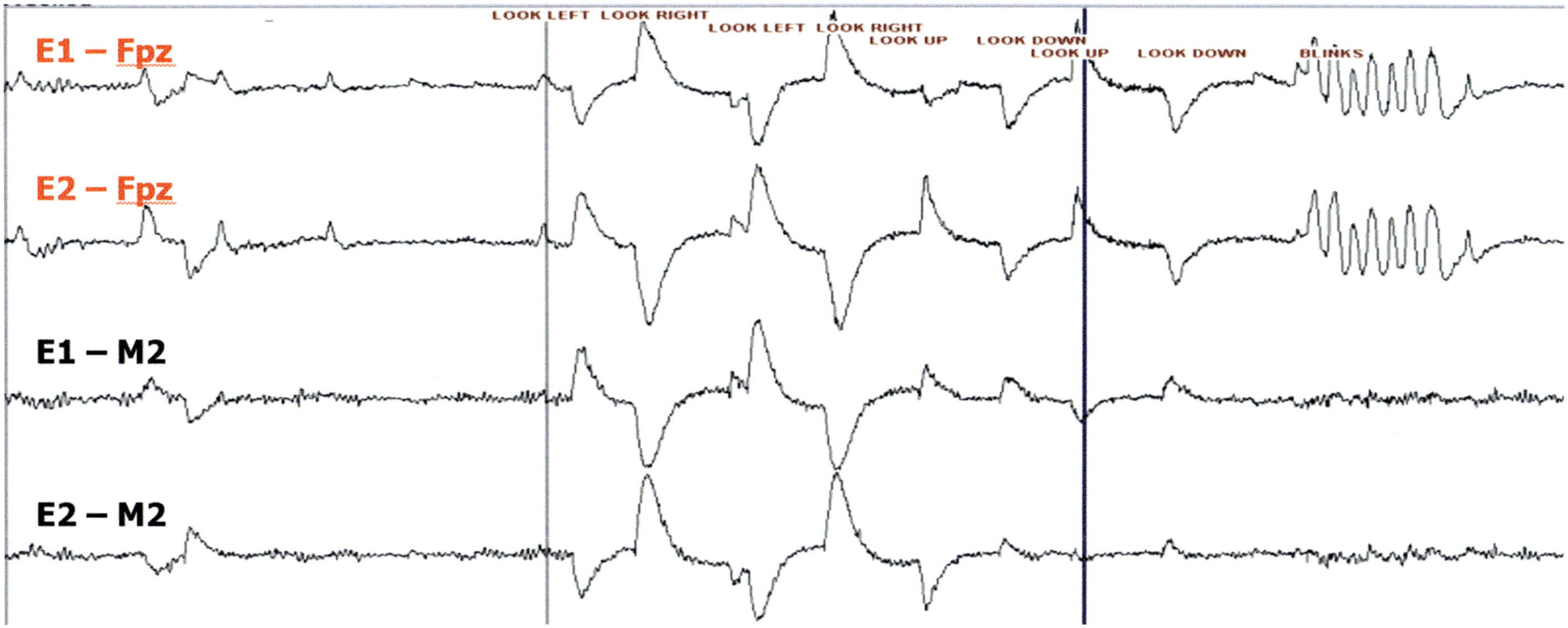

A

Recommended EOG		Alternative EOG	
E1-M2 E2-M2	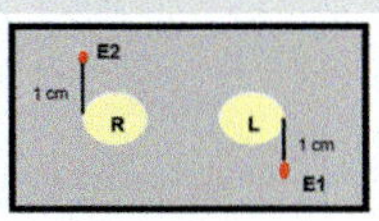	E1-FPz E2-FPz	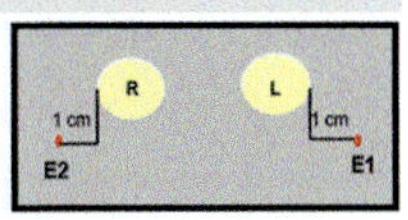
Do NOT show direction of eye movements		Show direction of eye movements	
Can miss low amplitude movements		Show all eye movements	
Easy to distinguish artifacts and EEG		Less easy to distinguish artifacts and EEG	

B

FIGURE 11.24: (A) American Academy of Sleep Medicine recommended and acceptable eye movement montages. (B) Comparison of the recommended and alternative EOG montages.

EOG, electrooculography.

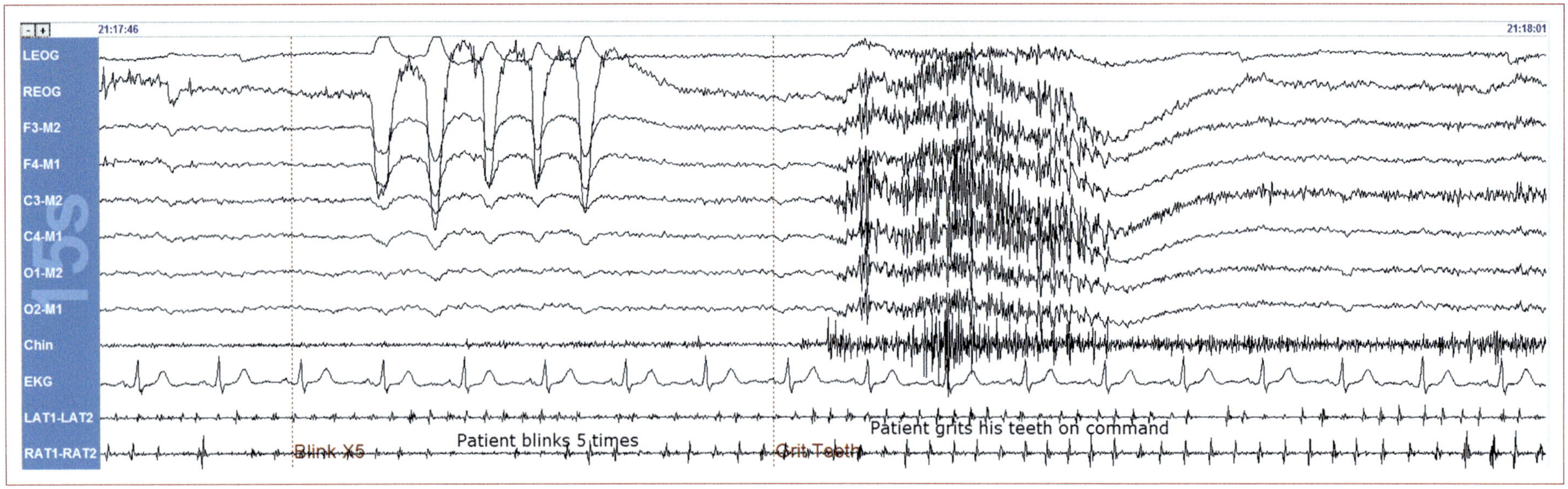

FIGURE 11.25: Recognizing the direction of eye movements by vertical eye blink artifact seen best with E1-FPz, E2-FPz.

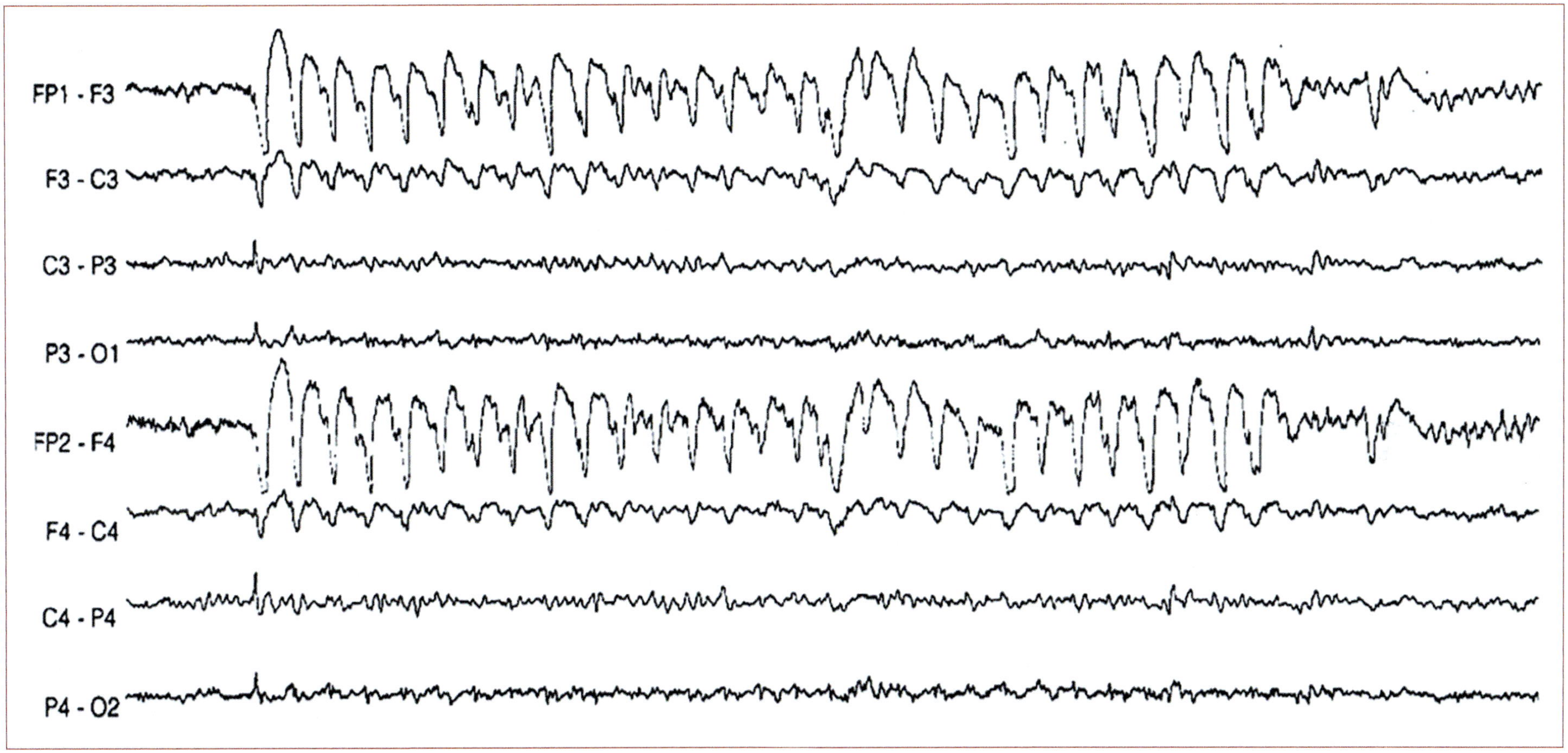

FIGURE 11.26: Eye flutter artifact in the EEG, most notable in FP1-F3 and FP2-F4 electrode derivations.

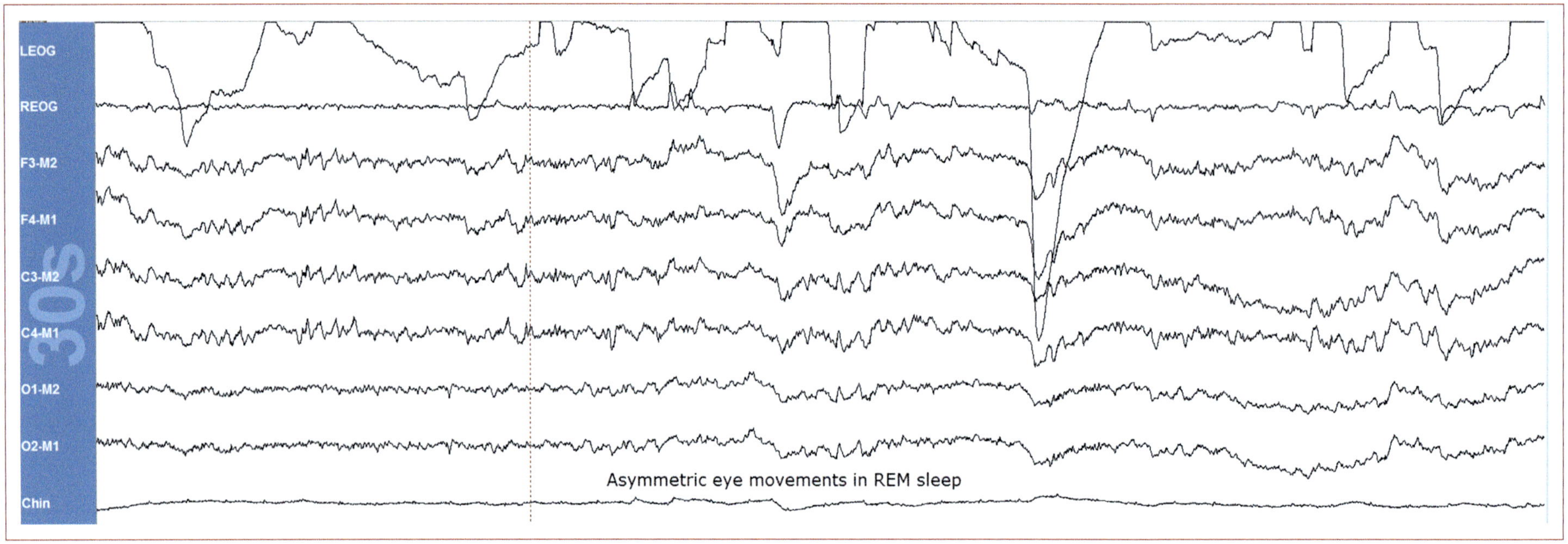

FIGURE 11.27: Asymmetric eye movements in REM sleep "aliased" due to the LLF on EOG set at 5.3 Hz.

EOG, electrooculography; REM, rapid eye movement.

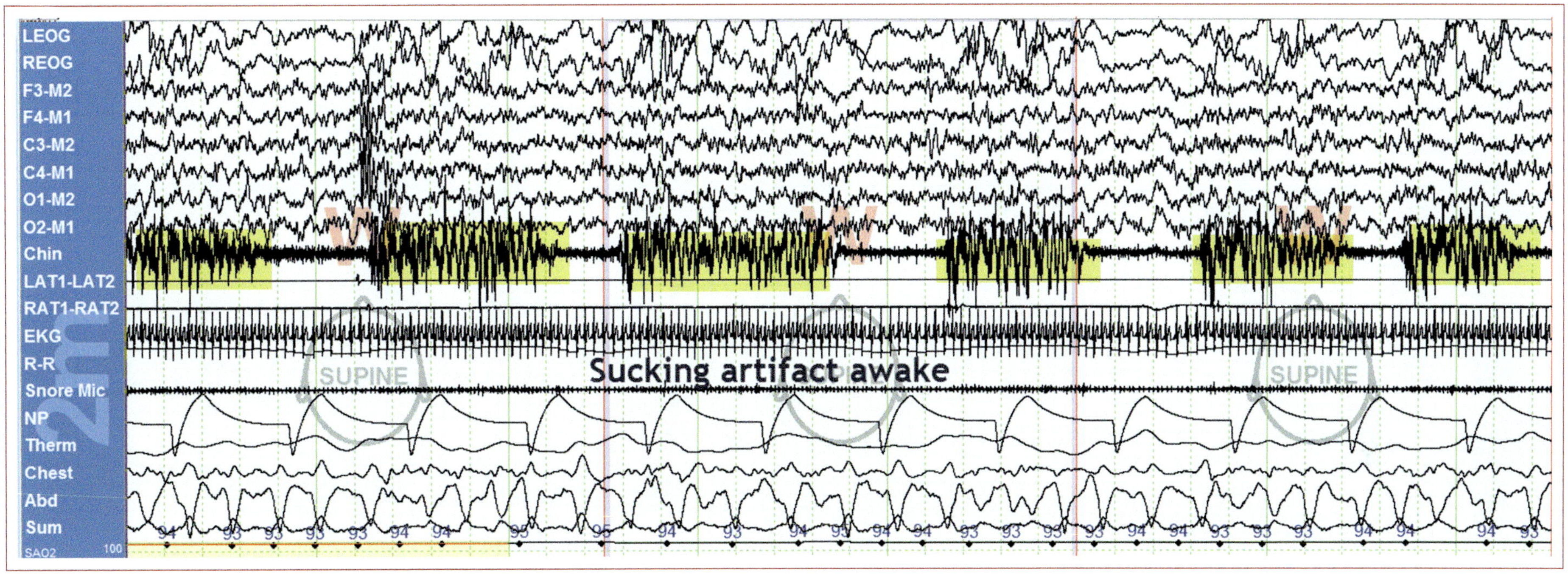

FIGURE 11.28: Sucking artifact (yellow) is present in the chin EMG reflecting perioral muscular involvement. Note the lack of periodicity, myogenic activity, and movement isolated to chin EMG during wakefulness, localizing movement to the face/mouth area.

EMG, electromyography.

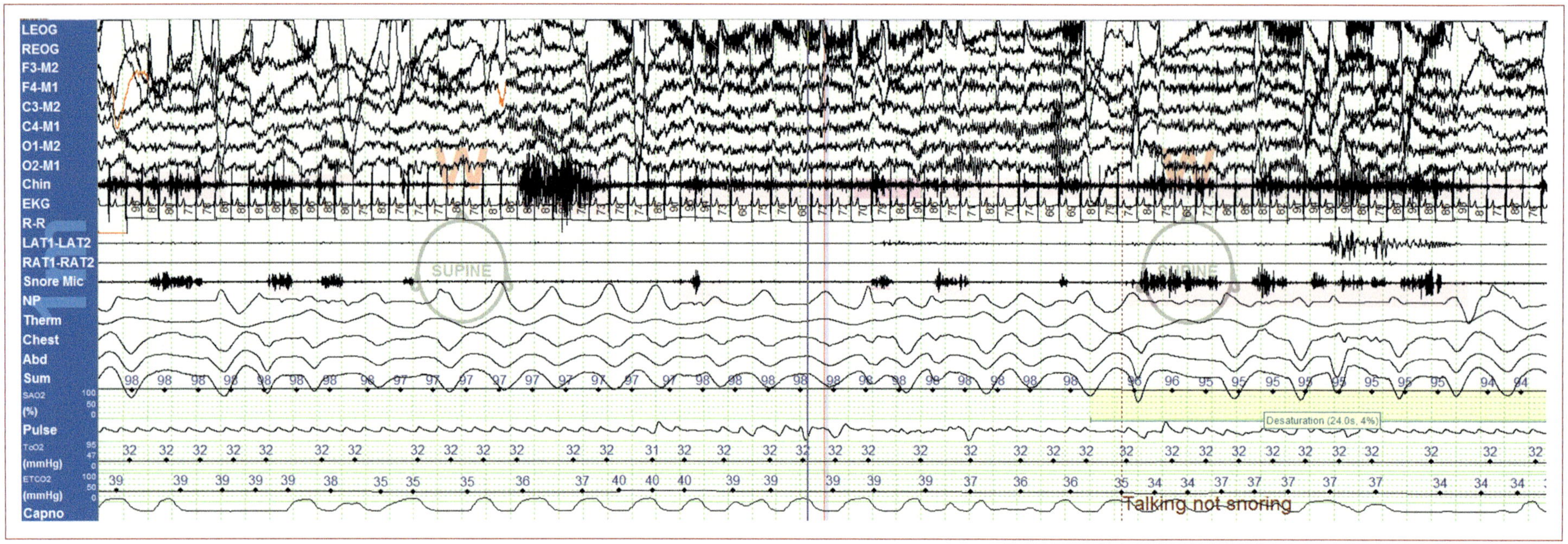

FIGURE 11.29: Talking artifact is reflected in multiple PSG channels. In this epoch of the PSG, the patient is awake. Muscle artifact is present in the chin and snore microphone channels because the patient is talking. Notice prominent eye movement artifact in the eye movement channels (L EOG, R EOG), which involve the left and right frontal EEG channels (F3-M2, F4-M1). The respiration is irregular because the patient is intermittently speaking.

Abd, abdominal respiratory effort; C3-M2, left central referenced to right mastoid; C4-M1, right central EEG referenced to left mastoid; chest, thoracic respiratory effort; ECG, modified lead II; F3-M2, left frontal EEG, left frontal-right mastoid; F4-M1, right frontal EEG, right frontal-left mastoid; L EOG, left extraocular muscles; NP, nasal pressure sensor; O2-M1, right occipital EEG, right occipital-left mastoid; R EOG, right extraocular muscles; SaO_2 (%), pulse oximetry signal; Snore Mic, snore microphone; Sum, summed signal of thoracic and abdominal respiratory effort signals; Therm, oronasal thermal sensor.

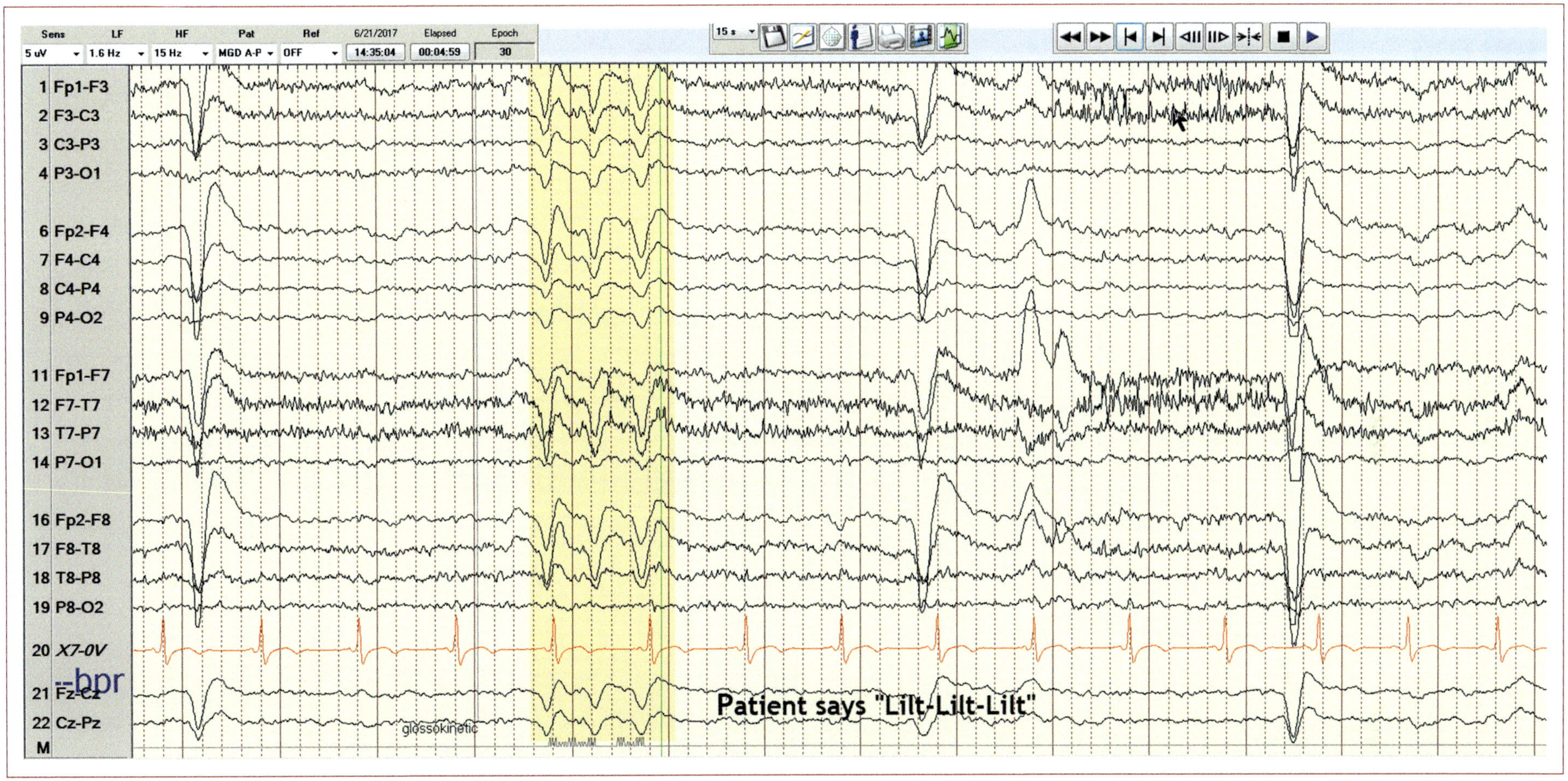

FIGURE 11.30: Glossokinetic artifact that appears similar in morphology to vertical eyeblink artifact. Note the production of the waveforms (highlighted in yellow) as the patient says "lilt."

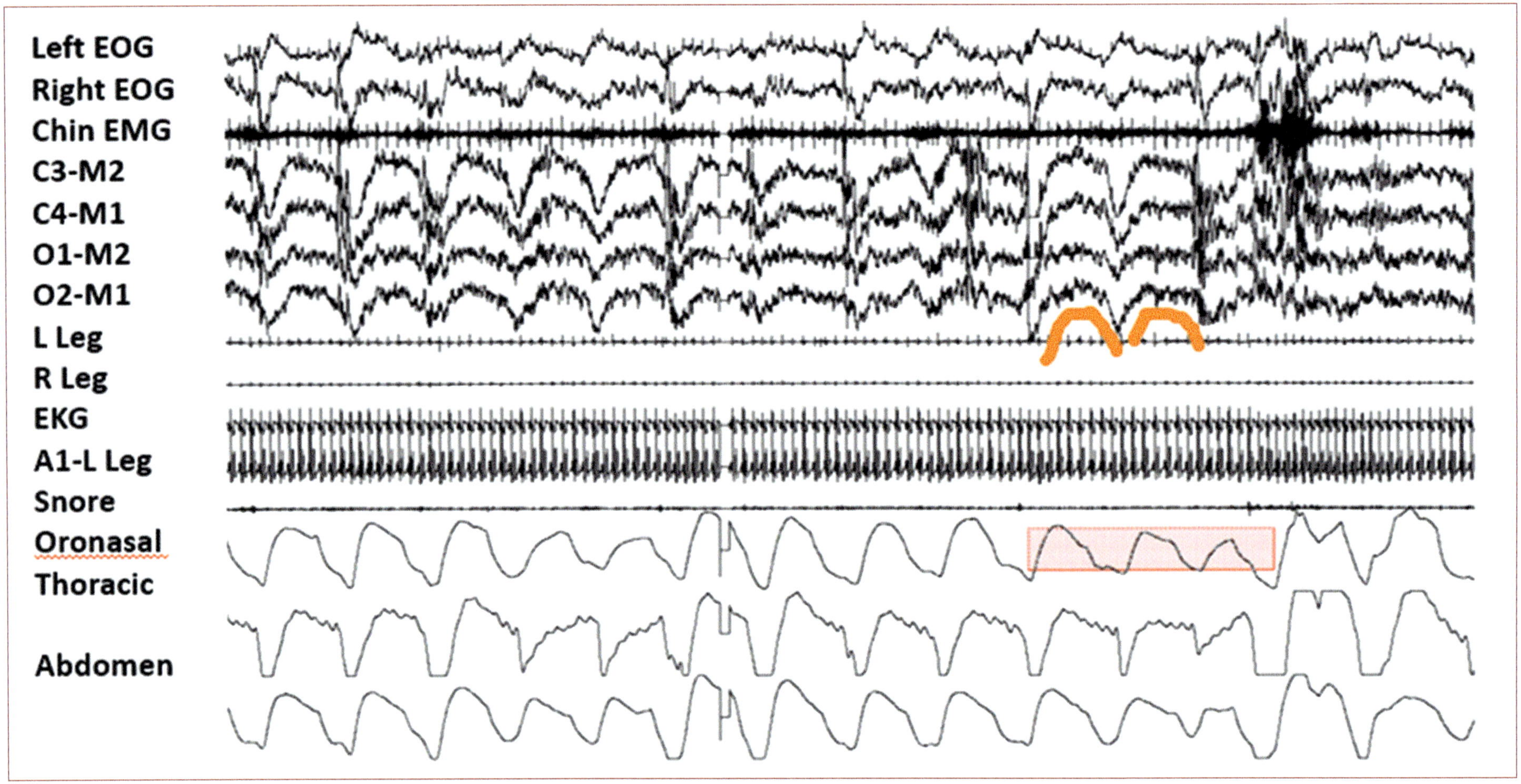

FIGURE 11.31: Respiratory artifact often intrudes into the EEG derivations. Respiration artifact appears here as slow sway in the baseline EEG (in orange) which is time-locked, occurring in-phase with the phases of inspiration and expiration (red rectangle).

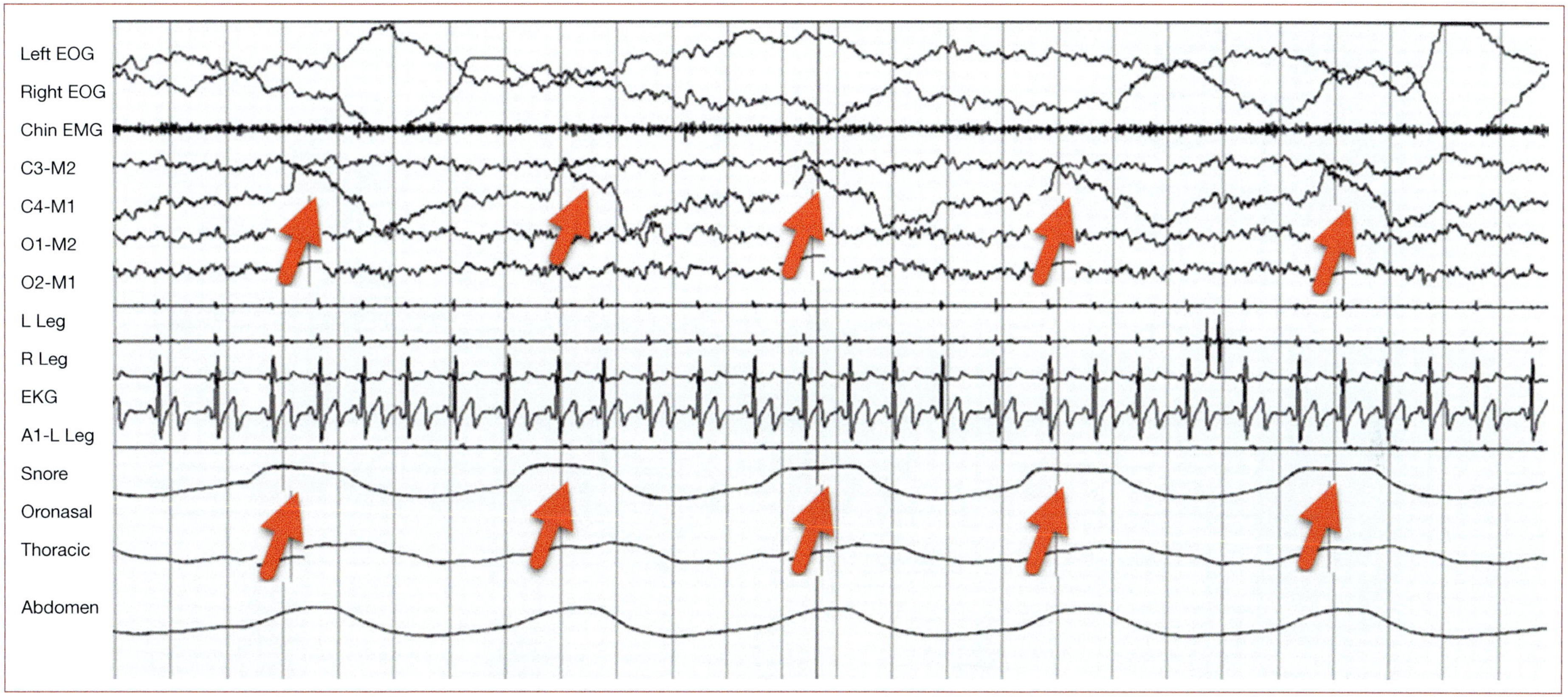

FIGURE 11.32: Respiratory effort-related artifact involves the right central EEG channel time-locked with inspiration only most likely because the patient is lying on the right central electrode. Arrows point to the artifact in the C4-M1 EEG channel and inspiration marked by an arrow in oronasal but also evident in the thoracic and abdominal respiratory effort channels.

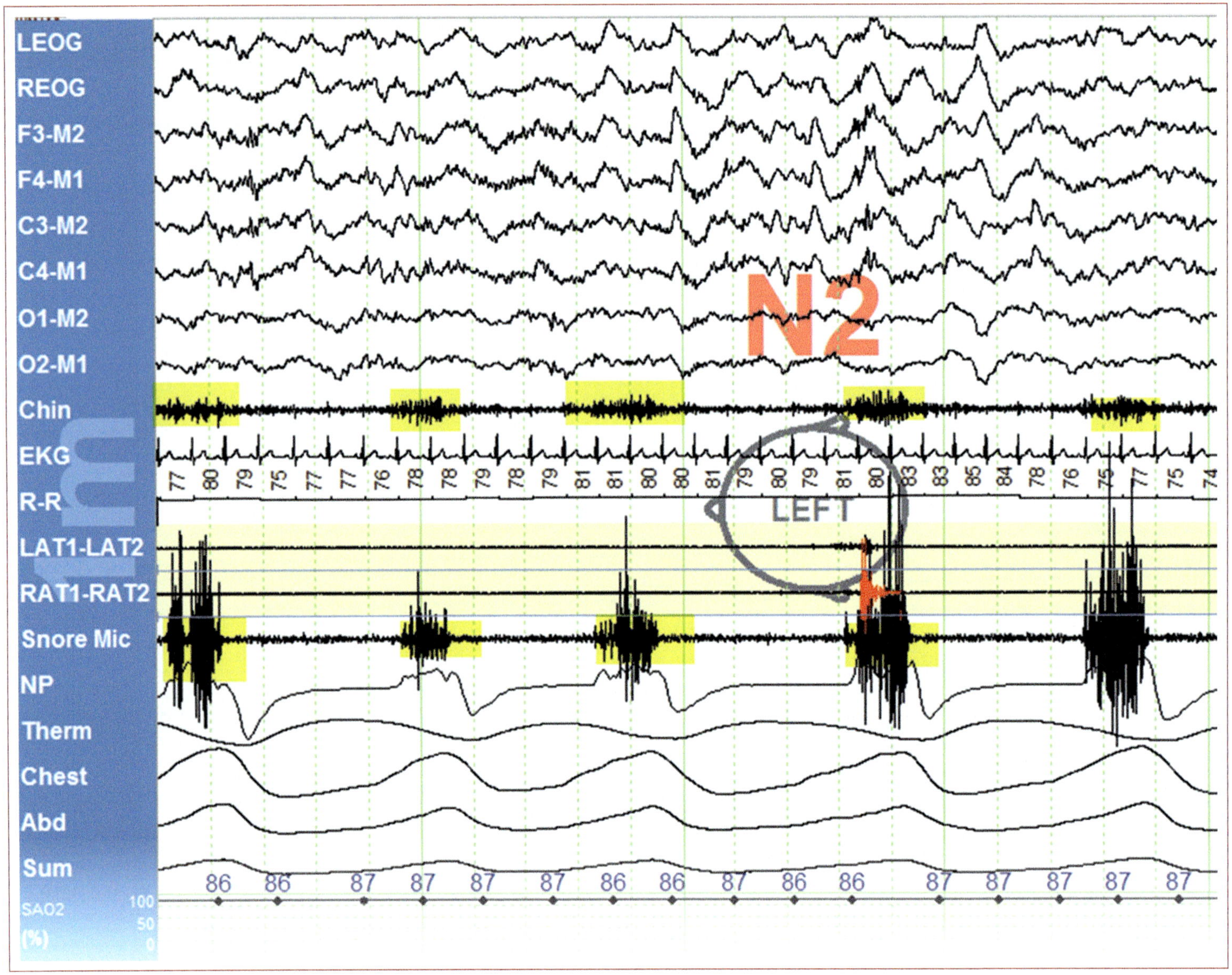

FIGURE 11.33: A different respiration-related artifact is snoring-related vibration captured by the snore microphone, which can cause high-frequency artifacts in other channels such as chin EMG (in yellow). This artifact cannot be removed but should be recognized as snoring related.

EMG, electromyography.

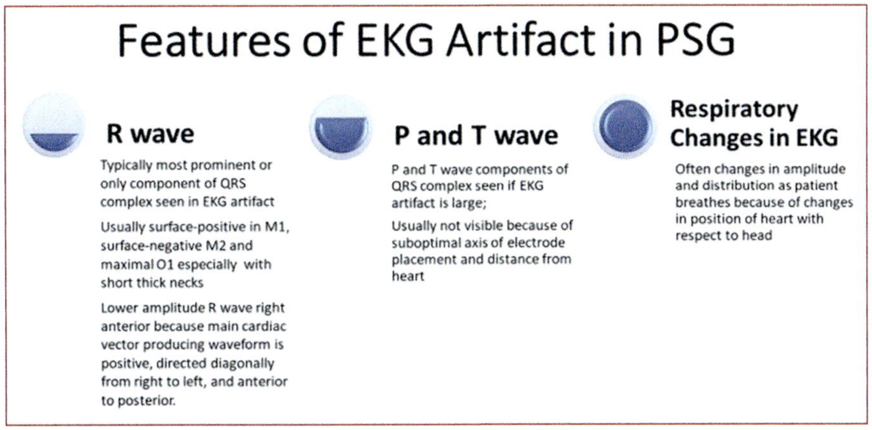

FIGURE 11.34: Features of ECG artifact present in the PSG.

PSG, polysomnography.

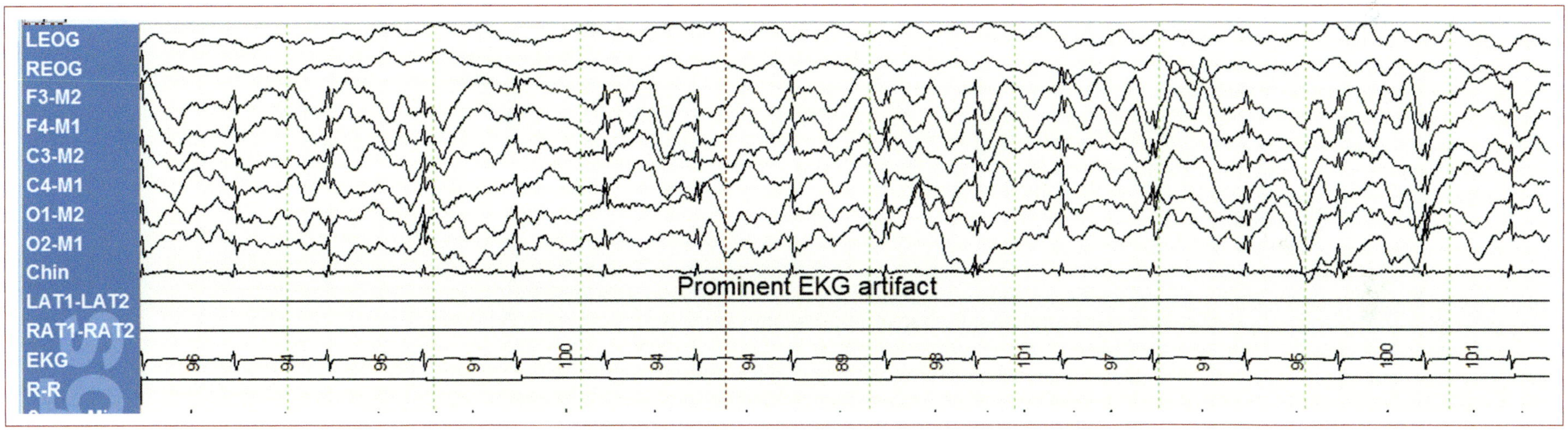

FIGURE 11.35: Prominent ECG artifact is often observed in adults with short thick necks. A 30-second epoch of PSG recorded in an infant. Note the fast heart rate in the ECG channel. The ECG artifact is often of higher amplitude over the left posterior head region but is variably present because the right EEG channels are linked to the left mastoid. Notice how ECG artifact is not seen in the EOG channels because these are linked to FPz.

EOG, electrooculography; PSG, polysomnography.

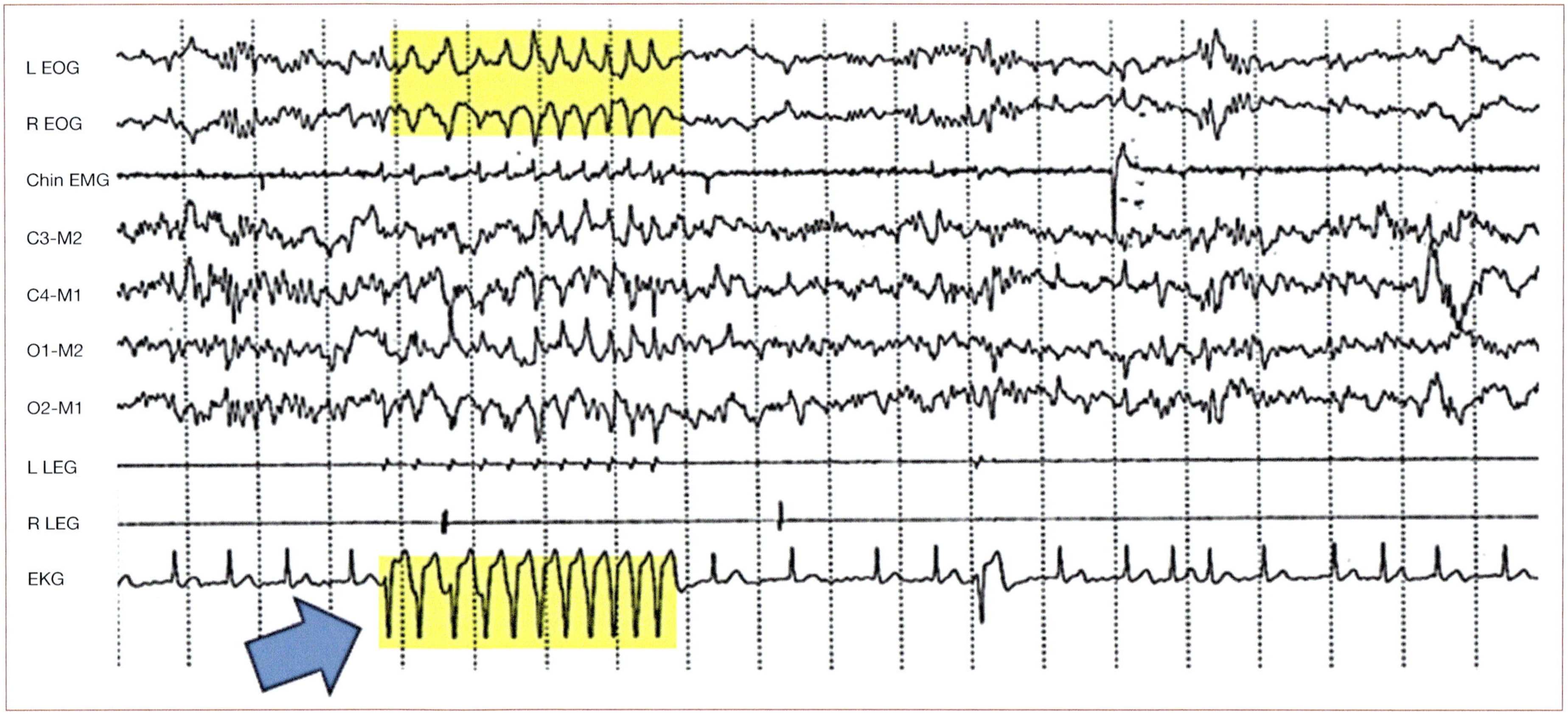

FIGURE 11.36: Ventricular tachycardia present in the ECG during PSG. A 20-second epoch of PSG recorded in an elderly patient during NREM 2 sleep. The electrical signal from the heart creates artifact that is diffuse but most prominent in the EOG during a run of ventricular tachycardia in the ECG (arrow). Always check whether each ECG artifact is time-locked to a QRS complex to determine the presence of artifact. The heart rate tends to increase slightly with inspiration and decrease with expiration. When the fluctuation is prominent, it is referred to as sinus arrhythmia. The presence of ventricular tachycardia (now known as wide-complex tachycardia) typically prompts concern when observed in overnight PSG.

EOG, electrooculography; NREM, nonrapid eye movement sleep; PSG, polysomnography.

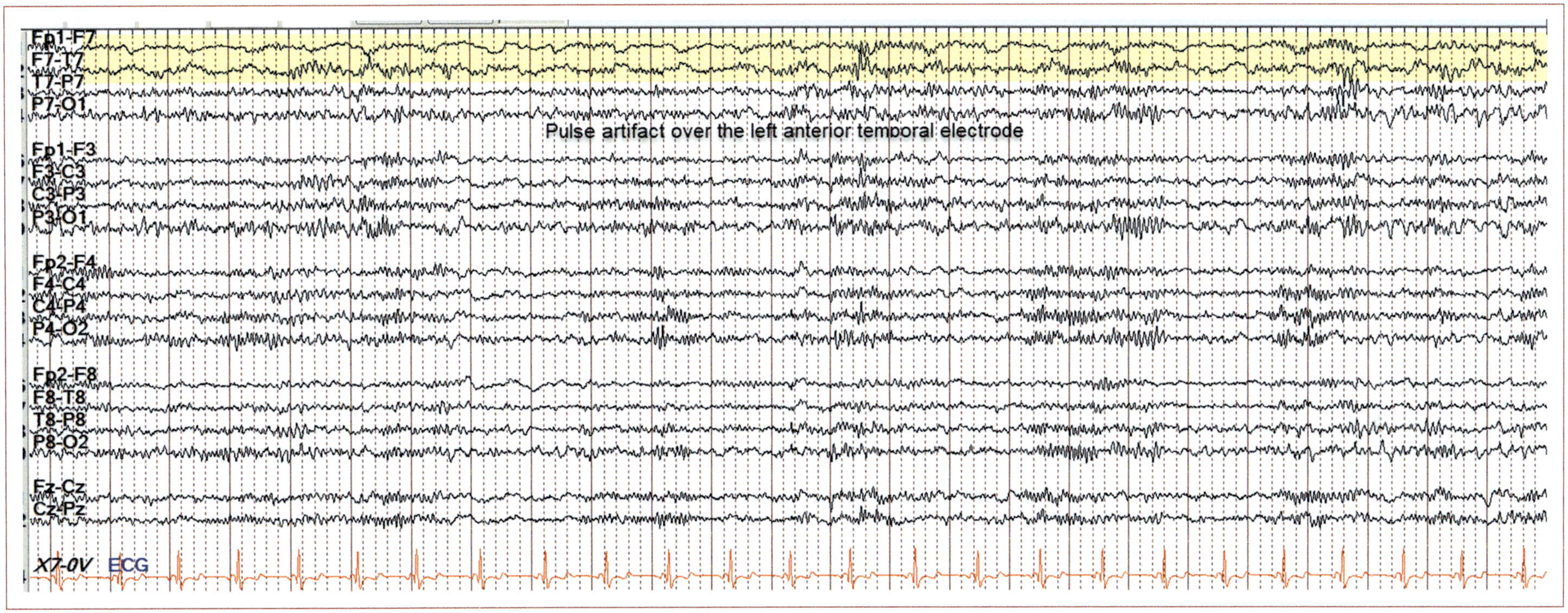

FIGURE 11.37: Pulse artifact. A 25-second epoch of EEG demonstrates pulse artifact in the left anterior temporal electrode (F7). Pulse artifact is caused by movement of an electrode when it rests over a pulsating artery. It appears as a smooth, periodic slow wave which follows the QRS ECG complex artifact by a slight delay (approximately 200 msec); delayed by the time it takes the blood to travel from the heart to the pulsating blood vessel. Sometimes, the pulse artifact is triangular or sharply contoured. Pulse artifacts are more likely to occur in frontal, central, or temporal head regions rather than occipital regions but may appear anywhere near a blood vessel. To eliminate or reduce pulse artifact in PSG, first try moving the patient's head slightly off the particular electrode; if the artifact persists, reapply the electrode a small distance away from the superficial artery.

PSG, polysomnography.

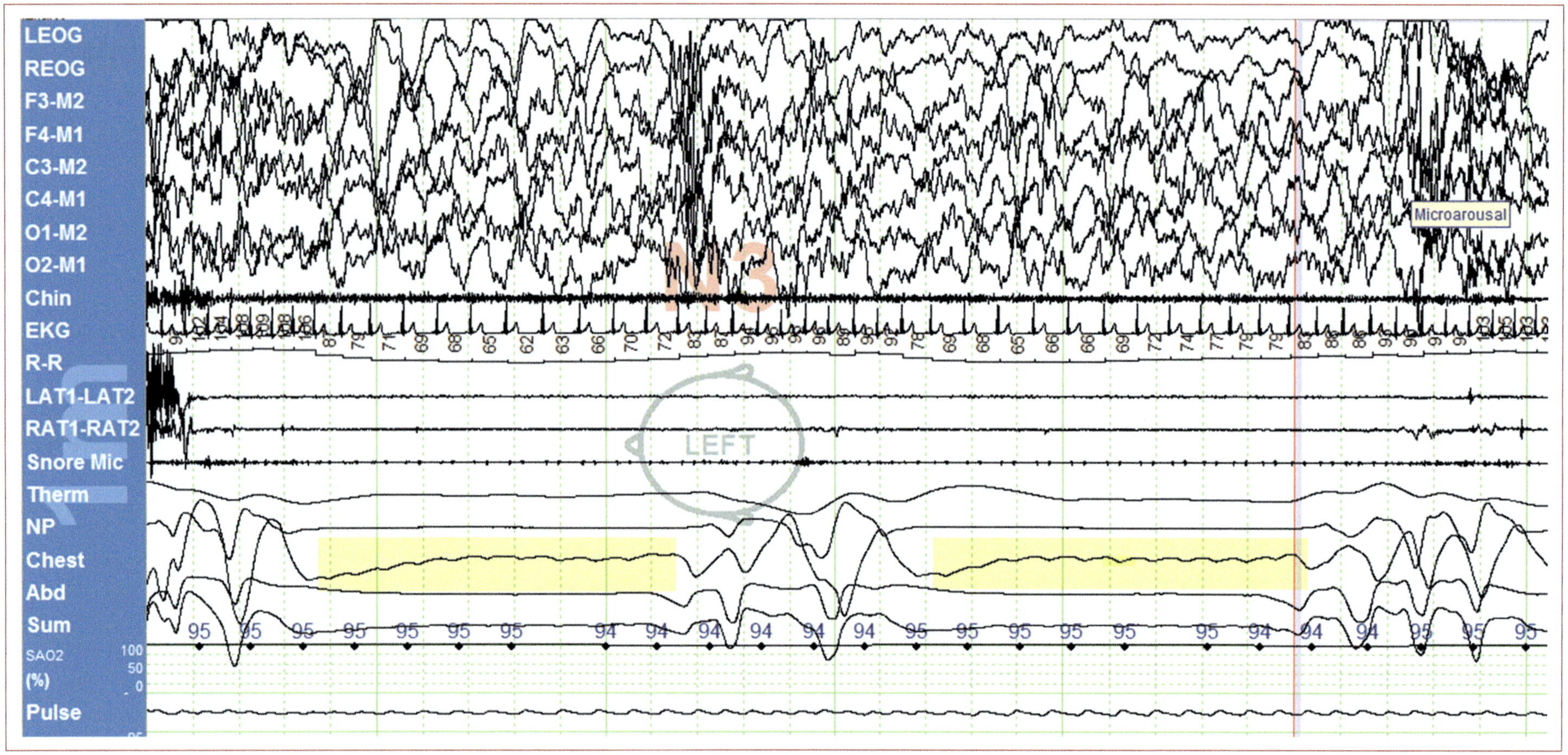

FIGURE 11.38: Ballistocardiographic artifact in the chest respiratory effort channel. This is a 36-second epoch of PSG showing two central apneas in a middle-aged adult. Note the ballistocardiographic artifact in the thoracic respiratory effort channels (chest). It typically occurs as small "pulse waves" that correspond to cardiac contractions in the ECG channel with a slight delay. It is caused by either (a) recoil movements of the patient's head or body as the blood pumps from the heart; (b) pulsatile force on the aortic arch from abrupt redirection of blood flow; and (c) changes in intrathoracic pressure produced with each heartbeat result in movement of air through the patent upper airway.

PSG, polysomnography.

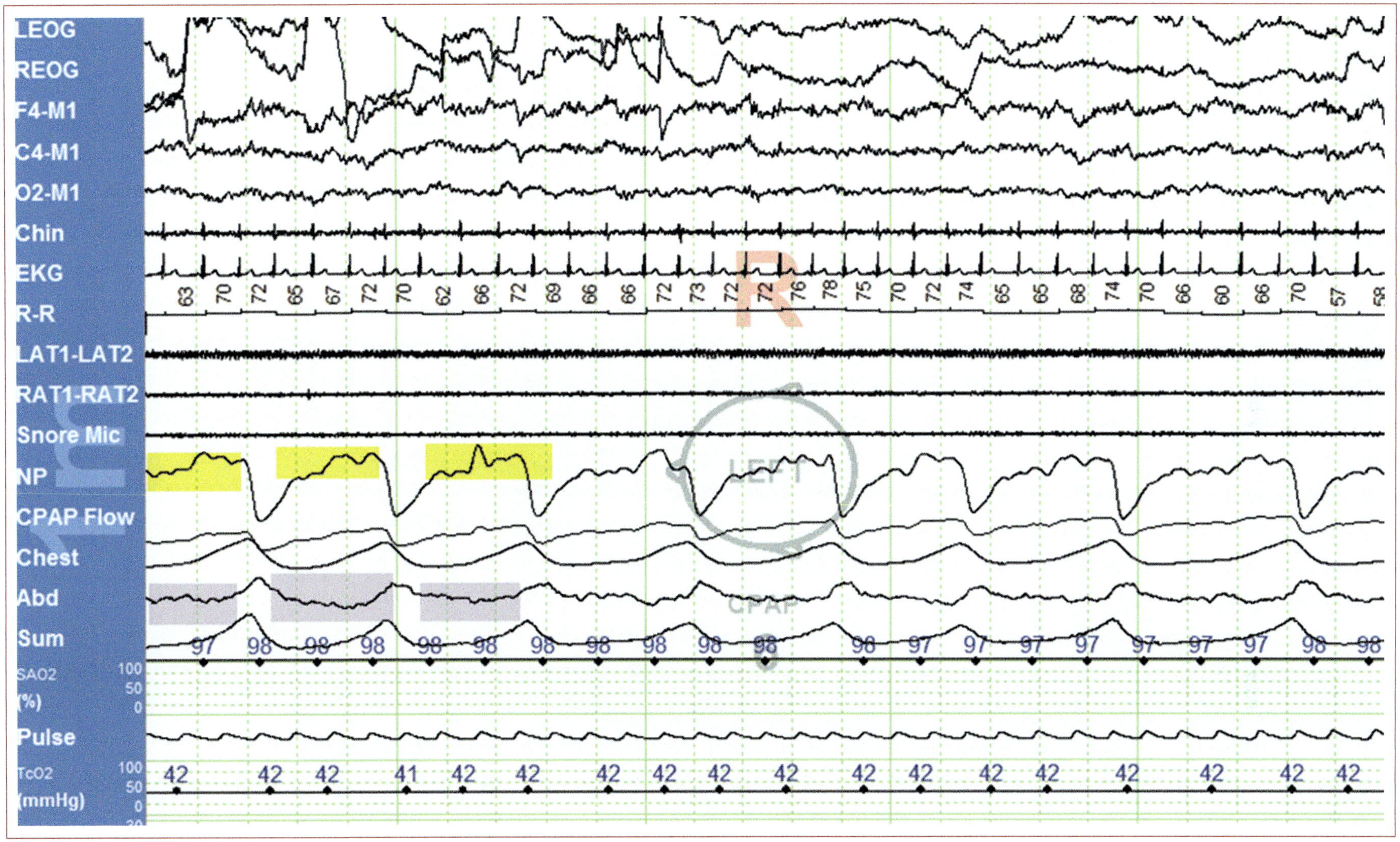

FIGURE 11.39: Ballistocardiographic artifact in nasal pressure and thoracic respiratory effort channels. A 30-second epoch of PSG recorded in REM sleep in an adult during titration of continuous positive airway pressure. The ballistocardiographic artifact here is seen in the NP and also the abdominal respiratory effort channels. It appears as small "pulse waves" that correspond to cardiac contractions in the ECG tracing with a slight delay. Prominent rapid eye movements are noted in the EOG (L EOG and R EOG). Ballistocardiographic artifact when seen on airflow channels often occurs during prolonged central apneas.

EOG, electrooculography; NP, nasal pressure; PSG, polysomnography; REM, rapid eye movement.

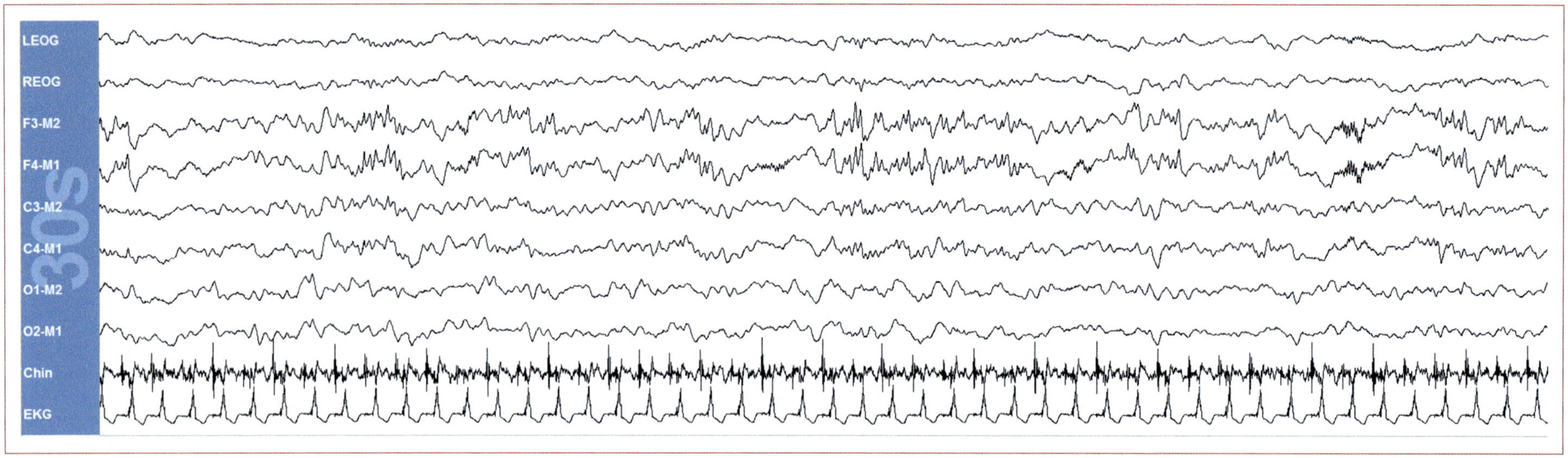

FIGURE 11.40: Cardiac pacemaker artifact. A 30-second epoch of PSG in an infant with complete heart block and requires ventricular pacing. The pacemaker artifact appears as a high-amplitude fast spike when the internal cardiac pacemaker delivers an electrical stimulus, which may be seen in the EEG and EOG channels and is time-locked with ECG. The pacing spike is of much shorter duration than ECG artifact. Usually there is no heart rate variability with respiratory events when the heart is paced because this form of artifact is regulated and cannot be eliminated.

EOG, electrooculography; PSG, polysomnography.

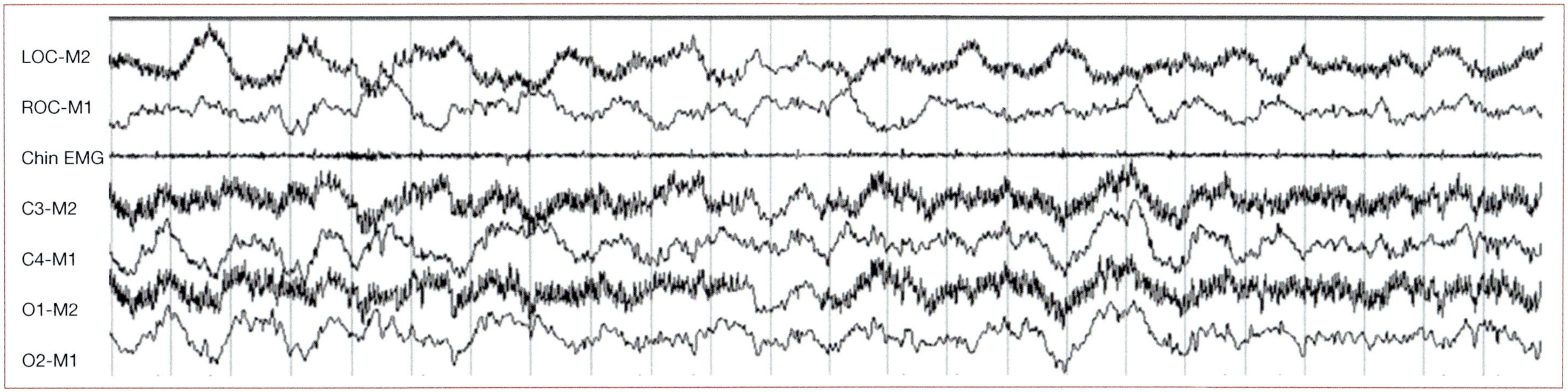

FIGURE 11.41: 60-Hz artifact. A 24-second epoch of PSG with electrical interference caused by 60-Hz artifact involving the right mastoid electrode (M2) and present in LOC-M2, C3-M2, and O1-M2. It is caused by a problem in continuity or grounding anywhere between the patient-to-digital polygraph circuitry. A 60-Hz artifact usually appears as a thick line in the channel of interest (undulations at a frequency of 60/sec can be counted if the epoch speed is changed to 1/sec per screen) and affects PSG channels recording AC.

AC, alternating current; PSG, polysomnography.

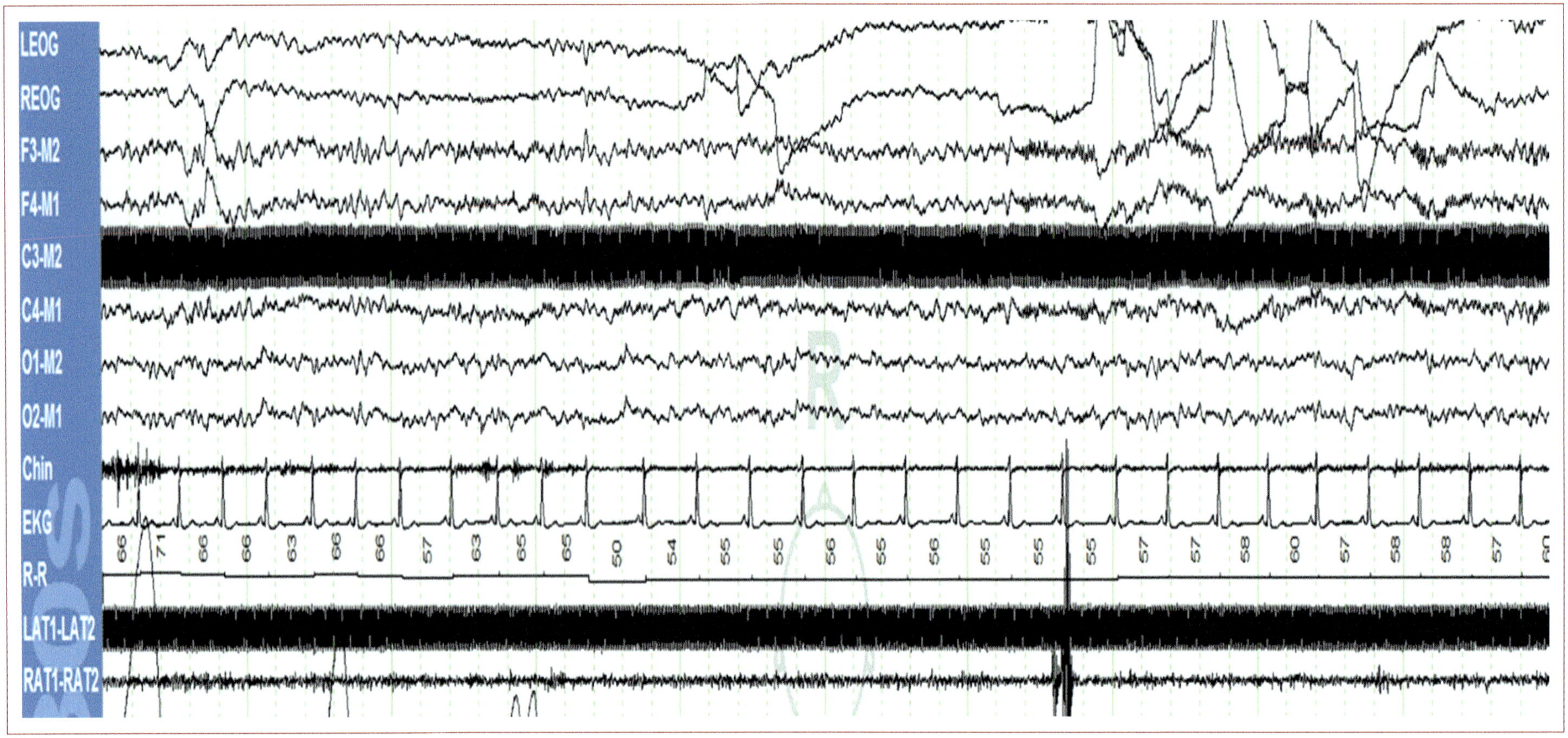

FIGURE 11.42: A 30-second epoch of PSG containing 60-Hz artifact present in the C3 electrode and channels recording movement in the left leg (LAT1-LAT2). When 60-Hz artifact affects only one or a few AC-recorded channels, it often reflects high or imbalanced electrode impedances. When observing 60-Hz artifact, first check electrode impedances for abnormality. Maximum electrode impedances for EEG and EOG in PSG need to be less than 5 kΩ and the difference between electrode pairs less than 1 kΩ. Unbalanced impedance between electrode pairs defeats the ability of the differential amplifier to cancel out electrical noise. Sixty-hertz artifact present in one electrode may also be due to a broken or disconnected wire, poor electrode contact, and/or nearby electrical equipment. Linking the left and right anterior tibialis EMG channels as was done here increases the likelihood for artifact.

AC, alternating current; EMG, electromyography; EOG, electrooculography; PSG, polysomnography.

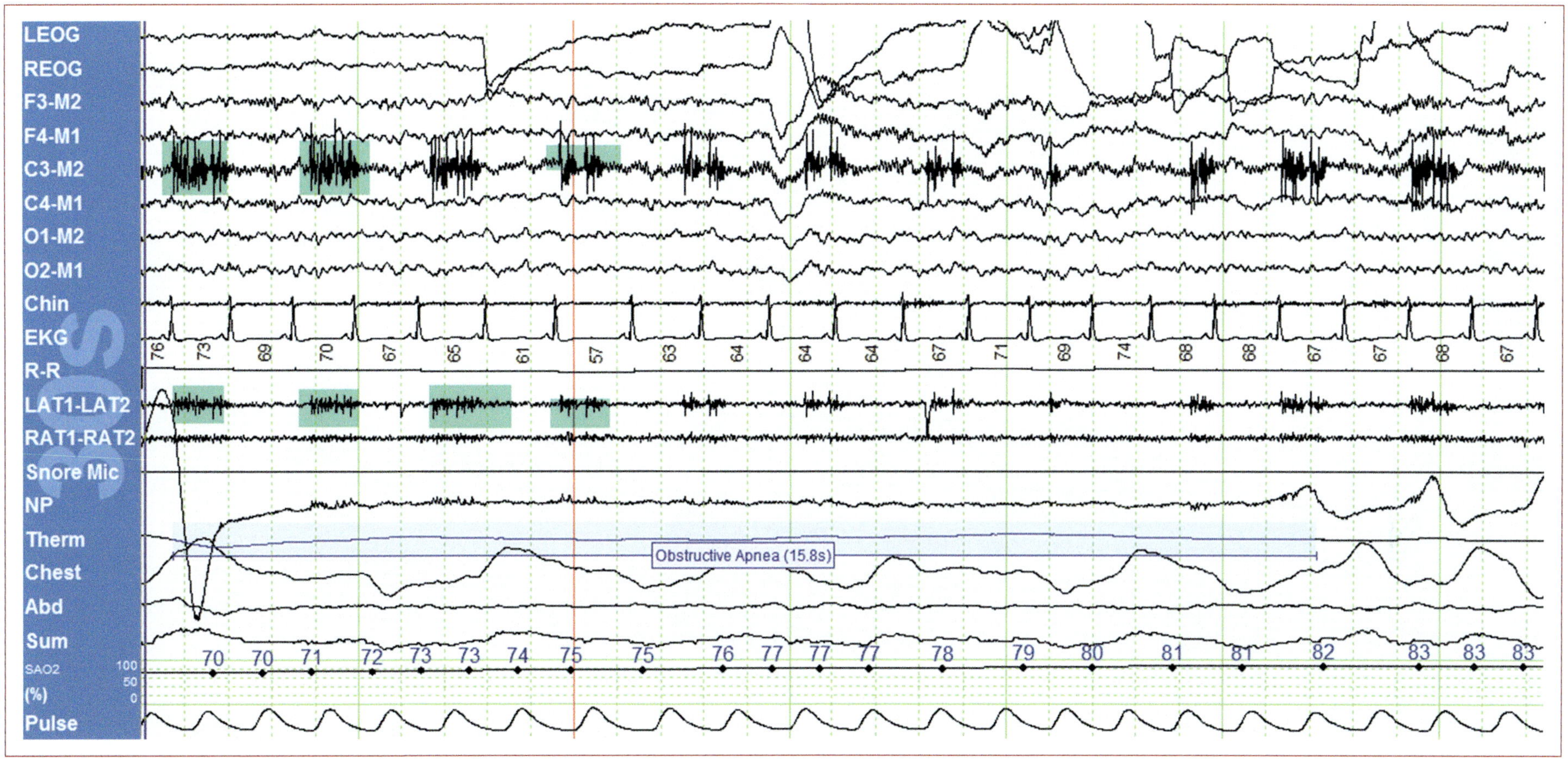

FIGURE 11.43: Electrode pop artifact. A 40-second epoch of PSG shows snore-related vibration artifact being detected in the left central EEG derivation (C3-M2) because the C3 electrode is poorly attached to the scalp surface. Turning off the 60-Hz notch filter for the C3 channel confirms the C3 electrode is poorly attached and demonstrates the continuous electrode artifact that requires fixing.

PSG, polysomnography.

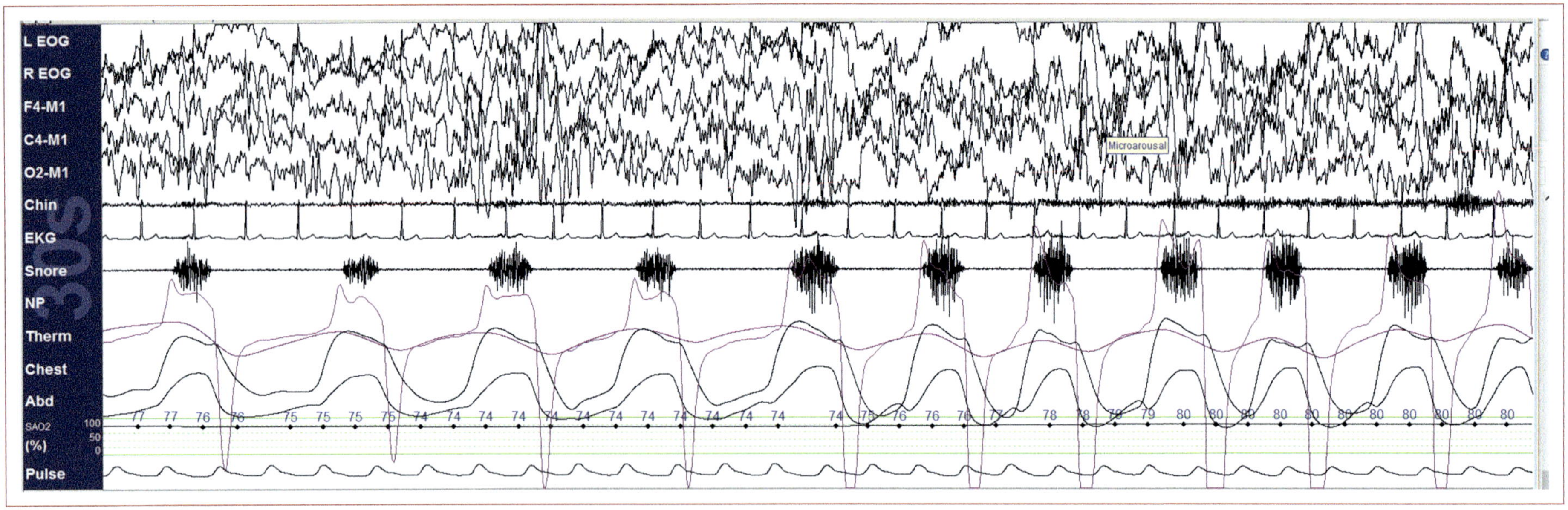

FIGURE 11.44: Overamplification of signals. A 30-second epoch of PSG showing overamplification of EOG and EEG channels and the nasal pressure sensor. Hard to identify sleep spindles (which may occur in lighter NREM 3 sleep). Also, it is difficult to appreciate flattening of the nasal pressure signal when overamplified.

EOG, electrooculography; NREM, nonrapid eye movement sleep; PSG, polysomnography.

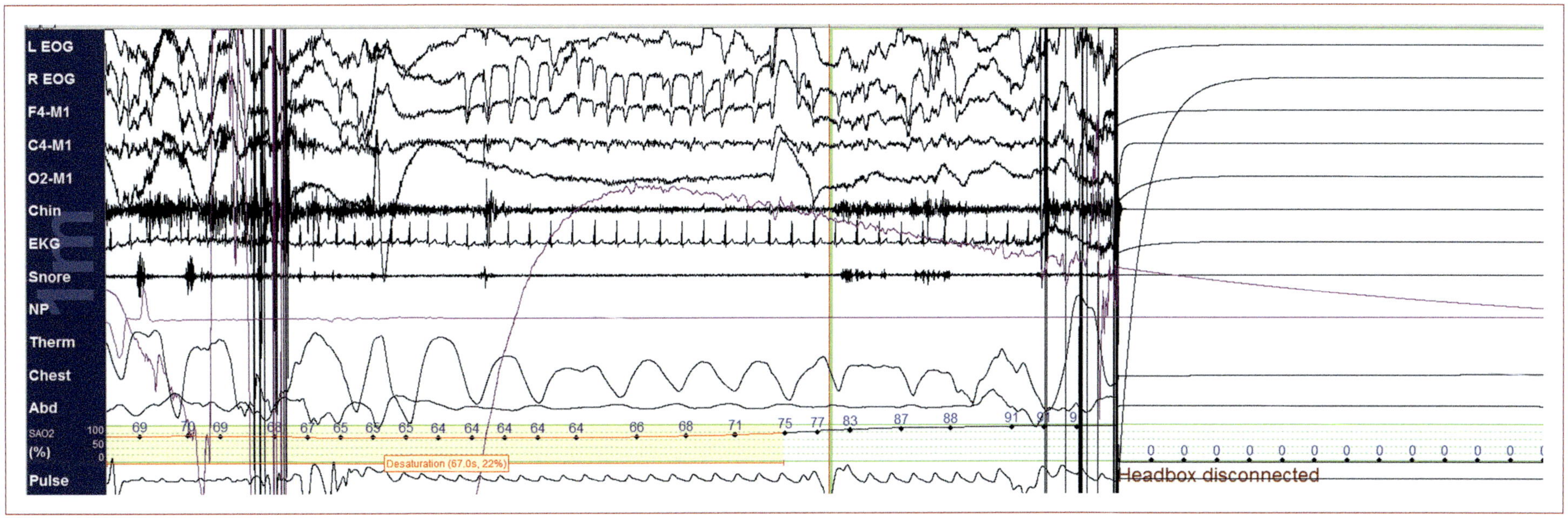

FIGURE 11.45: A 60-second epoch of PSG showing all the PSG signals have flattened when the patient is disconnected from the jack box, in this case to use the bathroom.

PSG, polysomnography.

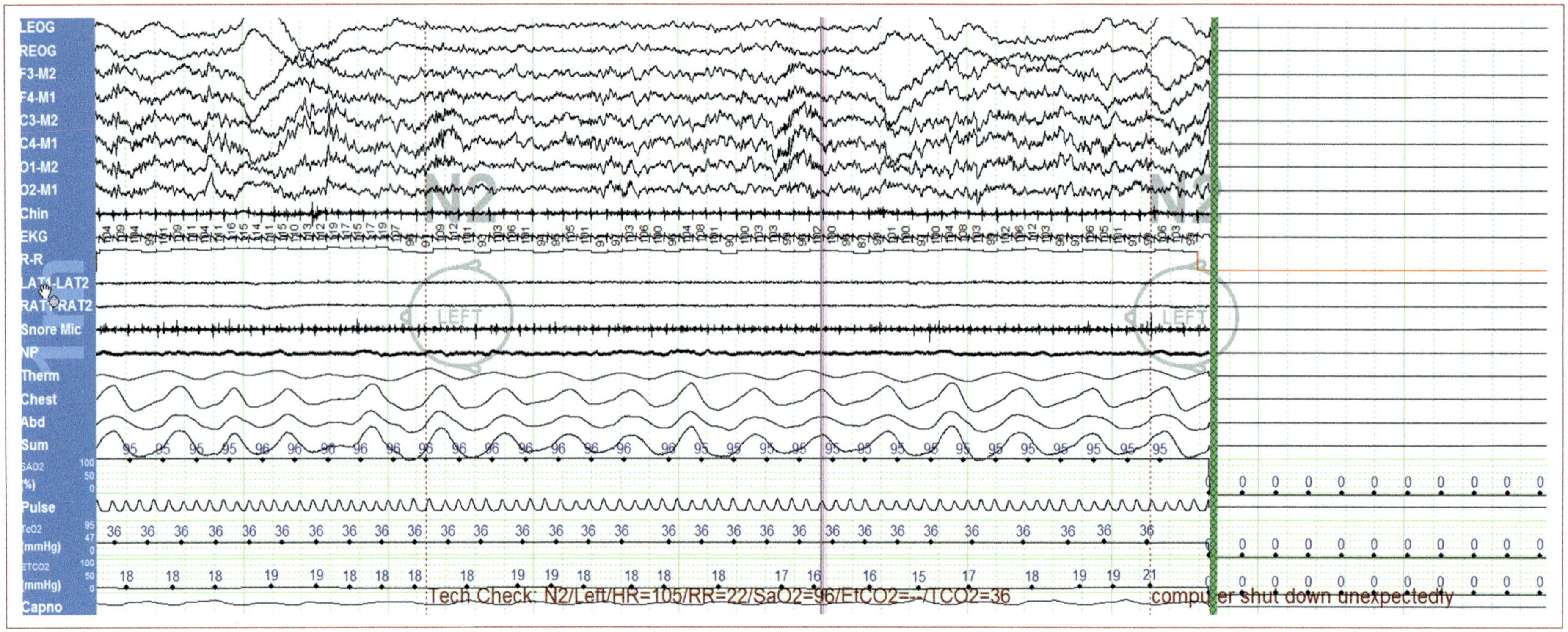

FIGURE 11.46: Computer shutdown. A 60-second epoch of PSG in NREM 2 sleep. Sudden flattening of all PSG signals (vertical green line) is observed in the last fourth of the figure because the polygraph recording computer shut down (when virus protection software programs were being automatically downloaded into the computer systems).

NREM, nonrapid eye movement sleep; PSG, polysomnography.

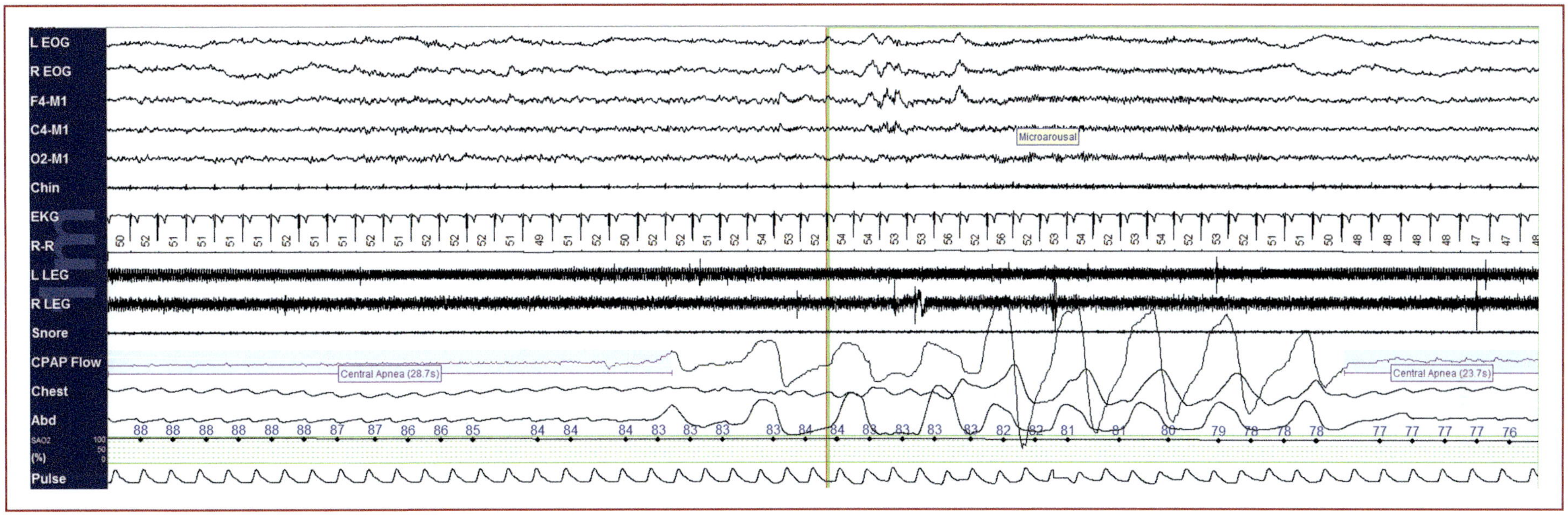

FIGURE 11.47: Inappropriate inversion in the ECG channel. A 60-second epoch of PSG showing ECG channel is inverted. Additionally noted is ballistocardiographic artifact in the chest and abdominal respiratory effort channel during central apneas. Sixty-hertz interference artifact is present in the right and leg channels.

PSG, polysomnography.

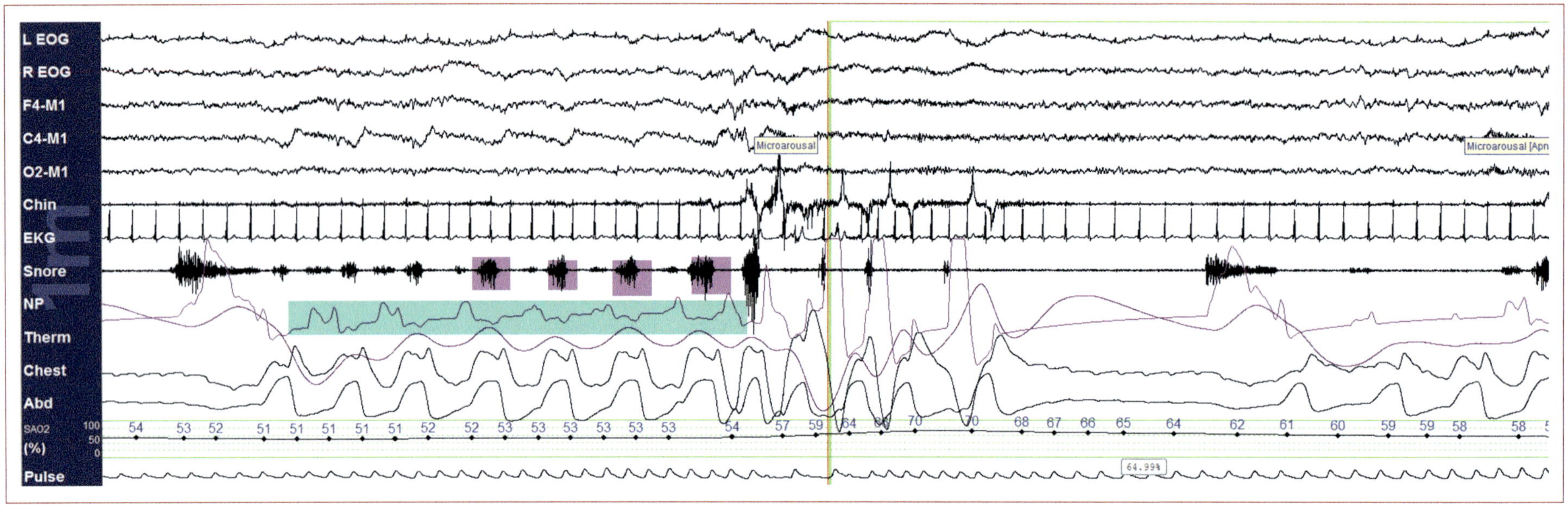

FIGURE 11.48: Inversion of nasal pressure transducer. The snore microphone (purple highlight) is in-phase with the thermal, thoracic, and abdominal respiratory sensors. The nasal pressure sensor is inverted. This can lead to erroneous interpretations of respiratory events. Note the ballistocardiographic artifact in the second respiratory event (a mixed apnea following an arousal). Observe the movement artifacts in the chin EMG during arousal and respiratory artifacts in the EEG channels.

EMG, electromyography.

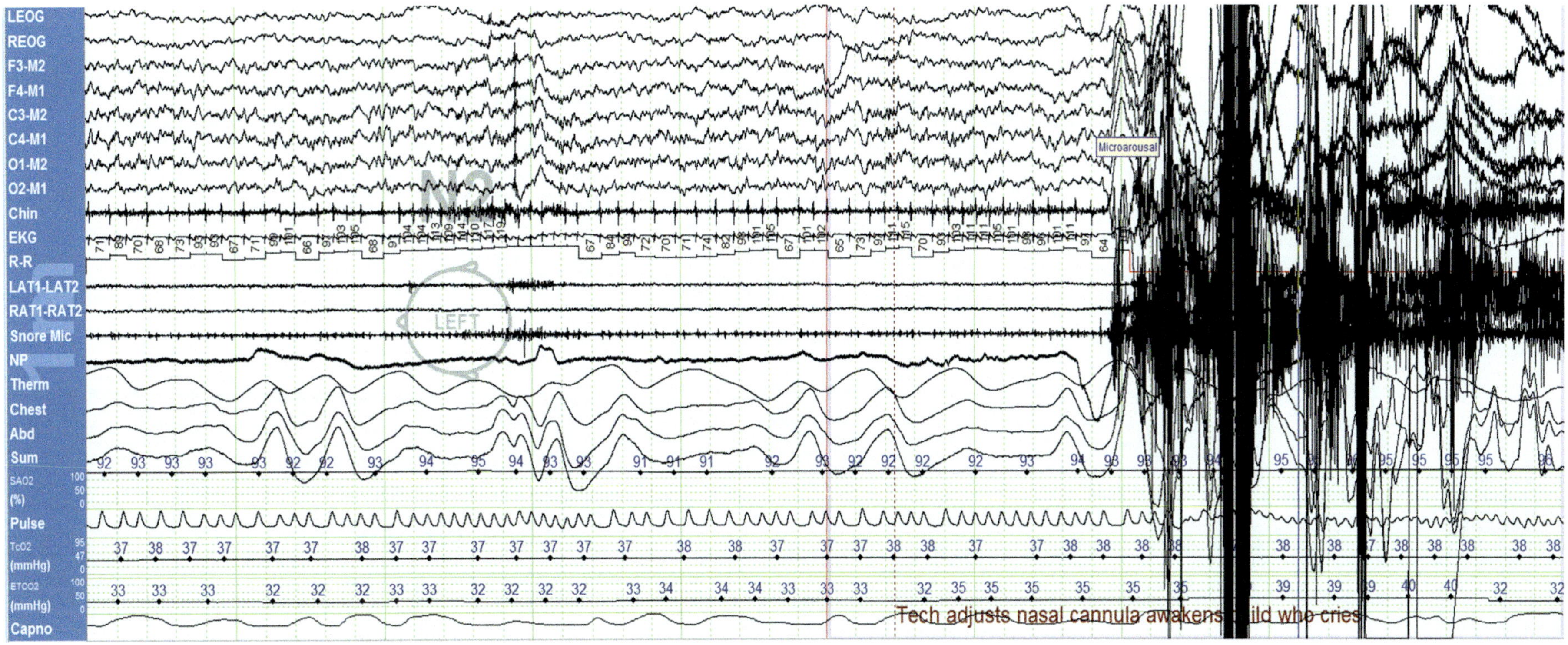

A

FIGURE 11.49: Nasal cannula unreliable. (A) During this 60-second epoch recorded in a child, the nasal cannula is dislodged (patient pulled it out of her nose). The technologist enters and adjusts the cannula, repositioning it in her nose. This prompts an arousal and whole body movement artifact (microarousal). ***(continued)***

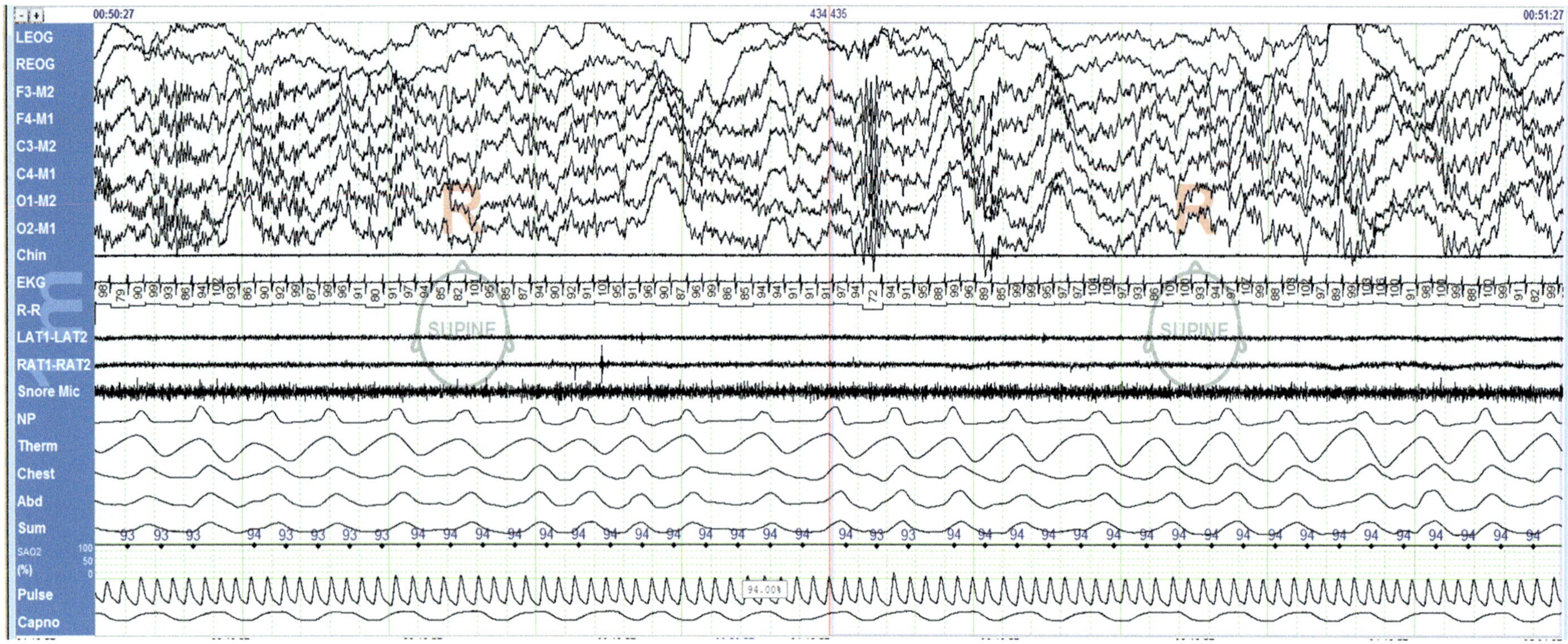

B

FIGURE 11.49: (*continued*) In (B), the nasal cannula is now functioning. Note the overamplification artifact in the EOG channels.

EOG, electrooculography.

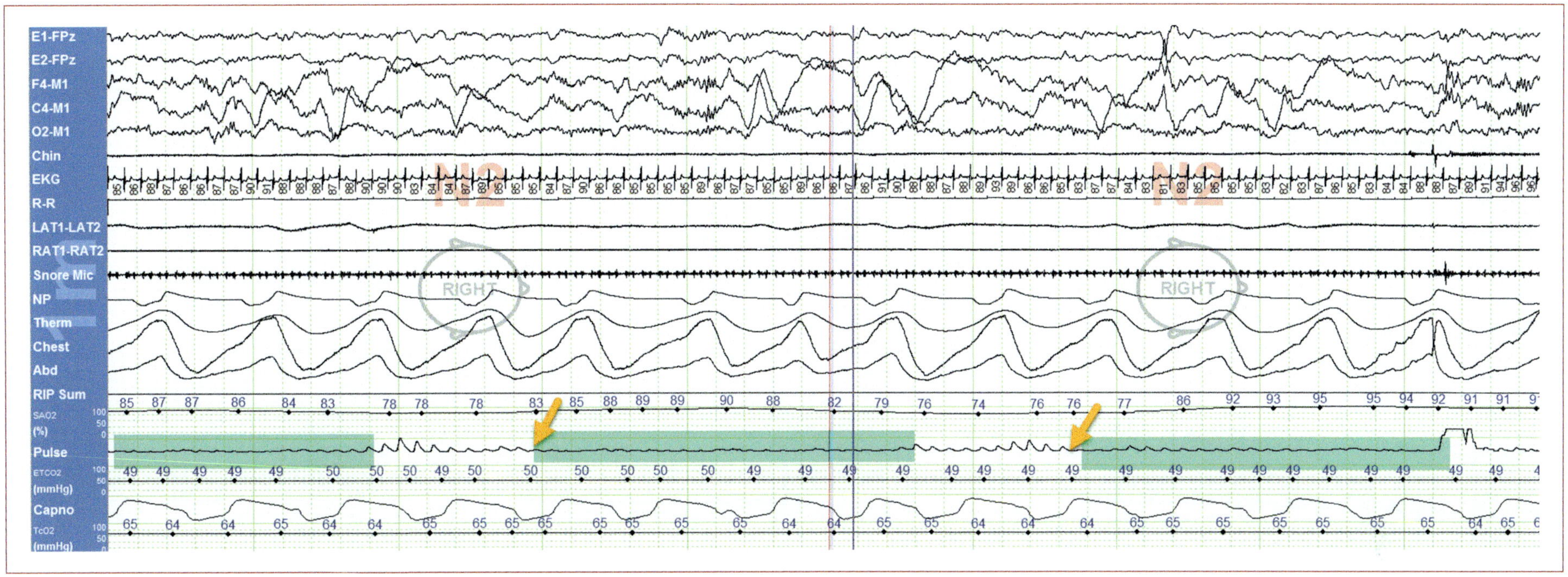

FIGURE 11.50: Pulse waveform blunted reflecting inaccurate recording. During this 60-second epoch of PSG, the nasal pressure sensor is inverted. Also observed are falsely low arterial oxygen saturations because of pulse oximeter signal, identified by flattening of the pulse waveform (pulse). Pulse waveforms are extraordinarily useful in confirming whether the pulse oximeter signal is "reliable." Observing a low SpO_2, one should confirm the pulse waveform is preserved. If it is blunted or absent, the SpO_2 signal is deemed unreliable.

PSG, polysomnography; SpO_2, peripheral capillary oxygen saturation.

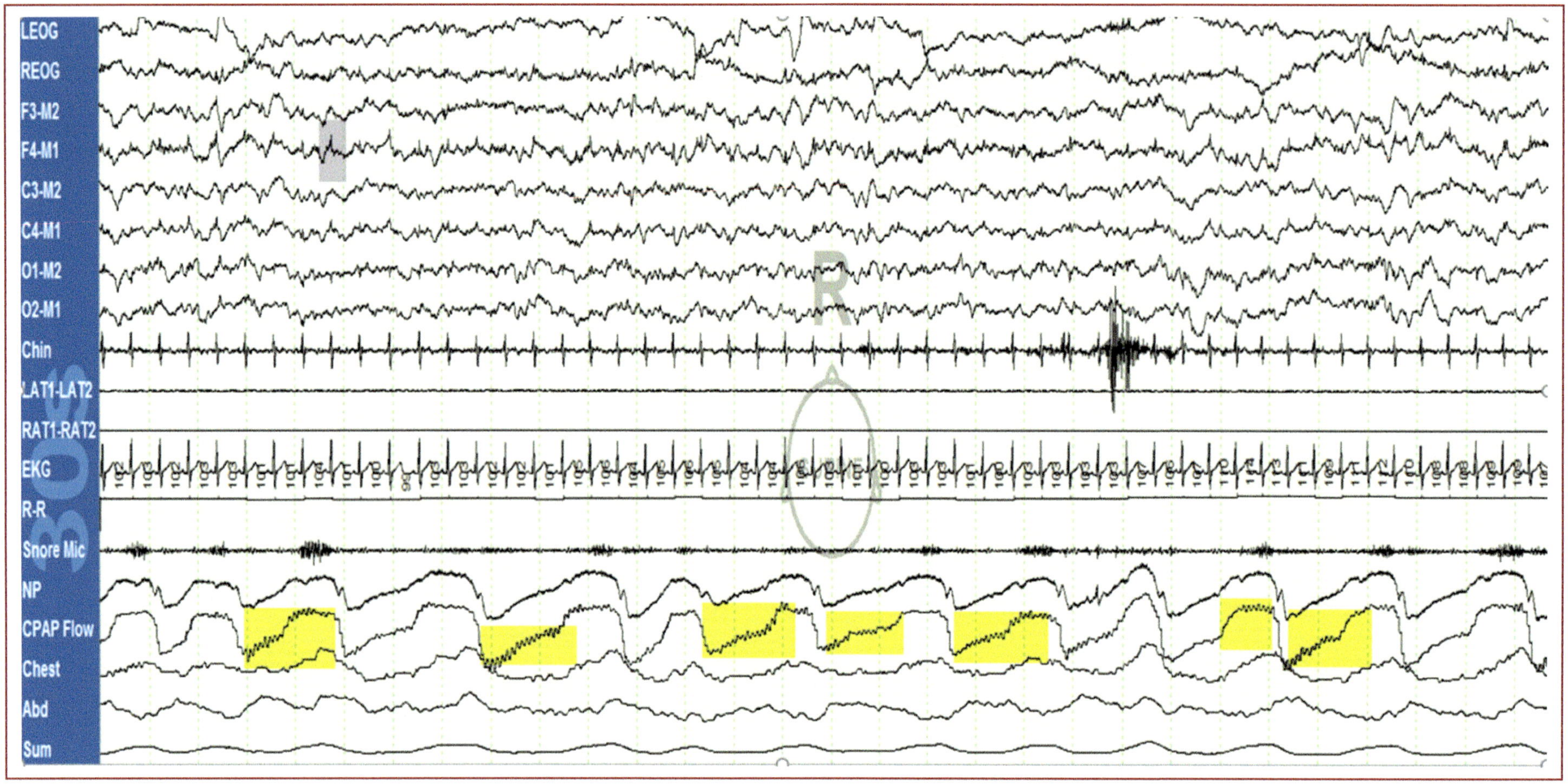

FIGURE 11.51: Water in nasal cannula tubing artifact. A 30-second epoch of PSG showing the impact of water in the nasal cannula tubing evidenced in the CPAP flow channel. It causes a fast undulating signal artifact. It appears as an M-shaped waveform with each breath as the water moves back and forth in the tubing. It occurs during diagnostic PSGs if the moisture gets into the cannula or the tubing connecting it to the nasal pressure sensor. This is often observed during CPAP titration if there is a mismatch between the room temperature and humidification in the CPAP circuit.

CPAP, continuous positive airway pressure; PSG, polysomnography.

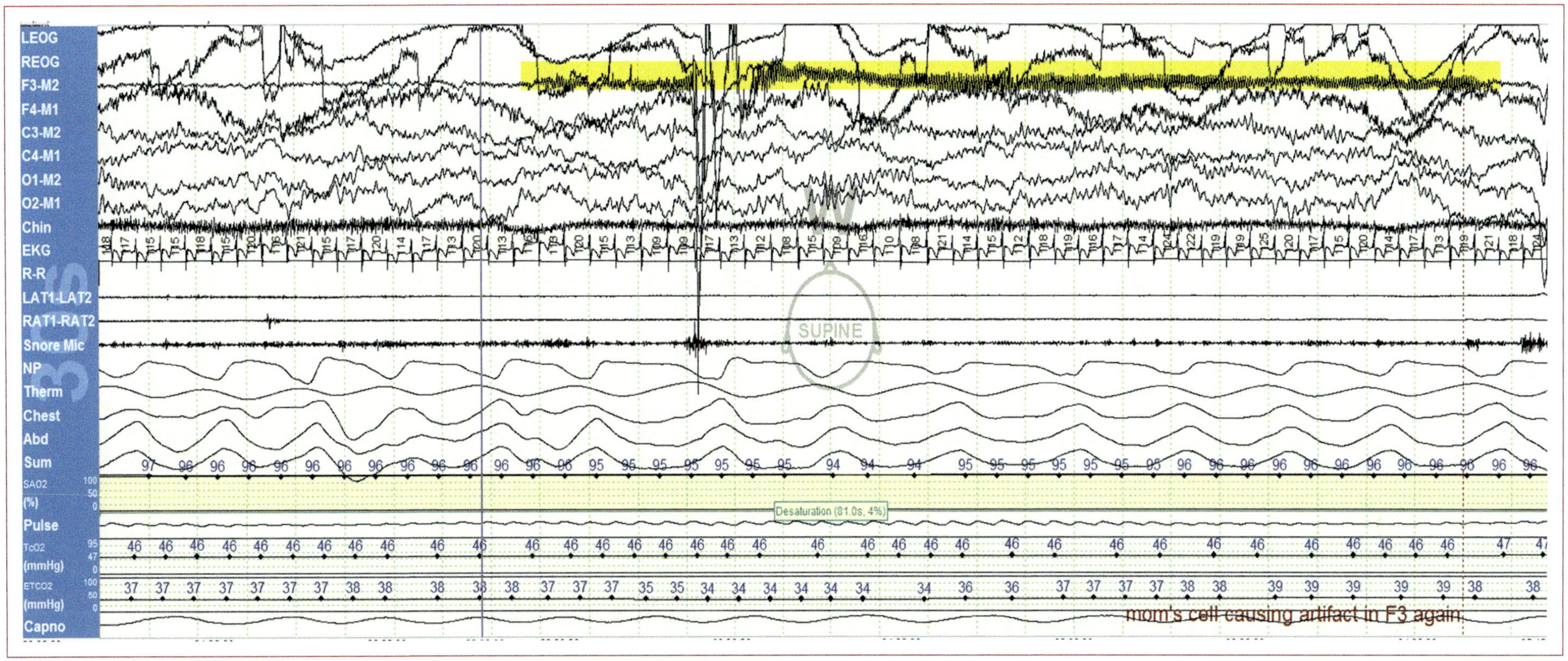

FIGURE 11.52: Cell phone artifact. A 40-second epoch of PSG shows the mother's cell phone ringing and causing artifact in the F3-M2 derivation. The mother was in bed with the child near the right side of the child's head. In response to recognizing the artifact, the technologist requested the mother place the cell phone at least 3 feet away from the bed.

PSG, polysomnography.

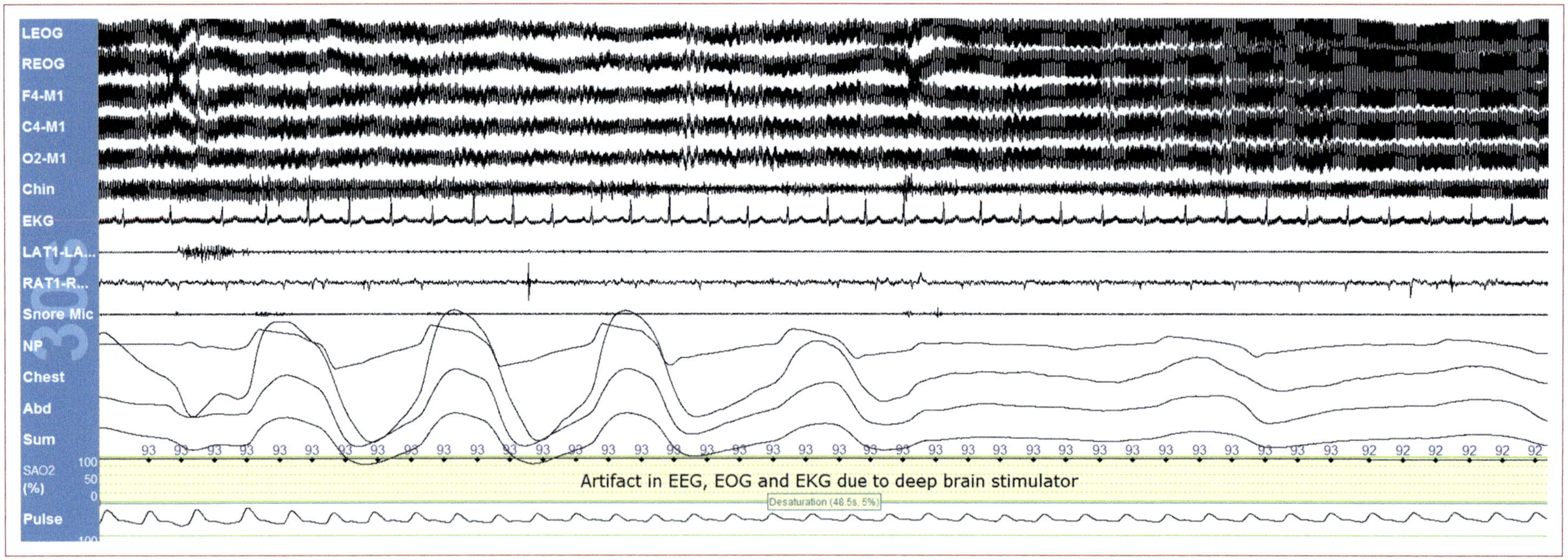

FIGURE 11.53: DBS artifact. A 30-second epoch of PSG showing 60-Hz interference artifact in the EOG, EEG, and ECG channels sparing the respiratory and limb EMG signals. This patient had a DBS and refused to turn it off. DBSs are used in the United States to treat Parkinson's disease, dystonia, neuropsychiatric disorders, and drug-resistant epilepsy. DBS generates electrical artifact which affects every PSG signal recorded using AC. Bipolar DBS cause fewer artifacts than unipolar DBS. Unfortunately, turning off the DBS during the recording often results in emergence of tremor artifact in patients with Parkinson's disease and may create a different type of artifact in the PSG. Bilateral monopolar DBS produces a high-frequency artifact which obscures most channels of EEG and is more pronounced in those channels with long interelectrode distances.

AC, alternating current; DBS, deep brain stimulator; EMG, electromyography; EOG, electrooculography; PSG, polysomnography.

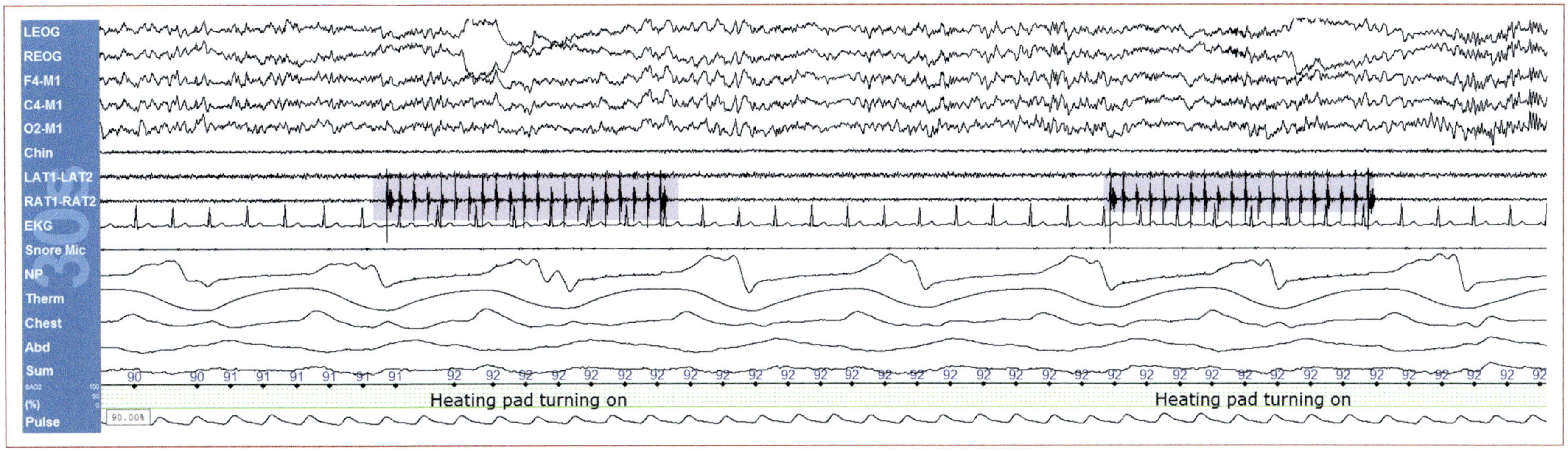

FIGURE 11.54: Heating blanket artifact. Repetitive electrical artifact present in the right leg EMG channels (RAT1-RAT2). This was not caused by hypnagogic foot tremor but a heating pad turning on and off.

EMG, electromyography.

REFERENCES

1. Epstein CM. Aliasing in the visual EEG: a potential pitfall of video display technology. *Clin Neurophysiol*. 2003;114(10):1974-1976. doi:10.1016/S1388-2457(03)00168-8.
2. Frysinger RC, Quigg M, Elias WJ. Bipolar deep brain stimulation permits routine EKG, EEG, and polysomnography. *Neurology*. 2006;66(2):268-270. doi:10.1212/01.wnl.0000194272.79084.7e.
3. Maher E, Epstein LJ. Artifacts and Troubleshooting. *Sleep Med Clin*. 2009;4:421-434. doi:10.1016/j.jsmc.2009.04.010.
4. Berry RB, Brooks R, Gamaldo CE, et al. for the American Academy of Sleep Medicine. *The AASM Manual for the Scoring of Sleep and Associated Events: Rules, Terminology and Technical Specifications. Version 2.4*. Darien, IL: American Academy of Sleep Medicine; 2017.
5. Muthukumaraswamy SD. High-frequency brain activity and muscle artifacts in MEG/EEG: a review and recommendations. *Front Hum Neurosci*. 2013;7:138. doi:10.3389/fnhum.2013.00138.
6. Wilde-Frenz J, Schulz H. Rate and distribution of body movements during sleep in humans. *Percept Mot Skills*. 1983;56(1):275-283. doi:10.2466/pms.1983.56.1.275.
7. De Koninck J, Lorrain D, Gagnon P. Sleep positions and position shifts in five age groups: an ontogenetic picture. *Sleep*. 1992;15(2):143-149.
8. Fisch BJ, Spehlmann R. *Fisch and Spehlmann's EEG Primer: Basic Principles of Digital and Analog EEG*. 3rd rev. and enl. ed. Amsterdam, the Netherlands; New York, NY: Elsevier; 1999.
9. Gwyther AR, Walters AS, Hill CM. Rhythmic movement disorder in childhood: an integrative review. *Sleep Med Rev*. 2017;35:62-75. doi:10.1016/j.smrv.2016.08.003.
10. Grigg-Damberger M, Ralls F. Primary sleep disorders and paroxysmal nocturnal nonepileptic events in adults with epilepsy from the perspective of sleep specialists. *J Clin Neurophysiol*. 2011;28(2):120-140. doi:10.1097/WNP.0b013e3182120fed.
11. Fish DR, Sawyers D, Allen PJ, et al. The effect of sleep on the dyskinetic movements of Parkinson's disease, Gilles de la Tourette syndrome, Huntington's disease, and torsion dystonia. *Arch Neurol*. 1991;48(2):210-214. doi:10.1001/archneur.1991.00530140106023.
12. Siddiqui F, Osuna E, Walters AS, et al. Sweat artifact and respiratory artifact occurring simultaneously in polysomnogram. *Sleep Med*. 2006;7(2):197-199. doi:1016/j.sleep.2005.11.013.
13. Silber MH, Ancoli-Israel S, Bonnet MH, et al. The visual scoring of sleep in adults. *J Clin Sleep Med*. 2007;3(2):121-131.
14. Klass DW. The continuing challenge of artifacts in the EEG. *Am J Electroneurodiagn Technol*. 1995;35:239-269. doi:10.5664/jcsm.5600.
15. Iwasaki M, Kellinghaus C, Alexopoulos AV, et al. Effects of eyelid closure, blinks, and eye movements on the electroencephalogram. *Clin Neurophysiol*. 2005;116(4):878-885. doi:10.1016/j.clinph.2004.11.001.
16. Tassinari CA, Cantalupo G, Hogl B, et al. Neuroethological approach to frontolimbic epileptic seizures and parasomnias: the same central pattern generators for the same behaviours. *Rev Neurol (Paris)*. 2009;165(10):762-768. doi:10.1016/j.neurol.2009.08.002.
17. Hoque R, Delrosso L. Persistent low oxygen saturation on polysomnogram. *J Clin Sleep Med*. 2013;9(9):967-969. doi:10.5664/jcsm.3006.
18. Rasquinha RJ, Moszczynski AJ, Murray BJ. A modern artifact in the sleep laboratory. *J Clin Sleep Med*. 2012;8(2):225-226. doi:10.5664/jcsm.1792.
19. Duan X. Electrocardiographic artifact due to a mobile phone mimicking ventricular tachycardia. *J Electrocardiol*. 2014;47(3):333-334. doi:10.1016/j.jelectrocard.2014.01.008.
20. Myers KA. Cell phone saccades: electroencephalographic artifact for the twenty-first century. *Pediatr Neurol*. 2016;63:82-83. doi:10.1016/j.pediatrneurol.2016.06.010.
21. Mahmoud Pashazadeh A, Aghajani M, Nabipour I, et al. An update on mobile phones interference with medical devices. *Radiat Prot Dosim*. 2013;156(4):401-406. doi:10.1093/rpd/nct091.
22. Marzec M, Edwards J, Sagher O, et al. Effects of vagus nerve stimulation on sleep-related breathing in epilepsy patients. *Epilepsia*. 2003;44(7):930-935. doi:10.1046/j.1528-1157.2003.56202.
23. Parhizgar F, Nugent K, Raj R. Obstructive sleep apnea and respiratory complications associated with vagus nerve stimulators. *J Clin Sleep Med*. 2011;7(4):401-407. doi:10.5664/JCSM.1204.
24. Zaaimi B, Grebe R, Berquin P, Wallois F. Vagus nerve stimulation induces changes in respiratory sinus arrhythmia of epileptic children during sleep. *Epilepsia*. 2009;50(11):2473-2480. doi:10.1111/j.1528-1167.2009.02190.x.
25. Zaaimi B, Héberlé C, Berquin P, et al. Vagus nerve stimulation induces concomitant respiratory alterations and a decrease in SaO_2 in children. *Epilepsia*. 2005;46(11):1802-1809. doi:10.1111/j.1528-1167.2005.00283.x.

CHAPTER 12

Artifacts in Evoked Potential Recordings

Alan D. Legatt

INTRODUCTION

Evoked potentials (EPs) are the electrical signals produced by the nervous system in response to external stimulation. The term was initially restricted to sensory EPs, elicited most often by visual, auditory, or somatosensory stimulation (1), but has more recently been expanded (2) to include motor evoked potentials (MEPs), which are signals generated in neural tissue (such as the spinal cord) or in muscles following electrical or magnetic stimulation of the descending motor tracts in the brain (3).

The recording electrodes placed on the subject pick up a variety of other signals in addition to the desired EP. These other signals, which may be labeled "artifacts," are the subjects of this chapter. Some of them are of physiologic origin, such as ECG, EEG, the electrooculogram (EOG), and electromyographic (EMG) activity from muscles near the recording electrodes. Others, such as the electrical stimulus artifact, are related to the stimuli used to elicit the EPs. Some degree of pickup of the power line frequency is almost inevitable. And during neurophysiologic intraoperative monitoring (NIOM) of EPs, there are many other possible sources of artifact from other equipment in the operating room. Some of these artifacts are orders of magnitude larger in amplitude than the EPs (4).

A voltage cannot be measured in isolation; all EP recordings measure voltage differences between pairs of electrodes. Some signals, such as line frequency artifact, are widely distributed over the patient's body and therefore are picked up at approximately the same amplitude by all of the recording electrodes. Ideally, the differential amplifiers in the recording equipment will amplify the voltage difference between the two amplifiers (the differential signal), whereas the signals that are present at both electrodes (the common-mode signal) will not appear in the amplifier output (a process called in-phase cancellation). The common-mode rejection ratio (CMRR) measures how well the amplifiers in the recording equipment approach that ideal; it is the ratio between the amplifier gain for the differential signal and that for the common-mode signal. EP guidelines call for a CMRR of at least 80 dB or 10,000:1 (5).

SIGNAL AVERAGING

In some cases, EPs are large enough to be clearly visible following a single stimulus, such as myogenic MEPs (recorded from muscles) (**Figure 12.1**). The relative sizes of visual evoked potentials (VEPs) to stroboscopic flash stimulation and the background EEG upon which they are superimposed determines whether the VEPs are visible in the raw data; when they are, they are labeled a "photic driving response" (**Figure 12.2**). In contrast, brainstem auditory evoked potentials (BAEPs) are a fraction of a microvolt in amplitude, and are never visible in scalp-recorded data. Signal averaging is used to extract them (**Figure 12.3**), as well as VEPs, somatosensory evoked potentials (SEPs), and D-waves (neurogenic MEPs recorded from the spinal cord) from the other electrical signals picked up by the recording electrodes. Each epoch or sweep of data can be regarded as the sum of the EP and of all the other unrelated electrical signals, which for the purposes of EP recording, can be regarded as "noise." In most cases, the EP is identical from trial to trial, since the same stimulus is being given to the same nervous system, and is therefore unaltered by the averaging process. The noise, in contrast, is random. Thus, at a given poststimulus latency, the noise polarity will sometimes be positive and sometimes negative, and will tend to cancel when the epochs are summated. Dividing the summed epochs by the number of epochs included in the average (*N*) further decreases the amplitude of the residual noise. Quantitatively, the amplitude of the residual noise in the average will approximate the typical noise amplitude in a single epoch divided by the square root of *N*. The signal-to-noise ratio is therefore multiplied by the square root of *N* (4). Even if VEPs are visible in the raw data (**Figure 12.2**), signal averaging is used to attenuate the superimposed EEG signal and therefore make the representation of the VEP waveform more accurate.

The number of epochs per average is a compromise. Increasing the number of epochs gives "cleaner" signals with a better signal-to-noise ratio but takes longer. During extraoperative diagnostic EP studies, this will require subject cooperation for a longer period of time; during NIOM, it may cause increased delay before the surgeons are notified about significant EP changes. Measures taken to decrease the amount of noise in the raw data, such as subject relaxation to decrease EMG noise from muscle tension in head and neck muscles during a clinical BAEP study, are useful. Epochs containing an unusually large amount of noise are identified by automatic artifact rejection and are excluded from the average.

Signal averaging is not an intelligent process; it selectively attenuates signals that do not correlate with stimulus delivery, while retaining those that are time-locked with stimulus delivery, such as the EPs. If the repetition rate of the stimulus is a submultiple of the line frequency (e.g., 2, 3, 5, 6, 10, or 12 per second in North America where the line frequency is 60 Hz), then the inevitable line frequency artifact will be phase-locked with stimulus delivery and will be identical in each sweep; therefore, it will be preserved in the average just as the EP is. Timing circuits can drift, causing the stimulus repetition frequency to become a subharmonic of the line frequency. Therefore, if line frequency artifact becomes troublesome (e.g., during NIOM) and the amount of line frequency artifact in the raw data does not appear to have increased, a small change in the stimulus repetition rate may be useful (6). The same principle applies to higher frequency sinusoidal artifact, to which the stimulus repetition rate may have become harmonically entrained (**Figure 12.4**). Whenever a sinusoidal artifact appears in EP data, the presence of line frequency or higher harmonic artifact should be suspected. The frequency of the artifact can be determined by measuring its period or peak-to-peak latency in milliseconds, and dividing this into 1,000 (6).

The one type of EP for which signal averaging is not used is myogenic MEPs because they often differ markedly from trial to trial (**Figure 12.5**), most likely because a different subset of motor units is recruited each time. Fortunately, myogenic MEPs are typically orders of magnitude larger than sensory EPs, with a signal-to-noise ratio that permits them to be easily identified in unaveraged recordings.

Physiologic Artifacts Arising From Signals Originating Within the Patient's Body

Electrocardiogram

Artifact from the ECG is most prominent at electrodes close to the heart, such as SEP recording electrodes at Erb's point or on the posterior part of the neck. ECG artifact may cause some sweeps to be rejected, but usually this is not problematic unless the stimulus repetition rate and the cardiac rate are harmonically synchronized, so that a large percentage of the epochs contain prominent ECG artifact and are rejected. If it seems that too many sweeps are being rejected because of the ECG, a small alteration in the stimulus repetition rate may eliminate that harmonic relationship and lead to more epochs being included in the average.

Electroencephalogram

EP recording electrodes on the head invariably pick up EEG activity, and signal averaging is used to reduce this. In patients with high-voltage EEGs, such as normal children, adolescents, and especially young children with an epileptic encephalopathy and abnormal high-voltage EEGs (e.g., hypsarrhythmia), the amount of EEG "noise" in the unaveraged EP raw data will be greater. Consequently, EP recordings may be noisier (**Figure 12.6**), and averaging a larger number of epochs may be necessary to produce sufficiently clean recordings. For typical SEP filter settings, slower frequencies of the EEG (e.g., theta and delta) will be removed by the filtering; however, it is the faster frequencies that contaminate the EP waveforms. High-voltage EEG activity in the alpha and beta frequency bands (**Figure 12.6B**), as well as the faster frequencies contained in EEG spikes, may have periods of tens of milliseconds, and thus may appear "slow" when viewed at the time window of the EP recording (**Figure 12.6A**).

Electrooculogram

The retina of the eye generates a corneoretinal potential, with the cornea electropositive with respect to the retina. The magnitude of this potential, which is in the millivolt range, is affected by ambient light levels. When the light level changes, it takes 10 to 15 minutes for the potential to change (7). Such slow (low-frequency) potential changes would be removed by bandpass filtering during standard EP recordings. However, when the eyes move, the equivalent dipole of the corneoretinal potential can shift rapidly, producing artifacts in the EOG that are commonly seen in the EEG. EP recording electrodes on the anterior part of the head can also pick up EOG signals, though these will mostly be removed from the recordings by filtering and artifact rejection.

Electromyogram

EMG artifact from muscle tension in the head and neck muscles may cause prominent artifact during EP recordings, especially when recording SEPs and BAEPs where the EPs are small in amplitude and the high-frequency filter setting is high enough so that the EMG artifact is not removed by filtering. Dorsal scalp electrodes may be located over an aponeurosis rather than muscle, so recordings of cortical SEPs tend to be less contaminated by muscle artifact. Increased noise levels in subcortical SEP channels can give an indication of a light depth of anesthesia during NIOM (**Figure 12.7**). During clinical, extraoperative recordings of SEPs and BAEPs, muscle relaxation is important to obtain "clean" recordings. In the past, sedative medications such as diazepam were used in some EP laboratories to facilitate patient relaxation. But, like the use of chloral hydrate for EEG recordings, this has largely been abandoned due to the many safety constraints and personnel and monitoring requirements for conscious sedation of patients (8,9).

Implanted Electrical Stimulators

Implanted electrical stimulators such as cardiac pacemakers and deep brain stimulation (DBS) systems can introduce artifact into the EP raw data. Like ECG artifact, cardiac pacemaker artifact is infrequent and individual epochs containing it can be eliminated by automatic artifact rejection. DBS stimulation is more pervasive and produces large artifacts that may be recorded from the head (**Figure 12.8B**) which can cause rejection of all epochs with the usual artifact rejection settings. Even if the artifact rejection window is widened and automatic artifact rejection is turned off, the SEP waveforms will be markedly contaminated by artifact (**Figure 12.8A**).

Stimulus Artifact

During recording of SEPs to stimulation of peripheral nerves and of MEPs to transcranial electrical stimulation, large electrical stimuli that may be many volts in amplitude are applied directly to the patient's body. While they may be substantially attenuated by distance, when they reach the recording electrodes they are still often as large as, or larger than, the EPs being recorded. These signals appear as electrical stimulus artifacts at the beginning of the data epoch (**Figures 12.9A** and **12.10**). Inductive or capacitive coupling between the wires carrying the stimuli to the patient and the recording electrode lead wires can also contribute to the stimulus artifacts. During BAEP recordings, no electricity is applied to the patient's body, but the transducer that converts the electrical square-wave pulse to the acoustic click typically contains a coil, and by inductive coupling can produce electrical signals in the patient recording transmitted by the lead wires to produce a stimulus artifact (**Figures 12.11A** and **12.12**). The use of shielded headphones and headphones with piezoelectric transducers rather than voice coil transducers can reduce the stimulus artifact in the BAEP waveforms (10).

BAEP stimuli can be compression clicks, in which a wave of increased air pressure is delivered to the patient's ear, or rarefaction clicks, in which the electrical signal delivered to the transducer is opposite in polarity and a wave of decreased air pressure is delivered. BAEPs to rarefaction and compression clicks may differ; therefore, a single click polarity is preferred for extraoperative diagnostic BAEP studies, unless alternating polarities are necessary for canceling the electrical stimulus artifact or the cochlear microphonic. During NIOM of BAEPs, where artifacts are often more problematic, alternating stimulus polarity can be used by default to (partially) cancel the electrical stimulus artifact. It will also tend to cancel the cochlear microphonic, which otherwise might hamper the identification of wave I (11).

Audiometric headphones are typically used for stimulus delivery during extraoperative diagnostic BAEP studies, but are not practical for NIOM. The electromechanical transducer that converts the electrical square pulses to clicks is housed in a small box that is located at some distance from the patient's ear, and conducted to the ear via plastic tube that is several centimeters long. This helps mitigate stimulus artifact problems in two ways. The BAEPs, including wave I, are delayed by the time required for the acoustic stimulus to propagate through the plastic tube (typically 0.9–1.0 milliseconds). However, the electrical stimulus artifact remains simultaneous with transducer activation and the increased temporal separation between them permits greater decay of the stimulus artifact prior to the onset of wave I. The increased separation between the electrical wires/transducer and the patient's head also serves to reduce the amplitude of the electrical stimulus artifact (11).

Since the stimulus artifact in an SEP waveform reflects the stimulation current that reaches the patient's body, it can be used to evaluate whether the stimulus is still being delivered. If SEPs deteriorate due to neurologic dysfunction (**Figure 12.9**), the stimulus artifact will remain unchanged. In contrast, the stimulus artifact will be altered if technical problems are interfering with delivery of the stimulus to the patient (**Figure 12.10**). With constant current stimulators, the EP recording system typically indicates an open circuit or impedance limit condition when it cannot deliver the preset stimulating current intensity, such as when lead wires are disconnected or stimulating electrodes are dislodged. In contrast, the SEP alterations shown in **Figure 12.10** were caused by a short circuit between the stimulating lead wires. In this case, the equipment was able to deliver the preset stimulating current intensity and therefore gave no error indication.

During BAEP recordings, an unchanged stimulus artifact only indicates an absence of problems with the recording equipment, the wire coil within the transducer, and the electrical connection between them. Technical problems with the conduction of the acoustic stimulus to the patient's ear can still alter the BAEPs without affecting the stimulus artifact (**Figure 12.12**).

Line Frequency Artifact

Line frequency artifact is ubiquitous, derived from the electrical wiring, the lights, and the various pieces of equipment connected to the patient or in the patient's vicinity. The scalp potentials induced by the electromagnetic field produced by the electrical wiring and room lighting can reach 100 mV. Fortunately, this is relatively uniform, and thus can be markedly reduced or eliminated by in-phase cancellation (4). Fluid warmers, used during surgery to avoid infusing cold intravenous fluids, can generate much larger amounts of 60-Hz artifact (**Figure 12.13**). The fluid warmer contains a coil of wire through which alternating current (AC) electricity is passed to generate heat. This acts as the primary coil of a transformer, and prominent 60-Hz artifact can be induced in nearby conductors, including the lead wires for the NIOM electrodes. Temporarily turning off the fluid warmer can identify it as the source of the artifact if it resolves. Rotating the fluid warmer or the pole to which it is attached can reduce the artifact by altering the electromagnetic coupling between the fluid warmer coil and the lead wires. Improperly grounded equipment connected to the patient can also produce line frequency artifact due to leakage currents. During NIOM, the operating table can be a prominent source of line frequency artifact; I have encountered situations in which this occurred because the ground lug of the operating table's power cord, or the ground lug in the socket in the operating table to which the (female polarity) end of the power cord plugged in, was broken off.

Line frequency notch filters are often used during EEG recordings to eliminate line frequency artifact. Line frequency notch filters should not be used for SEP recordings, for two reasons (6): (a) spectral analysis demonstrates that the SEP waveform itself contains frequencies around 50 to 60 Hz, thus, use of the notch filter will substantially distort the SSEPs; (b) the notch filter may prolong the electrical artifact arising from the SEP stimulus into a long-lasting oscillation which will markedly obscure the SEP waveform (12) (**Figure 12.14**).

A notch filter is of limited utility for BAEP recordings, in which line frequency is already markedly attenuated by the high-frequency filter setting (typically 100–150 Hz). Higher harmonics of the line frequency, which might not be removed by band-pass filtering, would also not be removed by the line frequency notch filter.

Additional Sources of Artifact in EPs During NIOM

Electrocautery

Electrocautery uses high-frequency electrical currents to heat and cut tissue and coagulate bleeding. The cautery currents can travel widely through the patient's body, be detected at substantially greater amplitude by the recording electrodes, and contaminate the EP waveforms (waveforms at 12:15 in **Figure 12.7**). They can also trigger automatic artifact rejection (**Figure 12.11B**), but this is not inevitable. Some EP recording systems incorporate sensors that can be placed over the lead wires from the cautery equipment, to detect when the cautery is active and block EP data acquisition even if the cautery artifact itself does not trigger automatic artifact rejection.

There are two types of electrocautery: bipolar and monopolar. In bipolar cautery, the current is passed between the two ends of a forceps that the surgeons place within the surgical field. In monopolar cautery, the surgeon uses an insulated wand with an uninsulated tip; the current return is a large pad, typically placed on the patient's leg. With monopolar cautery, the cautery currents spread widely through the patient's body, and are more likely to trigger artifact rejection. The artifact from monopolar cautery may be large enough to saturate the amplifier input stages of some EP recording systems, so EP acquisition is blocked for several seconds after the cautery current stops. Since direct current (DC) and low frequencies are removed by band-pass filtering, the amplifier outputs rapidly return to near zero, and the data epochs are not rejected as artifactual. This may result in the incorporation of many sweeps of essentially zero data into the averages. EP latencies will not be altered but amplitudes may appear to be significantly attenuated. To manage this problem, averaging must be paused until the amplified and digitized raw data have clearly recovered, which may take several seconds (13).

With monopolar cautery, the amount of current passing through the current return pad is the same as the current passing through the wand tip; no injury occurs under the pad because the area is large and the current density is low. If the pad were to become dislodged so that only a small area was contacting the patient, the current density would be high and a burn could result. Also, if the electrical connection to the current return pad was interrupted (e.g., due to broken or disconnected lead wires), the cautery current could return through other paths, such as parts of the operating table touching the patient's body or the NIOM electrodes, causing burns there. In order to avoid this, many monopolar cautery systems incorporate a return electrode quality monitoring system, in which the return electrode is split into two halves (both of which return the high cautery current) and the resistance of the circuit for passing a small monitoring current between the two halves of the pad is measured (14). Although the monitoring current is small, it can cause artifact in recording electrodes near the ground pad (Figure 12.15).

Ultrasonic Aspirators

Ultrasonic aspirator devices use ultrasonic vibrations to pulverize tissue into a form that can be washed away by saline irrigation and suctioning, without traction on underlying structures. The irrigation and suction ports are incorporated into the same surgical instrument as the ultrasonic vibrator. The ultrasonic vibrations can cause high-frequency artifact which may not be large enough to trigger automatic artifact rejection (Figure 12.11C) and thus can be incorporated in the EP data, causing high-frequency artifact (Figure 12.16), or creating an apparent lower frequency artifact because of aliasing (Figure 12.17).

Other Sources of Artifact During NIOM

Voltages are generated when dissimilar metals (e.g., surgical instruments, retractors, and NIOM electrodes) are in contact with an electrolyte (e.g., the patient's blood and tissue fluids), forming battery half-cell potentials. Electrostatic potentials can also be generated close to or within the surgical field (e.g., by surgical gloves rubbing against drapes) or more remotely by other mechanisms (e.g., by the surgeons' shoes rubbing on the floor) with intermittent transmission of the static electricity to the patient's body. The latter would be many orders of magnitude smaller than the thousands of volts in a typical static shock from touching a doorknob when the absolute humidity of the air is low and thus would not be visible or tactile, yet could still be many orders of magnitude larger than an EP. Artifacts from dissimilar metal potentials and electrostatic discharges are typically brief, though they may recur, and are usually mitigated by automatic artifact rejection.

Some operating microscopes (e.g., those with arc light sources) may generate artifacts that recur at the second harmonic of the line frequency as the alternating current through the arc stops and starts in either direction. Such artifacts may be sharply contoured (Figure 12.11D), with frequency spectra containing higher harmonics, so that a line frequency notch filter would not remove them.

Drills may also produce rhythmic artifacts, as the cutting edges on a rotating drill bit or bur repetitively contact tissue, due to dissimilar metals and/or electrostatic potentials (Figure 12.18). Drilling of the skull or of the roof of the internal auditory canal may interfere with BAEP recordings in another way: the high noise levels that are bone-conducted to the cochlea can attenuate the BAEPs due to acoustic masking (15,16).

Electric shavers can cause artifacts at the line frequency (Figure 12.19) since the blades are moved using a coil through which the line frequency AC is passed. As in the case of the fluid warmer, this may form the primary coil of a transformer. Shaver artifact may be problematic while attempting to establish baselines as the anesthetized patient is being prepped for surgery, but would not occur later on during the surgery after shaving is complete.

Measures to Prevent and Ameliorate Artifacts

Several measures to reduce artifacts during EP recordings, such as patient relaxation during extraoperative diagnostic EP studies or rotation of the fluid warmer during NIOM, have already been discussed. There are additional measures that can be taken to reduce artifact during EP recordings.

Electrodes that are making poor electrical contact with the subject are another source of artifact; impedances should be checked and kept below 5 kΩ when possible. Electrode impedances should be similar across the array of recording electrodes, since mismatched electrode impedances impair the rejection of common-mode signals (17) and may increase the degree to which widespread artifact (such as line frequency artifact) is present in the EP waveforms. Using various types of recording electrodes (e.g., needles, cup electrodes with electrode paste, and sticky pads) simultaneously and recording differentially between different types of electrodes will increase the chances of impedance mismatches.

In-phase cancellation removes signals present at the two inputs to a channel, such as ECG picked up by two electrodes on the head but not appearing in the differential recording between them. As the distance between the two electrodes that are inputs to the same recording channel is increased, the amount of artifact in that recording channel that is not in-phase canceled will increase. This may make it desirable to use alternative recording derivations, such as recording the P14 component of the median nerve SEP between two electrodes on the head rather than between an electrode on the head and a noncephalic electrode (18) (**Figure 12.20**).

Artifact may be picked up by the EP recording lead wires (in contrast to artifact coming from the patient's body) when they are acting as the secondary coil of a transformer. If the lead wires are located close to each other, the artifact they pick up will be very similar and can be reduced or eliminated by in-phase cancellation. Thus, use of twisted pair recording lead wires or braiding together of recording lead wires can help to reduce artifact.

In paired stimulation lead wires, the currents in the two wires are equal and opposite and therefore the magnetic fields that they produce will largely cancel out if the wires are located close to each other. Since stimulation lead wires can act as the primary coil of a transformer, inducing stimulus artifact in the recording lead wires, use of twisted pair stimulation lead wires can help to reduce the electrical stimulus artifact.

REPLICATION OF EP WAVEFORMS

Although signal averaging decreases noise (**Figure 12.3**), it does not eliminate it completely. Residual artifact in the averaged EP waveform could be misinterpreted as an EP peak. Therefore, during clinical diagnostic EP studies, all waveforms should be replicated (5) at least twice, and more times if it seems appropriate. For example, in the SEP waveforms in **Figure 12.20**, the N20 component in the first channel replicates nicely and represents a true EP signal; the deflections in the second channel, while equally large, do not replicate and represent artifact.

If there were no noise, the EP signals in the two replications would overlap exactly. Therefore, the spacing or difference between the two replications gives a visual estimate of the amount of residual noise remaining in the EP waveforms. Since noise peaks in the two repetitions could occasionally overlap by coincidence, replicating peaks that are as small as the difference between the two replications should be interpreted with caution.

During NIOM of EPs, serially recorded waveforms provide the replications needed to distinguish reproducible EP peaks from artifacts. If the amount of noise in the waveforms is similar to the amplitude of the EPs themselves, measures should be taken to identify the causes of the artifacts and try to reduce them. If necessary, the number of sweeps in the average can be increased. Alternatively, measures can be taken to increase the size of the EPs and therefore improve the signal-to-noise ratio. This may involve increases in the stimulus intensity, decreases in the stimulus rate, and changes in the anesthetic regimen to lessen anesthetic-related attenuation of the EPs that are prominently affected by anesthesia.

CONCLUSION

Understanding of the sources and mechanisms of artifacts and ways in which they can be eliminated or reduced can lead to an improvement in the quality of EP recordings, both during NIOM and during extraoperative diagnostic EP studies.

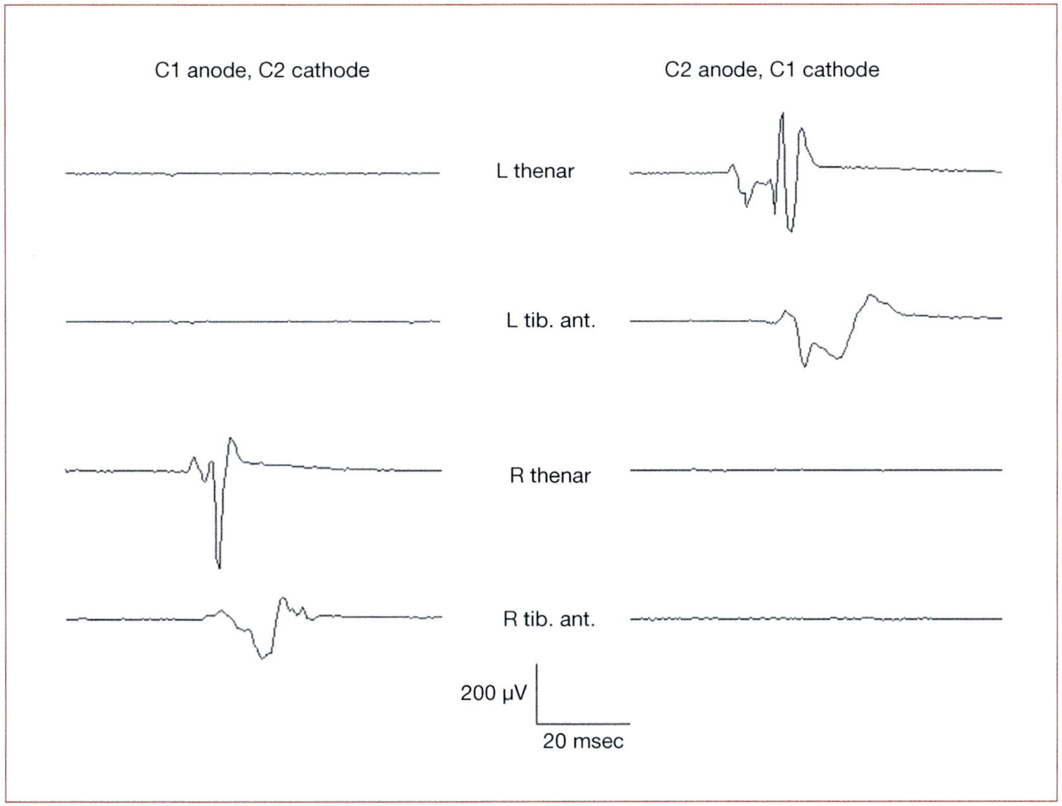

FIGURE 12.1: Myogenic MEPs derived from TES appear between electrodes at scalp positions C1 and C2 using both TES stimulus polarities. MEPs were recorded bilaterally from thenar and tibialis anterior muscles during an occipitocervical fusion. These are the responses to stimulation with a single stimulus train; no signal averaging was done (19).

MEP, motor evoked potential; TES, transcranial electrical stimulation.

Source: From Legatt AD, Emerson RG, Epstein CM, et al. ACNS guideline: transcranial electrical stimulation motor evoked potential monitoring. *J Clin Neurophysiol.* 2016;33(1):42-50. doi:10.1097/WNP.0000000000000253, with permission.

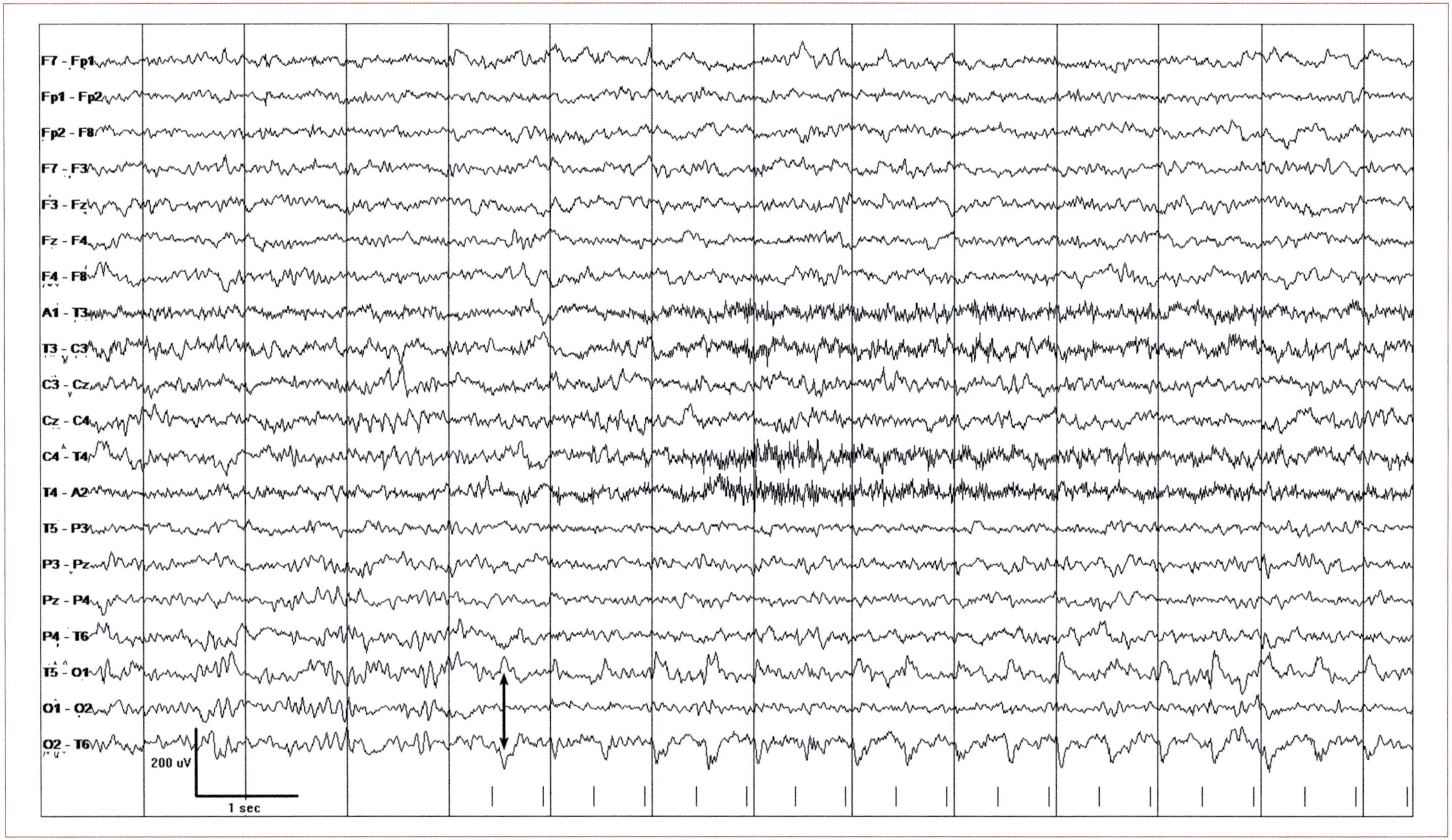

FIGURE 12.2: A prominent occipital photic driving response is shown in a transverse bipolar montage following stroboscopic flash stimulation at a rate of 2 per second in a 9-year-old girl. The vertical bars at the bottom, beginning in the fifth second, mark the timing of the strobe flashes. The double-headed arrow indicates the driving response (VEP) to the first strobe flash. The EEG, performed because of syncope, was normal for the girl's age in the awake and drowsy states.

VEP, visual evoked potential.

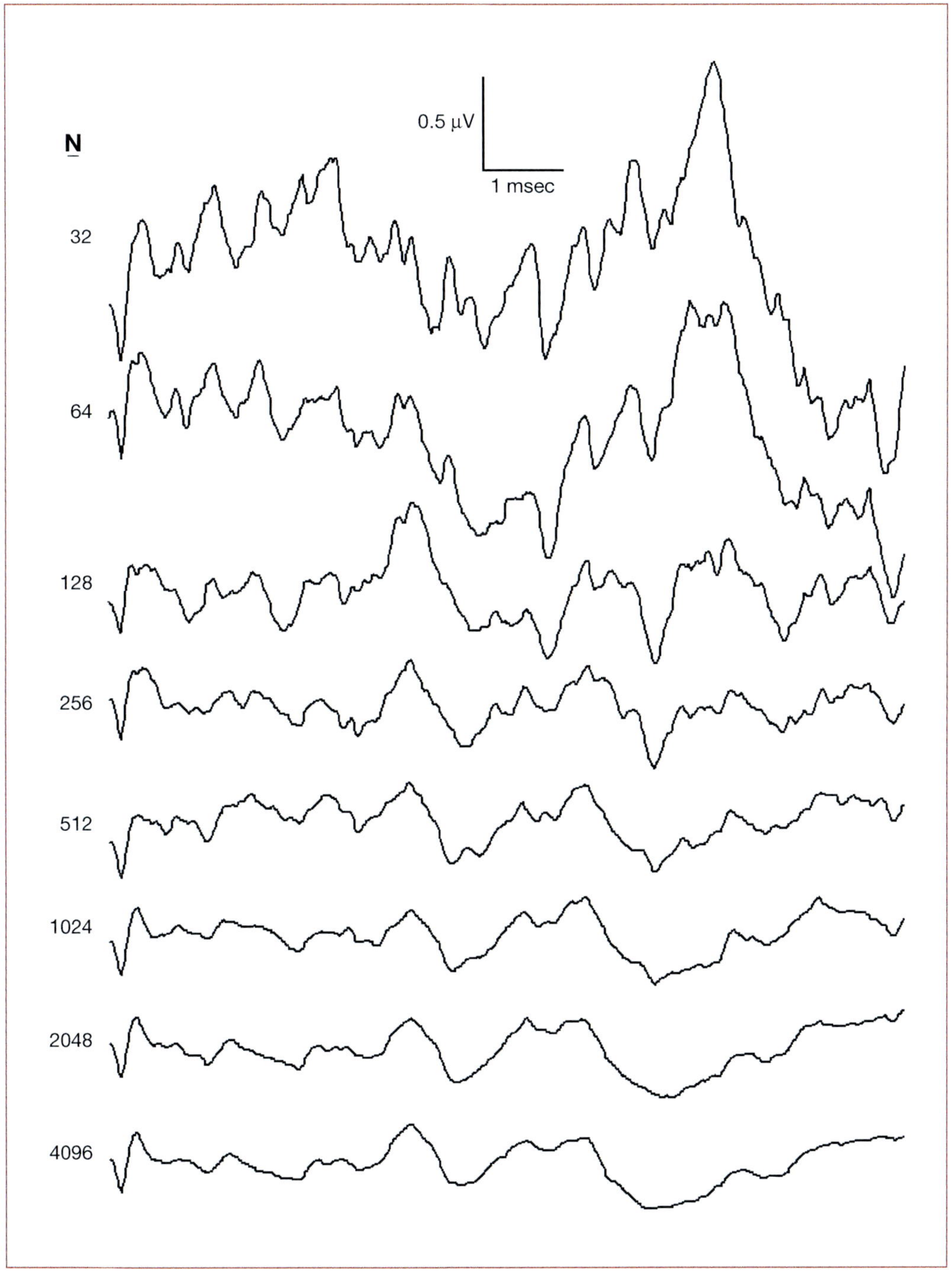

FIGURE 12.3: BAEPs to right-ear stimulation are demonstrated with a progressively increasing number of stimuli included in the averages. In this figure, the effect of signal averaging in improving the signal-to-noise ratio is evident. *N* = the number of sweeps in the average. Vertex-to-right mastoid recording is utilized. In this and subsequent BAEP figures, positive polarity at the vertex is plotted as an upward deflection (20).

BAEP, brainstem auditory evoked potential.

Source: From Legatt AD. Evoked potentials (EPs). In: Aminoff MJ, Daroff R, eds. *Encyclopedia of the Neurological Sciences*. 2nd ed. San Diego, CA: Elsevier Science; 2014:228-231, with permission.

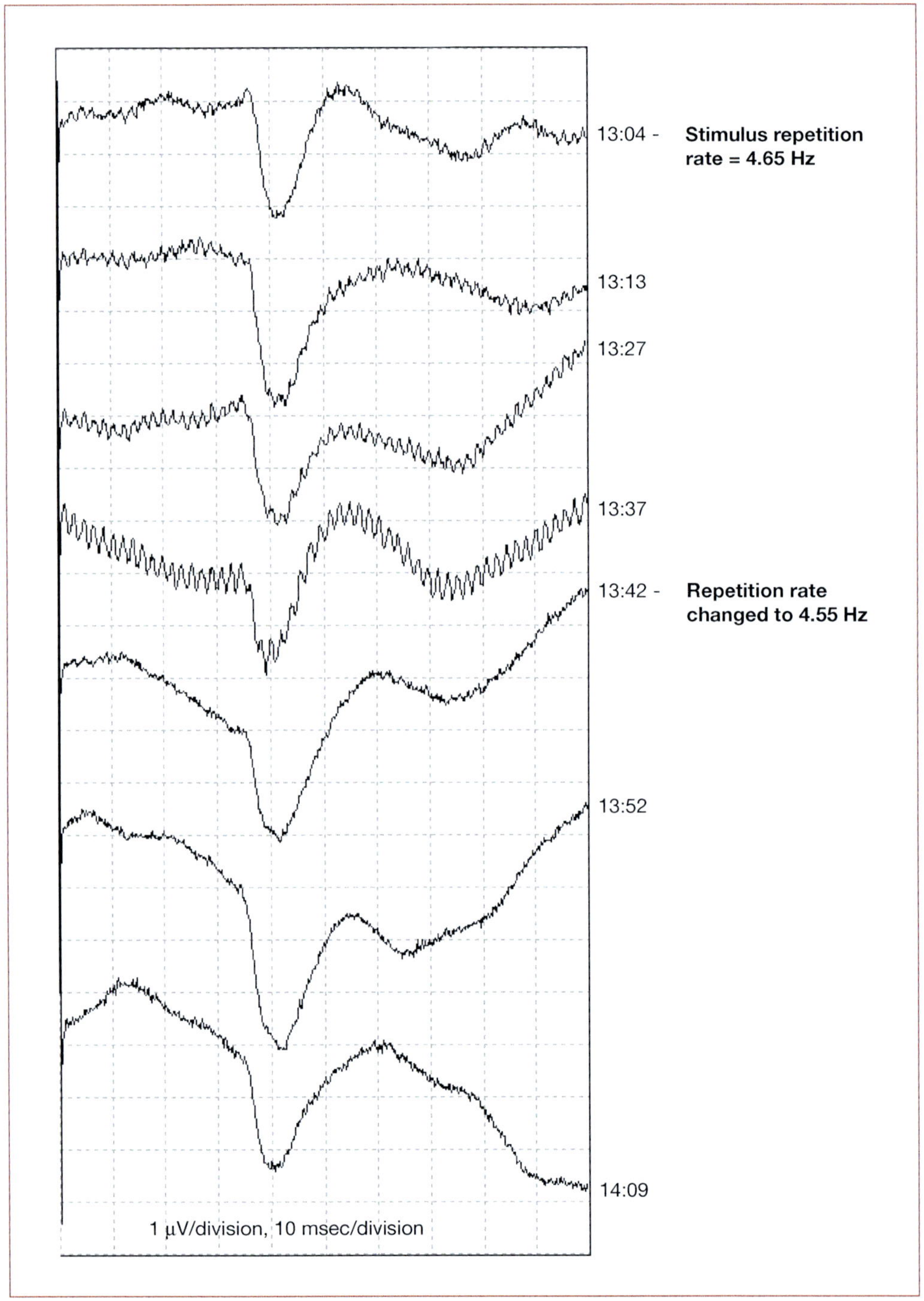

FIGURE 12.4: Cortical SEPs to right posterior tibial nerve stimulation recorded during surgery for removal of spinal instrumentation hardware that had become infected in a patient with scoliosis. Sinusoidal artifact with a calculated frequency of 540 Hz became increasingly prominent, but was eliminated from the averaged SEP waveforms by changing the stimulus repetition rate from 4.65 to 4.55 Hz. In this and subsequent SEP figures, negativity at input 1 is plotted as an upward deflection.

SEP, somatosensory evoked potential.

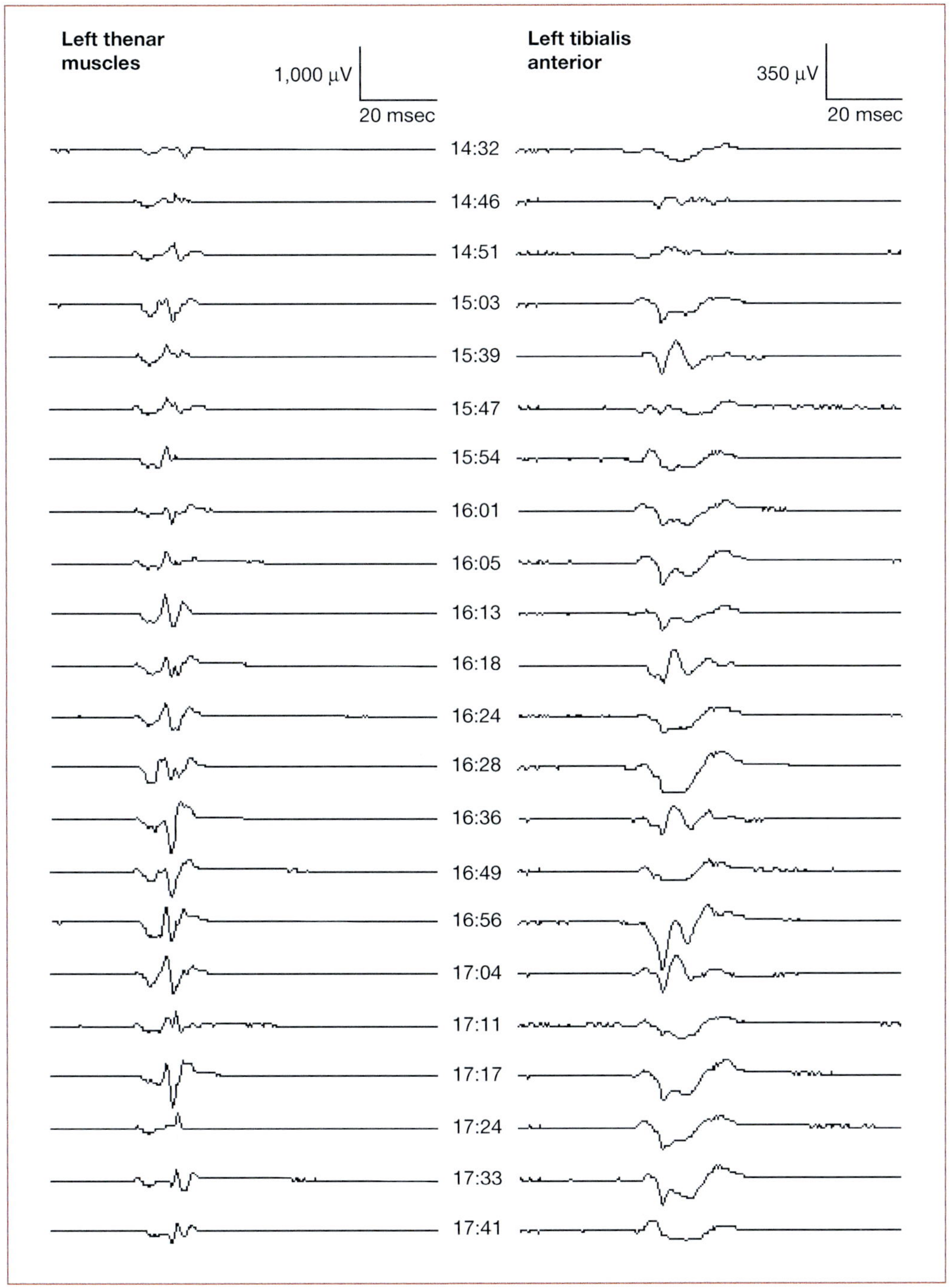

FIGURE 12.5: Myogenic MEPs recorded from the left tibialis anterior and thenar muscles following pulse-train transcranial electrical stimulation with the anode at C2 and the cathode at C1 over a 3-hour period during an occipitocervical fusion. Note the large run-to-run variability of the MEP amplitudes and waveforms. The numbers in the middle are the clock times of each run (21).

MEP, motor evoked potential.

Source: From Legatt AD. Ellen R. Grass lecture: motor evoked potential monitoring. *Am J Electroneurodiagn Technol*. 2004;44(4):223-243. Reprinted by permission of the publisher Taylor & Francis Ltd.

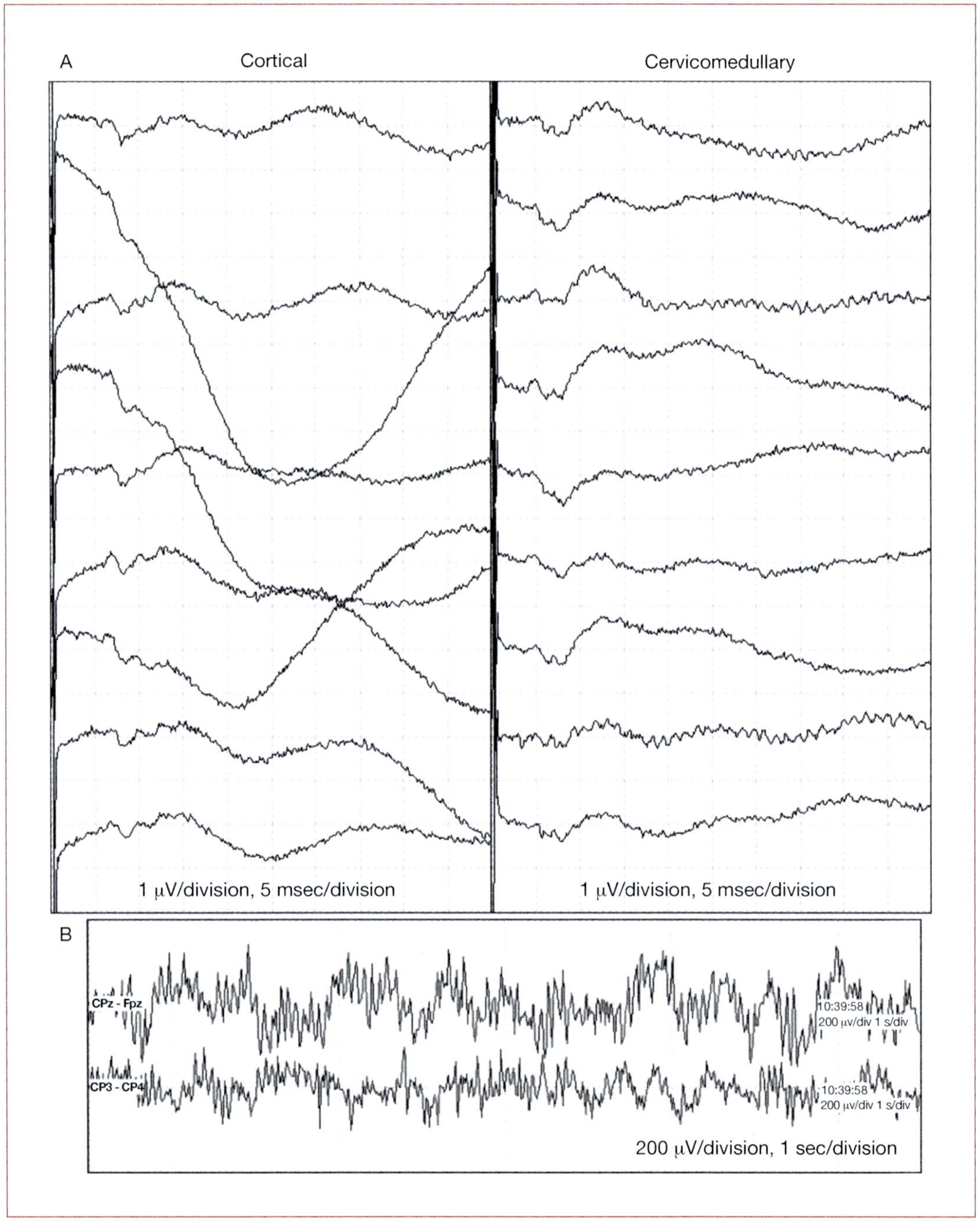

FIGURE 12.6: (A) Consecutive left ulnar nerve SEP runs recorded during surgery for release of tethered spinal cord and resection of sacral lipoma in a 2-year-old girl with a history of lipomeningomyelocele repair, sacral dysgenesis, microcephaly, diffuse polymicrogyria, developmental delay, and epilepsy. The SEPs themselves are visible between 5 and 15 millseconds post-stimulus. Large, variable, and much slower deflections derived from the faster frequencies of the EEG are seen prominently in the cortical SEP recording channels but do not contaminate the cervical SEP recording channels as much. (B) Two-channel EEG recorded during surgery, showing the high-voltage EEG with prominent alpha and beta frequency activity. Routine EEG in this patient in the unanesthetized state showed excessive beta activity as well as right and left central spikes.

SEP, somatosensory evoked potential.

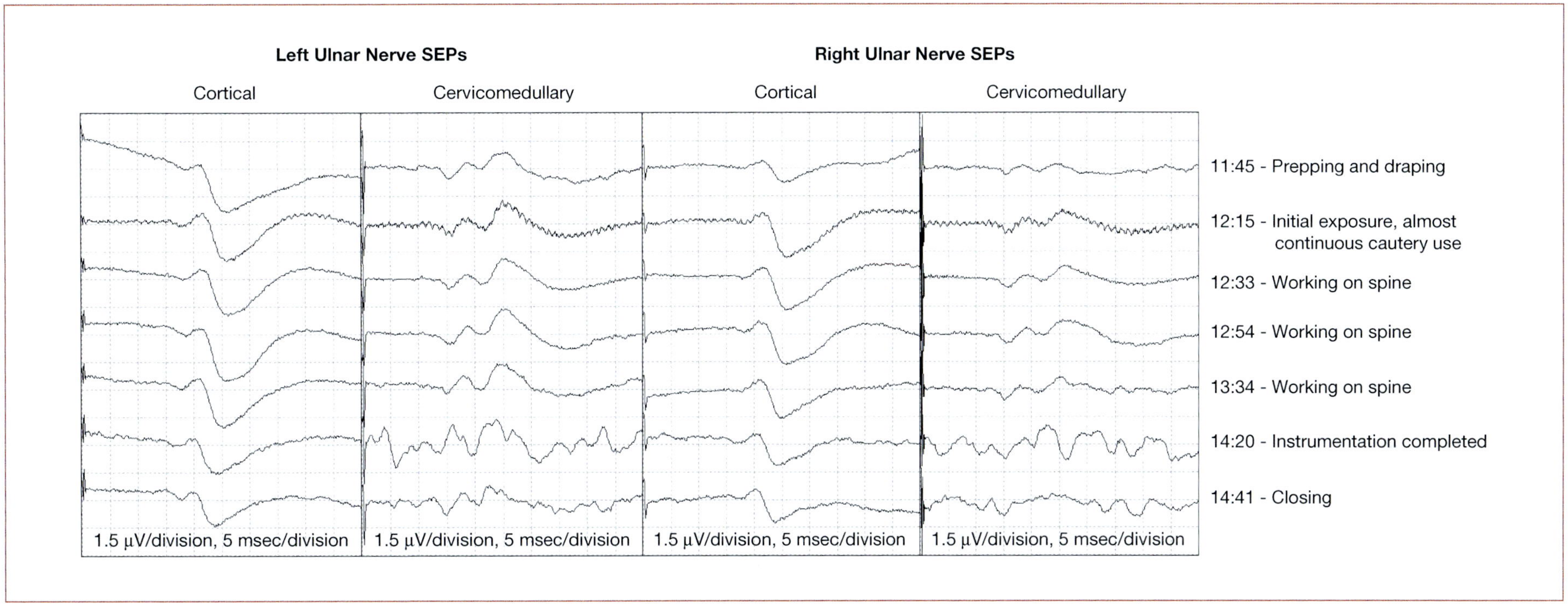

FIGURE 12.7: Ulnar nerve SEPs recorded during lumbar decompression and fusion surgery in a 39-year-old man. During the initial exposure, some data epochs containing cautery artifact escaped automatic artifact rejection and contaminated the waveforms at 12:15 with sinusoidal interference. During the latter part of the operation, the neuromuscular blockade had worn off, the depth of anesthesia was lighter, and some muscle tone was present. The resultant EMG contamination of the SEP waveforms at 14:20 and 14:41 was most prominent in the cervicomedullary SEP recording channels.

EMG, electromyography; SEP, somatosensory evoked potential.

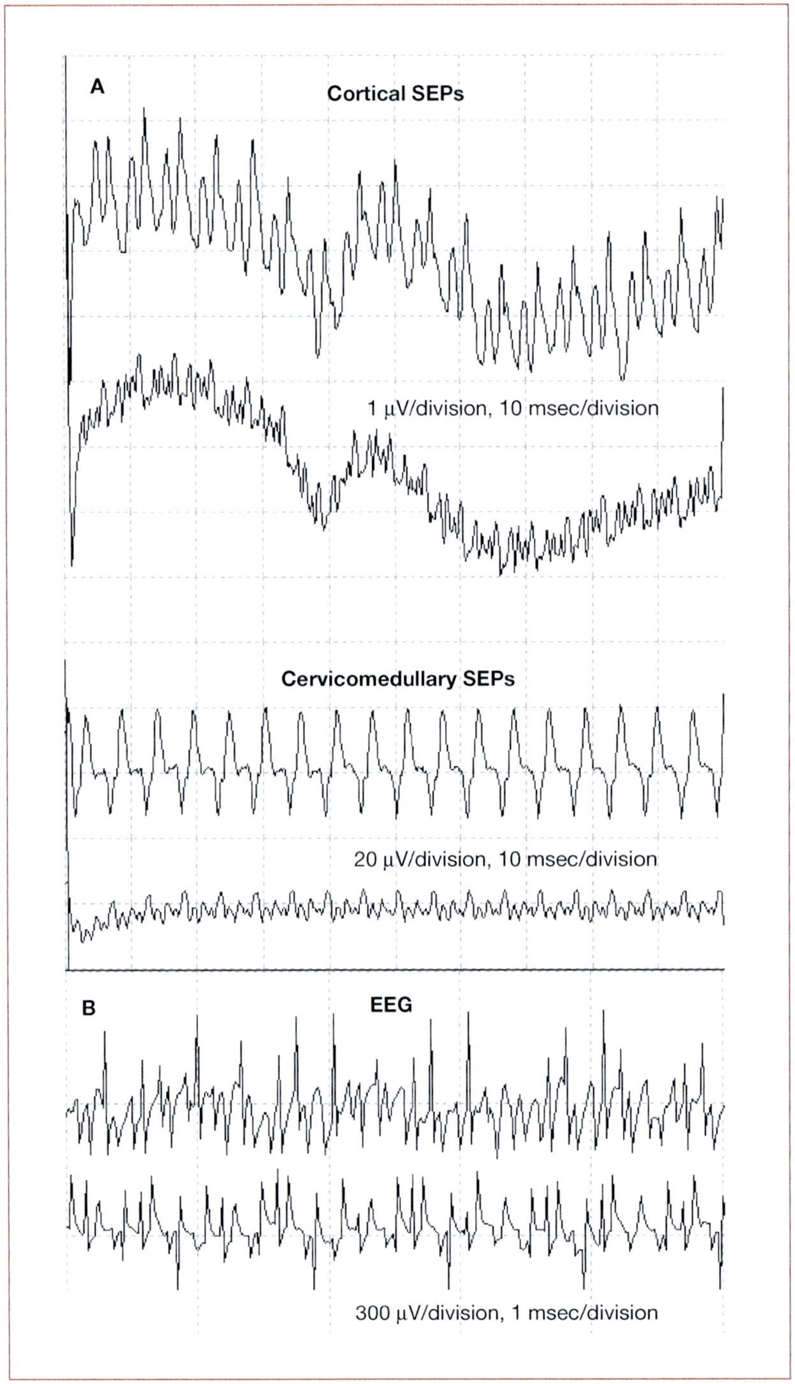

FIGURE 12.8: Artifact generated by a DBS in a patient with Parkinson's disease having surgery for a compression fracture of the L3 vertebra is shown. (A) SEPs to left posterior tibial nerve stimulation. Note the artifact is much larger in the cervicomedullary recording channel (note the different calibrations) and completely obscures the cervicomedullary SEP component even when the number of epochs per average is increased to 1,000 (lower SEP waveform in each pair). (B) A high-voltage artifact is also visible in the EEG. For the SEP recordings, the artifact rejection window was widened substantially to 500 μV for the cortical SEP recordings and to 2,000 μV for the cervicomedullary SEP recordings. At the usual setting of 100 μV, all data epochs were rejected. The EEG channels are CPz-Fpz and CP3-Cp4.

DBS, deep brain stimulator; SEP, somatosensory evoked potential.

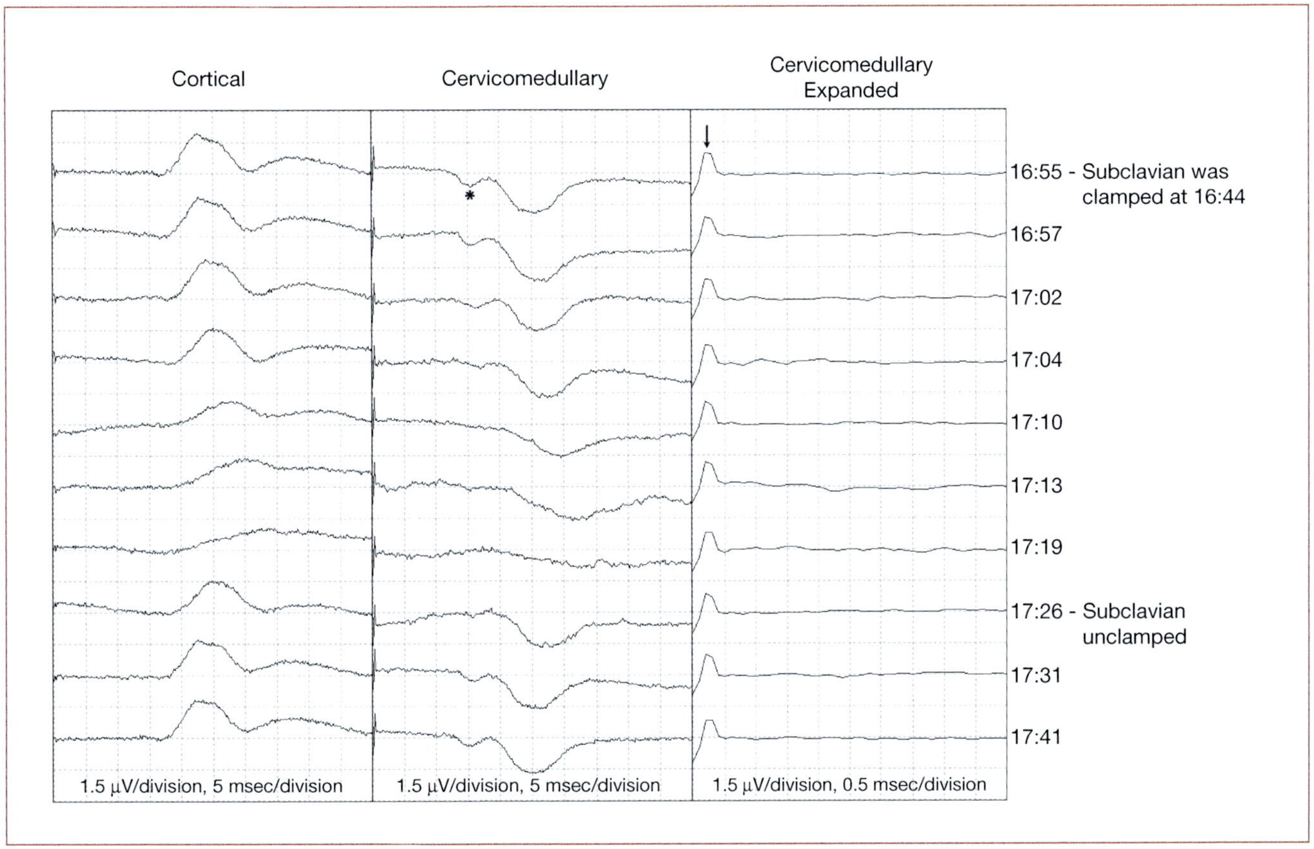

FIGURE 12.9: SEPs to left median nerve stimulation recorded during surgery to create a bypass graft between the left carotid artery and the left subclavian artery in a patient with a thoracic aortic aneurysm. Grafting was performed as a precursor to endovascular aneurysm repair that would occlude the origin of the left subclavian artery. There were no immediate SEP changes when the subclavian artery was cross-clamped, but there was a delayed deterioration of both the cortical and the cervicomedullary SEPs to left median nerve stimulation due to arm ischemia, which was reversed when the subclavian artery was unclamped. There was no change in the electrical stimulus artifact during these SEP changes. The asterisk indicates the P14 SEP component generated in nucleus cuneatus. The cervicomedullary SEP waveforms also contain longer latency peaks reflecting volume-conducted cortical SEPs. In the rightmost column of waveforms, the cervicomedullary SEPs are shown with an expanded timescale so the electrical stimulus artifact (arrow) is clearly visible.

SEP, somatosensory evoked potential.

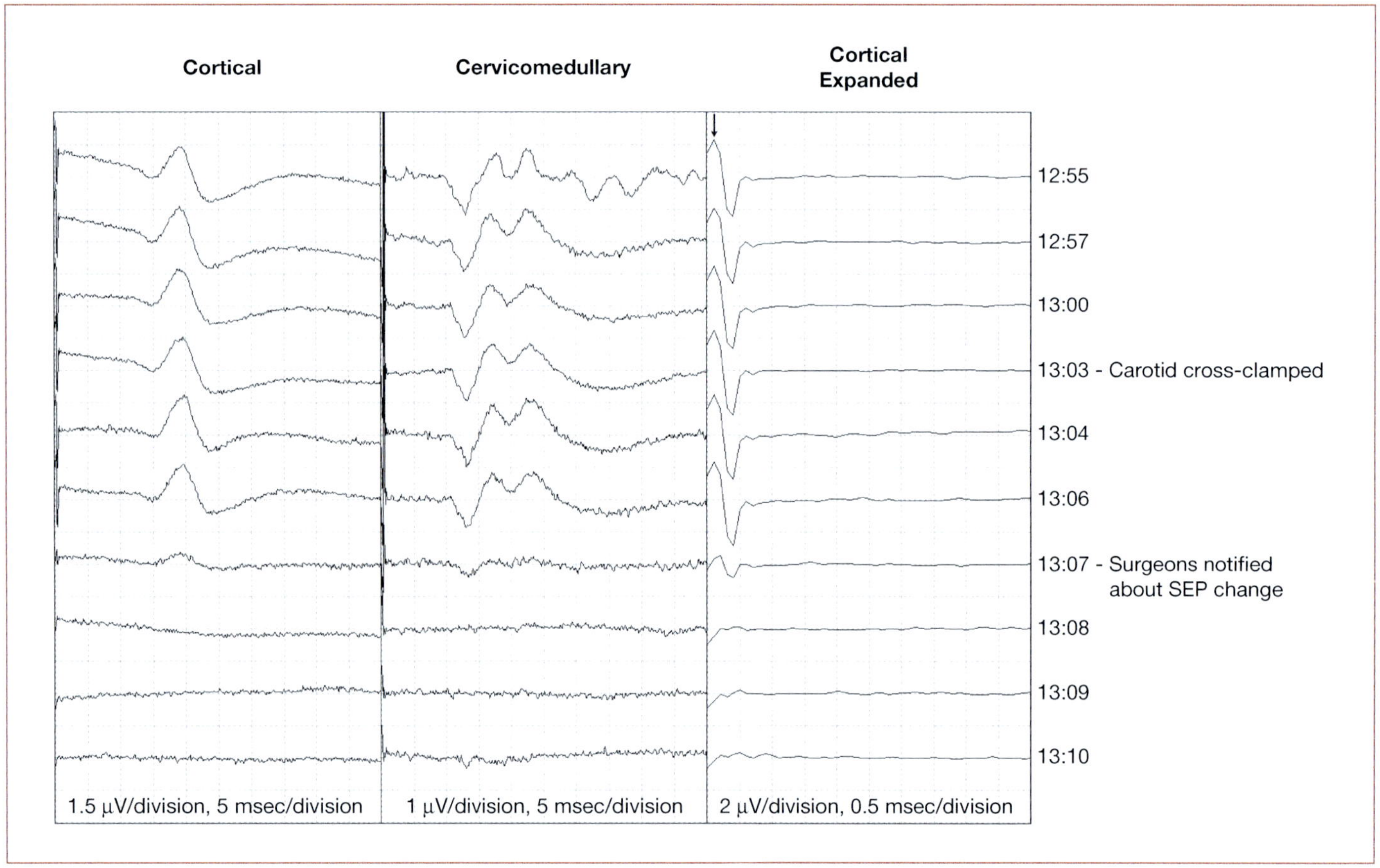

FIGURE 12.10: SEPs to left median nerve stimulation recorded during right carotid endarterectomy. In the rightmost column of waveforms, the cortical SEPs are shown with an expanded timescale so that the electrical stimulus artifact (arrow) is clearly visible. There were no immediate SEP changes when the carotid artery was cross-clamped, but then both the cortical and the cervicomedullary SEPs to left median nerve stimulation disappeared. The electrical stimulus artifact also disappeared. Switching the left and right stimulator outputs showed that the stimulators were working properly. Further investigation revealed that the paired wires carrying the stimulus to the left median nerve had been squeezed in a clamp attached to the operating table. The clamp broke the insulation and short-circuited them so together the stimulus current was not reaching the patient. Left ulnar nerve stimulating electrodes were placed, and stimulation elicited clear cortical and cervicomedullary SEPs, which were used for monitoring. The SEPs to right median nerve stimulation did not change during this time (22).

SEP, somatosensory evoked potential.

Source: Modified from Legatt AD. *Intraoperative Neurophysiology: Interactive Case Studies*. New York, NY: Demos Medical Publishing; 2015, case 50.

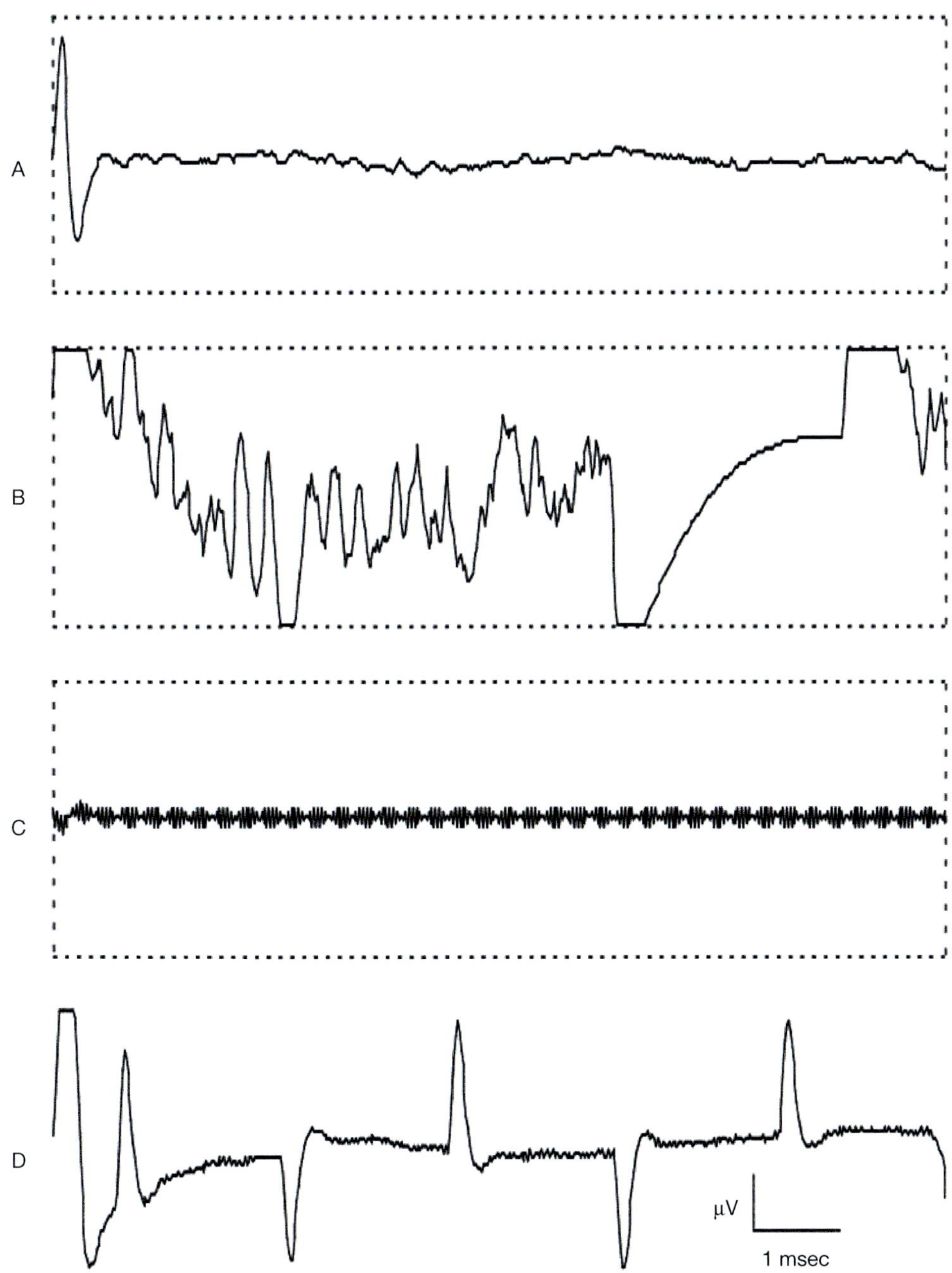

FIGURE 12.11: Single (unaveraged) data epochs recorded during intraoperative BAEP monitoring. (A) An electrical stimulus artifact is present at the beginning of the epoch. The BAEP, which is less than 1 µV in amplitude, is not visible in this single epoch of raw data. (B) Bipolar cautery produces a large artifact that would trigger automatic artifact rejection. (C) The ultrasonic aspirator device produces a very high-frequency but low-voltage artifact that would not trigger automatic artifact rejection. (D) This artifact from the light source of the operating microscope recurs at a harmonic of the line frequency but is composed of higher frequencies that would not be removed by a line frequency notch filter. In A, B, and C, the horizontal dotted lines show the input window of the analog-to-digital converter and the threshold for automatic artifact rejection. In D, the amplifier gain was reduced to show the light source artifacts in their entirety. Voltage calibration bar: 10 µV in A, B, and C, and 40 µV in D (16).

BAEP, brainstem auditory evoked potential.

Source: From Legatt AD. Mechanisms of intraoperative brainstem auditory evoked potential changes. *J Clin Neurophysiol*. 2002;19(5):396–408. doi:10.1097/00004691-200210000-00003, with permission.

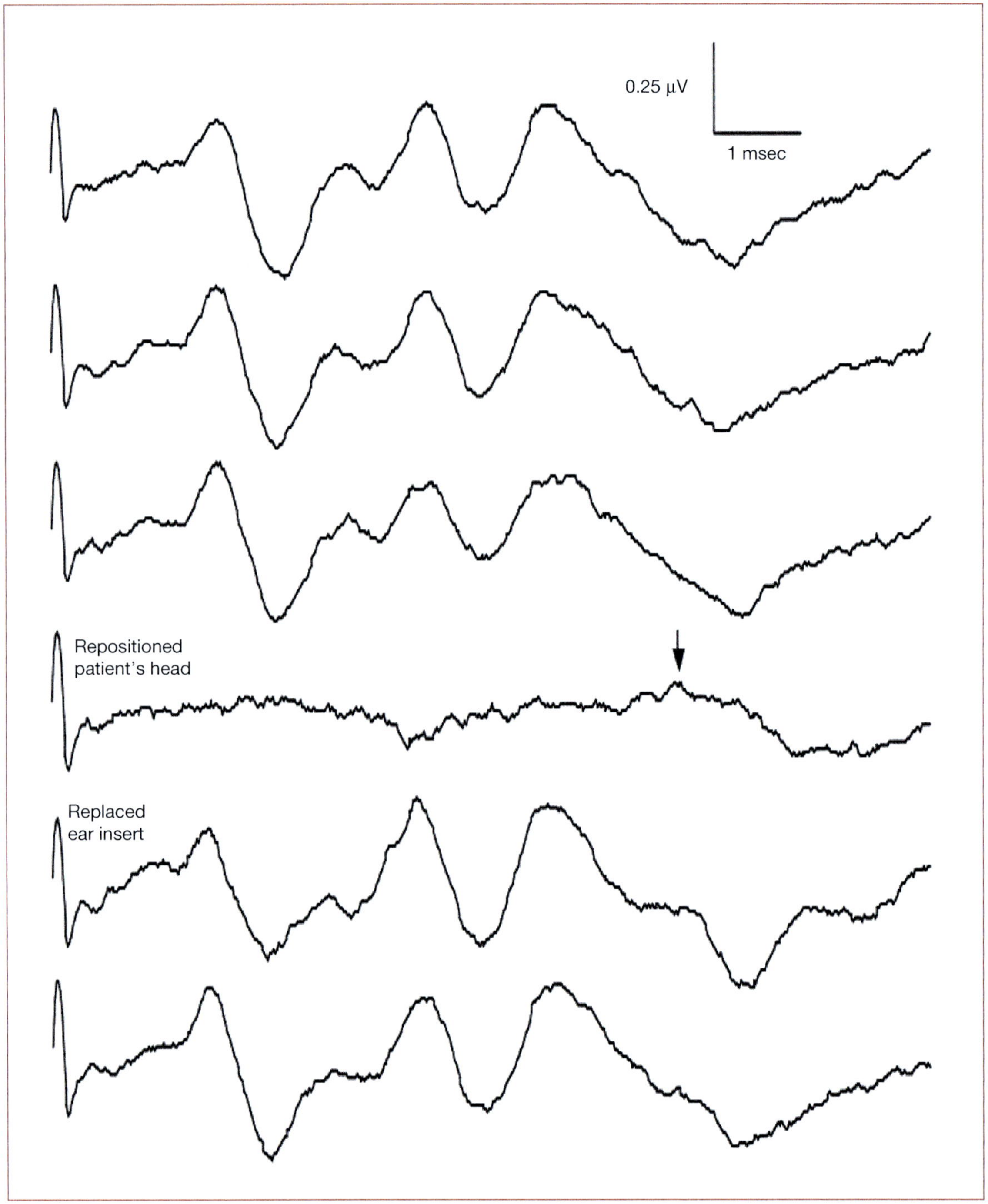

FIGURE 12.12: Loss of BAEPs due to technical problems in a patient operated for a left-sided vestibular schwannoma. Consecutive BAEPs (Cz-A2 recording) to right-ear stimulation are shown with the earliest waveform at the top. During positioning of the patient's head, these BAEPs disappeared. Investigation revealed that the tube carrying the acoustic stimulus had been accidentally pulled out of the patient's right ear. The tube was replaced and the BAEPs reappeared. The arrow indicates a possible delayed BAEP peak when the tube was dislodged, reflecting acoustic stimulation that reached the ear at a reduced intensity. BAEP stimuli with alternating stimulus polarity were used (16).

BAEP, brainstem auditory evoked potential.

Source: From Legatt AD. Mechanisms of intraoperative brainstem auditory evoked potential changes. *J Clin Neurophysiol*. 2002;19(5):396-408. doi:10.1097/00004691-200210000-00003, with permission.

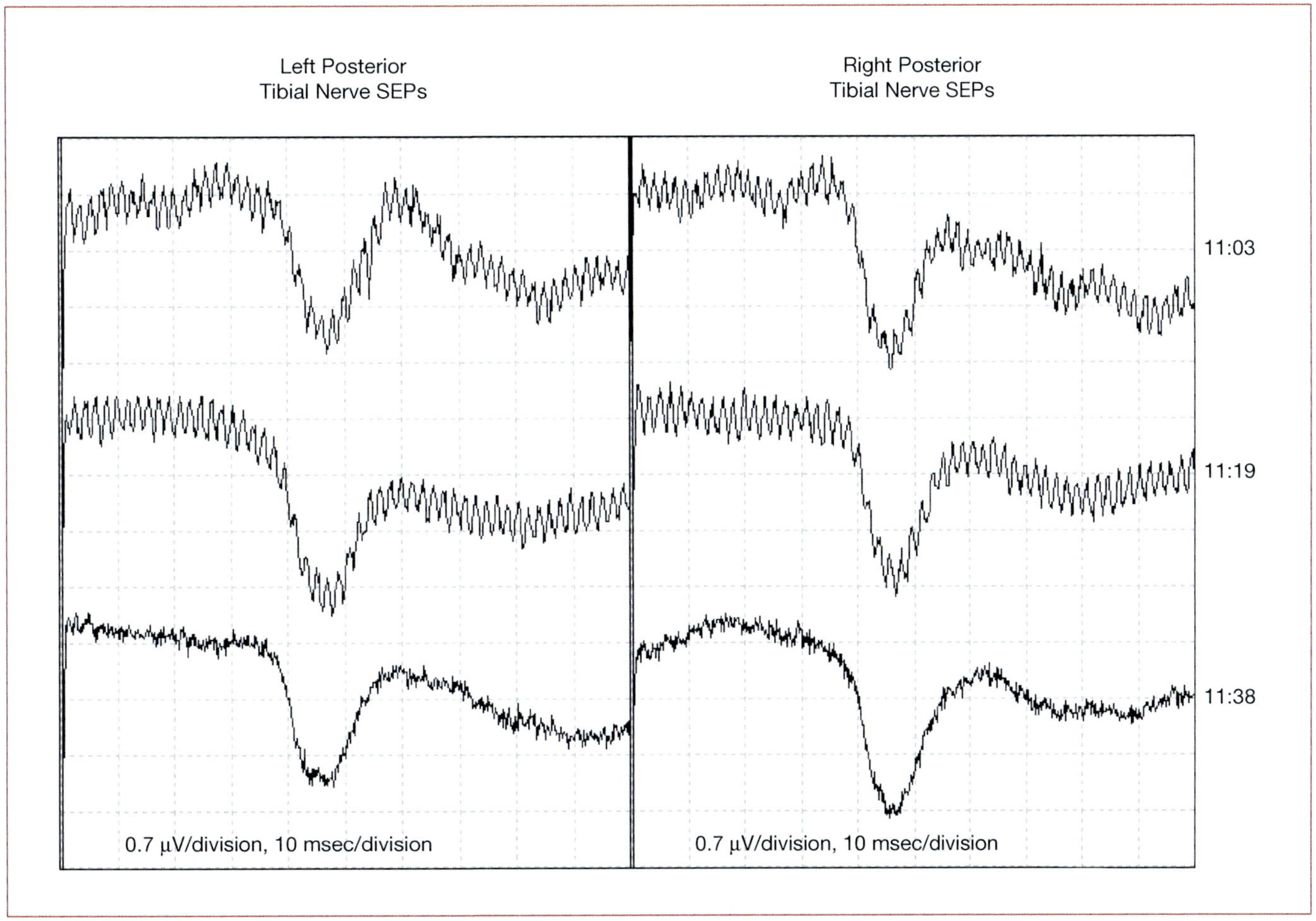

FIGURE 12.13: Three successive posterior tibial nerve SEP runs (CPz-Fpz recording, showing the cortical P37 components) during surgery for repair of a thoracoabdominal aortic aneurysm. The first two runs show prominent 60-Hz artifact from the fluid warmer which was turned off during the third run. The number of epochs per average was 1,000 for all three runs. The number had been increased in an attempt to improve the signal-to-noise ratio of the SEPs. The 60-Hz artifact returned when the fluid warmer was turned back on later.

SEP, somatosensory evoked potential.

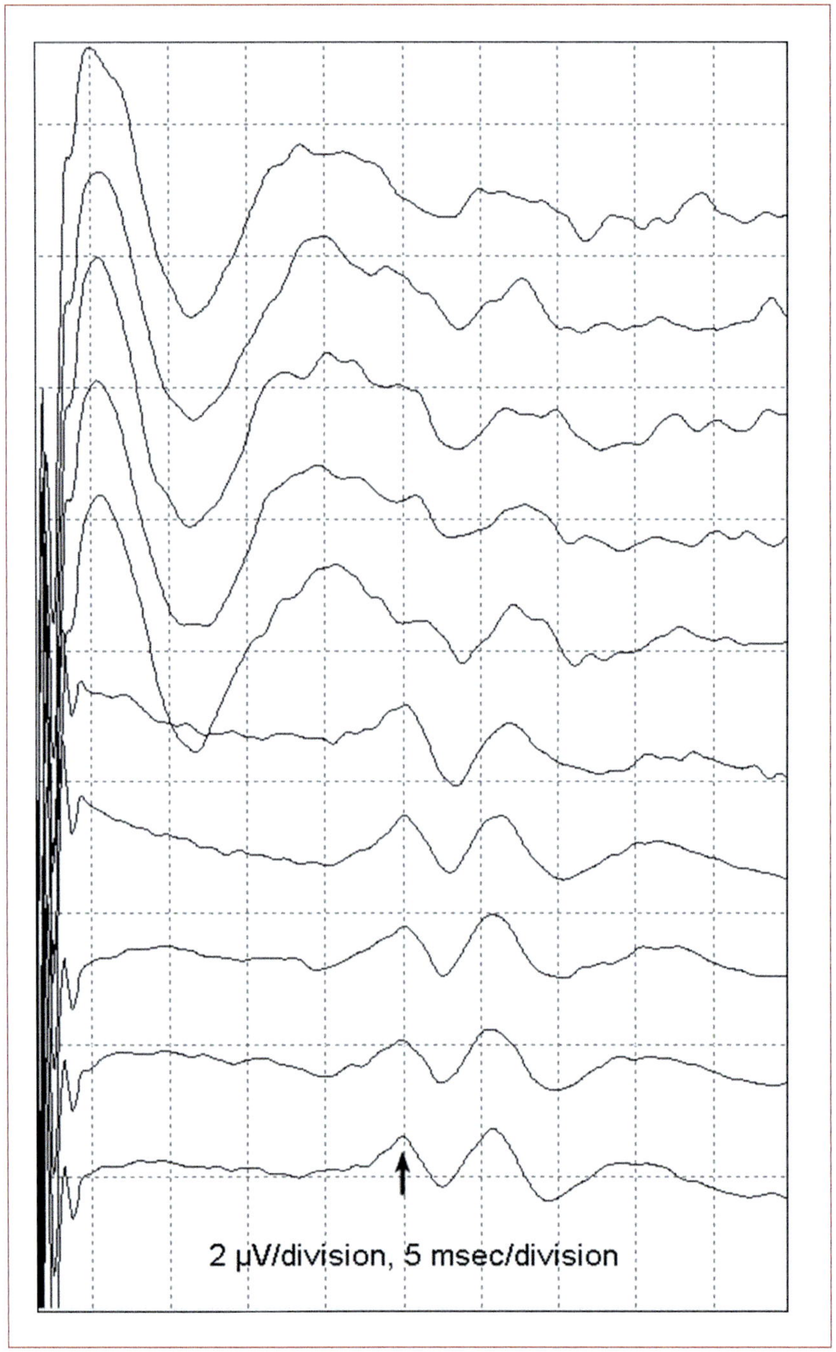

FIGURE 12.14: Ten consecutive recordings of cortical SEPs elicited by right ulnar nerve stimulation during spinal instrumentation and fusion surgery for scoliosis. The 60-Hz notch filter was turned on during the first five runs (top) and was turned off during the last five runs. The arrow indicates the N20 component, which was obscured when the notch filter was on.

SEP, somatosensory evoked potential.

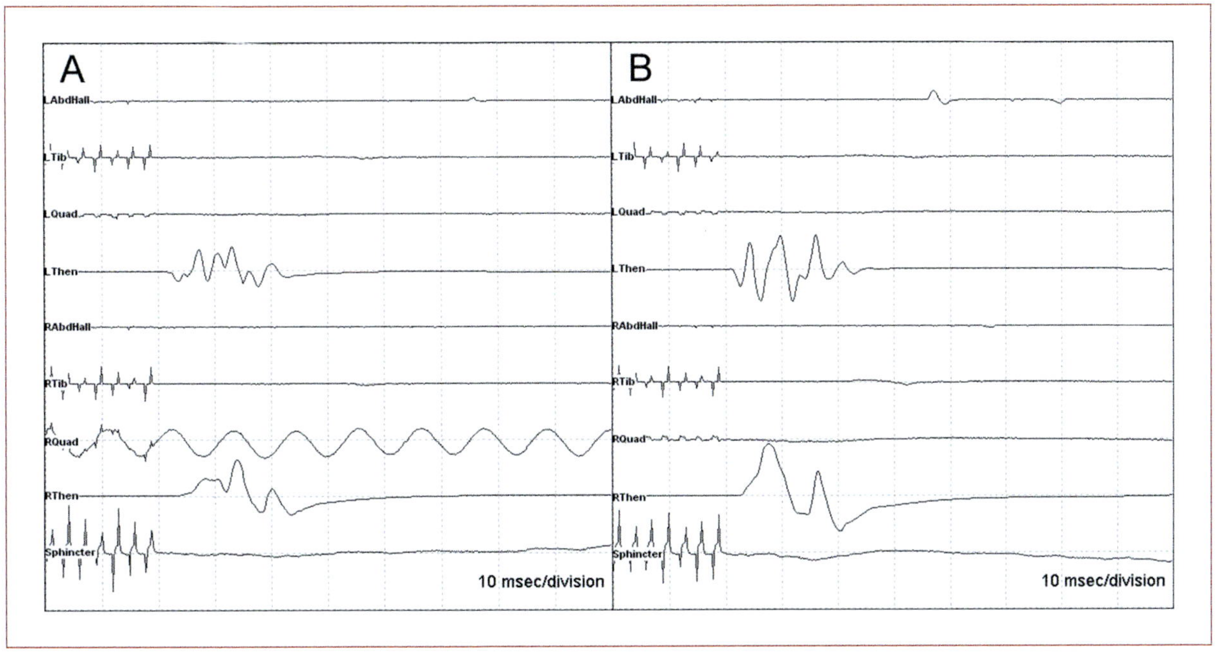

FIGURE 12.15: MEPs to TES with the anode on the right during surgery in a patient with a herniated thoracic disc, spinal cord compression, and paraparesis. There were large MEPs in both hands but no consistent lower limb MEPs. The vertical calibration is 5,000 μV/division for both left and right thenar muscles and 200 μV/division for the other recording channels. (A) A prominent sinusoidal artifact derived from the monopolar cautery's return electrode quality monitoring system is visible in the right quadriceps femoris recording channel (the current return electrode was on the patient's right thigh). (B) During closing, the cautery return electrode was disconnected and the cautery machine was turned off; this eliminated the artifact from the right quadriceps femoris recording channel.

MEP, motor evoked potential; TES, transcranial electrical stimulation.

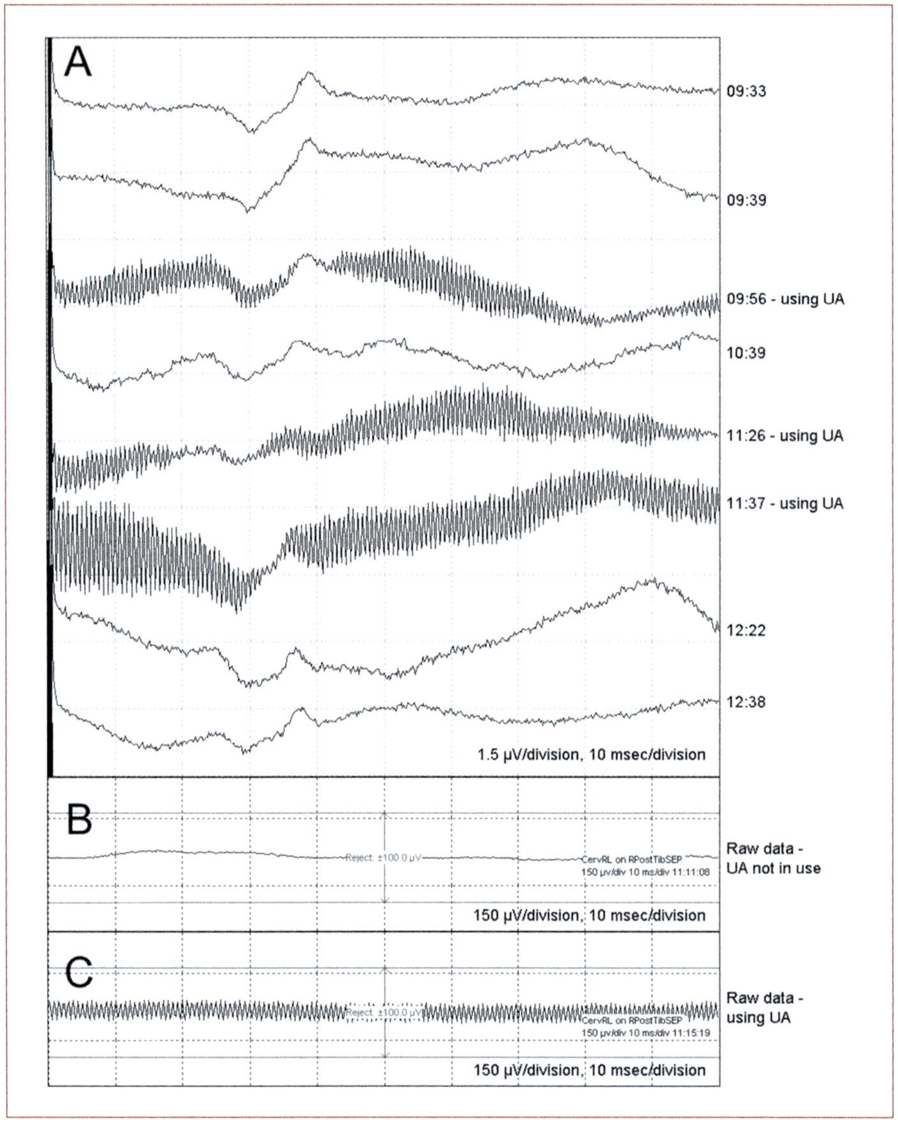

FIGURE 12.16: (A) Intraoperative cervical SEPs to right posterior tibial nerve stimulation during surgery for resection of a meningioma of the falx cerebri with three runs (at 09:56, 11:26, and 11:37) contaminated by artifact produced by an ultrasonic aspirator. (B) Unaveraged raw data (single sweep) when the device was not being used. (C) Unaveraged raw data showing the artifact.

SEP, somatosensory evoked potential.

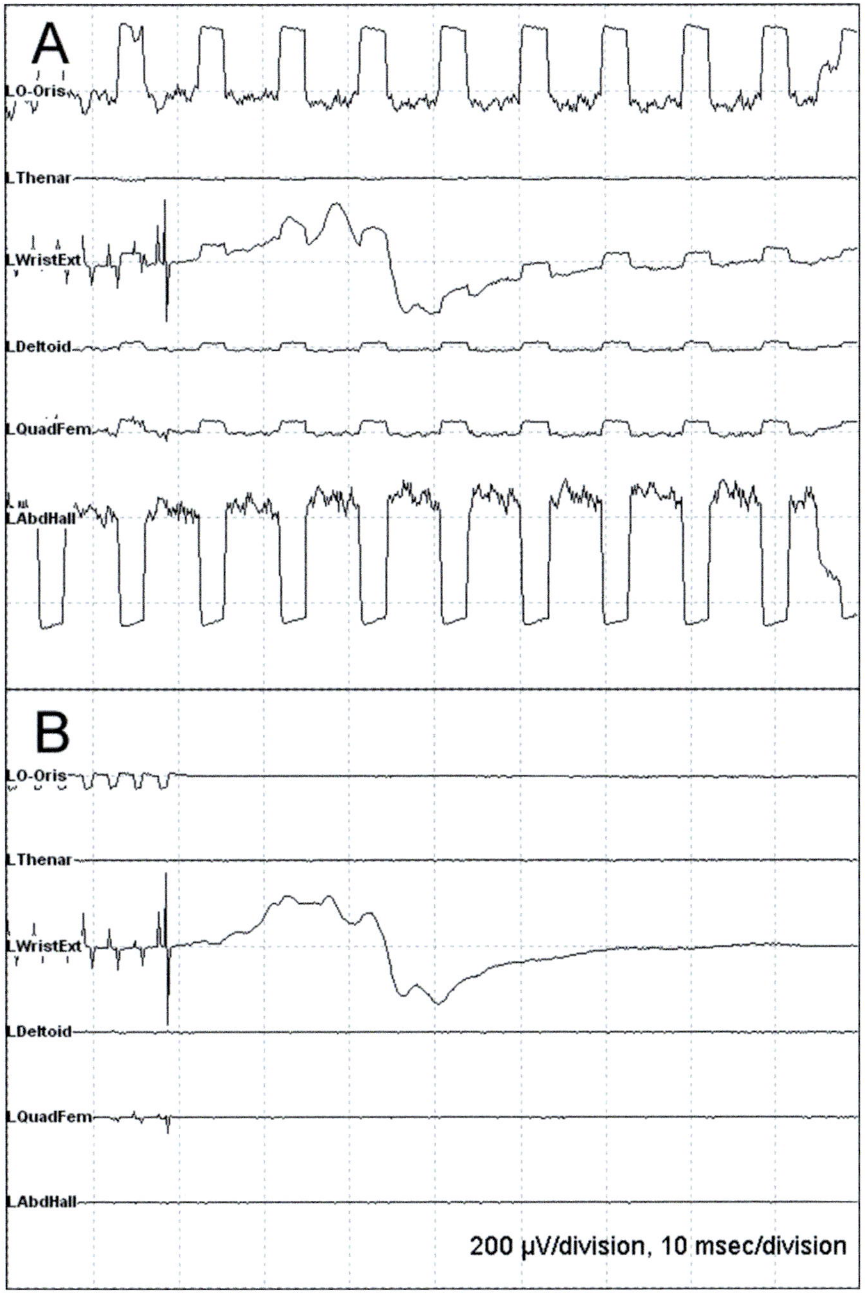

FIGURE 12.17: Single-sweep MEPs from multiple left body muscles to direct cortical stimulation using an electrode strip placed over the right motor cortex. MEPs were recorded to monitor the integrity of the corticospinal tract during resection of a lung cancer metastasis within the right hemisphere. (A) The ultrasonic aspiration device was activated during this run. (B) The run was repeated after the use of the device was temporarily discontinued with an MEP visible in the left wrist extensor recording channel.

MEP, motor evoked potential.

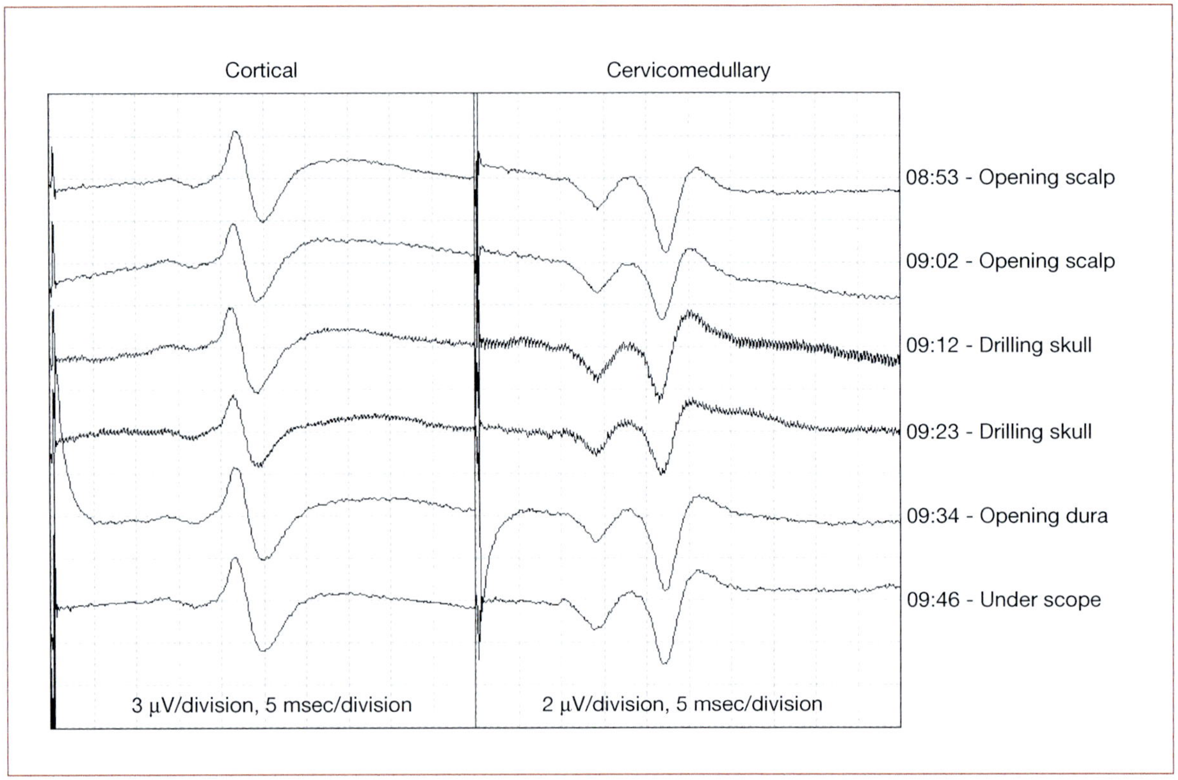

FIGURE 12.18: SEPs to right median nerve stimulation recorded during clipping of aneurysms of the right middle cerebral artery and the ophthalmic segment of the right internal carotid artery in a patient who had suffered a subarachnoid hemorrhage. Artifact from drilling of the skull is visible in the waveforms at 09:12 and 09:23.

SEP, somatosensory evoked potential.

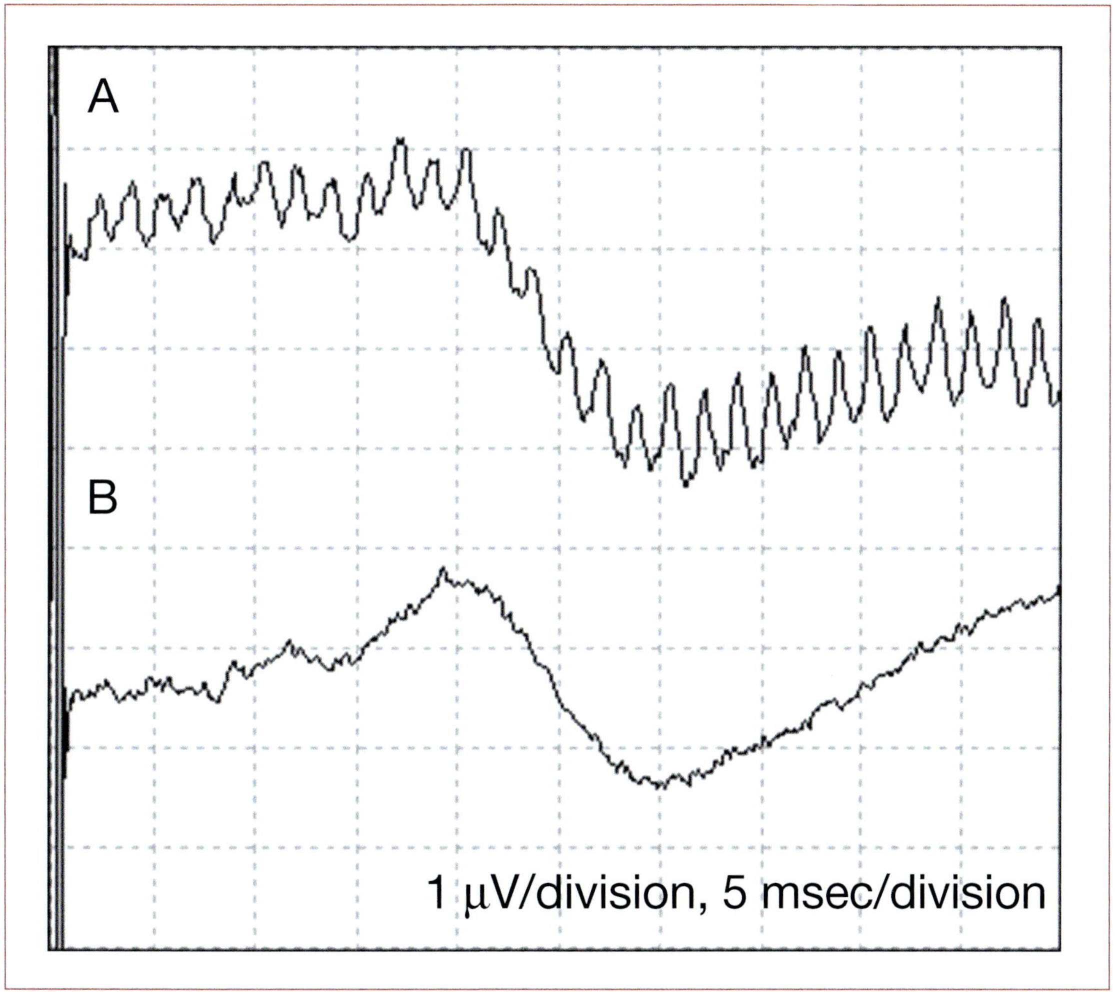

FIGURE 12.19: Cortical SEPs to left median nerve stimulation recorded during surgery for resection of an area of cortical dysplasia in the right frontal lobe in a patient with drug-resistant focal epilepsy. (A) A 60-Hz artifact from an electric shaver being used on an anesthetized patient. (B) Cortical SEP recorded after prepping and draping but before the initial incision, when the shaver was not being used.

SEP, somatosensory evoked potential.

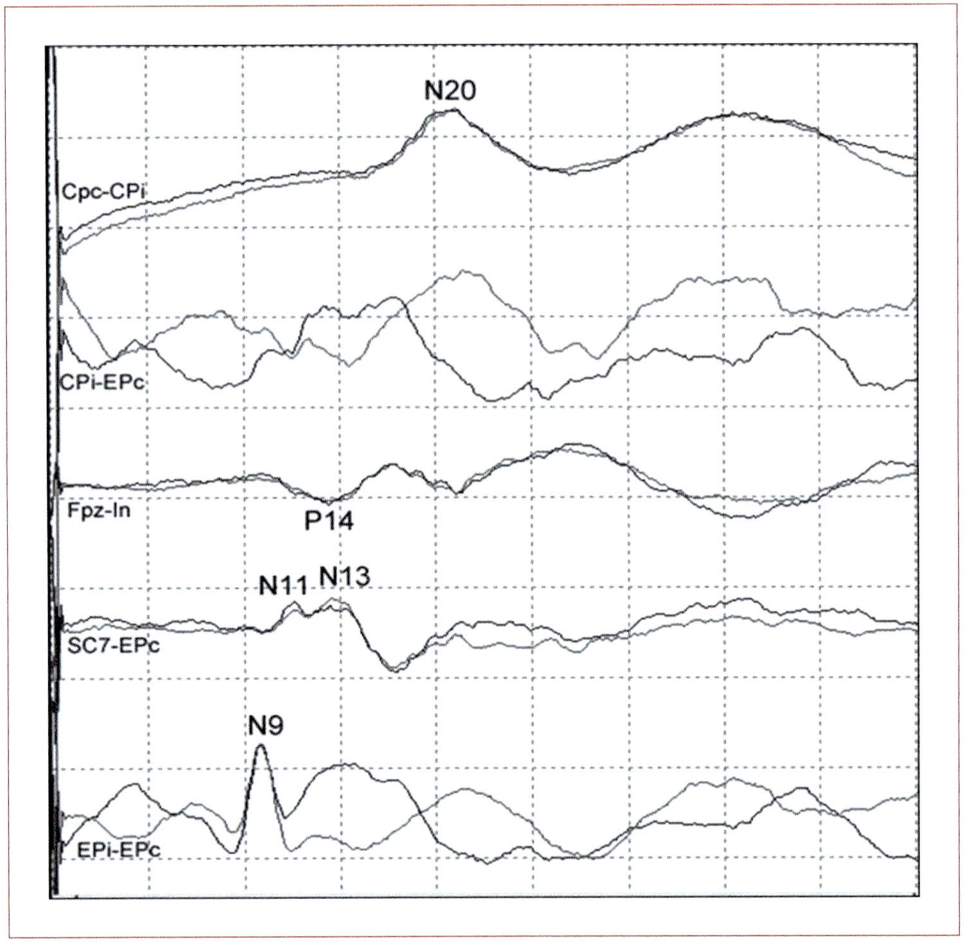

FIGURE 12.20: SEPs to right median nerve stimulation recorded during a diagnostic study in a 56-year-old man. The CPi-EPc recording channel usually used to record the P14 component (23) was compromised due to artifact. The P14 was not identifiable in it, but was identifiable when recording between the forehead (Fpz) and the inion (In). The EPi-EPc recording channel also shows the interference introduced by the noncephalic electrode. Calibrations: 3 μV/division vertical and 5 msec/division horizontal (18).

CPi, centroparietal electrode ipsilateral to the stimulated median nerve; EPc, contralateral Erb's point; EPi, ipsilateral Erb's point; SEP, somatosensory evoked potential.

Source: Fried SJ, Legatt AD. The utility of a forehead-to-inion derivation in recording the subcortical far-field potential (P14) during median nerve somatosensory-evoked potential testing. *Clin EEG Neurosci*. 2012;43(2):121-126. doi:10.1177/1550059411433613, with permission.

REFERENCES

1. Chiappa KH, ed. *Evoked Potentials in Clinical Medicine*. 2nd ed. New York, NY: Raven Press; 1990.
2. Chiappa KH, ed. *Evoked Potentials in Clinical Medicine*. 3rd ed. New York, NY: Lippincott-Raven; 1997.
3. Legatt AD, Pascual-Leone A, Rotenberg A. Technical aspects of transcranial magnetic and electrical stimulation. In: Schomer DL, Lopes da Silva F, eds. *Niedermeyer's Textbook of Electroencephalography: Basic Principles, Clinical Applications, and Related Fields*. 6th ed. Philadelphia, PA: Lippincott William & Wilkins; 2010:1129-1138.
4. Epstein CM, Boor DR. Principles of signal analysis and averaging. *Neurol Clin*. 1988;6(4):649-656.
5. American Clinical Neurophysiology Society. Guideline 9A: guidelines on evoked potentials. *J Clin Neurophysiol*. 2006;23(2):125-137. doi:10.1097/00004691-200604000-00010.
6. Legatt AD. Intraoperative neurophysiologic monitoring: some technical considerations. *Am J EEG Technol*. 1995;35:167-200 doi:10.1080/00029238.1995.11080516.
7. Lins OG, Picton TW, Berg P, et al. Ocular artifacts in EEG and event-related potentials. I: scalp topography. *Brain Topogr*. 1993;6(1):51-63. doi:10.1007/BF01234127.
8. American Academy of Pediatrics; American Academy of Pediatric Dentistry, Coté CJ, et al. Guidelines for monitoring and management of pediatric patients during and after sedation for diagnostic and therapeutic procedures: an update. *Pediatrics*. 2006;118(6):2587-2602. doi:10.1542/peds.2006-2780.
9. American Society of Anesthesiologists Task Force on Sedation and Analgesia by Non-Anesthesiologists. Practice guidelines for sedation and analgesia by non-anesthesiologists. *Anesthesiology*. 2002;96(4):1004-1017.
10. Hughes JR, Fino J. Usefulness of piezoelectric earphones in recording the brain stem auditory evoked potentials: a new early deflection. *Electroencephalogr Clin Neurophysiol*. 1980;48:357-360. doi:10.1016/0013-4694(80)90272-2.
11. Legatt AD. Brainstem auditory evoked potentials: methodology, interpretation, and clinical application. In: Aminoff MJ, ed. *Aminoff's Electrodiagnosis in Clinical Neurology*. 6th ed. New York, NY: Churchill Livingstone; 2012:519-552.
12. Yamada T. The anatomic and physiologic bases of median nerve somatosensory evoked potentials. *Neurol Clin*. 1988;6(4):705-733. doi:10.1016/S0733-8619(18)30839-9.
13. Legatt AD. Intraoperative neurophysiologic monitoring. In: Frost EAM, ed. *Clinical Anesthesia in Neurosurgery*. 2nd ed. Boston, MA: Butterworth-Heinemann; 1991:63-127.
14. Chan AYK. *Biomedical Device Technology: Principals and Design*. 2nd ed. Springfield, IL: Charles C. Thomas; 2016.
15. Levine RA, Ronner SF, Ojemann RG. Auditory evoked potential and other neurophysiologic monitoring techniques during tumor surgery in the cerebellopontine angle. In: Loftus CM, Traynelis VC, ed. *Intraoperative Monitoring Techniques in Neurosurgery*. New York, NY: McGraw-Hill; 1994:175-191.
16. Legatt AD. Mechanisms of intraoperative brainstem auditory evoked potential changes. *J Clin Neurophysiol*. 2002;19(5):396-408. doi:10.1097/00004691-200210000-00003.
17. Legatt AD. Impairment of common-mode rejection by mismatched electrode impedances: quantitative analysis. *Am J EEG Technol*. 1995;35:296-302. doi:10.1080/00029238.1995.11080527.
18. Fried SJ, Legatt AD. The utility of a forehead-to-inion derivation in recording the subcortical far-field potential (P14) during median nerve somatosensory-evoked potential testing. *Clin EEG Neurosci*. 2012;43(2):121-126. doi:10.1177/1550059411433613.
19. Legatt AD, Emerson RG, Epstein CM, et al. ACNS guideline: transcranial electrical stimulation motor evoked potential monitoring. *J Clin Neurophysiol*. 2016;33(1):42-50. doi:10.1097/WNP.0000000000000253.
20. Legatt AD. Evoked potentials (EPs). In: Aminoff MJ, Daroff R, eds. *Encyclopedia of the Neurological Sciences*. 2nd ed. San Diego, CA: Elsevier Science; 2014:228-231.
21. Legatt AD, Ellen R. Grass lecture: motor evoked potential monitoring. *Am J Electroneurodiagn Technol*. 2004;44(4):223-243. doi:10.1080/1086508X.2004.11079491.
22. Legatt AD. Intraoperative neurophysiology: interactive case studies. New York, NY: Demos Medical Publishing; 2015.
23. American Clinical Neurophysiology Society. Guideline 9D: Guidelines on short-latency somatosensory evoked potentials. *J Clin Neurophysiol*. 2006;23(2):168-179. doi:10.1097/00004691-200604000-00013.

CHAPTER 13

Artifacts in Neurophysiologic Intraoperative Monitoring

Aatif M. Husain, Stephanie L. Schwartz, and Emily B. Kale

INTRODUCTION

Neurophysiologic intraoperative monitoring (NIOM) involves recording low-amplitude neurophysiologic signals in the operating room (OR). NIOM brings all disciplines in clinical neurophysiology together in the OR, a particularly challenging environment that can produce a lot of artifacts. Artifacts are defined as unwanted signals that arise from sources that are not the ones of primary interest (1).

Neurophysiology laboratories are carefully designed and shielded to minimize extraneous artifacts from contaminating the neurophysiologic signal that is to be recorded. In the OR, such shielding is not available; rather, the OR is an environment that is "hostile" to neurophysiologic recordings (2). There are many electrical devices, movement of personnel, other simultaneous procedures, and lack of ready access to the patient that make the neurophysiologic data acquired in the OR particularly susceptible to artifacts. Also, removing objects or disconnecting equipment from power supplies cannot be readily done in the OR, making troubleshooting and eliminating artifacts more difficult.

In this chapter, artifacts commonly encountered in NIOM will be discussed. An overview of artifacts from the perspective of NIOM will be presented first, followed by the classification of these artifacts. Thereafter, the common types of artifacts encountered in NIOM will be described and examples presented where appropriate. How artifacts are recognized, differentiated, and eliminated (or avoided) will be discussed.

OVERVIEW

NIOM involves recording many types of neurophysiologic signals. EEG, electromyography (EMG), and evoked potentials (EPs) are often recorded simultaneously. Artifacts that appear in one type of monitoring modality may be the activity of interest in another type of monitoring. For example, EMG activity in the EEG channels confounds its interpretation, but there may be simultaneous EMG monitoring to assess peripheral nerve function. Eliminating some artifacts is sometimes not possible or desirable, making managing artifacts challenging in NIOM.

Recognizing artifacts in NIOM and deciding between surgery-induced changes and artifacts is a primary responsibility of the neuromonitoring team. Artifacts can mimic significant changes and they can make recognition of these changes difficult. Misinterpreting artifacts can lead to adverse patient consequences in all of clinical neurophysiology, but it can have particularly devastating consequences in NIOM (3).

Artifacts in NIOM can be thought of as continuous and intermittent types. Continuous artifacts are ones that are continuously present with some variability in waveform shape or amplitude. Ongoing 60-Hz electrical artifact can appear as a continuous artifact while trying to record EPs. Intermittent artifacts may occur as single or runs of independent waveforms that disrupt the background activity. Bursts of EMG activity may appear intermittently while recording EEG. At times, intermittent artifacts may appear superimposed on continuous ones. Recognizing artifact as continuous or intermittent helps to identify the source and may help to intervene and eliminate it.

At times artifacts are called "interference" or "noise," as they interfere with the signal of interest. In most cases, artifacts are to be avoided and eliminated when encountered. This can be done by changing the head or limb position, administering medications (like neuromuscular junction blocking drugs, paralytics), and use of filters and other amplifier settings. Some of these manipulations may not be possible during surgery. The limitations and changes in signals caused by changing amplifier settings should be appreciated. Occasionally, artifacts cannot be eliminated and should simply be recognized and mentally discounted (1).

CLASSIFICATION

Artifacts in NIOM, as in most of clinical neurophysiology, can be classified based on whether they are physiologic or nonphysiologic (**Table 13.1**). Physiologic artifacts are electrical potentials that originate from the patient from a source other than the one of primary interest. The physiological artifacts seen in NIOM are different than those seen in other types of neurophysiologic tests. In EEGs, extraocular movements and glossokinetic artifacts frequently contaminate the recording. These do not typically occur in anesthetized patients undergoing NIOM. Similarly, ECG artifact is seldom an issue in EP and EMG data, though occasionally it can be seen when recording EEG in the OR.

Nonphysiologic artifacts arise from sources external to the patient. There are many nonphysiologic sources of artifact that are unique to NIOM and not seen in other neurophysiologic procedures. There are many machines in the OR that can produce a continuous or intermittent electrical artifact. The electrocautery, patient warming devices, operating microscope, x-ray equipment, operating table, and other electrical items are only seen in the OR and produce a unique type of artifact. Sometimes a device that produces nonphysiologic artifact in one monitoring modality looks different than the artifact it produces in another modality.

DESCRIPTION

There are many types of artifacts that can be seen in NIOM, and new ones are routinely discovered with the introduction of new devices and machines. The more common types of artifacts encountered in NIOM, along with examples, are discussed in the following sections.

TABLE 13.1: Classification of Common Artifacts Seen in NIOM

A. Physiologic
  a. EMG
  b. EEG
  c. Respiration
  d. ECG and pulse
  e. Other physiologic signals
B. Nonphysiologic
  a. NIOM system
    i. Electrodes
    ii. Wires
    iii. NIOM machine
  b. Other equipment
    i. Electrical power lines
    ii. Electrocautery
    iii. Temperature management systems
    iv. Operating microscope
    v. Ultrasonic surgical aspirator
    vi. Brain stimulator
    vii. x-Ray equipment
    viii. Surgical drill
    ix. Cardiopulmonary bypass machine
    x. Other sources

EMG, electromyography; NIOM, neurophysiologic intraoperative monitoring.

Physiologic Artifacts

In NIOM, physiologic electrical signals may be artifacts or the signal of interest, depending on the modality being recorded. For example, during spinal surgery, EMG activity is considered physiologic artifact in the somatosensory evoked potential (SEP) recording, but it is the signal of interest when recording EMG activity to monitor for spinal root irritation. Thus, in NIOM it may be undesirable to completely eliminate some physiologic signals, rather it is best to manage them depending on what is being monitored. The common types of physiologic artifacts seen in NIOM are discussed in the following sections.

Electromyogram

EMG artifact is a very common physiologic artifact encountered in NIOM. In an anesthetized patient, while there is little movement, muscle tone is still present, unless paralytics are used. EMG artifact is of high frequency and may be seen as a continuous or intermittent discharge (4). A continuous EMG discharge may occur when the patient's anesthesia is inappropriately light or if there is a subconscious perception of pain. Intermittent EMG activity may be noted with unexpected movement or irritation of nerves and muscles. As noted earlier, although EMG artifact can make averaging EPs and interpreting EEG more difficult, it is the primary signal of interest when peripheral nerves or roots are at risk of injury. At times EMG may be noted with motor evoked potentials (MEPs) as well, appearing as random waveforms on the screen when an MEP is acquired. An example of this is presented in Figure 13.1.

When EMG artifact becomes excessive, elimination attempts can include moving the patient's head or limbs if possible. Using paralytics will help, but it may affect other types of monitoring and is usually avoided. A lower high-frequency filter (HFF) can also help, but it may distort other high-frequency signals of interest (such as various EPs). When recording EPs, increasing the number of repetitions averaged may help improve the signal as well. At times, the EMG artifact must simply be recognized and discounted.

Another type of EMG artifact is seen when muscle contraction occurs with peripheral nerve stimulation that is used during SEP monitoring. Ulnar and median nerve stimulation causes contraction of hand muscles, and this can be seen as regular motor potentials on free-running EMG recorded from the same muscles. Similarly, tibial nerve stimulation causes contraction of foot muscles, and regular motor potentials are seen in the free-running EMG from foot muscles. An example of this type of artifact is presented in Figure 13.2. These discharges are easy to identify; they cannot be eliminated but should be recognized and not confused with abnormal, spontaneous EMG activity from the same muscle groups.

Electroencephalogram

In many types of NIOM cases, EEG is the signal of interest. However, when recording various types of EPs, EEG activity becomes a continuous type of artifact that may reduce the reproducibility of the EPs. The frequency of EEG activity is usually between 0.5 and 30 Hz, though with craniotomies, higher frequencies may be noted. An example of EEG activity becoming artifact is when visual evoked potentials (VEPs) are recorded in OR. VEPs are highly sensitive to anesthetics, particularly inhalational ones, so total intravenous anesthesia (TIVA) with propofol is desirable. If the propofol dose is kept low, EEG activity may obscure the VEPs, as EEG is of much higher amplitude.

Eliminating all EEG activity is often not desirable or possible. Usually, reducing EEG activity involves increasing the anesthetic dose. The higher anesthetic dose may make obtaining the signal of interest more difficult. In the preceding example, EEG can be reduced by increasing the dose of propofol. However, if the depth of anesthesia increases considerably, obtaining VEPs may become impossible. In this example, the EEG artifact is best dealt with by increasing the number of repetitions averaged with each EP.

Respiration

Respiration can produce a slow-frequency artifact that occurs at the same frequency as the patient's breathing, about 5 to 15 per minute. In the OR, the patient's respiration is controlled by a ventilator, so the respiratory rate can easily be determined. Respirations can cause mild head movements, which causes mechanically induced impedance changes in the EEG leads (5). This manifests as artifact in the EEG channels as a continuous, very slow undulating wave. When diaphragmatic or intercostal EMG is monitored with needle electrodes, respiratory artifact may appear as a high-frequency, phasic burst of activity during inspiration when the muscles of respiration contract. Although this is considered an artifact, it also is useful as it confirms appropriate placement of the recording electrodes.

Respiratory artifact often cannot be entirely eliminated, and this may not be desirable either. Movement-induced respiratory artifact noted on EEG can usually be corrected by repositioning the patient's head if it is recognized before the patient is draped. Increasing the low-frequency filter (LFF) can also help, but it may distort other physiologic activity of interest. Respiratory artifact seen in diaphragmatic EMG cannot be easily eliminated, but it may serve a useful purpose and can easily be ignored.

Electrocardiogram and Pulse

The ECG artifact is seen as a regular, continuous artifact occurring at the same frequency as the heart rate. In the OR, it appears occasionally in EEG recordings and can be easily recognized and discounted. When ECG artifact appears in free-running EMG channels, it may be harder to recognize as typically only 1 second of EMG activity may be seen per screen (sweep of free-running EMG is usually 100 msec/division). Related to ECG artifact is pulse artifact. This occurs at the same frequency as the heart rate, though there is a slight lag in the pulse artifact compared to the QRS complex of the ECG. A pulse artifact is seen when the recording electrode is over or near a blood vessel. Though this is seen usually in EEG electrodes, it can also be seen in other modalities as well. If possible, the recording electrode should be moved slightly, but if that cannot be done, it is easy to ignore. An example of ECG and pulse artifact is presented in Figure 13.3.

Other Physiologic Signals

Several other types of physiologic artifacts can occur during NIOM, but they are much more common in EEG, EP, or EMG recordings. They are discussed in more detail in their respective chapters, and only a brief summary is presented here. Eye movements are a common type of physiologic artifact seen in the EEG laboratory. They produce an artifact in the frontal leads that can have a slow (slow eye movement) or fast (rapid eye movements) upslope, followed by a slow wave. Eye movements are seldom an issue when patients are under general anesthesia. Glossokinetic artifact from tongue movement produces a high-amplitude slow wave better seen in the temporal channels of the EEG. Like eye movement artifact, glossokinetic artifact is seldom a source of problems in the OR.

Sweat can cause artifacts in recording electrodes. Sweat itself can cause low-amplitude slow discharges due to its electrically charged nature. It can also cause electrode impedance issues and formation of salt bridges between electrodes, making recording signals difficult. The very slow sweat artifact can often be eliminated by increasing the LFF or by cooling off the patient. In the OR the temperature is often fairly low, and sweating is usually not a problem.

Nonphysiologic Artifacts

There are many possible sources of nonphysiologic artifacts that can occur during NIOM. They can be thought of as related to the monitoring system, from electrodes to the NIOM machine. Alternatively, they can be due to sources external to the NIOM system and the patient and originate from the environment, devices, and machines located in the OR.

NIOM System

Artifacts related to the NIOM system may come from the electrodes, wires, and electrode interface with the patient or from an NIOM machine.

Electrodes and Wires

Electrodes attached to a patient can produce many types of artifacts. Electrode artifacts are often limited to a single channel, making their identification easier. The commonest are "electrode pops." These are intermittent, sharp waveforms. Their morphology can mimic epileptiform spikes. They can occur in runs and mimic a rhythmic discharge. These artifacts occur more commonly when electrodes of different types are combined in a single channel, such as a needle electrode referenced to a surface electrode of a different metal (4). Electrode pops and other electrode artifacts are more common when the interface between the electrode and patient is impaired, such as when the conductive paste has dried or the electrode has become loose.

Wires that connect the electrodes to the headbox can also be a source of artifacts. Movement of the wires causes electrostatic artifacts that can mimic intermittent slow waves. In the OR, personnel movement around a patient cannot be controlled, and this movement may result in wire movement-related artifact. Damage to the wire may also be a source of artifact. Such damage may introduce electrical noise from other sources. Such an example is presented in Figures 13.4A to C.

Electrode and wire artifacts are best managed before they happen. Good technique in electrode application, headbox positioning, and wrapping the wires of the electrodes can help in preventing artifacts from appearing. This is very important in NIOM as once the patient has been draped, access to the patient to adjust electrodes is very limited. Once electrode artifacts appear, checking impedance can help determine if the electrodes are at fault. Often the impedance will be high. If a redundant electrode is available, it should be substituted for the electrode not making good contact with skin. Wire movement artifact can be reduced by using a LFF. Although electrode artifact that cannot be corrected can be ignored, it often foretells problems with reliability of monitoring as the recording electrodes are likely unable to faithfully reproduce the signal of interest.

NIOM Machine

Internal noise of the NIOM machine can also produce a variety of artifacts. Such artifacts are mostly due to problems with the headboxes or amplifiers in the machine. Movement of electrical charge through the input contacts on the headbox to the various components of the NIOM machine can produce these artifacts. Modern NIOM machines are made of components of very low inherent noise, and machine-related artifacts generally do not occur unless there is a machine failure. These artifacts can be of many types and may be continuous or intermittent. Their morphology is usually not similar to that of usual neurophysiologic signals and are easy to differentiate from the activity of interest. Unlike electrode artifacts, these artifacts usually occur in many channels simultaneously. An example of artifact related to bad inputs in the headbox is presented in Figures 13.5A and B.

Unfortunately, NIOM machine artifacts are difficult to eliminate other than by replacing the offending component of the NIOM machine (headbox, amplifier, etc.) or using alternate parts of the same equipment (using different inputs of the headbox, if available). Because components of an NIOM machine are difficult to change during a surgery (except for the headbox), when machine-related artifacts are seen, a different machine is used if available. Regular maintenance of equipment can prevent machine failure in the OR, and biomedical checks of all NIOM machines should be conducted according to the manufacturer's instructions.

Environment

Environmental artifact is one of the most common types of artifact seen in NIOM. Electrical line artifact is the most common, but there are many devices and equipment in the OR that can also produce environmental artifact (6).

Electrical Power Line

Alternating current (AC) in electrical power lines is a common source of artifact in NIOM. In the United States, AC is at 60 Hz, while in some European countries it is 50 Hz. Electrical power lines can produce a 60-Hz artifact in two primary ways (5). The common way this artifact appears is through electrostatic induction. Capacitance between the AC mains wiring and another conductor acting as a capacitor (such as electrodes and wires) can generate capacitive voltages. If these capacitive voltages reach the differential amplifier, they will be amplified if they are unequal in inputs 1 and 2. This will produce a 60-Hz artifact.

Electrical power line artifact can also occur through electromagnetic effects. This is caused by nearby electrical equipment, such as lamps, television screens, and other medical devices. These devices generate an electrical field that is inductively coupled with wires attached to a patient. At 60 Hz, or more frequently a harmonic of 60 Hz, such as 120 Hz, artifact is produced. An example of this type of artifact is in Figure 13.6.

The 60-Hz artifact is a very regular, continuous artifact. Its amplitude varies depending on the position of the patient in relationship to a variety of electrical equipment in the vicinity, as this will change the strength of the electrical field causing the artifact. At times, a 60-Hz or 120-Hz artifact can mimic an EMG discharge. They can be differentiated by increasing the sweep of the monitor to count the sinusoidal waveforms. Using a 60-Hz notch filter will almost entirely eliminate a 60-Hz artifact, but it will not change EMG activity or a 120-Hz (or other harmonic of 60) artifact very much. The presence of a 60-Hz artifact may also indicate poor electrode contact with the patient.

Good electrode application technique minimizes the chance of seeing excessive 60-Hz artifact. Many modern buildings have electrical lines grounded to the same earth ground, minimizing electrostatic interference. Using a 60-Hz notch filter can greatly reduce this artifact, but if this filter is applied after baseline data have been acquired, there may be a significant change in waveform latencies and amplitudes. These changes should be recognized as induced by the addition of a filter. Sometimes possible sources of electromagnetic interference can be eliminated by turning off various machines in the OR. Of course, a discussion with the surgeon and circulating nurse must occur before this is done to prevent disconnection of a vital piece of equipment. Temperature management systems and other such equipment can be turned off for at least a few minutes to help isolate the source of the artifact. If such a source is found and cannot be permanently disconnected, moving the headbox and NIOM machine as far away as possible from the offending machine may help reduce the artifact.

Electrocautery

Electrocautery causes a large-amplitude, high-frequency discharge (7). This discharge is easy to identify due to its large size and distinct morphology. It is intermittent and occurs only when the electrocautery is used by the surgeon. To the technologist in the OR, an audible sound may be associated with this discharge. The electrocautery discharge disrupts EEG and EMG signals by saturating amplifiers, which may take a few seconds to recover and start displaying physiologic signals again. An example of this is presented in Figure 13.7. It can also overwhelm the EPs if averaging is not paused. This is a commonly encountered artifact due to the frequent, necessary use of electrocautery during surgery.

Electrocautery artifact cannot be completely avoided. Modern amplifiers that are rated for OR use have rapid recovery times so little EEG and EMG data is missed from amplifier saturation. Artifact rejection software in the NIOM machine may prevent electrocautery artifact from being averaged with the EPs. However, despite using such software, it is best to pause the averaging because if the artifact is below the threshold value of the artifact rejection parameters, it can disrupt the EP average.

Temperature Management Systems

Temperature management systems, such as the Bair Hugger, help prevent the patient from becoming hypothermic during surgery. These systems can introduce a significant artifact in NIOM. The artifact produced by the temperature management system is a continuous 100-Hz artifact (8). Elimination of the artifact when the temperature management system is turned off positively identifies it as the cause. Averaging SEPs and brainstem auditory evoked potentials (BAEPs) can be very difficult with this type of artifact as the amplitude of the artifact is often not large enough for it to be eliminated by the artifact rejection software (it is within bounds of the artifact rejection parameters).

Artifact from the temperature management system can be reduced by moving electrode wires away from the device. Moving the NIOM equipment away from the temperature management system is also helpful in reducing the artifact. Increasing the number of repetitions in the EP average may help as well. If absolutely necessary, the surgery and anesthesia teams may allow it to be turned off, at least during critical periods in surgery.

Operating Microscope

The operating microscope can be a major source of artifact in NIOM. Different operating microscopes produce different degrees of artifact. The artifact is usually of high frequency, typically continuous, and a harmonic of the 60-Hz electrical power line artifact (9). SEPs and BAEPs are most affected by this type of artifact. An example is shown in Figures 13.8A and B.

Elimination of artifact induced by the operating microscope may be challenging. It is not removed by the 60-Hz notch filter as it has a harmonic frequency. Ensuring that the operating microscope is grounded to the same earth ground and has no leakage current is important. Moving the NIOM machine to a position in the room away from the operating microscope may help.

Cortical Stimulator

Cortical stimulators, such as the "Ojemann cortical stimulator," are used to deliver biphasic electrical stimuli, usually at 50 to 60 Hz, directly to the cortex for 1 to 5 seconds to disrupt underlying neural networks and validate eloquent cortical function. It is used after a craniotomy has been performed when mapping the brain for language and motor areas of the cortex are desirable. Simultaneous electrocorticography (ECoG) is often recorded to monitor for after discharges. When stimulation is performed at 60 Hz, a 60-Hz artifact is seen in the ECoG, and this may saturate the EEG amplifiers. Modern amplifiers recover quickly and register ECoG almost immediately after stimulation ceases. The amplitude of the artifact depends greatly on the position of the recording electrode in relation to the stimulator.

Although this artifact is due to brain stimulator activation, it is not necessary to eliminate. In fact, seeing the stimulation artifact alerts the NIOM team about when stimulation is performed so that they can be vigilant about reporting after discharges. Figure 13.9 shows an example of such an artifact.

Ultrasonic Surgical Aspirator

An ultrasonic surgical aspirator allows simultaneous tissue fragmentation, suction, and irrigation and is commonly used in neurosurgical and many other surgical procedures. It produces a very high-frequency, low-amplitude continuous artifact. Because the ultrasonic surgical aspirator artifact is of low amplitude, it is not eliminated by the artifact rejection software (9). If averaging of SEP and BAEP is not paused during the use of the aspirator, the artifact overwhelms the EP average and greatly reduces the amplitude of the signal of interest.

The ultrasonic surgical aspirator artifact may not be possible to eliminate entirely. Pausing the averaging during EPs is the most effective way of reducing this type of artifact. Repositioning the NIOM equipment and the aspirator may help as well.

X-Ray Equipment

Many ORs have x-ray equipment, such as the C-arm, that is intermittently used during surgery. The C-arm produces high-frequency artifact at 100 Hz, similar to the temperature management systems (8). This artifact may be present continuously while the C-arm is being used, but may also be present when it is not being used but still left on and in the OR.

Artifact from the C-arm can be reduced by moving the electrode wires away from the imaging device, and if possible, moving the NIOM equipment away as well. Increasing the number of repetitions averaged also helps. Finally, turning the C-arm off and disconnecting it from power when it is not in use will help, if allowed by the surgical team.

Surgical Drill

Surgical drills are used in many neuro and orthopedic surgeries. When in use, the surgical drill produces a high-frequency, continuous artifact. Typically, the amplitude is not very large, however it is much larger than SEP and BAEP waveforms.

Artifact from the surgical drill is very hard to eliminate. Because of its low amplitude, it is typically not eliminated by artifact rejection software. The best way to eliminate this artifact is to avoid it by not averaging EPs while drilling is ongoing. If averaging is not suspended when the drill is being used, the EP average can be overwhelmed. This is particularly the case in cerebellopontine angle surgeries. When the surgical drill is used during exposure, if averaging BAEPs is attempted, there may appear to be a reduction of amplitude compared to baseline. This can lead to false alerts to the surgical team.

A surgical drill placed directly on a limb may touch the needle electrodes in the muscle underneath. This can produce a high-frequency discharge in the EMG channels and can mimic spontaneous activity. Removing the drill will eliminate the artifact. An example of this type of artifact is presented in Figure 13.10.

Cardiopulmonary Bypass Machine

A cardiopulmonary bypass (CPB) machine is often used in aortic surgeries. A CPB machine is often used when EEG and/or EP monitoring is being performed. It can produce many types of artifacts that can interfere with NIOM, including electrical equipment interference, mechanical movements, static electricity, and piezoelectric effects (10). When EEG is being used to determine electrocerebral inactivity (ECI) in cases of deep hypothermic circulatory arrest, the artifact can make determination of ECI challenging. The high sensitivity of the EEG recording makes the artifacts more prominent (6). Additionally, the artifact can look like ECG, making it seem as if cardioplegia has not occurred. This latter issue is more problematic for the surgical and anesthesiology teams, but the NIOM team should also be aware of this effect.

Several techniques can be used to help eliminate CPB artifact. Moving the EEG or EP machine to the opposite side of the room as the CPB machine may help reduce the artifact. Proper grounding of the NIOM equipment, the CPB machine, and the patient can help reduce the electrical artifact as well.

Others Sources

There are many other devices and electrical equipment in the OR that can produce nonphysiologic artifacts during NIOM. Though these may be encountered less often than those already discussed, they are no less important to identify and try to eliminate.

Devices like the operating table may produce an electrical artifact which may be challenging to identify. Consumer electronics, such as cellular phones, are now increasingly used in the OR. Sometimes they can produce an artifact that can be identified by virtue of it appearing only when the device is in use. Interventions by the surgeon in the surgical field, such as hammering hardware, can cause intermittent artifacts as well. Generally, continuous artifacts are harder to identify and eliminate with averaging than intermittent ones. Intermittent artifacts can often be isolated by virtue of their relationship to a particular event or piece of equipment being turned on, cycling, or brought into the room.

CONCLUSIONS

Artifacts are ubiquitous during NIOM. Avoiding artifacts is better than eliminating them; this can be done most effectively with good electrode application and setup for the monitoring. When artifacts appear, identifying them and trying to eliminate or minimize them is important to preserve the integrity of the underlying neurophysiologic signal. In some instances, artifacts cannot be eliminated and do not impede recording the activity of interest. In these cases, it is best to recognize the artifact and mentally adjust interpretation appropriately.

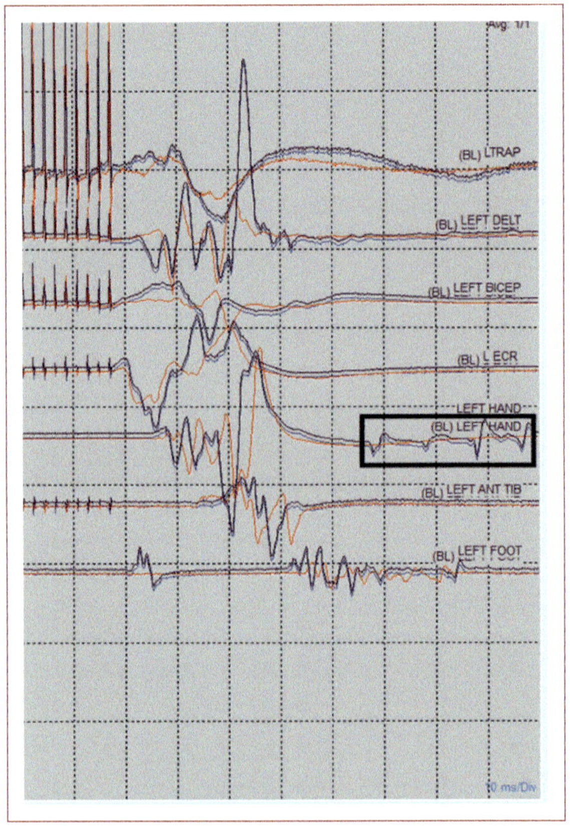

FIGURE 13.1: This is an MEP tracing obtained from a 71-year-old man undergoing an anterior cervical decompression and fixation for cervical spinal stenosis. This tracing occurred during the discectomy portion of the procedure. There is EMG artifact in the MEP (box). This is an example of an intermittent physiologic artifact. Free-running EMG activity can be present in any muscle from which MEP is obtained. In this figure, the hand MEP channel shows the EMG activity. These waveforms may be mistaken for MEP potentials from that muscle. EMG activity in this case is easy to identify as artifact because the earlier response from the hand muscle looks to clearly be the true MEP waveform. The latency of the artifact is longer than MEP responses recorded from the right foot, which would be unlikely for a true response. The morphology of the waveforms is also unusual. Obtaining more MEP trials will help to resolve the issue of artifact versus true MEP response. A true response will still be present, whereas random EMG activity will be absent or change in latency and amplitude. If this artifact is present, it is often not possible to eliminate it totally. Rather it is best to recognize it as artifact and not allow it to interfere with interpretation of the MEPs.

EMG, electromyography; MEP, motor evoked potential.

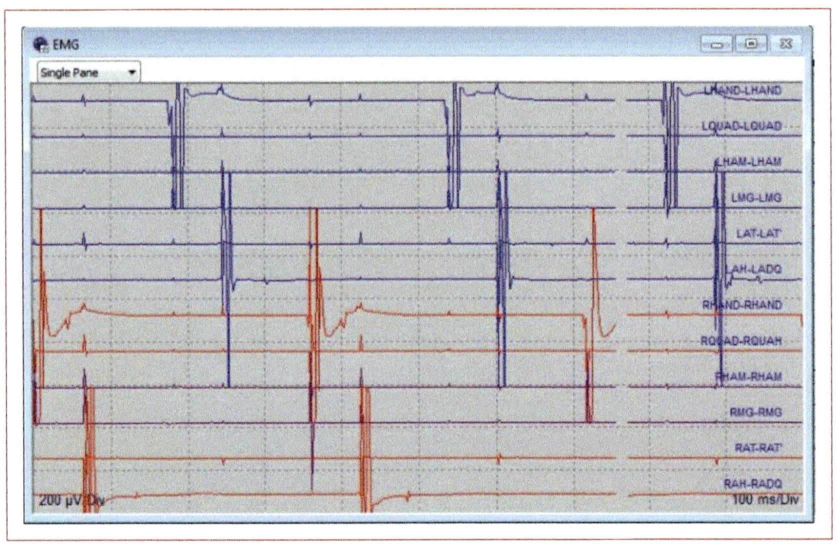

FIGURE 13.2: This is a free-running EMG tracing obtained from a 14-year-old girl undergoing posterior spinal fusion for neuromuscular scoliosis. The figure shows regular, high-amplitude discharges in bilateral hand and foot channels of the free-running EMG. This artifact is caused by bilateral ulnar and tibial nerve stimulation used to obtain SEPs. This is an example of a continuous physiologic artifact caused by muscle contraction induced by SEP stimulation. SEP and free-running EMG monitoring are frequently performed together. When SEP stimulation is turned on, contraction of the relevant target muscles occurs, producing muscle action potentials in the free-running EMG. Since the SEP stimulation is regular and continuous, the muscle action potentials are also regular and continuous. The resultant waveform is seen only in the muscle group innervated by the nerve being stimulated. In the example, stimulation of the right ulnar nerve results in artifact in the right-hand muscles (open arrow), whereas stimulation of the right tibial nerve results in artifact in the right-foot muscles. The regular nature, high amplitude, and presence in selected muscle groups differentiate these potentials from abnormal spontaneous activity that may also occur in free-running EMG. This type of artifact cannot be eliminated, but it is easy to recognize and account for during interpretation.

EMG, electromyography; SEP, somatosensory evoked potential.

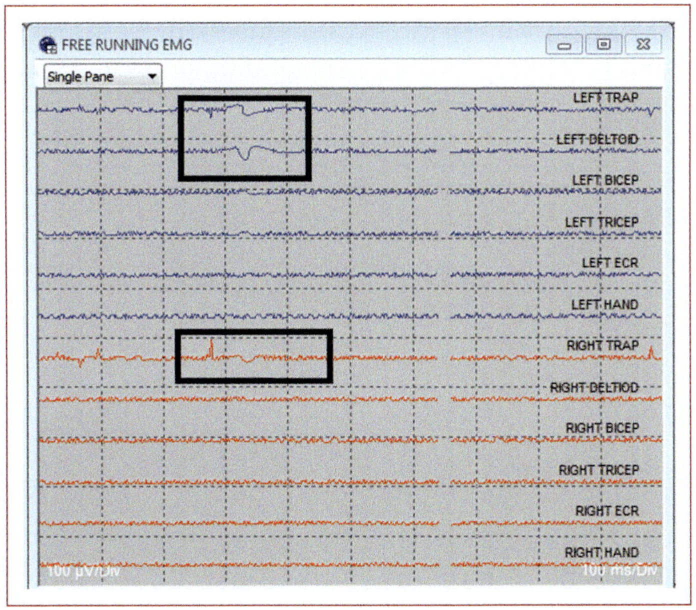

FIGURE 13.3: This is a free-running EMG tracing from a 51-year-old woman undergoing anterior cervical decompression and fusion for cervical stenosis. This image was recorded soon after exposure was complete. In bilateral trapezius and left deltoid muscle channels, there is a single upgoing potential followed by a slower wave (boxes). One such discharge was seen per screen, but the location of the discharge on the screen changed. This discharge is ECG followed by pulse artifact seen in several of the EMG channels. It is an example of a continuous physiologic artifact. This artifact can be confused with spontaneous activity from the muscles. It is identified as artifact by virtue of its consistent morphology and by determining its frequency (usually 50–70 beats per minute). Comparing this discharge to the ECG seen on the OR room monitors can help identify its source. Good electrode placement technique with low and matched impedances helps reduce the chance that such artifact will be seen. However, once it is present, it cannot be completely eliminated. It is best to recognize it and account for it during interpretation.

EMG, electromyography; OR, operating room.

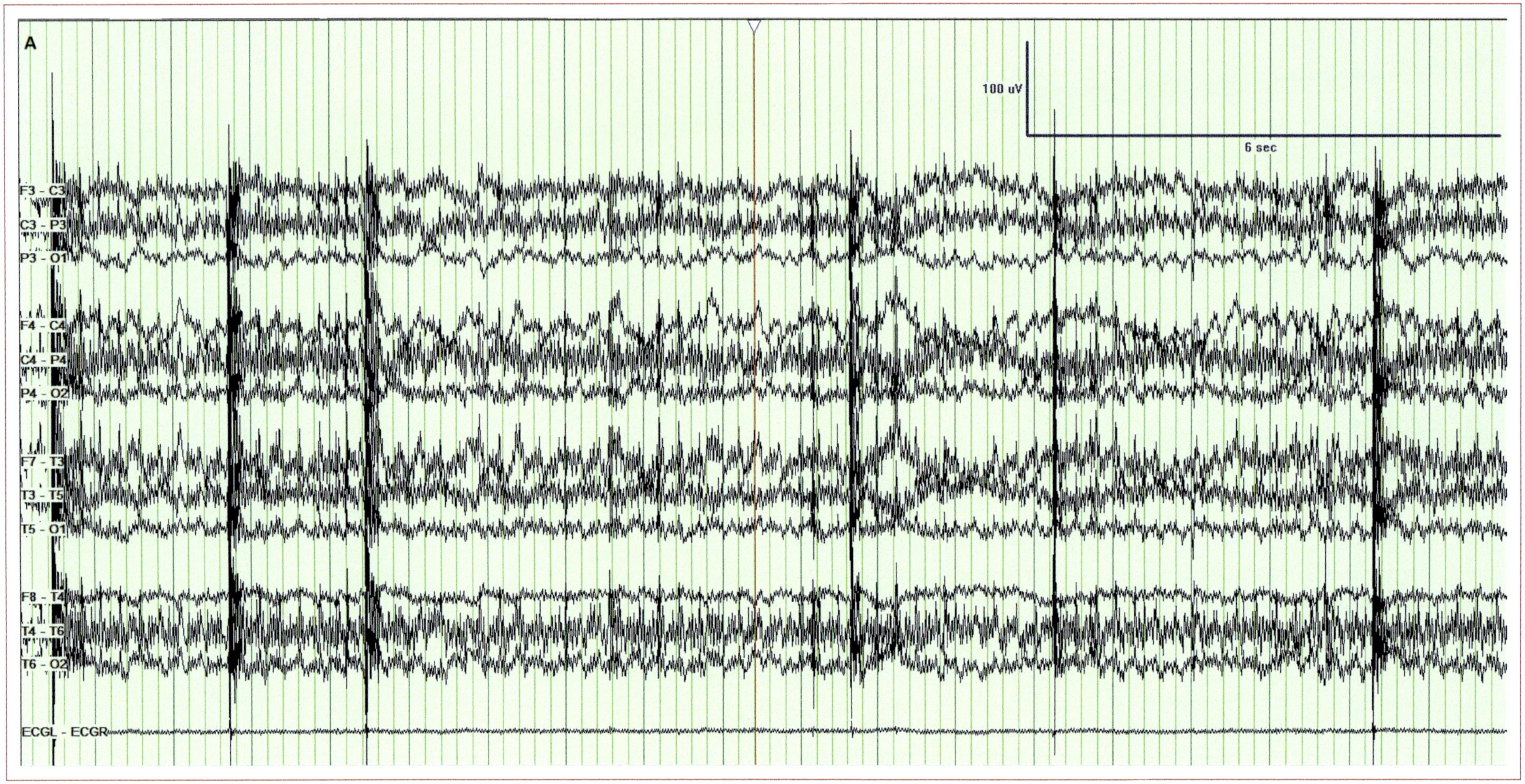

FIGURE 13.4: This is an EEG recording from a 53-year-old man undergoing thoracotomy for ascending hemi aortic arch repair. This EEG was recorded a few minutes prior to initiation of cardiopulmonary bypass (panel A). ***(continued)***

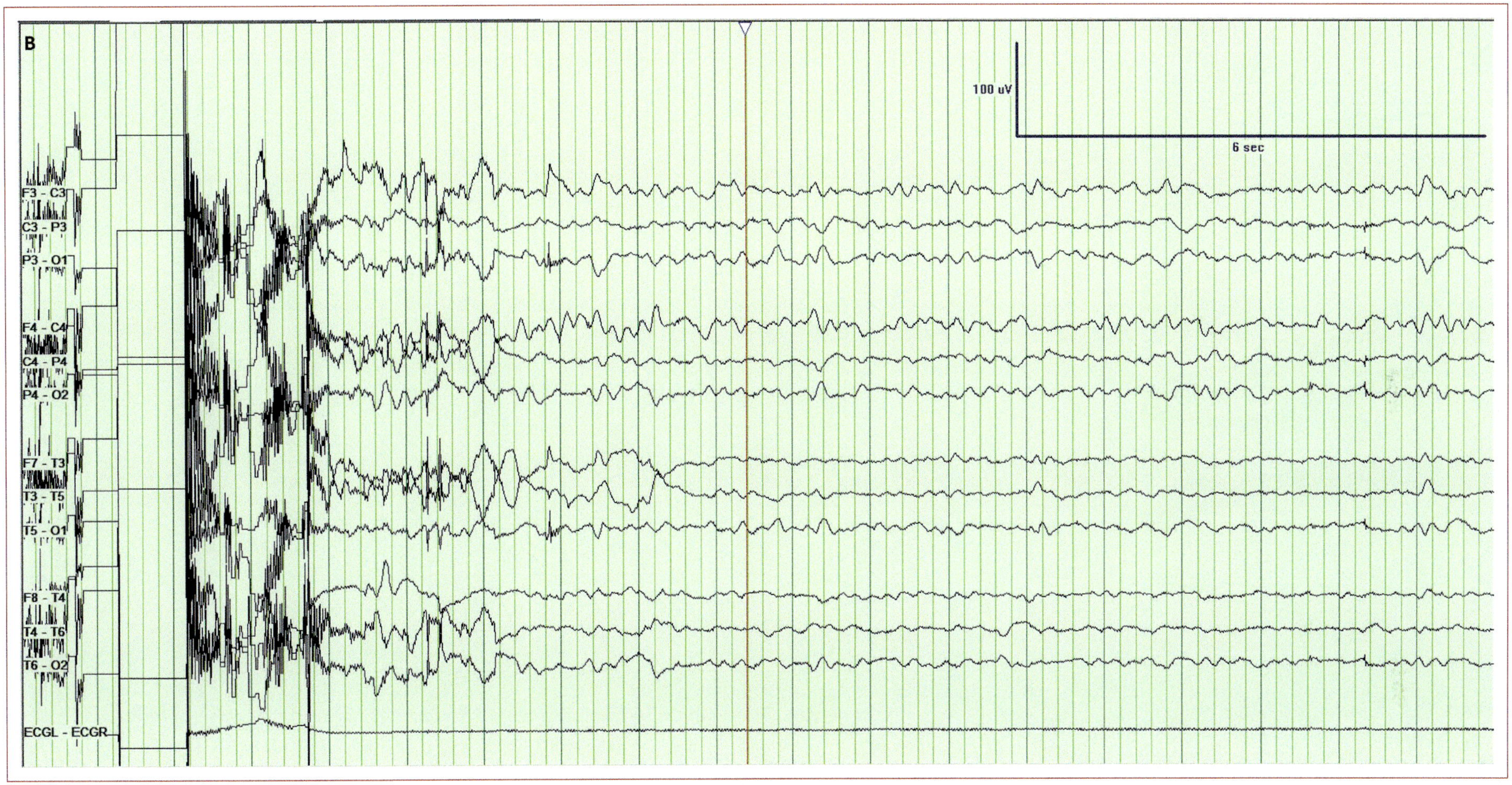

FIGURE 13.4: (*continued*) Widespread high-frequency artifact is noted. This discharge is electrical noise that did not improve with a 60-Hz filter. It is caused by a damaged and compromised EEG system reference electrode. This is a type of continuous nonphysiologic artifact from the NIOM wires. This artifact is pervasive and makes interpretation of the EEG impossible. As cooling progresses, changes in underlying EEG will not be possible to identify. A problem with the electrodes can cause this type of artifact. Because all the channels have the artifact, if this is an electrode problem, either all electrodes have been damaged or the system reference electrode has been damaged. It is more likely for a single electrode to be the cause of the problem. Replacing the system reference electrode (a cork screw electrode in this case) resulted in elimination of the artifact (panel B). **(*continued*)**

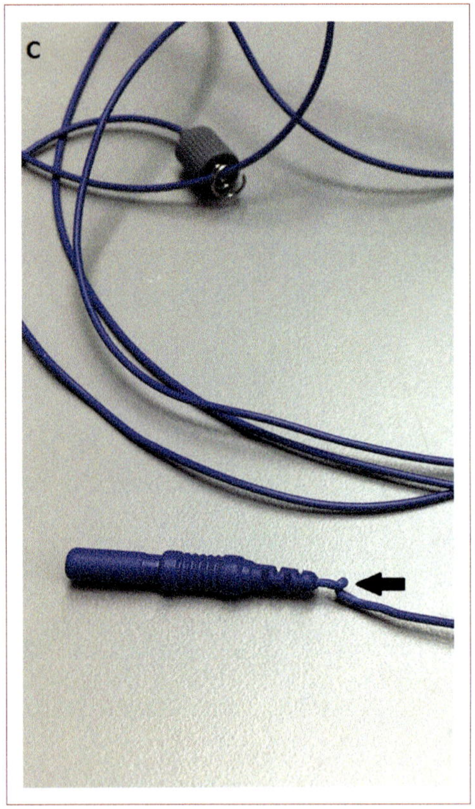

FIGURE 13.4: (*continued*) After the surgery, examination of the removed electrode revealed that indeed it had been damaged (panel C). Damaged electrodes cause problems with common mode rejection and result in lack of cancellation of various types of artifact by the differential amplifier. Correcting this artifact was essential for successful interpretation of the EEG.

NIOM, neurophysiologic intraoperative monitoring.

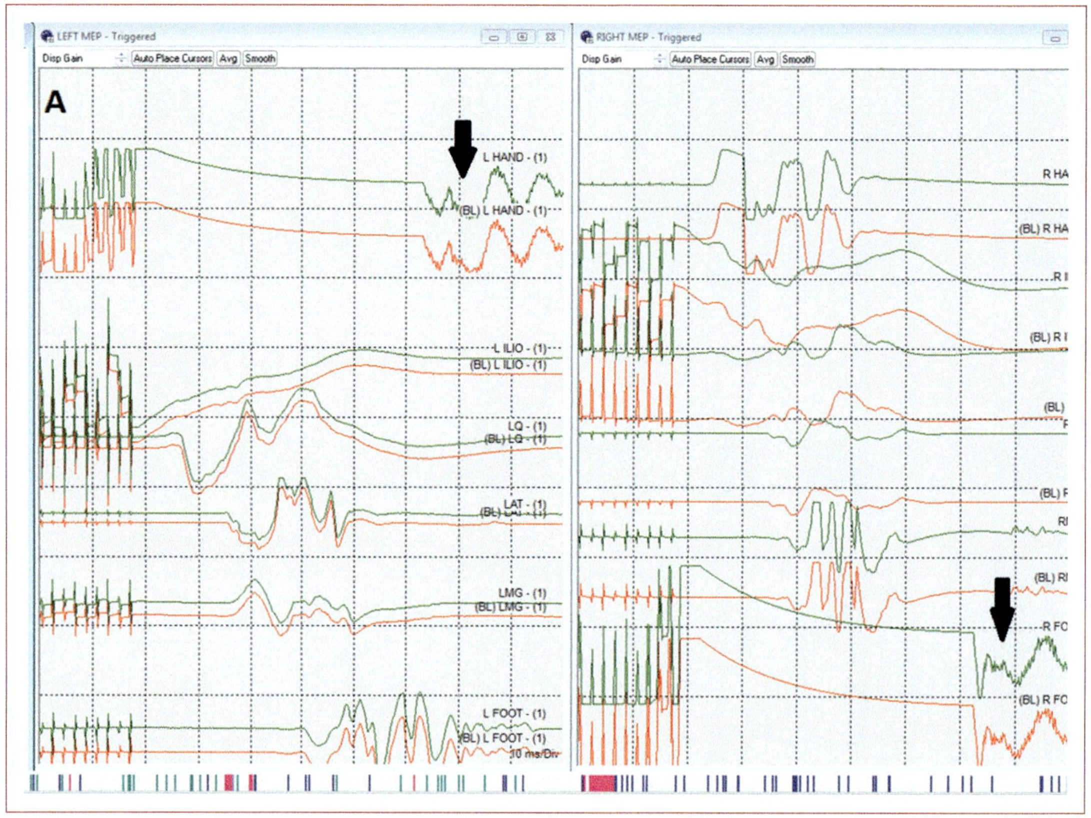

FIGURE 13.5: This is an MEP tracing from a 16-year-old girl undergoing posterior spinal fusion for scoliosis. MEPs from the left and right side are shown (panel A). (*continued*)

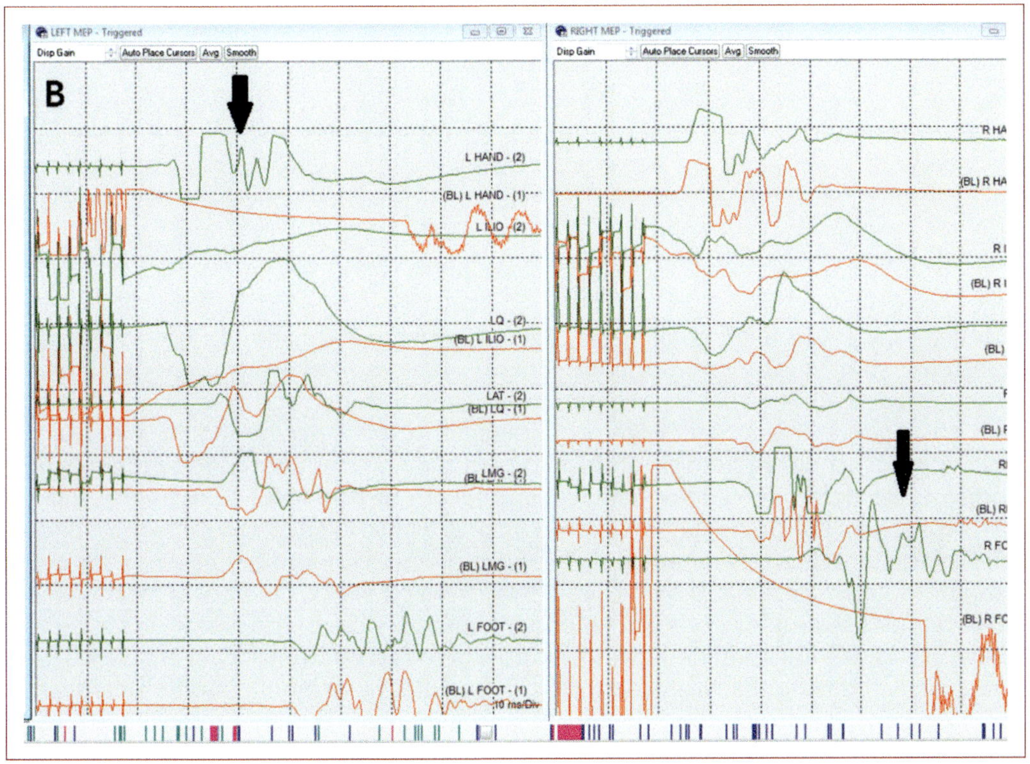

FIGURE 13.5: The MEPs from the left hand and right foot appear to have a prolonged latency and unusual morphology and appear to be an artifact (arrows). This artifact is caused by bad inputs in the headbox of the NIOM equipment. This is an example of intermittent nonphysiologic artifact from the NIOM machine. The MEP from the left hand is easier to identify as an artifact. It occurs at a latency which is longer than the left foot MEP, making it unlikely to be a physiologic response. The right foot response also occurs later than the left foot response, making it suspicious for artifact. Moreover, the morphology of the left-hand and right-foot responses is similar. It is important to identify these responses as artifact as the real MEP from these muscles is not being monitored. The headbox inputs should be suspected since only a few of the channels have the artifact. Changing the input jacks of the left hand and right foot in the headbox resulted in appearance of reliable MEPs in those muscle groups (panel B, arrows pointing to the improved MEPs).

MEP, motor evoked potential; NIOM, neurophysiologic intraoperative monitoring.

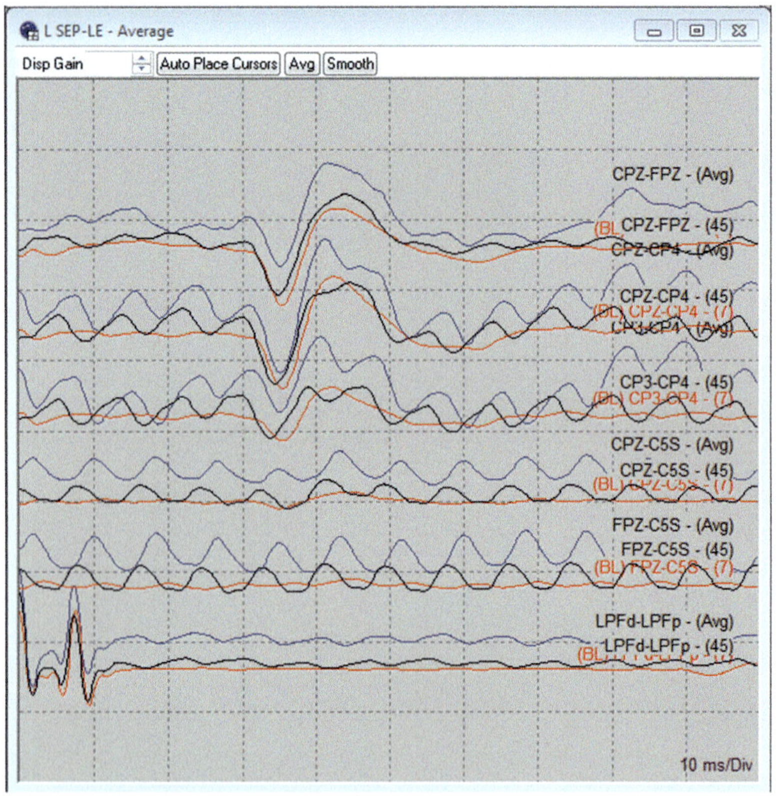

FIGURE 13.6: This is a left tibial nerve SEP tracing from a 14-year-old boy undergoing posterior spinal fusion for idiopathic scoliosis. A sinusoidal artifact is noted in all channels and appeared 4 hours into the procedure during rod placement. This is an electrical power line artifact from some piece of surgical equipment. It is an example of continuous nonphysiologic artifact. One of the first steps in trying to identify this artifact is to determine its frequency; it appears to be 120 Hz (12 waves in a 100-msec screen). Since this is a harmonic of the line noise (60 Hz), it is most likely to be an electrical power line artifact. The exact piece of equipment causing this artifact can be isolated by moving or, if possible, turning off various electrical machines. If this cannot be done or does not help identify the source of the artifact (as was the case in this example), maneuvers to reduce the effects of the artifact are used. This can involve moving the wire electrodes or the NIOM machine to a different location in the room away from other electrical equipment. Appropriate grounding of the patient and NIOM machine should be ensured. Increasing the number of repetitions to average can also reduce the effects of the artifact.

NIOM, neurophysiologic intraoperative monitoring; SEP, somatosensory evoked potential.

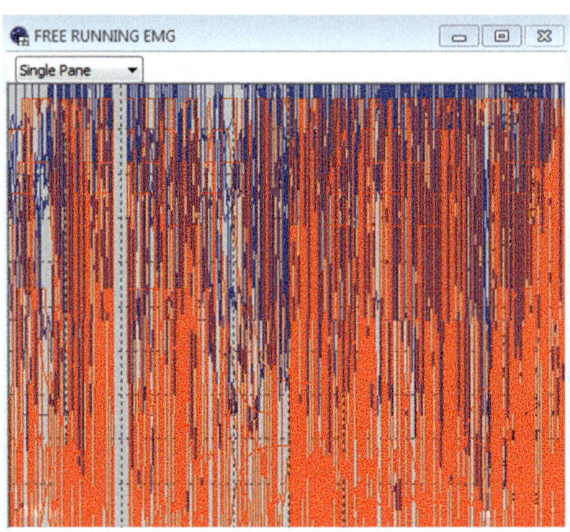

FIGURE 13.7: This is a free-running EMG tracing from a 61-year-old man undergoing lumbar decompressive laminectomy for lumbar spinal stenosis. This EMG image recording is taken during the surgical exposure. High-amplitude and high-frequency activity is abundant and obscures the entire screen. A loud sound can be heard each time this activity occurs as well. This artifact is caused by the electrocautery. This is an example of intermittent nonphysiologic artifact from surgical equipment. Electrocautery is frequently used during surgical exposure, and it causes artifact that can obscure the entire screen or parts of it. A loud sound clearly identifies the source of the artifact. However, if the sound is turned off, and the artifact is limited to only a few channels, it may appear like spontaneous EMG activity. However, its association with use of the electrocautery can clearly identify the source of the artifact. This artifact is not avoidable in surgery; rather, it must be recognized and interpretation of underlying EMG activity appropriately adjusted.

EMG, electromyography.

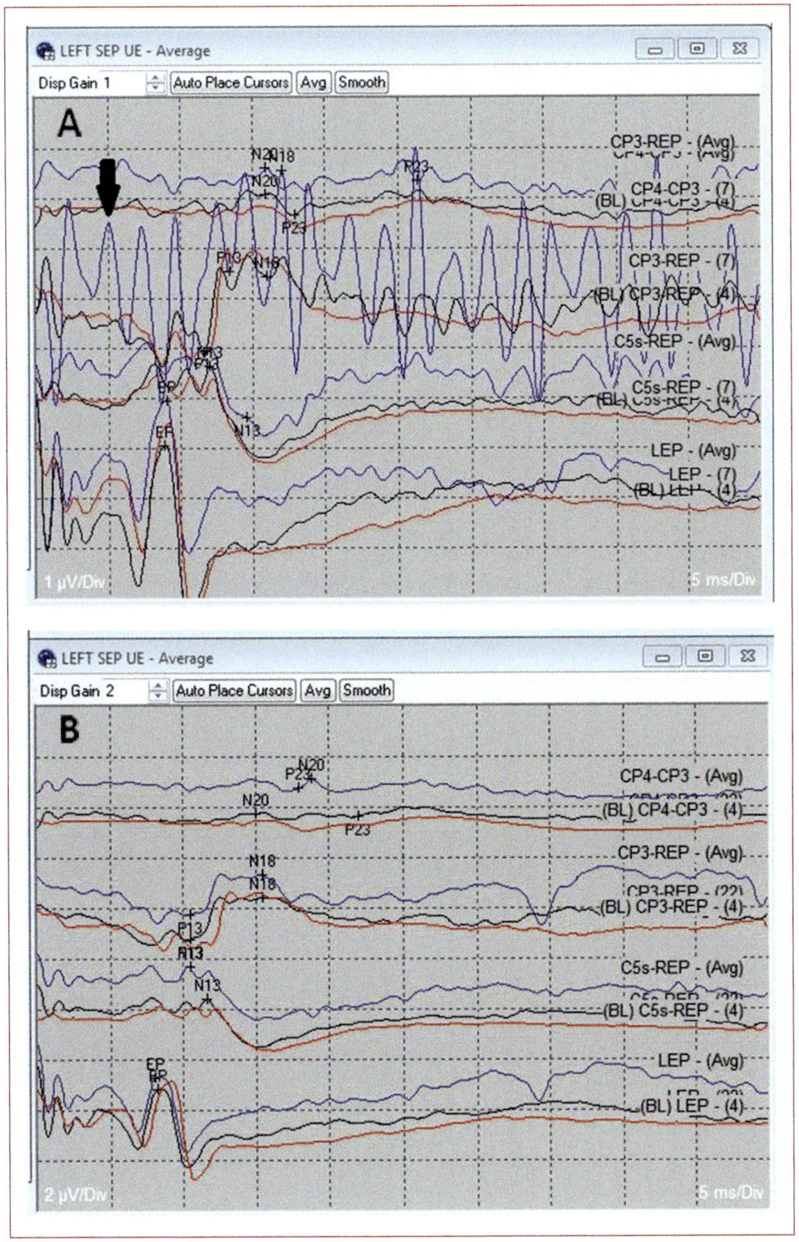

FIGURE 13.8: This is a median nerve SEP tracing of a 47-year-old woman undergoing a transcondylar approach for resection of a right-sided brainstem tumor. The left median SEP is shown in panel A. A high-frequency, high-amplitude artifact is noted in the second channel (arrow). This artifact appeared when the operating microscope was brought into the surgical field. This artifact is caused by the operating microscope. It is an example of continuous nonphysiologic artifact from surgical equipment. The operating microscope and other surgical equipment can cause electrical artifact. Often this electrical artifact is a harmonic of 60 Hz. In panel A, the artifact occurs at a frequency of 420 Hz (21 waveforms in a 50-msec screen). It was identified as operating microscope-related artifact because it appeared when the operating microscope was brought into the operating field. However, at times such an association may not be obvious. In those situations, the technologist must identify other causes of electrical artifact and try to eliminate them. In panel B, the electrical artifact has disappeared; the improvement was coincident with removal of the operating microscope. In this case, the artifact could not be eliminated as the operating microscope had to be used during the surgery. This makes averaging SEPs and BAEPs more difficult, but still possible. Attention to electrode application technique, proper grounding, and reducing all other sources of electrical noise can help reduce some of the artifact.

BAEP, brainstem auditory evoked potential; SEP, somatosensory evoked potential.

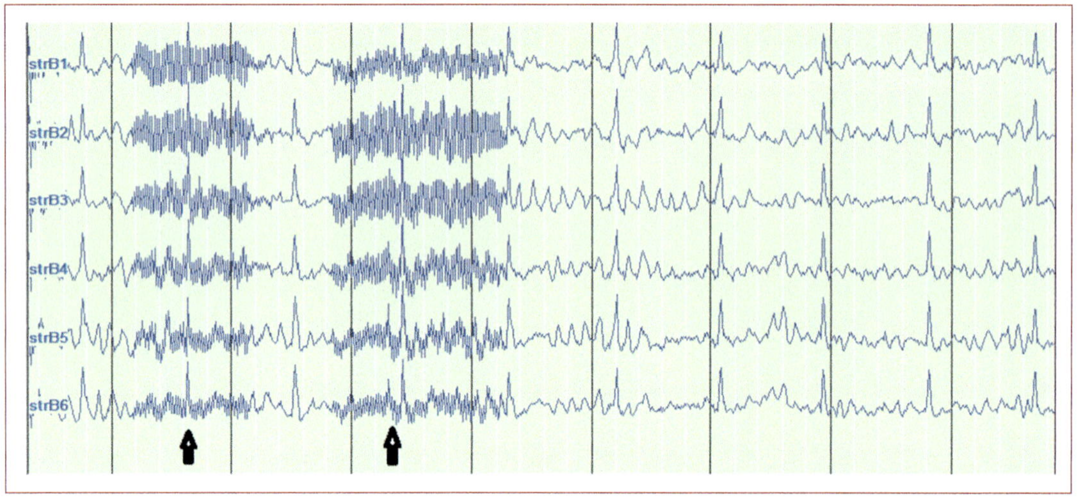

FIGURE 13.9: This is an ECoG recording from a 6-contact strip electrode placed directly on the cortex of a 63-year-old woman undergoing a left-sided craniotomy for resection of a brain tumor. Language mapping was performed prior to the resection. A discharge is noted on the screen intermittently (arrows). This artifact is caused by the Ojemann cortical stimulator. It is an example of intermittent nonphysiologic artifact from surgical equipment. The Ojemann brain stimulator is used to disrupt eloquent brain areas to identify their function. The electrical impulse is usually a 50- to 60-Hz stimulus that is delivered in bursts of 1 to 5 seconds. Often there is a sound produced whenever the stimulus is applied. The association with the sound and the characteristic morphology of the artifact make it easy to identify the source of this artifact. The actual waveforms embedded in the artifact can also be counted, and they will be of the same frequency as the stimulation frequency. This is a desirable artifact as afterdischarges can occur after this discharge ends. Thus, this discharge helps identify what the surgeon is doing and when to look for the activity of interest.

ECoG, electrocorticography.

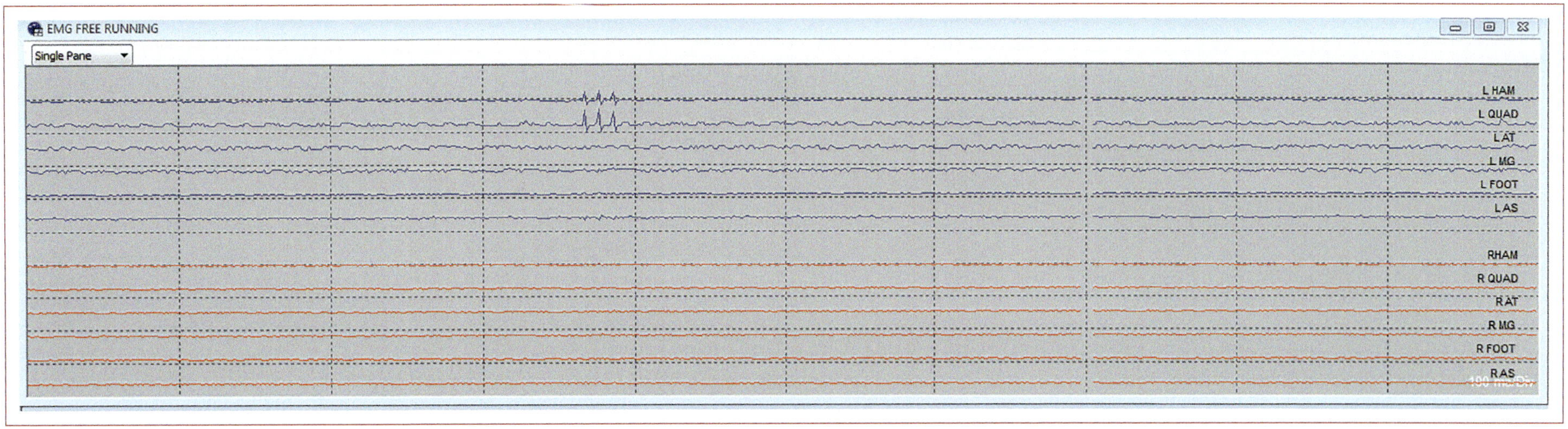

FIGURE 13.10: This is a free-running EMG tracing from a 73-year-old man undergoing lumbar decompressive laminectomy and fusion for severe lumbar spinal stenosis. This EMG image recording is obtained soon after exposure. It shows a burst of three waveforms in the left hamstring and quadriceps femoris muscles. This discharge occurred intermittently, and the morphology and latency remained the same for several minutes. This discharge is electrical artifact from the surgical drill lying in close proximity to the recording needle electrodes in the left hamstring and quadriceps femoris muscles. It is an example of an intermittent nonphysiologic artifact from surgical equipment.

This artifact can be confused with spontaneous activity from the muscles. It is identified as artifact by virtue of its unchanging morphology and latency in a free-running EMG window. Physiologic activity would change in both morphology and latency. The discharge appears and disappears depending on whether the drill is in the ON or OFF position. Also, a physiologic spontaneous discharge occurring in only the left hamstring and quadriceps femoris muscles would be unlikely as they are supplied by different nerve roots. Identifying and eliminating this artifact can be done by asking the surgical team to move the drill from the patient's leg to a different location.

EMG, electromyography.

REFERENCES

1. Daube JR. Waveforms and artifacts. In: Daube JR, Rubin DI, eds. *Clinical Neurophysiology*. New York, NY: Oxford University Press; 2009:103-114.
2. Tatum WO, Dworetzky BA, Freeman WD, et al. Artifact: recording EEG in special care units. *J Clin Neurophysiol*. 2011;28:264-277. doi:10.1097/WNP.
3. Tatum WO, Dworetzky BA, Schomer DL. Artifact and recording concepts in EEG. *J Clin Neurophysiol*. 2011;28:252-263. doi:10.1097/WNP.0b013e31821c3c93.
4. Cooper R, Osselton JW, Shaw JC. *Operational Techniques. EEG Technology*. London, UK: Butterworths; 1969: 74-96.
5. Tyner FS, Knott JR, Mayer WB. *Artifacts. Fundamental of EEG Technology: Vol 1: Basic Concepts and Methods*. New York, NY: Raven Press; 1983: 280-311.
6. Kale EB, Swisher CB. Introduction to the operating room. In: Husain AM, ed. *A Practical Approach to Neurophysiologic Intraoperative Monitoring*. New York, NY: Demos Medical Publishing; 2015:3-17.
7. Zielinski P, Furtak J. Influence of intraoperative neurophysiologic monitoring on the development of surgical dissection techniques. *Expert Rev Med Devices*. 2012;9:571-575. doi:10.1586/erd.12.52.
8. Farajidavar A, Seifert JL, Delgado MR, et al. Electromagnetic interference in intraoperative monitoring of motor evoked potentials and a wireless solution. *Med Eng Phys*. 2016;38:87-96. doi:10.1016/j.medengphy.2015.11.007.
9. Legatt AD. Mechanisms of intraoperative brainstem auditory evoked potential changes. *J Clin Neurophysiol*. 2002;19:396-408. doi:10.1097/00004691-200210000-00003.
10. Saied NN, Helwani MA, Comunale ME, et al. A simple solution for electrocardiographic artifacts during cardiopulmonary bypass and in the intensive care unit. *J Cardiothorac Vasc Anesth*. 2007;21:572-573. doi:10.1053/j.jvca.2006.12.003.

CHAPTER 14

Artifact Reduction

Tasneem F. Hasan and William O. Tatum, IV

INTRODUCTION

Many simple and complex sources of artifact exist when attempting to record physiological signals from the nervous system. Unwanted artifact is common and may be due to physiological and extraphysiological causes. When artifact obscures the ability to record the targeted neurophysiologic signal, reduction is an important goal to facilitate an accurate interpretation (**Figure 14.1**). Denoising is a challenge to optimize the physiological signal of interest prior to processing and analysis. All clinical neurophysiological (CNP) procedures use variations of scalp or indwelling electrodes to measure electrical potential and monitor neuronal activity. Signals are often composed of a mixture of frequencies recorded at each electrode site, amplified, and compared to comprise neuronal electrophysiological activity that is interpreted over a predetermined duration (1). Artifact reduction requires preparation during the initial stages of recording to ensure optimal electrical integrity. During the performance of the procedure, it is critical for an experienced technologist to have a heightened awareness of artifact to identify, localize, and eliminate artifact that serves as "interference" to interpretation of the physiological signal. Finally, artifact reduction techniques are essential for online and post hoc signal analysis to remove artifacts from the recorded signal of interest. Some artifacts are common to several CNP procedures (e.g., cardiac, ocular, and myogenic sources), whereas others are procedure-specific, requiring individual techniques (e.g., demagnetizing efforts for magnetoencephalography). Some require simple behavioral maneuvers such as asking the patient to relax their jaw during EEG to eliminate myogenic artifact. Others require simple techniques such as warming an extremity during electromyography (EMG). Electrophysiological techniques (e.g., averaging during recording of evoked potentials [EPs]) may be required to optimally record other CNP waveforms. Nevertheless, innovations in software development using automated techniques have improved our ability to optimize the signal-to-noise ratio (SNR) during CNP recordings. Although many forms are proprietary and evolving, the most common techniques that have been attempted to use or are using for artifact reduction are discussed in this chapter.

ARTIFACTS

Artifact occurs when there is a mismatch of physiological to nonphysiologic signal that is recorded. The presence of artifact may at times be helpful to facilitate interpretation. Ocular and myogenic artifact, for example, may provide insight into the stages of sleep during polysomnography (PSG) and help differentiate wakefulness and rapid eye movement (REM) sleep during EEG and PSG (2). Artifacts are classified according to their source of origin. Those arising from the subject's body are physiological, whereas those arising externally are nonphysiological (extracerebral) artifacts.

Physiological Artifacts

The common physiological artifacts reflect myogenic, ocular, and cardiac generators. Other complex signals seen during movement may reflect a combination of sources.

Myogenic

The impact of myogenic artifact that results from chewing/swallowing, tongue movement (glossokinetic), grimacing, and generalized muscular contraction range from rendering a CNP procedure useless to analyzing patterns that may have usefulness. It is the context of recording that reflects the significance. Muscle frequency may range from 10 to more than 100 Hz and occur with large amplitudes over 100 μV (3). Myogenic artifacts can be easily identified based on their characteristic nonoscillatory morphology and very brief duration (<20 msec), which reflect motor unit potentials (4). Excessive movement by patients during a CNP can substantially contaminate the recording. Physiological signals may closely resemble those artifacts arising from movement disorder patients. Slow (4–6 Hz), rhythmic, and sinusoidal signals in an EEG seen with Parkinson's disease may be distinguished from faster frequencies (7–12 Hz) typically encountered with essential tremor. Differentiating artifactual from physiologic signals may at times be challenging for the clinician (**Figure 14.2**). However, similar to sleep staging, patterns of myogenic artifact may be useful in diagnosing psychogenic movement disorders, chiefly movements comprising tremors, jerks, spasms, and dystonia using EEG time-locked with EMG (5). Surface EMG characteristics can differentiate between a convulsive epileptic seizure and a nonepileptic behavioral event even in the absence of rhythmic clonic movements (6). A photomyoclonic response that generates myogenic artifact appearing 50 to 60 milliseconds following intermittent photic stimulation may mimic a seizure and lead to overtreatment (7).

Ocular

Eye movements during CNP procedures such as EEG can disturb the electric fields in electrodes placed in the frontal head regions by generating large-amplitude alternate currents with fields that create artifact (8). Ocular artifacts range between 0 and 16 Hz and contaminate the physiological activity by introducing stronger deflections within the target signal (9). This may impact interpretation of neural signals produced during EEG, magnetoencephalography (MEG), and PSG. The amount of eye movement helps signify the stage of sleep and level of alertness reflecting a valuable contribution of artifact to overall interpretation of the recording. Fluttering of the eyelids generates a signal frequency in the theta bandwidth, while slower infrequent repetitive eyeblinking occurs within the delta range in the EEG. When excessive eye movements are encountered, they can obscure the CNP recording and interfere with the physiological signal. Challenging aspects of identifying ocular artifact may involve correct identification of the source (**Figure 14.3**). Therefore, monitoring eye movements and artifact reduction of intrusive eye movements during CNP recordings is essential.

Cardiac

Cardiac artifacts are common and may be divided into mechanical and electrophysiological artifact. They may be identified by sharp, regular waveforms synchronized to QRS complexes on the ECG channel. During various types of CNP recording, cardiac artifacts may limit interpretation of the recording or even beguile the interpreter into misinterpreting a nonphysiological cardiac signal as an abnormal one derived from the brain. These artifacts may mimic periodic discharges (PDs; lateralized or generalized) in EEG but can be distinguished by the presence of recurrent time-synched intervals between artifactual discharges and ECG while PDs lack precise periodicity of intervals between discharges (10). Cardiac artifacts may also contaminate MEG, PSG, and EP. Additionally, the presence of arrhythmia may complicate the signal further due to irregular intervals between discharges. Cardiac pacemakers produce a distinct artifact. They can be identified in electrodes as high-frequency, polyphasic potentials of short duration (10). Ballistocardiographic artifact is mechanical artifact from head/body movement during cardiac contractions that is introduced into a CNP recording (11).

Nonphysiological Artifacts

Motion

Movement of the head, body, and limbs is complex and generates high-voltage signals at irregular intervals and can occur simultaneously during an act of seizure or may be due to hyperventilation/respiration, movement disorders, ocular movements, and cardiac activity.

Electrode

The electrode–tissue junction is the most critical interface for generating a high-quality physiological signal. Electrode artifacts arise from contact impedance between the electrodes and tissue which may be due to excessive or dried out gel paste. Dry electrodes are superior to their gel counterpart due to patient comfort and ease of setup (e.g., minimal skin preparation time or conductive gel) and have demonstrated better utility during home-EEG recording, long-term monitoring, and during emergencies due to expedited setup (12). However, dry electrodes are subjected to contact impedance and can substantially contaminate the signal. When dry electrodes are preferred, constant monitoring of the electrode–tissue contact is warranted to minimize motion artifact during CNP (12).

Artifact may also arise from change in resistance or electrode potential between the electrode and the tissue, or can be due to a broken lead.

Electrodes may "pop" and introduce artifact that is characterized by a sudden discharge or change in the electrical potential between the electrode and the tissue and give rise to a distinct waveform with a steep rise and slow fall (10). When several pops result over a few seconds, this suggests technical pitfalls in the recording environment (e.g., loose or nonadherent electrode). Salt bridge artifact results from excessive gel paste in between the electrodes and is channel specific, and appears as attenuated waveforms (10).

Instrumental

The power main artifact is typically produced at 50 or 60 Hz (60 Hz in the United States). Avoiding patient contact with nearby machines, electrical devices, and connectors or cables should be followed to prevent 50/60 Hz alternating current (AC) interference. Unplugging nearby machines in the ICU or the operating room (OR) may help eliminate the source so digital notch filters are not required. The frequencies associated with the power main are not static at a single frequency. Notch filters may produce "ringing" in the time domain and obscure the target signal using an overly narrow filter (seen during EP recording).

QUANTIZATION ERROR ARTIFACT

The ICU and the OR are common settings for quantization error artifact caused by an interaction of sampling rate and high-amplitude periodic patterns, most commonly 50- to 60-Hz artifact. The sampling rate and the high-amplitude signal have to share a common divisor. In the presence of high-amplitude 60-Hz waveforms, it is manifested as 20-Hz activity when the sampling rate is 200/sec, or as 4, 12, and 20 Hz activity when the sampling rate is 250/sec. It occurs more extensively in the ICU setting when the acquisition machine uses a sampling rate of 200/sec (**Figure 14.4A**). It can be present in a large percentage of recordings, especially as the recordings become increasingly contaminated with high-amplitude, 60-cycle activity (Mark Scheuer, personal communication, March 14, 2018). It may be mistaken as excess cerebral beta activity by EEG readers. Quantization artifact can contaminate both the original waveforms and quantitative EEG (QEEG) metrics and augment beta power or interfere with the alpha delta ratio when the artifactual patterns hit at 4 and 12 Hz at 256/sec sampling rates (**Figure 14.4B**). However, it is usually easy to recognize in trends because it generates a narrow continuous band of activity to stand out at a precise frequency bandwidth unlike cerebral activity composed of more variation. Quantization artifact is not eliminated through the use of a notch filter because it occurs as an independent signal resulting from the digitization process. It can be eliminated using independent component analysis (ICA) or similar techniques, through the use of narrow notch filters at the appropriate frequency, or by using a sampling rate that does not share a common divisor between the sampling rate and the high-amplitude signal, 60 Hz (or 50 Hz in non-U.S. areas) (**Figure 14.5**).

APPLICATION OF ARTIFACT TO PATIENT CARE

Most CNP recordings are subject to numerous artifacts. Contamination of CNP recordings with artifact can greatly hamper accurate interpretation and fail to differentiate between neuronal activity and artifact. This can result in compromised interpretation of the procedure and interfere with patient management. A minimum duration of artifact-free recording is suggested to evaluate baseline activity when performing a CNP procedure (13). Current advancements in technology aimed at artifact reduction help facilitate automatic detection and removal of artifact.

TECHNIQUES OF ARTIFACT REDUCTION

Artifacts arising on CNP procedures can be discarded by the use of various techniques; these may be behavioral, manual, or automated methods. Prior to utilizing these methods, employing appropriate preparation technique prior to the CNP procedure is crucial to limit the occurrence of nonphysiological artifact. The American Clinical Neurophysiology Society (ACNS) has established minimum criteria to obtain a technically sound and standardized recording in EEG, EPs, and neurophysiologic intraoperative monitoring (NIOM) that can be interpreted with consistency (14). The American Association of Neuromuscular and Electrodiagnostic Medicine (AANEM) provides evidence-based practice guidelines to enhance the diagnostic accuracy and efficiency of electrodiagnostic studies during the assessment and treatment of muscles and nerve disorders (15). The Standards of Practice Committee of the American Sleep Disorders Association (ASDA) sets practice parameters and indications for PSG in the diagnosis of sleep disorders (16), whereas the American Clinical Magnetoencephalography (MEG) Society (ACMEGS) provides minimum standard practice guidelines for the routine clinical recording and analysis of MEG and EEG in all age groups in attempt to standardize procedures and allow for exchange of recordings/reports among facilities (17).

The electrode–tissue junction, for instance, is the most critical interface for electrical conduction and is most often subjected to high impedance. Although electrodes have evolved with time and are relatively simple to use, they are responsible for significant artifact on CNP recordings. Electrode caps may be used during CNP procedures (e.g., EEG and EP). They may also be useful during ICU or ambulatory EEG monitoring for clinical and research purposes (18). Technicians fitting electrode caps must also have prior experience with cap placement to avoid the occurrence of artifact (19). When comparing individual electrodes with cap electrodes, they were found to be of similar quality in one study (18). For most routine CNP recordings, 1-cm diameter, cup-shaped electrodes with a flat rim are utilized and offer good contact in the presence of electroconductive gel (20). Collodion helps maintain electrode attachment for prolonged use and a piece of gauze is used to cover the electrode to establish firm contact (20). Additionally, technologists abrade the skin using an abrasive detergent to remove debris and oil from the surface of the scalp prior to attaching the electrodes. A long-standing understanding that electrodes must have low impedance (i.e., less than 5 kΩ) to eliminate unwanted electrode artifact during the recording is a fallacy. Good recording may be achieved even with high electrode–scalp impedances (21), and subdermal and PressOn electrodes can sustain even higher impedances. Thus, when artifact is difficult to overcome (e.g., in the OR and ICU), subdermal needle electrodes may be helpful to reduce artifact (22). The choice and location of the reference electrode may affect the integrity of the recording and introduce artifact (Figure 14.6). Scalp references are often more subject to artifact than an intracranial source during invasive EEG recording. Signals from the scalp are much lower in voltage than those recorded directly from the brain. Therefore, if a scalp reference is chosen, a secure scalp–electrode interface is essential to provide adequate recording. When a "noisy" scalp reference is present (Figure 14.7), data may be lost. We prefer an intracranial reference to eliminate artifact introduced by scalp recording. The location should be remote from the anticipated region of interest in a "silent" area. Some place an intracranial electrode reference on a subdural strip (usually a 1 × 4) separately at implantation of clinical electrode placement to ensure optimal integrity of the recording.

BEHAVIORAL TECHNIQUES

Behavioral maneuvers are the first line of defense against artifact. Subjects are asked to lie still, close their eyes, breathe regularly, and focus on stimuli when the CNP procedure is performed while awake. On the contrary, provocative behavioral techniques such as sleep deprivation may be used to increase the yield of abnormalities on CNP procedures. For EEG recording, to reduce myogenic artifact, subjects may be asked to relax their jaw or reposition their head. During EMG and nerve conduction studies, temperature-evoked artifact is common due to fluctuation in skin temperature from anxiety, especially in children, or due to air conditioning (23). Measuring limb temperatures and rewarming to 34°C to 36°C for upper limbs and 31°C to 34°C for lower limbs should be done to limit slowing nerve conduction velocities (24). Further, recording external cues during MEG recording can help with artifact reduction, while preserving the spectra and time domain waveforms of the neuromagnetic activity and without reducing the rank of the data (25).

MANUAL TECHNIQUES

Manual or offline rejection methods may be labor intensive for continuous and multichannel EEG recordings, but are most reliable. The American Society of Electroneurodiagnostic Technologists (ASET) Inc. has defined criteria which technologists must meet to standardize the approach to performing various neurodiagnostic procedures (e.g., EEG, EP, nerve conduction study [NCS], PSG, NIOM) in the clinic or ICU setting (26). During EEG recording, the technologist will manually inspect and eliminate or reduce artifact-affected epochs simultaneously. Manual methods are useful for offline analysis, but cannot be utilized during real-time recording. During EEG monitoring, video recording often sheds light on suspicious artifacts to elucidate waveforms that mimic abnormality.

AUTOMATED TECHNIQUES OF ARTIFACT REDUCTION

Artifact Subtraction

Automated techniques utilize mathematical algorithms for artifact removal. In automated *subtraction*, short epochs or segments of recordings are rejected when exceeding a predetermined threshold has been met. This technique can be used online or offline. However, this method is both time-consuming and results in loss of significant physiological signal. Regression software methods can help focus on specific artifacts (e.g., eye movements, cardiac artifacts) and target them to be subtracted from the CNP recording (27). However, myogenic and electrode artifacts are less amenable to reduction by regression methods due to contamination of several reference channels.

Conventional Trial Rejection

Conventional trial rejection (CTR) is a method that can be used to eliminate high-amplitude artifacts from CNP recordings. It is desirable to perform CTR when there are numerous trials such as during EP and CNP procedures performed during NIOM, as those trials containing artifact across all electrodes are eliminated from each channel. Consequently, CTR can be effectively used during procedures when a large number of trials require fewer artifacts. This has more limited use in the pediatric setting.

ARTIFACT REJECTION AND DIGITAL FILTERS

Artifact *rejection* via digital recording involves montage manipulation, filter adjustments, and speed alterations for artifact reduction (28). Algorithms, including least mean squares (LMS), use adaptive filters and require obtaining a suitable reference signal. This reference is then used against the artifact of interest to estimate the acquired signal. Further, commercially available digital filters are available for standard use, eliminating artifacts with cutoff filters varying from direct current (DC) to 512 Hz. During the preprocessing stage of the data for analysis, filtering out data in the frequency range of interest is fundamental for minimizing artifact. Nonetheless, overuse of digital filters, particularly high-frequency low-pass filters, can modify true neurophysiological signals. This is achieved by removing sharp peaks and altering the signal rhythmicity. In this case, after undergoing several degrees of filtration, some artifacts (e.g., muscle) may falsely appear as a physiologic or even pathological signal (e.g., periodic discharges). This warrants documentation and understanding filter use during CNP recordings to ensure the neurophysiologist is aware of the potential for false representation of the signal (**Figure 14.8**) that might be present during interpretation (27,29). Similarly, high-frequency filters may reduce artifact composed of compound muscle action potentials (CMAP) yet it also eliminates the sensory nerve action potential (SNAP) (23). Consequently, these limitations and loss of significant amounts of data during artifact rejection discourage the routine use of digital filters and warrants development of superior automated techniques.

BLIND SOURCE SEPARATION

The blind source separation (BSS) algorithm is most widely used for artifact reduction in CNP procedures (e.g., EEG, EMG, EP, PSG, MEG). It can use ICA, principal component analysis (PCA), and canonical correlation analysis (CCA) to identify waveform components. Maximum noise fraction (MNF), a relatively new technique, has also demonstrated utility in artifact reduction during EEG recording (30,31). BSS-based algorithms assume that the observed CNP recording signal is linear, composed of a mixture of different sources, and the total number sources are less than or equal to the signal of interest (32). These methods of BSS isolate the observed complex signal and separate it into source-based components. Myogenic, electrode, and ocular movement artifacts when present may obscure important portions of the CNP tracing (**Figure 14.9**). An effective source separation technique will avoid mixed components comprising physiological and artifactual signals (**Figure 14.10**). Second-order as opposed to higher-order statistics have been shown to be more effective in removing sources involving ocular artifact (33,34). Additionally, random breaks of the source component into several components should be avoidable by the algorithm when combining ICA with PCA as the preceding step for dimensional reduction (35). ICA and PCA have reported success in artifact removal because artifactual signals tend to be much stronger and therefore easier to isolate when compared to neuronal activity (36). When extracting P300 source components, ICA was not superior to PCA or MNF, and no distinguishable differences were noted between the three methods (37). By contrast, PCA was found to be the simplest technique and required the shortest computation time, whereas MNF was an order of magnitude greater than PCA and ICA (37).

Some proprietary methods of artifact reduction (Persyst Corporation, Prescott, Arizona) use advanced waveform analysis technology (e.g., P13) where BSS divides the original signal into independent source components and subsequently applies advanced machine learning to neural network signals to recognize artifactual components for removal (**Figure 14.11**) (38). Usage of digital filters may alter the original waveform (**Figure 14.12**). These algorithms involved with initial BSS continuously analyze recordings and identify common artifact waveforms channel by channel, with subsequent and automated artifact removal (38). Using BSS methods to remove myogenic artifact and neural network identification algorithms to remove eye movement artifact can effectively reduce artifact to facilitate interpretation (**Figure 14.13**). Because digital filters result in distortion of the original signal, complex BSS algorithms characterize a novel method of artifact reduction. Applying these techniques produces a gray ghosting of frequencies to allow the interpreter to track changes in scalp EEG and QEEG to facilitate greater accuracy in analysis of simple artifacts (**Figures 14.14** and **14.15**) and those that are more complex (**Figures 14.16** and **14.17**) (38).

One validation study compared spike detection performance of P13 to three skilled experts and demonstrated comparable results on pairwise evaluation. Mean, pairwise human sensitivities of the three skilled experts were 40.0%, 42.1%, and 51.5%, and the false-positive rates (per minute) were 0.80, 0.97, and 1.99/min, respectively. By contrast, P13 demonstrated a comparable sensitivity of 43.9% ± 29.4% and a false-positive rate of 1.65 ± 2.37/min. The authors concluded that P13 had a sensitivity in the range of human expert assessment and was statistically noninferior in criteria (39). Three iterations of Persyst® spike detector, 2004 (P11), 2012 (P12), and 2016

(P13) were used in this study, and by contrast, each subsequent iteration also demonstrated improvement in the computational methodology for artifact detection and neural network technology. Twenty feedforward neural network rules (NN rule), where each NN rule is composed of additional 40 individuals' NNs, help describe the spike morphology. Each NN is further composed of one to three hidden layers, depending on the complexity of the event. The NN rule takes into account the "expert-derived concept," such that, if the morphology (e.g., amplitude and sharpness) of the spike exceeds that of background activity, it will be identified as a spike. Additionally, NNs are organized in a hierarchy pattern with three absolute thresholds built within to help fasten the removal of nonphysiological events or artifact. Unclear events are assigned a perception value, varying between 0 and 1, where uncertain events will have a value near 0.5 (39). Further, spike activity can be identified based on morphology of half-wave segments (e.g., six-half-wave model). The first two half waves refer to the activity preceding immediately after the spike, the middle two half waves describe negative or positive deflection of the spike, and the last two half waves describe the slow wave, if present. Each half wave is described by its amplitude, duration, and curvature, and can help distinguish spikes from artifact composed of rhythmic activity (39). Spikes from different channels are combined to determine the electric field of the event. Electrodes that include artifact arising from muscle, cardiac, and ocular sources are identified and eliminated (39).

Independent Component Analysis

ICA operates with the principle that all CNP recorded signals are generated by independent frequency components (IC) forming a linear pattern. ICA decomposes the original signal using the fast Fourier transformation, estimates statistically ICs, and then extracts them. This facilitates quantitative analysis, identification of different source components, and thus facilitates differentiation of artifact from true neuronal activity for removal (40). After eliminating the artifactual ICs, a clear CNP recording is rendered for interpretation. Further, traditional ICA can only be used on multichannel EEG recordings. Recently, a single-channel ICA, with time-embedded data, was introduced and has demonstrated success in separating the signal into source components (41,42).

ICA is widely used for EEG artifact reduction and can be combined with other methods for superior results (e.g., Bayesian classifier, high-order statistics) (43,44). It is frequently used for processing motion artifacts, including those arising from ocular movements, and has also demonstrated utility in reducing myogenic artifact when combined with EMG data (45). The application of ICA to EMG signal for contraction classification demonstrated that the statistical ICs extracted were more prominent and statistic variation was much less as opposed to using EMG alone, thus making ICA-EMG ideal for feature extraction (46). Further, ICA is less reliable when extracting EP data (e.g., P300), as it extracts P300, but also non-P300 components. Nonetheless, a constrained ICA (cICA) algorithm for extracting EPs and relevant components has reported to be fast, reliable, inexpensive, with an accuracy of 98.3% in detecting P300 (47). Additionally, ICA has shown success in differentiating between somatosensory and auditory brain responses during vibratory tactile stimulation (48). Further, extracting essential data from MEG recording is difficult due to large-amplitude artifacts contaminating the signal, but when combined with ICA, particularly FastICA, isolate eye-blinking/movement, cardiac, myogenic, and other artifacts from the MEG signal is made possible (48).

ICA has been effectively used with PSG for analyzing sleep disorders. When PSG data are visually analyzed, epochs grossly containing artifact observed in a sleep disorder such as sleep apnea can be identified and extracted from the data set. However, when these data are subjected to ICA, other sources of electrophysiological signals contributing to the sleep disorder may be encountered that could provide further insight into the overall mechanism of a specific disorder (49).

EEGLAB is a Matlab toolbox that works interactively in processing continuous and event-related EEG data through ICA, time-frequency analysis, or other standard methods. This open-source platform allows researchers to contribute EEGLAB "plug-ins" or extensions that can be added to the EEGLAB toolbox (50). Using these plug-ins, users can build new data processing/visualization functions using structures and conventions of EEGLAB data (51). Several EEGLAB plug-ins are currently available. For example, FIRfilt for applying linear filters to data and automatic artifact removal (AAR) toolbox, which combines state-of-the-art artifact removal methods for ocular and myogenic artifact reduction in EEG recordings. However, they should be used with caution as not all plug-ins have been assessed by EEGLAB developers. Automatic artifact detection based on the joint use of spatial and temporal features (ADJUST) is an ICA-based, automated algorithm that works as an EEGLAB plug-in and is used for artifact identification (51). ADJUST identifies artifactual ICs and combines stereotyped, artifact-specific spatial and temporal features together. By contrast, IC classification by ADJUST was comparable to a manual, expert classification (95.2% agreement of data variance), and reconstructed visual and auditory event-related potentials (ERPs) were recovered from a profoundly artifact-laden EEG recording (51). Further, Fully Automated Statistical Thresholding for EEG artifact Rejection (FASTER) is another ICA-based technique that works as an EEGLAB plug-in and has demonstrated success in detecting and eliminating artifact components from EEG recordings arising from functional MRI (fMRI) scanning (52). It was tested on 47 simulated and real-time EEG recordings each, and was compared to expert artifact detection and to a variant of statistical control for dense arrays of sensors (SCADS) method. FASTER demonstrated greater than 90% sensitivity and specificity for detecting ocular and myogenic artifact and identifying contaminated channels (52).

Principal Component Analysis

PCA is a multivariate technique that aims to analyze and extract statistical data by identifying a set of correlated variables; this analysis is focused on second-order statistics (53). Lower-order statistics utilize conventional techniques comprising constant, linear, and quadratic terms such as zeroth, first, and second powers, and are used in the arithmetic mean as first order and variance as second order (54). Higher-order statistics involve functions of the third or higher power of a sample and are used for estimating *skewness* (measure of asymmetry that can be positive or negative) and *kurtosis* (sharpness of the peak) in a normal distribution. Unexpectedly, higher-order statistics tend to be less robust than lower order statistics (54). Further, during artifact reduction, singular value decomposition is used to derive principle or major components, which are multiple linear independent components (temporally and spatially noncorrelated) from the CNP recording by finding the greatest variance within the signal. The original signal is then reconstructed by linearly combining these components together and by subtracting the artifactual components to render a new and clean CNP recording. However, PCA may not effectively isolate each signal source into separate components, especially when they have comparable amplitudes (55,56). Thus, ICA is often more effective than PCA in isolating independently active sources for artifact reduction (40). By contrast, when PCA and ICA were compared for ocular artifact reduction, PCA was capable of reducing but not eliminating the artifact, with significant loss in underlying CNP data. In contrast, ICA effectively eliminated the ocular artifact in EEG, including low-frequency ocular activity, with minimal loss in data. In addition, it preserved the theta, alpha, and beta band rhythmic activities in the original EEG signal. When used in EEG, a significant amount of theta activity (4–6 Hz) was removed and false alpha activity (8–10 Hz) was observed after PCA (40). Further, PCA was tested on 800 simulated ERPs, randomly weighted combinations of three 64-point components using covariance PCAs, varimax rotations, and univariate analysis of variance (ANOVAs). Results indicate that PCA was inferior and incorrectly allocated variance across the components, leading to potentially serious misinterpretation (57).

Canonical Correlation Analysis

CCA is a multivariate analysis technique to test relationships between two sets of variables. *Canonical* is a term specifically used in statistics to describe the analysis of latent variables that are not directly observed but which characterize multiple variables that are directly observed. CCA has been used in CNP procedures and may be especially useful for EP recording. This includes steady-state visually evoked potential–brain computer interface to detect frequency components present in EEG. It has also been suggested for the creation of spatial filters to improve SNR of EEG, in addition to analyzing ERPs (58,59). One study proposes an algorithm combining CCA and wavelets with *random forests* (an ensemble approach to improve performance) for the automatic removal of muscle artifact from continuous EEG recording, and report excellent performance using this approach, which eliminates the need for expert marking, reference signal recording, and visual inspection (60). When techniques of BSS are compared, ICA-based techniques appear to be widely used in CNP procedures and have demonstrated reliable and consistent results for artifact reduction (40,61–63).

EMPIRICAL MODE DECOMPOSITION

Empirical mode decomposition (EMD) is a time–frequency analysis tool used to decompose nonlinear, nonstationary signals into a set number of *intrinsic mode functions* (IMFs), which are basic modes directly derived from the data (64). Irregular components and artifact in the CNP recording are identified as IMFs. IMFs are composed of a large number of artifacts, on a scale from fine to coarse, are statistically determined and removed, and the remaining IMFs are combined together to recreate a clear signal (64). Traditional methods, including wave-based techniques, rely on a priori knowledge to effectively utilize these techniques, while the same is not true for EMD. One study simulating EMD-based algorithms on several different cases demonstrated success in reducing muscle artifact and those that were related to power interference (reference). Additionally, results from various other experimental studies conclude that EMD-based techniques are data driven, adaptive, highly efficient, and can be effectively applied to complex data (64). Although EMD and ICA algorithms have been utilized in analyzing MEG single-trial data and have demonstrated high performance in reducing artifact (65), EMD has also shown success in frequency band analysis of MEG data during volitional sensorimotor tasks, where extraction of IMFs has provided insight into cognitive activity, often limited by classic methods of frequency band analysis (66).

Wavelet-Based Techniques

Wavelet Transform

Several wavelet techniques exist, including wavelet transform (WT), discrete wavelet transform (DWT), wavelet packet transform (WPT), and stationary wavelet transform (SWT). WT is performed under the assumption that time complexity is linear, and the wavelet is an oscillatory waveform with a limited duration of low value or zero (67). The input signal undergoes wavelet decomposition where the low-pass filter produces a waveform called *approximation* and the high-pass filter produces a waveform called *detail*. The "multiresolution decomposition" role of WT thus separates the input signal into *details* at various scales and *approximations* (67). Artifact reduction can be achieved by setting a threshold for wavelet coefficients and then separating these coefficients, while preserving important data (67). MEG data from 274 sensors were effectively subjected to wavelet decomposition using three different types of wavelets (daubechies, coiflet, and adjusted Haar). Results indicated this technique to be robust for MEG denoising (68). Further, another study reported using wavelet-based technique as an adjunct to PSG to extract the correct stage of sleep for diagnosis of sleep disorder from EEG data, in addition to assisting the diagnosis of an arousal by correlating wavelet-extracted data from various CNP procedures (e.g., oximetry in PSG, EMG) (69).

Several wavelet-based techniques, developed in combination with other reduction techniques to target specific artifacts (e.g., ballistocardiographic artifact), or special studies like pervasive EEG recording, where monitoring takes place in a more natural environment with greater degrees of movement, are discussed in the following sections.

Wavelet-Based Nonlinear Noise Reduction

EEG and functional MRI (EEG–fMRI) are collectively used to achieve spatiotemporal resolution of the neuronal activity. However, interference occurs between both systems and poses challenges for its routine use. Good spatial, but poor temporal resolution can be obtained on fMRI, while the reverse is true with EEG (70). Thus, combining both systems together provides the ideal spatiotemporal resolution required for auditory perception studies (70). Although artifact-free fMRI is easy to obtain, the same is not true with EEG–fMRI recordings because the EEG system is highly sensitive to magnetic fields within the machines used to obtain fMRI (11). fMRI has the tendency to induce cardiac pulsation within a highly static magnetic field, and thus, can severely compromise EEG recordings when performed simultaneously (70).

Wavelet-based nonlinear noise reduction (WNNR) method has demonstrated success in reducing ballistocardiographic artifact during EEG–fMRI use, with preservation of a temporal relationship to the EEG signal (11). WNNR is composed of three components: (a) wavelet transformation, (b) nonlinear noise reduction, and (c) spatial average subtraction, and undergoes two stages of analysis. During the first stage, wavelet transformation separates EEG data in each channel into multiple bands. This is followed by embedding wavelet coefficients on each individual band (11). Wavelet transformation utilizes a multiresolution decomposition system to separate the data, while simultaneously preserving the local time–frequency features (11). Ballistocardiographic artifact undergoes nonlinear noise reduction through manipulation on space embedding, and after achieving reduction, the data are inversely transformed back within the time domain (11). In the second stage, the residual artifacts in the corrected data across all EEG channels are reduced using spatial average subtraction (11).

WNNR is limited by its slow speed; it requires nearly 2 hours for processing the data on MATLAB 6.0 (11). However, the use of fast K-D tree algorithm may be helpful in reducing the computational time required for WNNR data processing (71).

Combined Artifact Reduction Techniques

Complex signals from multiple sources are present in EEG and contain artifacts that have more recently been approached through combined techniques for artifact reduction. In one study, a framework for automatic rejection for eyeblink, hand movement, and head shaking artifact was developed and used an SNR-like metric calculating signal cleansing performance (72). Results indicate that the hybrid algorithms were more effective in reducing artifact compared to individual techniques alone. As per the SNR-like criterion, WPT–EMD hybrid was superior to WPT–ICA for artifact reduction in all subjects (72).

Linear techniques through adaptive filtering, including finite/infinite impulse response (FIR) filters, can be used when the source of artifact is able to be measured (e.g., electrooculogram for eye movement artifact or EMG for muscle artifact) (73–75). In pervasive EEG recording, artifact source measurement is not possible and linear techniques cannot be employed. Thus, BSS-based methods, including ICA and PCA, have demonstrated success and have been utilized in combination with WPT for artifact reduction (72).

In both WPT–ICA and WPT–EMD, WPT is first applied to all EEG channels where both the *approximation* and *detail* space are further decomposed into frequency sub-bands. Although WPT cannot extract single-frequency components, it brings it to the frequency of interest. The wavelet coefficients of all channels are then considered and the maximum standard deviation of the wavelet energy is used to identify the node with the maximum captured artifact within the decomposition (72). The coefficients of the identified node are rejected and a clean signal is thus produced, which is then analyzed by ICA or EMD.

In WPT–ICA, artifact components contaminating the EEG have channels separated via fast-ICA algorithm. Within an area of artifact, the temporal standard deviation of each component as identified by the amplitude threshold is used as a baseline to detect components composed of the artifact. The highest standard deviation of the artifact component is the most powerful constituent and is thus removed from the signal (72). In WPT–EMD, irregular oscillations and large-amplitude signals, which are features of all artifacts, are matched with the nonlinear signals from EMD for decomposition. Similar to ICA, the IMF with the highest temporal standard deviation and greatest entropy is considered for evaluating the hybrid index of each channel in the decontaminated and resting state EEG. The IMF with the greatest hybrid index (most significant area with artifact) is rejected during signal reconstruction to reduce artifactual interference in interpretation (72).

PEDIATRIC CLINICAL NEUROPHYSIOLOGY

CNP procedures in children are fraught with numerous challenges regarding artifact. Electrode placement during EEG in a child requires an experienced, well-trained technologist to affix electrodes using collodion (76,77). Wrapping the child's head after electrode attachment may be done to reduce high sensor impedances during a CNP procedure (78). ACNS recommends the use of inverted silver–silver chloride disc electrodes in the pediatric setting (79). During EMG, limited tolerance to pain may necessitate topical anesthetic creams, sedation, or even general anesthesia during the procedure. The smallest commercially available needle (30-gauge, 25-mm disposable concentric needle) is often used (80). Children may be referred to sleep specialists for the evaluation of sleep disorders using PSG. Although PSG is a painless, noninvasive technique in adults, it may be terrifying for children and requires a child-friendly sleep laboratory (81). NIOM in children follows the same basic principles as in adults; however, the effect of the inhalant anesthetics can be more profound in children and produce a greater reduction in the amplitude of cortical potentials than in adults (82).

Significant artifact on CNP recording is commonly encountered in children and therefore, conventional artifact-reduction techniques used in adults cannot be extrapolated to the pediatric setting. This is due to limited duration of time in cooperating for CNP procedures, and heavy contamination of physiological signals caused by prominent motion artifact. Two automated artifact-reduction techniques, independent channel rejection (ICR), and artifact blocking (AB) algorithm, have demonstrated success in children and are discussed further.

EVENT-RELATED POTENTIALS

ERPs measure the cerebral response to various stimuli (e.g., sound, speech, and music) in preverbal infants and populations where obtaining verbal response may be challenging (83). ERP estimation is obtained as an average value over numerous trials. However, the ERP amplitude is classically less than 5 μV and approximately 10 times smaller than background EEG activity and poses a challenge during ERP extraction and assessment (84). Background EEG activity in pediatrics consists of high-amplitude, slow-frequency waveforms, chiefly compromised by motion artifact (83). During ERP estimation, artifact removal is necessary but results in the loss of a large number of trials and rejection of data.

ARTIFACT REDUCTION

Sudden and continuous movement during EEG recording generates high-amplitude artifact, disrupts the electrode–tissue interface, and frequently introduces artifact. Challenges caused by limited monitoring time warrants usage of alternate techniques for artifact reduction in the pediatric setting. During pediatric nerve-conduction studies, stimulus artifact is obtained in nearly every SNAP recording. The absence of artifacts suggests a technical pitfall such as disconnection of the recording leads from the amplifier (23).

Furthermore, children are more susceptible to stimulus artifact due to the short distance between the recording and stimulating leads, which can be reduced by isolating the stimulator and shielding the cables, as seen with modern EMG machines (23). Additionally, avoiding short distances, drying the skin to limit impedance prior to testing, changing the electrode, and using a ground electrode between the recording and stimulating leads can help limit artifact during EMG (23). Additionally, myogenic artifact or compound motor action potential (CMAP) during EMG is common in children due to smaller limbs and close proximity of nerves to muscles and can contaminate the true signal or SNAP. Reducing the stimulating current or performing orthodromic sensory nerve testing can help remove the CMAP artifact from the recording (23).

PSG in children is not only challenging, but subjected to artifact. Pulse oximetry, used to assess oxygenation, may be contaminated with motion artifact during unattended periods overnight. Thus, correlating the pulse waveform with the saturation value would be insightful in differentiating motion artifact from true desaturation (81). Further, oximeters incorporating artifact reduction algorithms have reported good accuracy and fewer false-positives due to motion artifact (85).

Conventional trial rejection (CTR) is often employed in adult CNP recordings and rejects trials that are composed of significant background artifact. Nonetheless, it is of limited use in the pediatric setting due to fewer trials and greater time constraint. Similarly, ICA is highly effective in eliminating ocular artifacts in adults, but due to ill-defined distribution of these artifacts in children, its utility is limited in the pediatric setting. Further, one study testing ICA on infant EEG recordings found that the ICA algorithm spread the artifacts across 14 different sources. These 14 independent sources were composed of both neuronal activity and artifactual signals at various points in time. After obtaining an ICA-corrected EEG, artifacts still persisted and removal of the 14 independent components resulted in loss of significant data (84). Similarly, utilization of other standard methods of artifact reduction in children is limited due to similar challenges. Fujioka et al. report two pediatric automated artifact-reduction techniques during CNP procedures, with favorable results (84).

INDEPENDENT CHANNEL REJECTION

Pediatric CNP procedures are subjected to significant artifact and tend to affect one or a few electrodes on any specific trial. ICR can eliminate artifact arising from a single electrode (e.g., FP1 and FP2 in EEG) or affecting a specific trial during EPs, and thus, data in the remaining channels can be further utilized (84). Thus, depending on the number of electrodes affected, each channel will offer a varied number of trials, and these trials are then averaged together. A drawback of this technique is spatial distortion due to electrode-specific elimination of trials, thus resulting in a mixed number of trials per electrode and selective representation of the EEG study (84). This effectiveness of ICR has been previously tested and has reported good results (86–89).

ARTIFACT BLOCKING ALGORITHM

An AB algorithm is largely data driven and does not depend on the number of components as in ICA (84). AB algorithms applied to EEG have two phases. The first is composed of developing a reference matrix from the data matrix and adjusts all samples of the EEG data matrix to zero as a baseline, with absolute amplitude levels surpassing a predetermined threshold. Choosing an appropriate threshold value would thus allow identification of high-amplitude artifacts. The second phase uses the reference and EEG data matrix to estimate a "smoothing matrix." When the smoothing matrix is multiplied by the initial EEG data matrix, a new EEG data matrix is produced, minimizing artifact (84). The smoothing matrix thus also blocks high-amplitude artifacts from the initial EEG data matrix. Further, AB algorithms are a linear transformation of the original data and are similar to interpolation methods. When the reference data matrix is projected onto the initial EEG data matrix, EEG data coinciding with zero is obtained (84). An AB algorithm can be applied to continuous data to study steady state activity, or activity in various frequency bands (as opposed to ICR), and is subjected to less spatial distortion (84). It has an advantage over other EEG interpolation methods because no previous knowledge of the volume conductor model or three-dimensional scalp surfaces is necessary (90–93). Finally, an AB algorithm is especially appropriate for infants with anatomical variations including open fontanelles, as the presence of a skull breach can significantly influence the degree of volume conduction of the electrophysiological signal leading to false representation (94).

CONCLUSION

Neurophysiological function in neurobiological disorders reflects age-specific and technology-based application of artifact reduction. Several techniques and methods of artifact reduction exist, applicable in different settings (Figures 14.18 and 14.19). None are perfect in eliminating every form of artifact for all CNP procedures and are especially challenging with complex and multiple source generators. Prior techniques of artifact subtraction and elimination are increasingly being replaced with state-of-the-art techniques for simple and complex artifact reduction. Technology is advancing our ability to reduce artifact in CNP procedures though it should not replace the technologist's and neurophysiologist's role for artifact prevention, identification, and elimination.

ACKNOWLEDGMENT

The authors thank Mark Scheuer MD, Persyst® for his review and comments to improve the manuscript and for his donation of selected examples of artifact involving QEEG and blind source separation.

GLOSSARY

ADJUST—Automatic artifact detection based on the Joint Use of Spatial and Temporal features (ADJUST) is an ICA-based, automated algorithm that works as an EEGLAB plug-in.

Approximations—A waveform produced when the input signal undergoes wavelet decomposition and is passed through a low-pass filter.

Blind Source Separation (BSS)—A widely used algorithm for artifact reduction during clinical neurophysiology procedures; comprises of ICA, PCA, and CCA.

Canonical Correlation Analysis (CCA)—A multivariate analysis technique to test relationships between two sets of variables.

Conventional Trial Rejection (CTR)—A method that can be used to eliminate high-amplitude artifacts from CNP recordings.

Detail—A waveform produced when the input signal undergoes wavelet decomposition and is passed through a high-pass filter.

EEGLAB—A Matlab toolbox that works interactively in processing continuous and event-related EEG data through ICA, time-frequency analysis, or other standard methods.

Empirical Mode Decomposition (EMD)—A time-frequency analysis tool used to decompose nonlinear, nonstationary signals into a set number of intrinsic mode functions.

FASTER—Fully Automated Statistical Thresholding for EEG artifact Rejection (FASTER) is an ICA-based technique, used for artifact reduction, that works as an EEGLAB plug-in.

Independent Component Analysis—A technique used for artifact reduction during CNP procedures by generating independent source components linearly and extracting the artifactual components from the original signal.

Intrinsic Mode Function (IMF)—Basic mode that arises from the application of EMD to CNP recordings for artifact reduction.

Kurtosis—The sharpness of a peak in a frequency-distribution curve.

Maximum Noise Fraction (MNF)—A blind source separation technique for artifact reduction.

Principal Component Analysis (PCA)—A multivariate technique that uses second-order statistics and aims to analyze and extract statistical data by identifying a set of correlated variables.

Random Forests—An ensemble approach or learning method to improve performance during classification, regression, and other tasks.

Skewness—A measure of asymmetry (positive or negative) of a frequency-distribution curve.

Wavelet-based Nonlinear Noise Reduction (WNNR)—Composed of three components, including wavelet transformation, nonlinear noise reduction, and spatial average subtraction for artifact reduction.

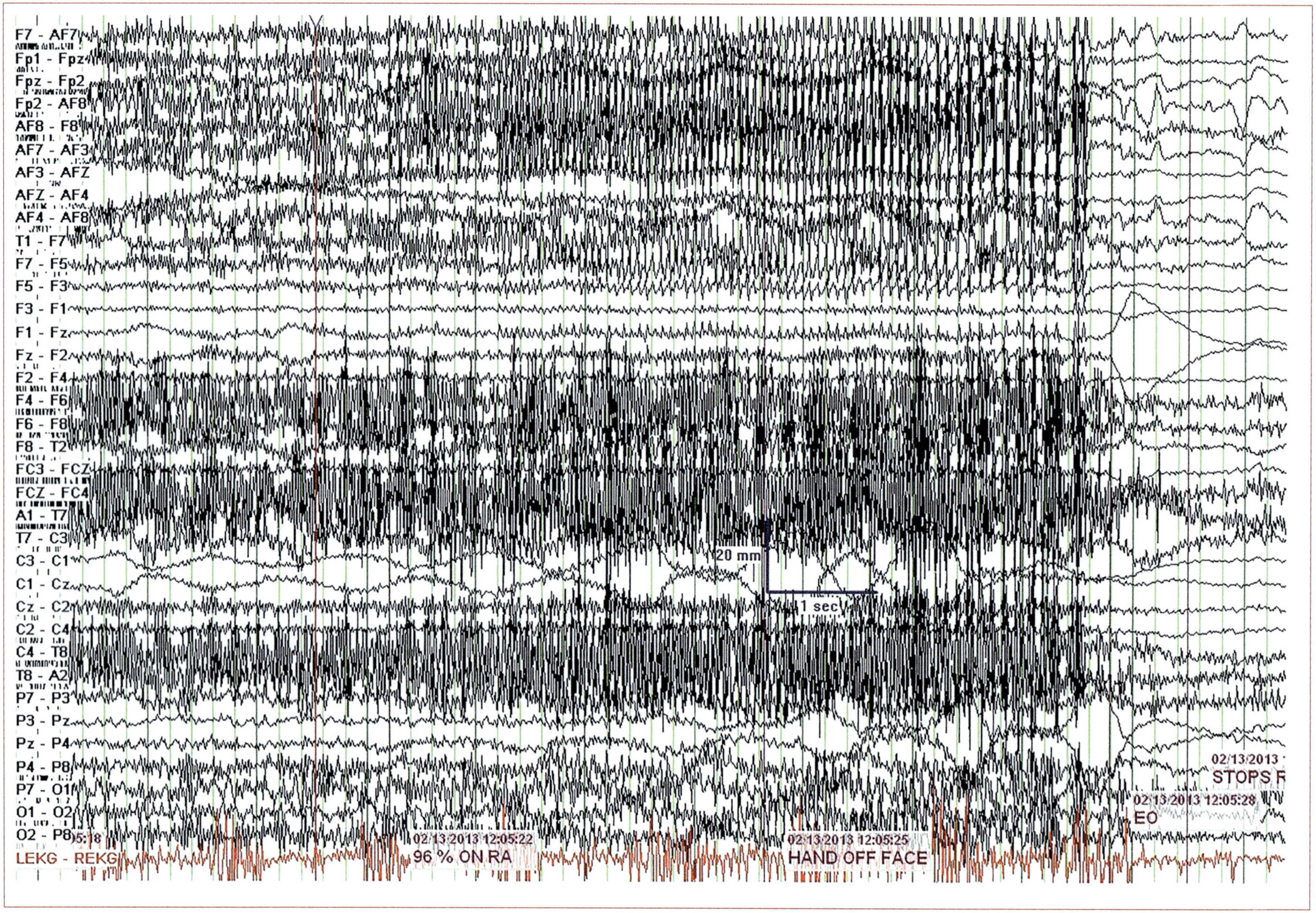

FIGURE 14.1: Myogenic artifact during a frontal lobe seizure obscuring the underlying ictal activity. However, note the brief 9-second evolving artifactual pattern that changes from initial confluence to crescendo as higher amplitude phasic myogenic artifact with abrupt termination, which suggests an ictal origin of the event.

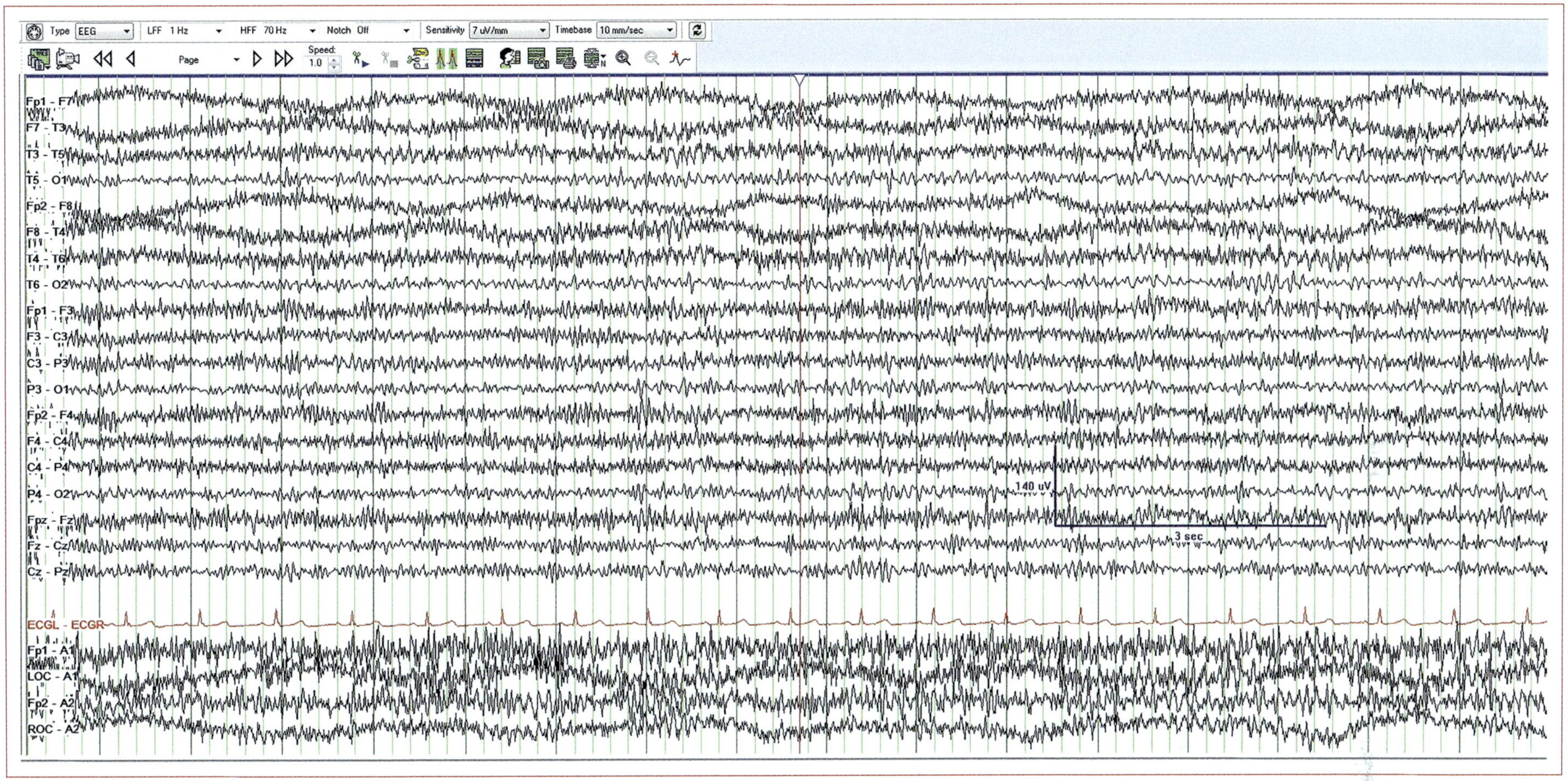

FIGURE 14.2: EEG obtained from a 32-year-old with anxiety. Continuous beta activity occurs with bitemporal myogenic artifact, making source separation of physiologic and artifactual high frequencies challenging to differentiate. However, note that the myogenic artifact appears slightly darker and spikier. Slow rolling eye movement artifact is visible and reflects the state of drowsiness.

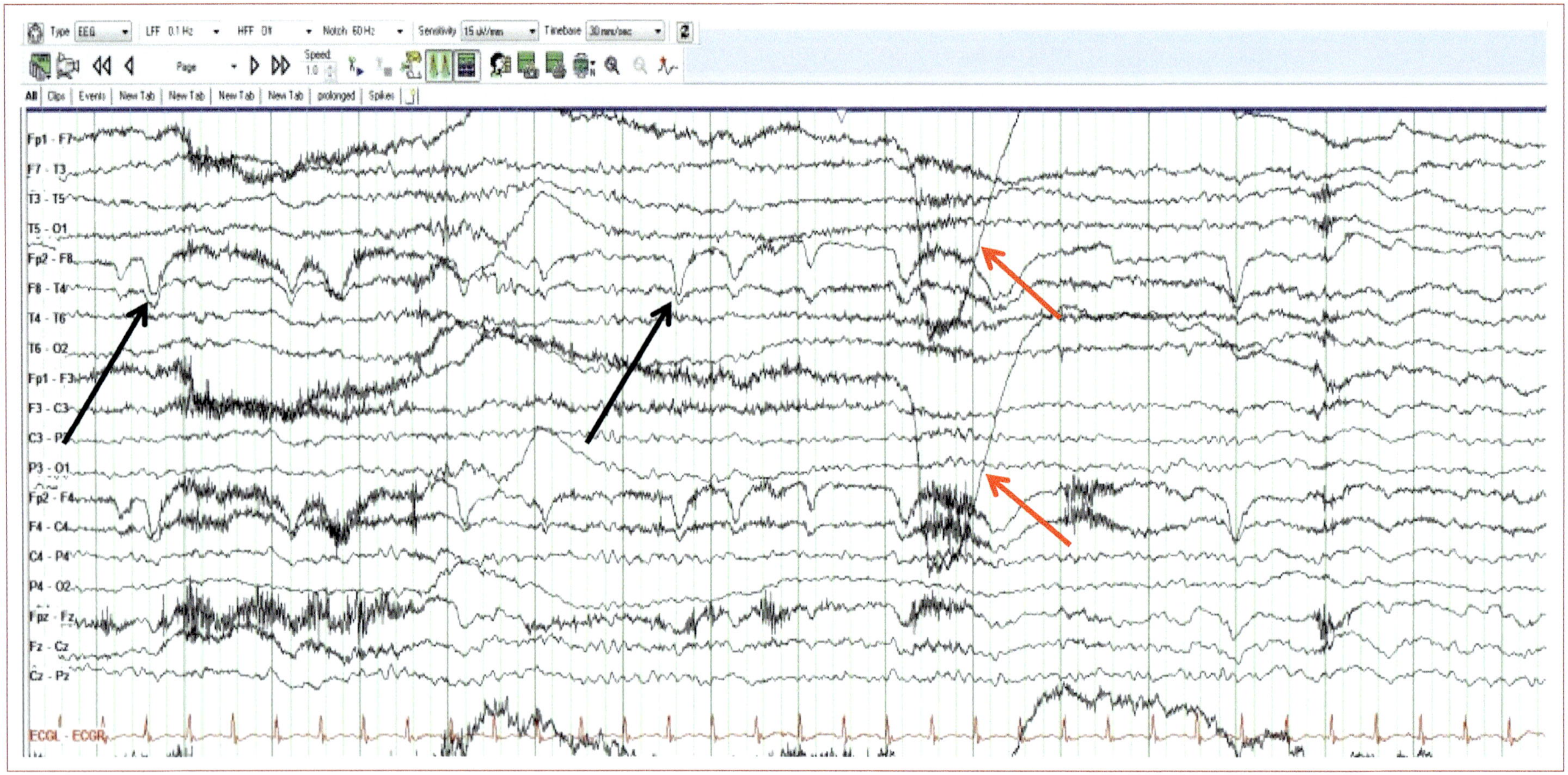

FIGURE 14.3: Unilateral vertical eyeblink artifact due to the physiological effect of left frontal, local scalp edema following head injury (black arrows). Later in the recording, the FP1 electrode was dislodged, leading to obvious artifact (red arrow). Note at the beginning of the epoch there is no believable spatial field of distribution despite a normal left eyeblink visible on video review.

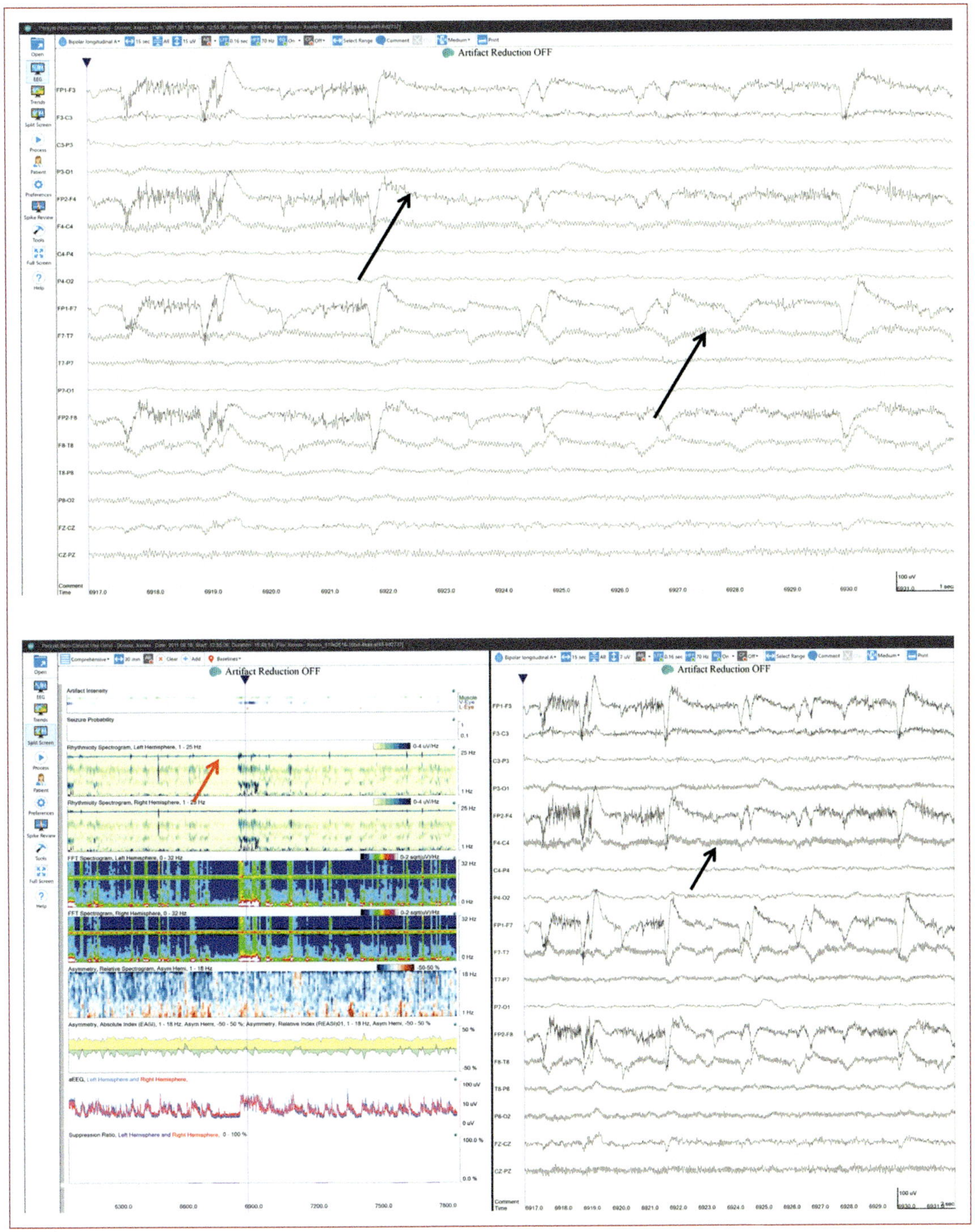

FIGURE 14.4: (A) Quantization error artifact due to misrepresentation of faster frequencies from limited sampling. Note the rhythmic artifact throughout the scalp EEG (arrows). Slide courtesy of Mark Scheuer, Persyst Corporation. (B) ICU-EEG (raw data on right) with panels displaying trend analysis (left) during quantization error artifact. Note the rhythmic artifact in F4-C4 in the raw EEG on the right (black arrow) in addition to a restricted bandwidth on QEEG in the rhythmicity spectrogram in the left trending panel (red arrow). Slide courtesy of Mark Scheuer, Persyst Corporation.

QEEG, quantitative EEG.

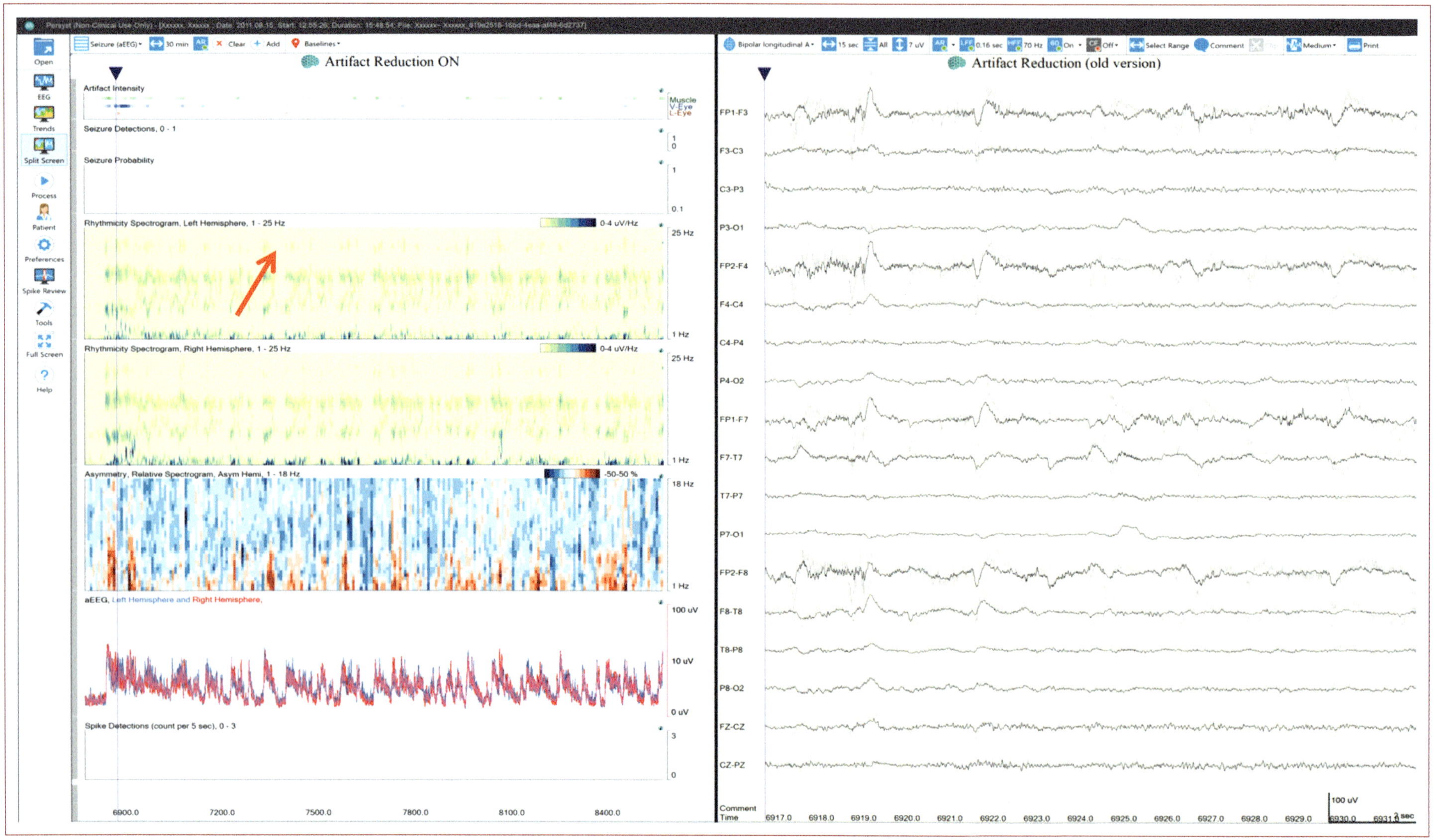

FIGURE 14.5: Quantization error artifact present in **Figure 14.4** is now eliminated with the artifact reduction "ON." Note the absence of the increase in narrowband high-frequency power now absent in the QEEG compared with the prior example (approximated by red arrow). The shadowing effect from artifact reduction is now visible in the F4-C4 derivation in the raw EEG on the right. Slide courtesy of Mark Scheuer, Persyst Corporation.

QEEG, quantitative EEG.

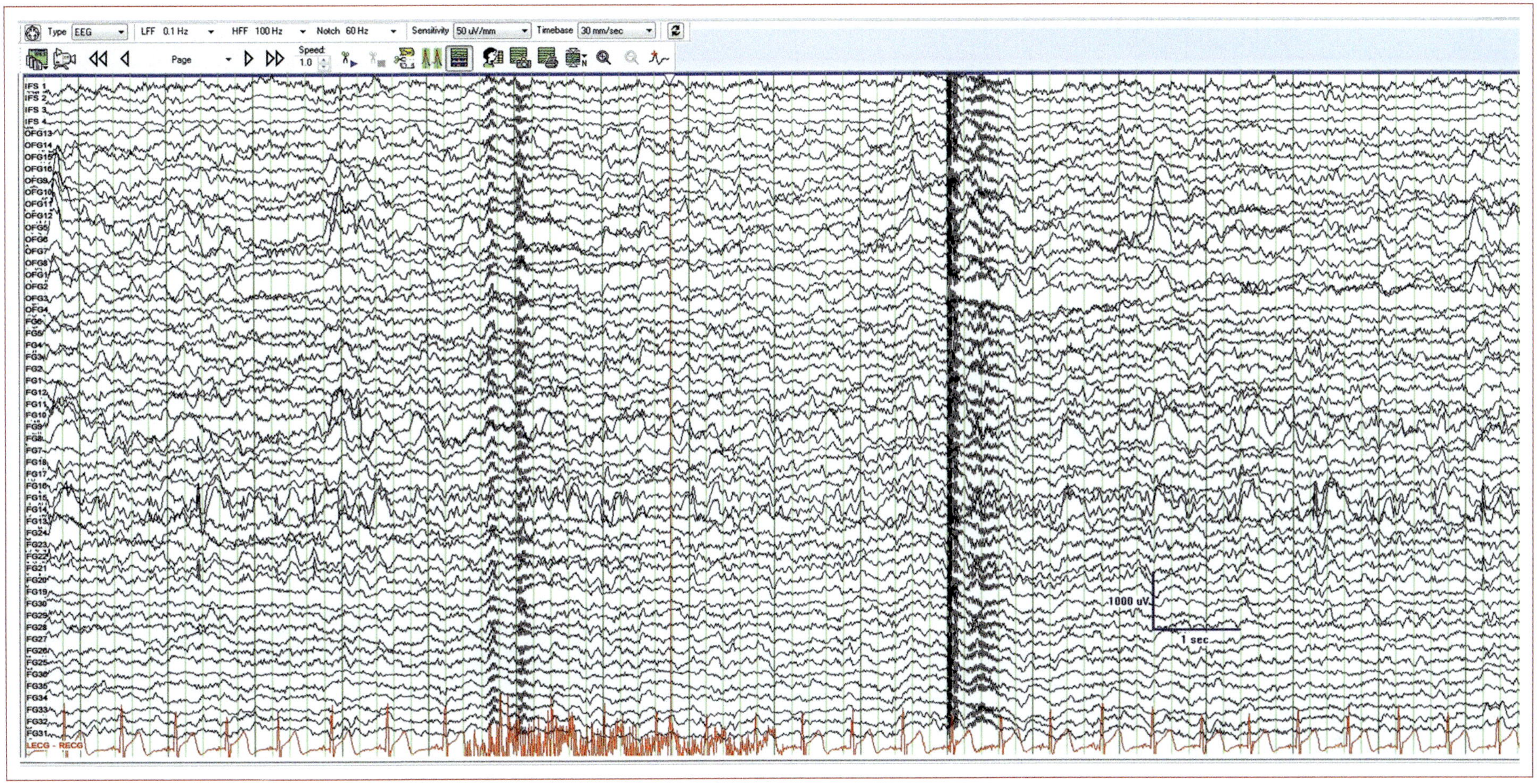

FIGURE 14.6: Intracranial EEG demonstrating intermixed artifact caused by using a scalp reference in seconds 5 and 11. Resolution was able to be accomplished by selecting an intracranial reference electrode at a site on the same grid removed from the area of interest.

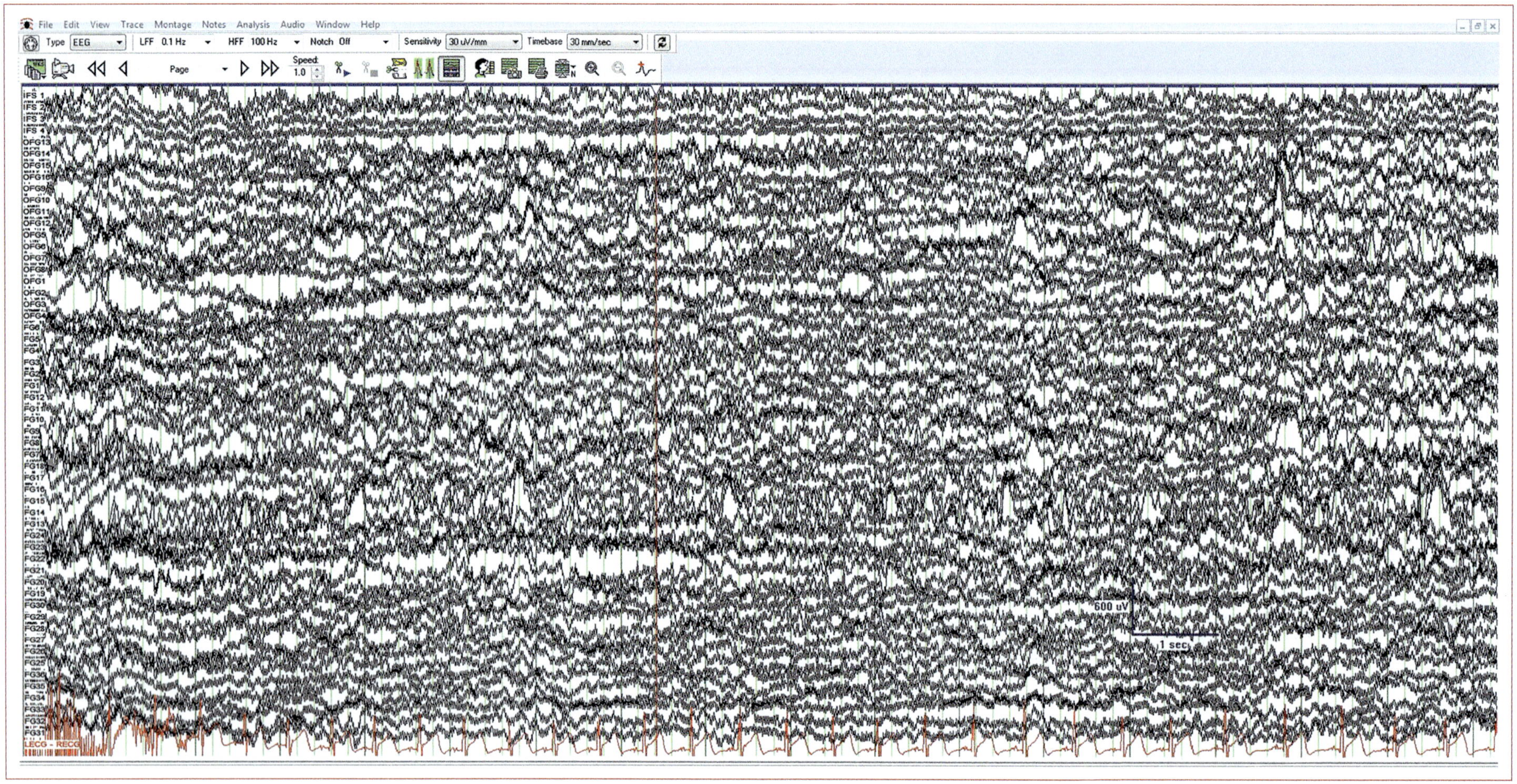

FIGURE 14.7: Another patient undergoing intracranial EEG with continuous intermixed artifact produced by a scalp reference and ground location that resolved following relocation to a different site on a distant subdural strip electrode.

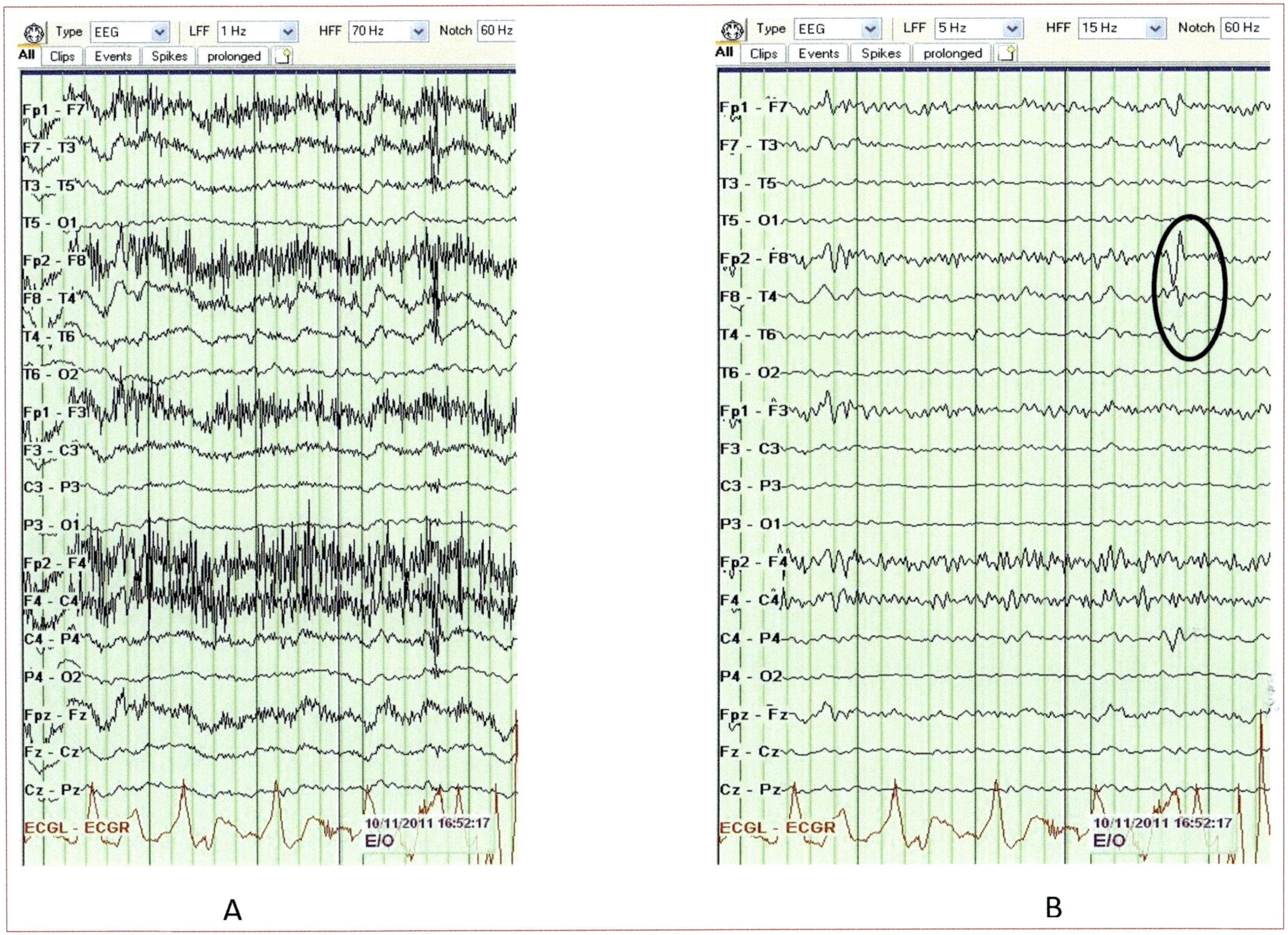

FIGURE 14.8: Overly aggressive use of digital filters in EEG. By modifying the EEG to increase the LFF and reduce the HFF and "clean up" the recording, misrepresentation of the muscle source of a signal in the fourth second in 8A occurs, which falsely appears as an abnormal right anterior temporal sharp wave in 8B (oval).

HFF, high-frequency filter; LFF, low-frequency filter.

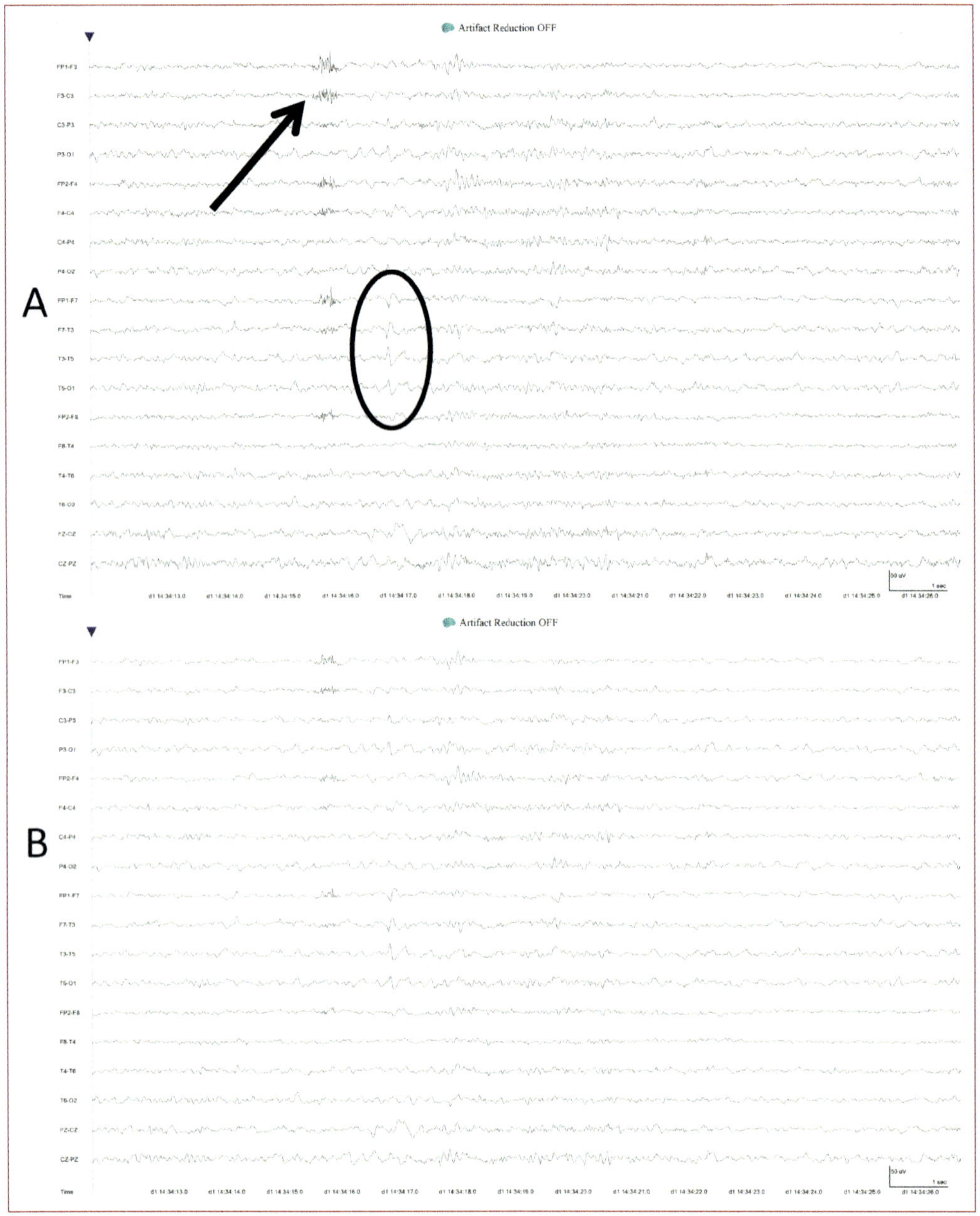

FIGURE 14.9: (A) A left temporal sharp wave (oval) and a brief burst of bifrontal myogenic artifact during sleep; original waveforms, HFF 70 Hz, LFF 1.0 Hz. Small burst of bifrontal EMG artifact evident at about 4 seconds. (B) Digital filters applied to the original waveforms, HFF 15 Hz, LFF 1.0 Hz. Note the 15-Hz filter reduced the EMG artifact to some degree but also made it appear more like frontal beta activity, and in addition attenuated cerebral beta patterns to some degree.

EMG, electromyography; HFF, high-frequency filter; LFF, low-frequency filter.

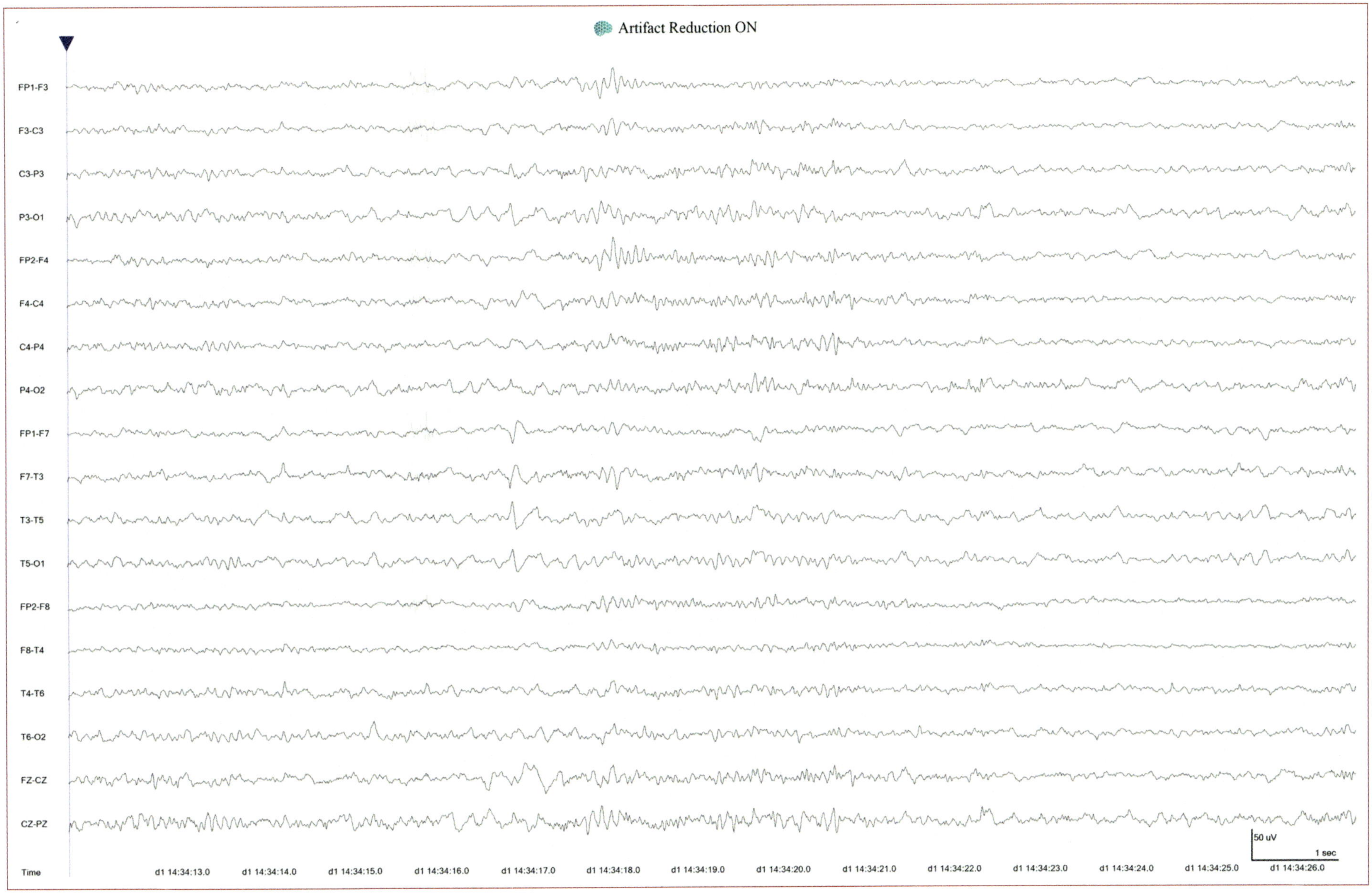

FIGURE 14.10: Gray ghost of the original EEG in **Figure 14.9A**. The AR markedly reduced the brief burst of EMG activity, but produced very little effect on the beta range cerebral activities or sharp wave discharge.

AR, artifact reduction EMG, electromyography.

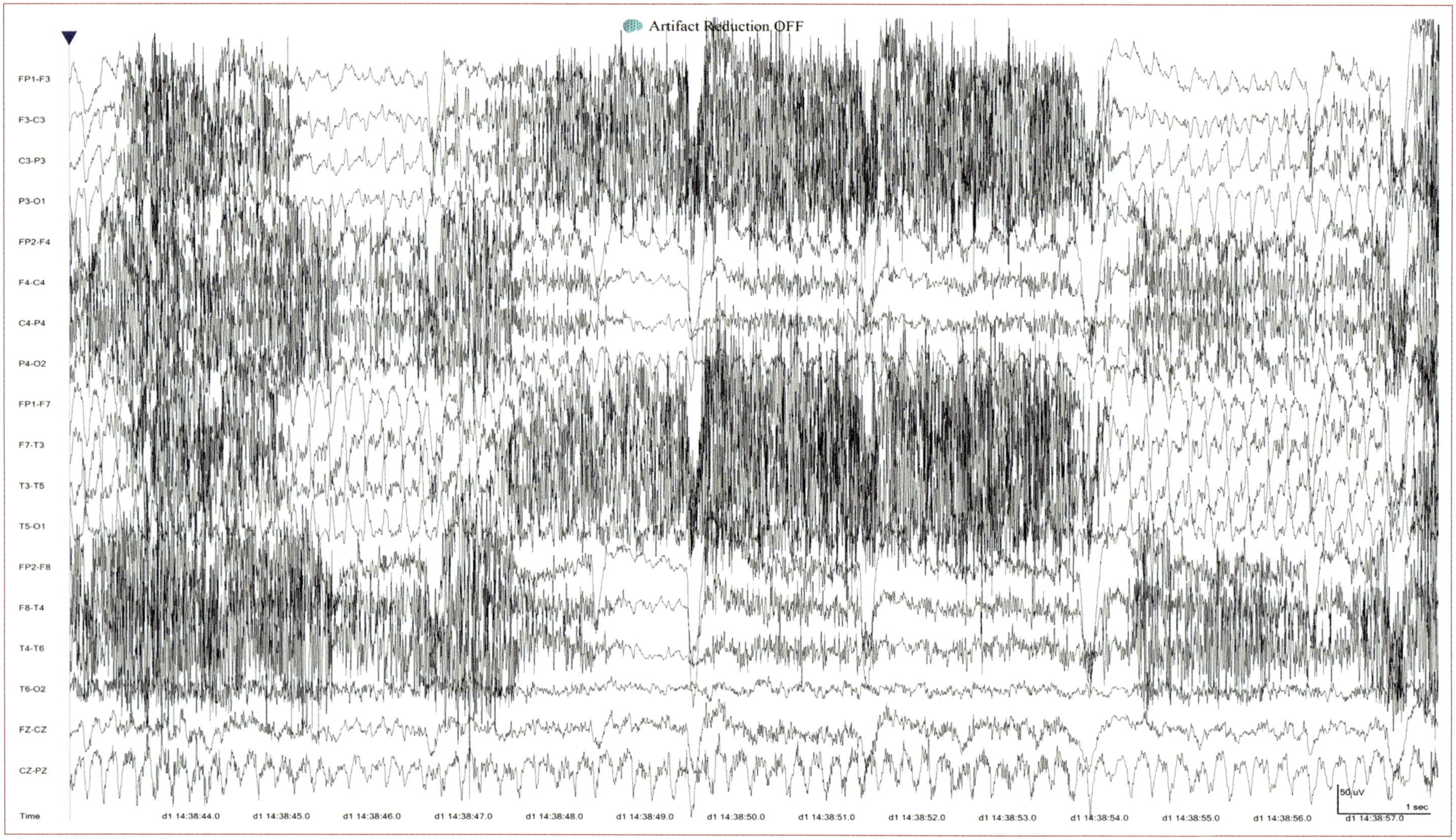

FIGURE 14.11: Myogenic artifact present in a sample of scalp EEG in **Figure 14.9A**. Right and left alternating high-frequency artifact is present that obscures the underlying electrocerebral activity.

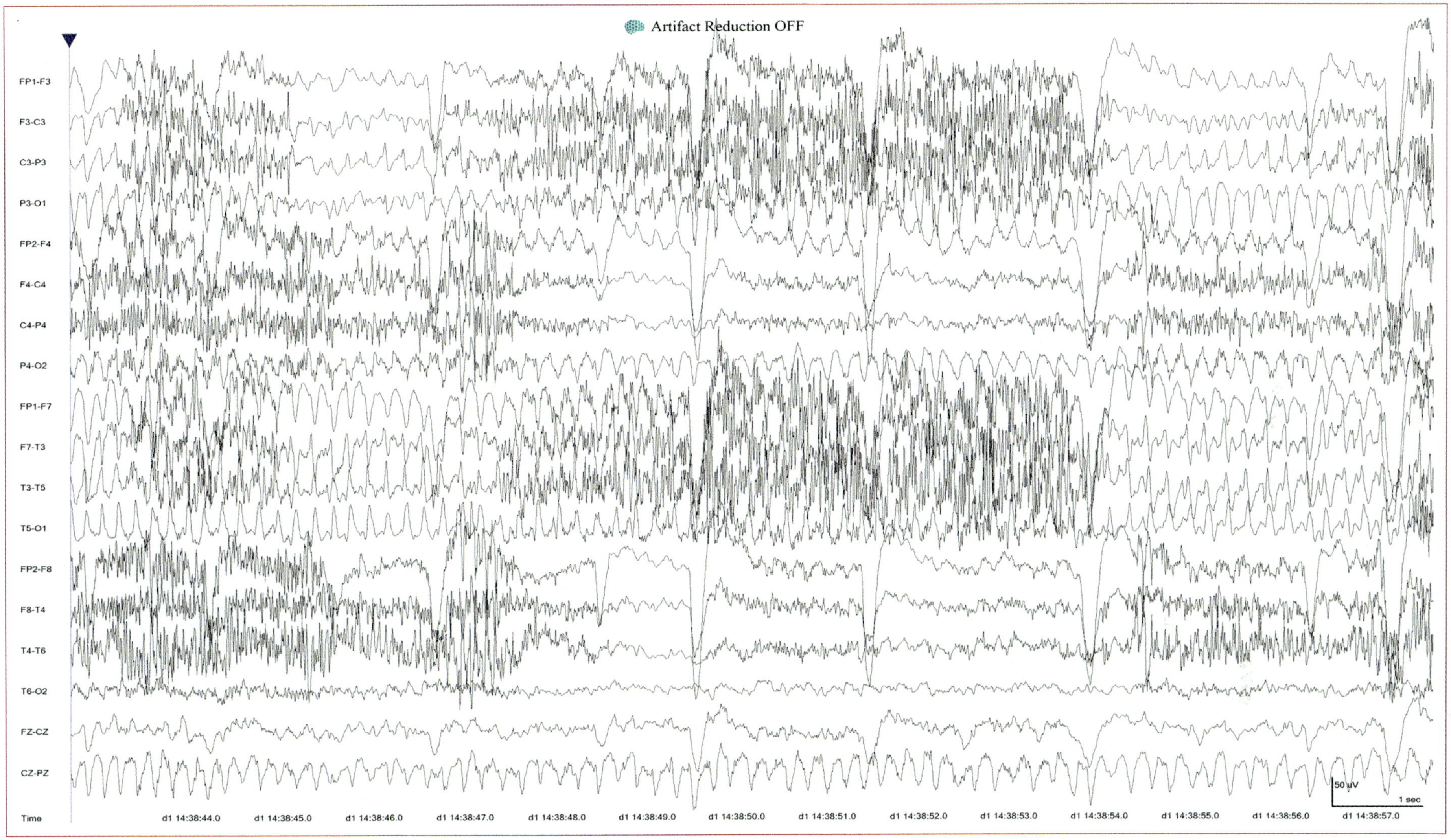

FIGURE 14.12: Muscle and eye movement artifacts during the same epoch during a left temporal onset seizure in **Figure 14.9** using digital filter settings of HFF 15 Hz, LFF 1.0 Hz to the original waveforms.

HFF, high-frequency filter; LFF, low-frequency filter.

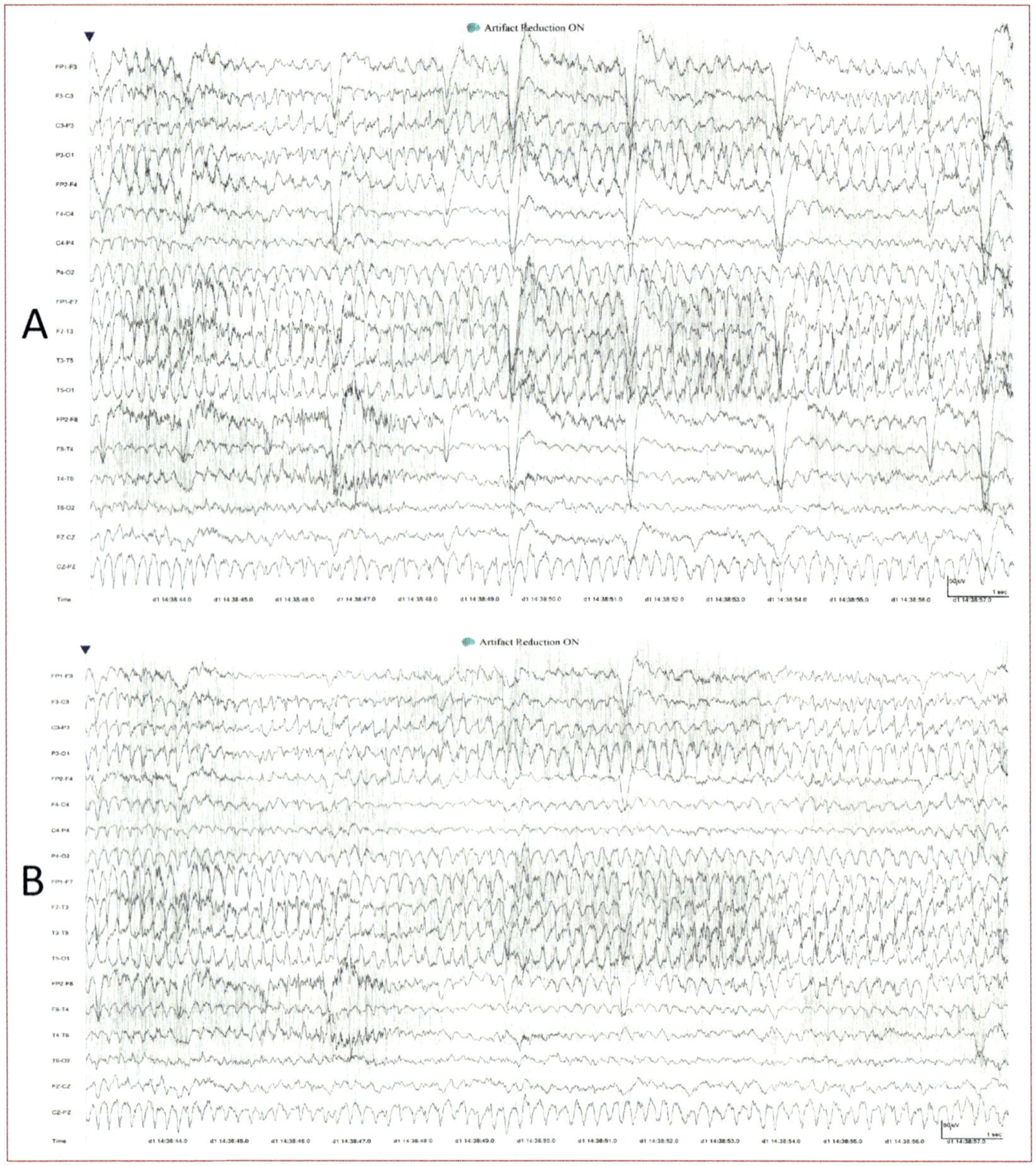

FIGURE 14.13: Muscle and eye movement artifacts during the same left temporal onset seizure in **Figures 14.9** and **14.10**. (A) Stage 1 of AR process, with blind source separation methods used to automatically extract muscle artifact, HFF 70 Hz, LFF 1.0 Hz; (B) Stage 2 of AR process, with neural network identification algorithms and blind source separation methods used to automatically extract much of vertical and lateral eye movement signal in addition, HFF 70 Hz, LFF 1.0 Hz. Gray ghost images of original EEG use blind source separation to shadow the artifact without altering the underlying brain-derived signal, permitting more complete visualization of the left temporal seizure. Slide courtesy of Mark Scheuer, Persyst Corporation.

AR, artifact reduction; HFF, high-frequency filter; LFF, low-frequency filter.

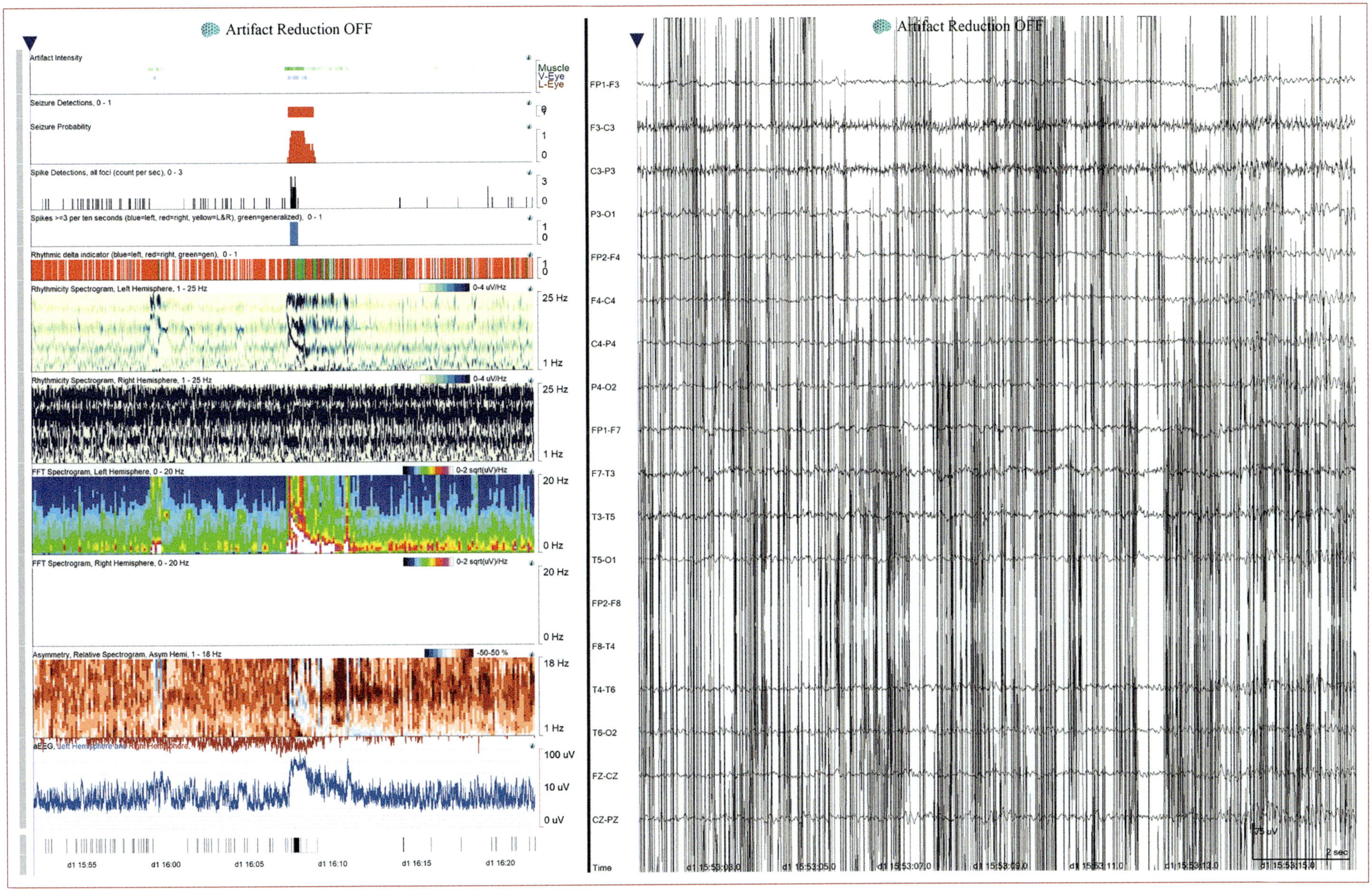

FIGURE 14.14: The effect of a bad F8 electrode on scalp EEG and the accompanying 30-minute QEEG trends, seizure, and spike-detection trends. Original EEG waveforms, HFF 70 Hz and LFF 1.0 Hz, shown with 30 minutes of trends AR OFF.

AR, artifact reduction; HFF, high-frequency filter; LFF, low-frequency filter; QEEG, quantitative EEG.

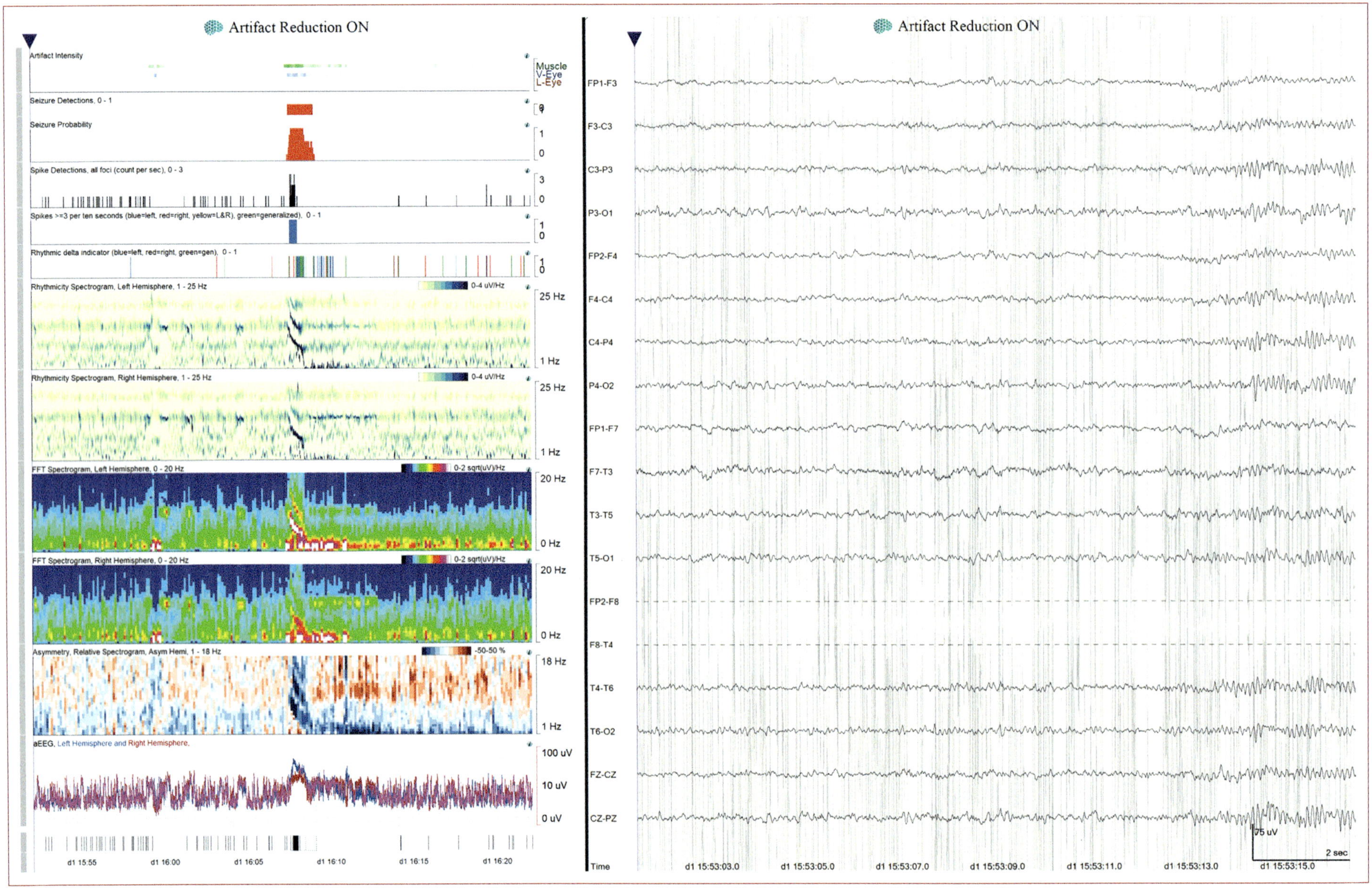

FIGURE 14.15: AR has dynamically and automatically removed the effect of the bad F8 electrode.

AR, artifact reduction.

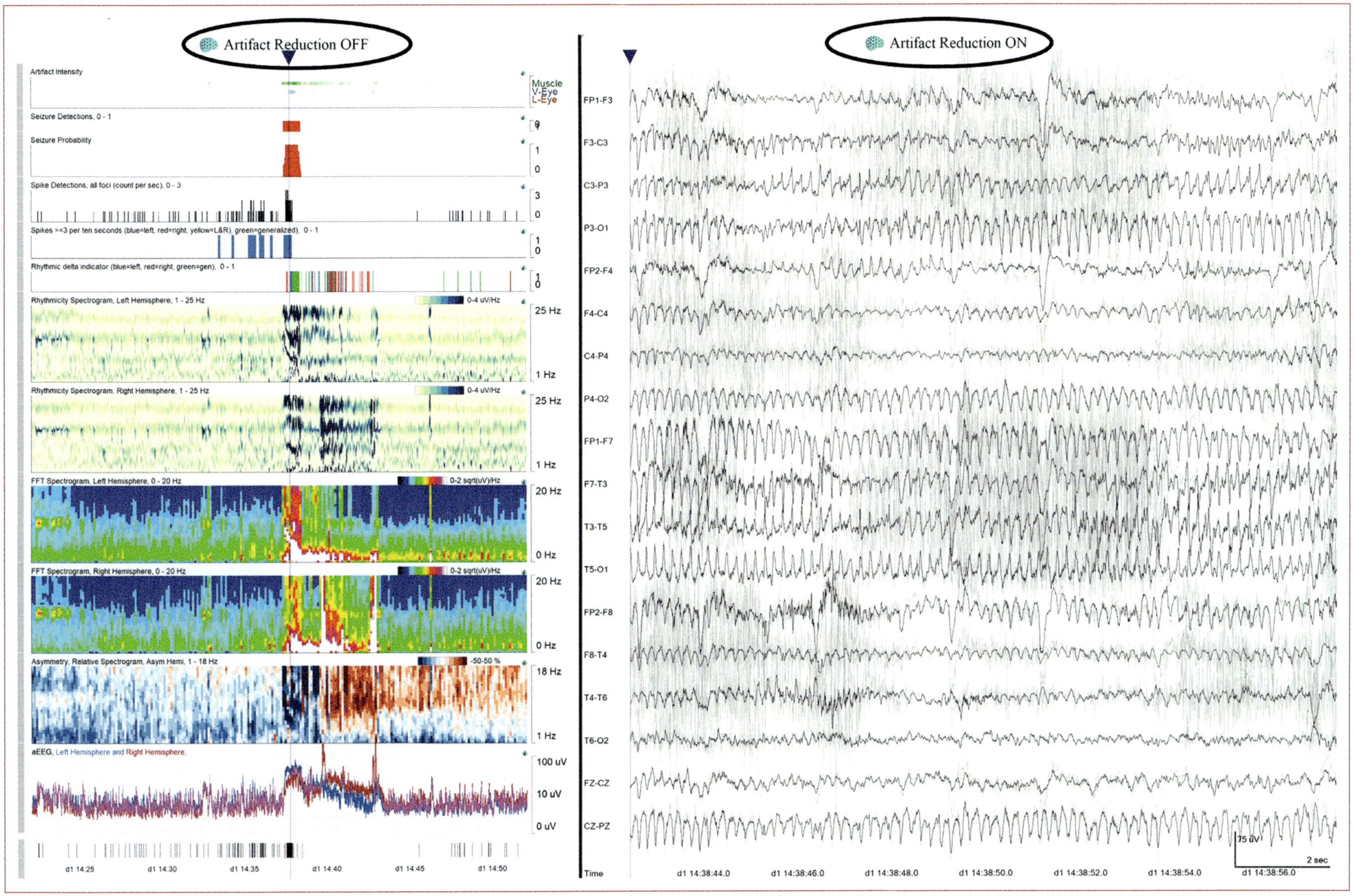

FIGURE 14.16: Artifact-reduced scalp EEG waveforms (right panel); HFF 70 Hz and LFF 1.0 Hz. Thirty minutes of trends (left panels) AR OFF for muscle and eye movement artifacts during a left temporal onset seizure accompanying 30 minutes of QEEG trends, seizure, and spike-detection trends (AR OFF). Note the difficulty discerning data, suggesting a seizure in the QEEG trends.

AR, artifact reduction; HFF, high-frequency filter; LFF, low-frequency filter; QEEG, quantitative EEG.

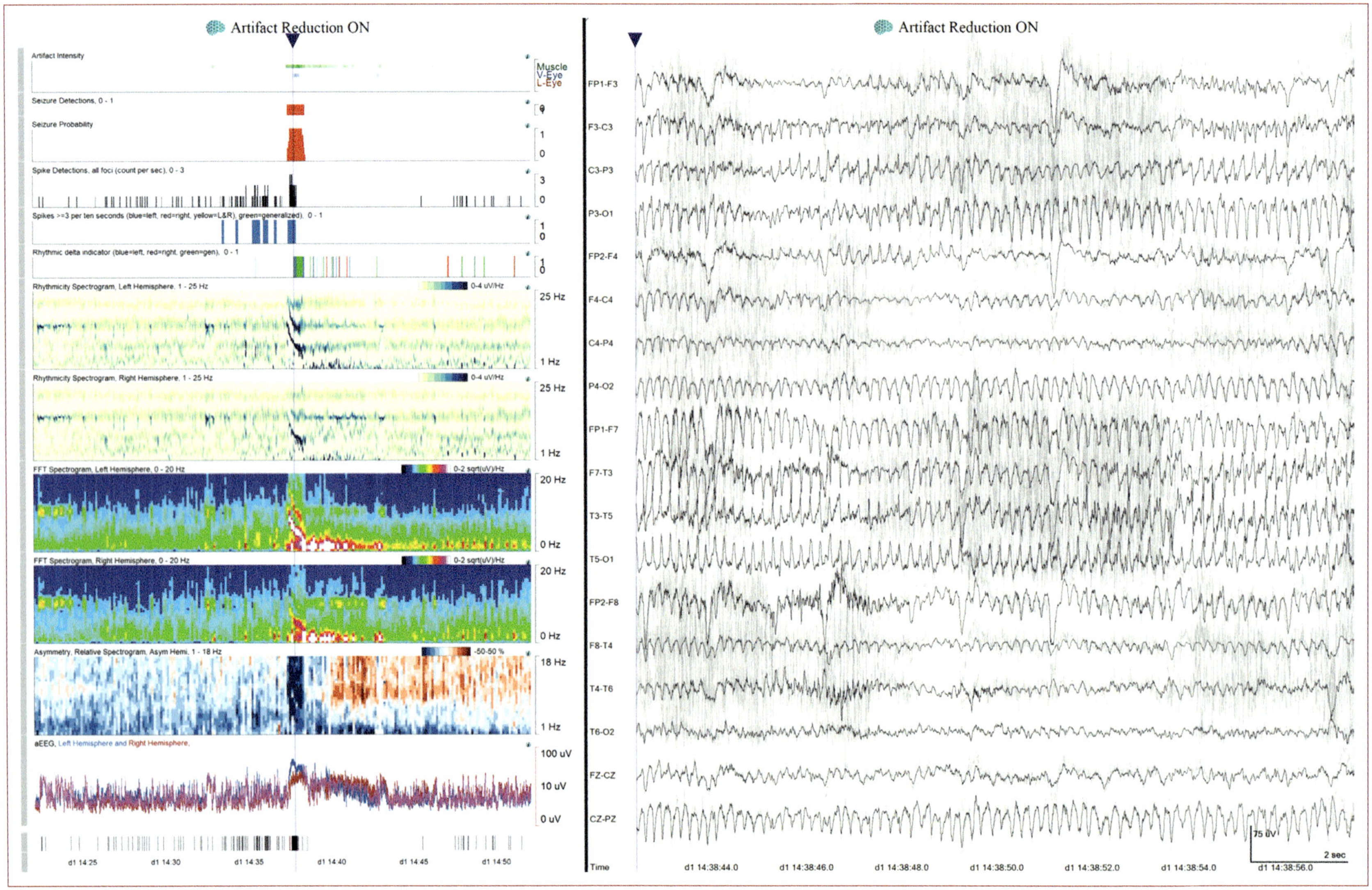

FIGURE 14.17: Artifact-reduced scalp EEG waveforms (right panel); HFF 70 Hz and LFF 1.0 Hz. Thirty minutes of trending (left panels) AR ON for muscle and eye movement artifacts during a left temporal onset seizure accompanying 30 minutes of QEEG trends, seizure, and spike-detection trends (AR ON). During the seizure, AR produces a marked reduction in noncerebral EEG signal caused by muscle activity, eye movements, and electrode artifacts and enhanced clarity of the QEEG for interpretation.

AR, artifact reduction; HFF, high-frequency filter; LFF, low-frequency filter; QEEG, quantitative EEG.

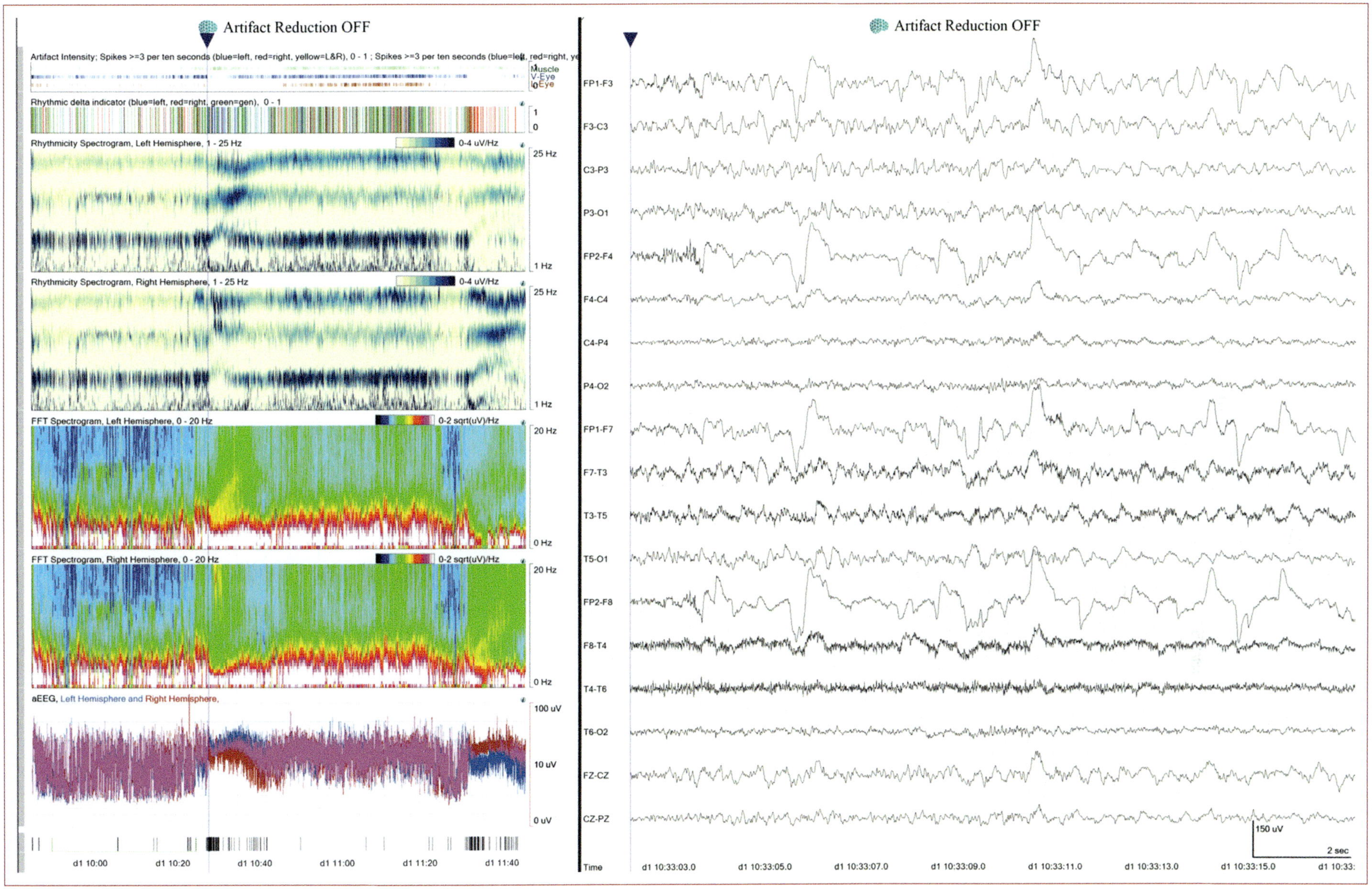

FIGURE 14.18: Two hours of trends (left panels) and 15 seconds of scalp EEG (right) show original waveforms, HFF 70 Hz and LFF 1.0 Hz, and QEEG trends with AR OFF. The vertical blue cursor shows the instant when the patient's right arm drops following left carotid injection.

AR, artifact reduction; HFF, high-frequency filter; LFF, low-frequency filter; QEEG, quantitative EEG.

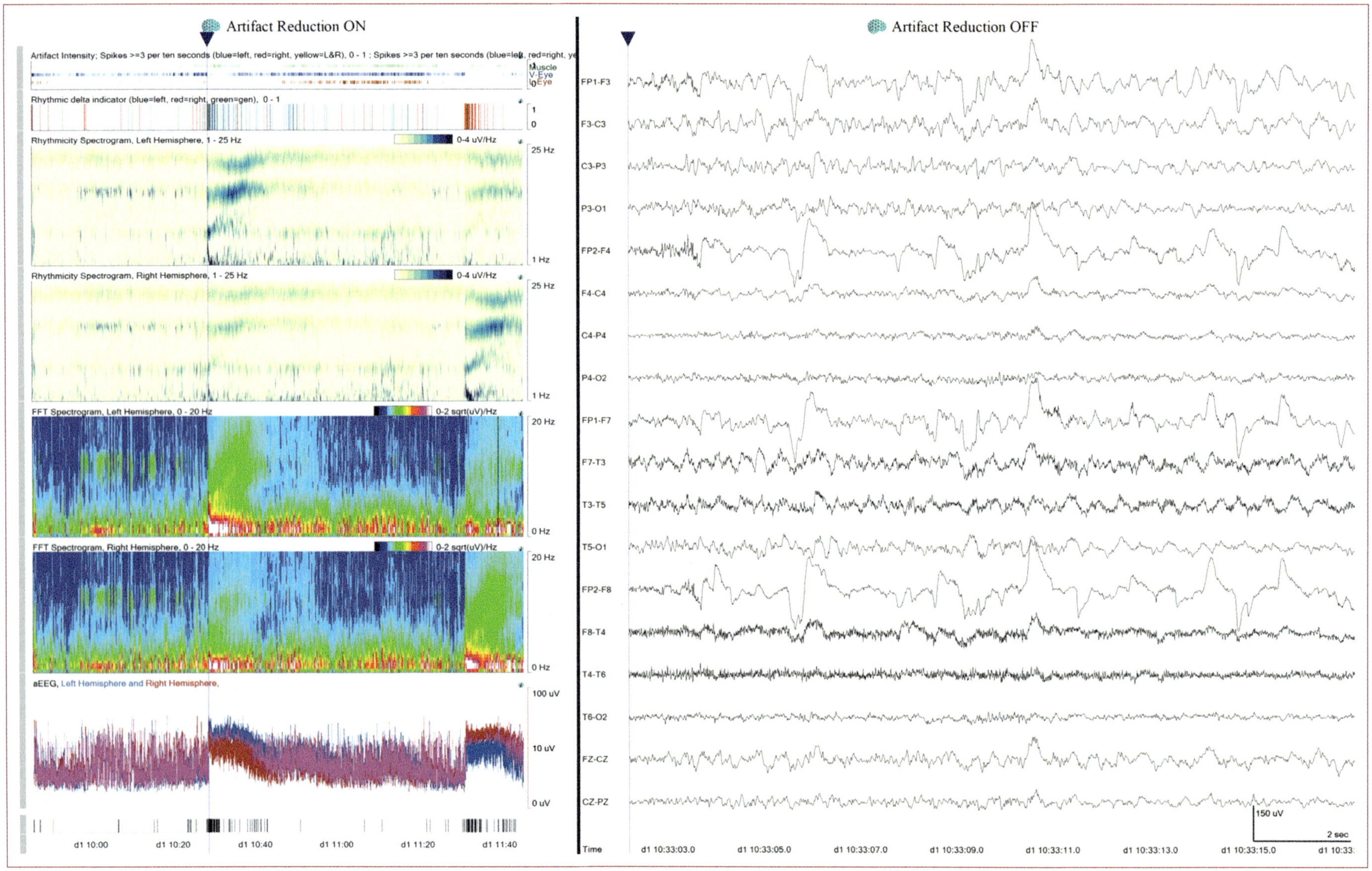

FIGURE 14.19: Effect of AR on QEEG trends during an intracarotid amytal test: 2 hours of trends (left panels) and 15 seconds of scalp EEG (right) show original waveforms, HFF 70 Hz and LFF 1.0 Hz with AR OFF and QEEG trends with AR ON. The vertical blue cursor shows the instant when the patient's right arm drops following left carotid injection. The trends during carotid amytal injection (left panels) are much more clearly delineated with AR ON.

AR, artifact reduction; HFF, high-frequency filter; LFF, low-frequency filter; QEEG, quantitative EEG.

REFERENCES

1. Magee P, Tooley M. *The Physics, Clinical Measurement and Equipment of Anaesthetic Practice*. Oxford, NY: Oxford University Press; 2005:xvii, 189.
2. Zhang Y, Wang B, Jing J, et al. A comparison study on multidomain EEG features for sleep stage classification. *Comput Intell Neurosci*. 2017;2017:4574079. doi:10.1155/2017/4574079.
3. O'Donnell RD, Berkhout J, Adey WR. Contamination of scalp EEG spectrum during contraction of cranio-facial muscles. *Electroencephalogr Clin Neurophysiol*. 1974;37(2):145-151. doi:10.1016/0013-4694(74)90005-4.
4. Muthukumaraswamy SD. High-frequency brain activity and muscle artifacts in MEG/EEG: a review and recommendations. *Front Hum Neurosci*. 2013;7:138. doi:10.3389/fnhum.2013.00138.
5. Pal PK. Electrophysiologic evaluation of psychogenic movement disorders. *J Mov Disord*. 2011;4(1):21-32. doi:10.14802/jmd.11004.
6. Beniczky S, Conradsen I, Moldovan M, et al. Quantitative analysis of surface electromyography during epileptic and nonepileptic convulsive seizures. *Epilepsia*. 2014;55(7):1128-1134. doi:10.1111/epi.12669.
7. da Silva EA, Muller RA, Chugani DC, et al. Brain activation during intermittent photic stimulation: a [15O]-water PET study on photosensitive epilepsy. *Epilepsia*. 1999;40(suppl 4):17-22. doi:10.1111/j.1528-1157.1999.tb00901.x.
8. Croft RJ, Barry RJ. Removal of ocular artifact from the EEG: a review. *Neurophysiol Clin*. 2000;30(1):5-19. doi:10.1016/S0987-7053(00)00055-1.
9. Kiamini M, Alirezaee S, Perseh B, et al. *Elimination of Ocular Artifacts from EEG Signals Using the Wavelet Transform and Empirical Mode Decomposition*. Pattaya, Chonburi, Thailand: IEEE; 2009:1094-1097.
10. Stern JM, Engel J. *Atlas of EEG Patterns*. 2nd ed. Philadelphia, PA: Wolters Kluwer/Lippincott Williams & Wilkins Health; 2013:ix, 457.
11. Wan X, Iwata K, Riera J, et al. Artifact reduction for EEG/fMRI recording: nonlinear reductionof ballistocardiogram artifacts. *Clin. Neurophysiol*. 2006;117(3):668-680. doi:10.1016/j.clinph.2005.12.015.
12. Bertrand A, Mihajlovic V, Grundlehner B, et al., eds. Motion artifact reduction in EEG recordings using multi-channel contact impedance measurements. In: *Biomedical Circuits and Systems Conference (BioCAS)*. Rotterdam, the Netherlands: IEEE; 2013.
13. American Clinical Neurophysiology Society. Guideline 1: Minimum technical requirements for performing clinical electroencephalography. *J Clin Neurophysiol*. 2006;23(2):86-91. doi:10.1097/WNP.0000000000000308.
14. American Clinical Neurophysiology Society. Guideline 8: Guidelines for recording clinical EEG on digital media. *J Clin Neurophysiol*. 2006;23(2):122-124.
15. AANEM. Proper performance and interpretation of electrodiagnostic studies. *Muscle Nerve*. 2015;51(3):468-471. doi:10.1002/mus.20493.
16. Kushida CA, Littner MR, Morgenthaler T, et al. Practice parameters for the indications for polysomnography and related procedures: an update for 2005. *Sleep*. 2005;28(4):499-521.
17. Bagic AI, Knowlton RC, Rose DF, et al. American Clinical Magnetoencephalography Society Clinical Practice Guideline 1: recording and analysis of spontaneous cerebral activity. *J Clin Neurophysiol*. 2011;28(4):348-354. doi:10.1097/WNP.0b013e3182272fed.
18. Blom JL, Anneveldt M. An electrode cap tested. *Electroencephalogr Clin Neurophysiol*. 1982;54(5):591-594. doi:10.1016/0013-4694(82)90046-3.
19. Shields SM, Morse CE, Applebaugh ED, et al. Are electrode caps worth the investment? An evaluation of EEG methods in undergraduate neuroscience laboratory courses and research. *J Undergrad Neurosci Educ*. 2016;15(1):A29-A37.
20. Greenfield LJ, Jr. Recording the EEG. In: Greenfield LJ, Jr., Geyer JD, Carney PR, eds. *Chapter 1*. 1st ed. Philadelphia, PA: Lippincott Williams & Wilkins; 2010:1-37.
21. Ferree TC, Luu P, Russell GS, et al. Scalp electrode impedance, infection risk, and EEG data quality. *Clin Neurophysiol*. 2001;112(3):536-544. doi:10.1016/S1388-2457(00)00533-2.
22. David RB. *Clinical Pediatric Neurology*. 3rd ed. New York, NY: Demos Medical; 2009:xvi, 622.
23. Hugh M, Peter K, eds. *Pediatric Electromyography: Concepts and Clinical Applications*. New York, NY: Springer Berlin Heidelberg; 2017.
24. Gooch CL, Weimer LH. The electrodiagnosis of neuropathy: basic principles and common pitfalls. *Neurol Clin*. 2007;25(1):1-28. doi:10.1016/j.ncl.2007.01.011.
25. Tal I, Abeles M. Cleaning MEG artifacts using external cues. *J Neurosci Methods*. 2013;217(1-2):31-38. doi:10.1016/j.jneumeth.2013.04.002.
26. American Society of Electroneurodiagnostic Technologists. Scope of practice for neurodiagnostic technology. http://www.aset.org/files/public/Scope_of_Practice_Approved_2011.pdf.
27. Tatum WO, Reinsberger C, Dworetzky BA. Artifacts of recording and common errors in interpretation. Chapter 11. Schomer DL, Lopes da Silva FH, eds. Niedermeyer's Electroencephalography: Basic Principles, Clinical Applications, and Related Fields. 7th ed. New York, NY: Oxford University Press; 2018:266-316.

28. Tatum WO. EEG interpretation: common problems. *Clin Pract*. 2012;9(5): 527-538. doi:10.1016/j.jneumeth.2013.04.002.

29. Connolly MB, Sharbrough FW, Wong PKH. Electrical fields and recording techniques. Chapter 4. Ebersole JS, Pedley TA, eds. *Current Practice of Clinical Electroencephalography*: Lippincott Williams & Wilkins; 2003:72-99

30. Knight J. *Signal Fraction Analysis and Artifact Removal in EEG*. Fort Collins: Colorado State; 2008.

31. Sun L, Rieger J, Hinrichs H. Maximum noise fraction (MNF) transformation to remove ballistocardiographic artifacts in EEG signals recorded during fMRI scanning. *Neuroimage*. 2009;46(1):144-153. doi:10.1016/j.neuroimage .2009.01.059.

32. Islam MK, Rastegarnia A, Yang Z. A wavelet-based artifact reduction from scalp EEG for epileptic seizure detection. *IEEE J Biomed Health Inform*. 2016;20(5):1321-1332. doi:10.1109/JBHI.2015.2457093.

33. Romero S, Mananas MA, Barbanoj MJ. A comparative study of automatic techniques for ocular artifact reduction in spontaneous EEG signals based on clinical target variables: a simulation case. *Comput Biol Med*. 2008;38(3): 348-360. doi:10.1016/j.compbiomed.2007.12.001.

34. Halder S, Bensch M, Mellinger J, et al. Online artifact removal for brain-computer interfaces using support vector machines and blind source separation. *Comput Intell Neurosci*. 2007:82069. doi:10.1155/2007/82069.

35. Winkler I, Haufe S, Tangermann M. Automatic classification of artifactual ICA-components for artifact removal in EEG signals. *Behav Brain Funct*. 2011;7:30. doi:10.1186/1744-9081-7-30.

36. Jung TP, Humphries C, Lee TW, et al., eds. Removing electroencephalographic artifacts: comparison between ICA and PCA. Neural Networks for Signal Processing VIII. In: *Proceedings of the 1998 IEEE Signal Processing Society Workshop (Cat No98TH8378)*; August 31, 1998 to September 2, 1998.

37. Cashero Z, Anderson C, eds. Comparison of EEG blind source separation techniques to improve the classification of P300 trials. In: *2011 Annual International Conference of the IEEE Engineering in Medicine and Biology Society*; August 30, 2011 to September 3, 2011. doi: 10.1109/IEMBS.2011.6091815.

38. Persyst. Persyst artifact reduction 2016. https://www.persyst.com/technology/artifact-reduction/.

39. Scheuer ML, Bagic A, Wilson SB. Spike detection: inter-reader agreement and a statistical Turing test on a large data set. *Clin Neurophysiol*. 2017;128(1): 243-250. doi:10.1016/j.clinph.2016.11.005.

40. Jung TP, Makeig S, Humphries C, et al. Removing electroencephalographic artifacts by blind source separation. *Psychophysiology*. 2000;37(2):163-178.

41. Davies ME, James CJ. Sour ce separation using single channel ICA. *Signal Process*. 2007;87(8):1819-1832. doi:10.1016/j.sigpro.2007.01.011.

42. James CJ, Wang S, eds. Performance analysis of a P300 BCI speller throug single channel ICA. In: *4th IET International Conference on Advances in Medical, Signal and Information Processing—MEDSIP 2008*; July 14–16, 2008.

43. LeVan P, Urrestarazu E, Gotman J. A system for automatic artifact removal in ictal scalp EEG based on independent component analysis and Bayesian classification. *Clin Neurophysiol*. 2006;117(4):912-927. doi:10.1016/j.clinph .2005.12.013.

44. Delorme A, Jung T-P, Sejnowski T, Makeig S. Improved rejection of artifacts from EEG data using high-order statistics and independent component analysis, 2018.

45. Gabsteiger F, Leutheuser H, Reis P, eds. ICA-based reduction of electromyogenic artifacts in EEG data: Comparison with and without EMG data. In: *2014 36th Annual International Conference of the IEEE Engineering in Medicine and Biology Society*; August 26–30, 2014.

46. Sueaseenak D, Chanwimalueang T, Sangworasil M, et al, eds. An investigation of robustness in independent component analysis EMG. In: *2009 6th International Conference on Electrical Engineering/ Electronics, Computer, Telecommunications and Information Technology*; May 6–9, 2009.

47. Khan OI, Sang-Hyuk K, Rasheed T, et al. Extraction of P300 using constrained independent component analysis. In: *2009 Annual International Conference of the IEEE Engineering in Medicine and Biology Society*. 2009: 4031–4034. doi:10.1109/IEMBS.2009.5333727.

48. Vigario R, Sarela J, Jousmiki V, et al. Independent component approach to the analysis of EEG and MEG recordings. *IEEE Trans Biomed Eng*. 2000;47(5): 589-593. doi:10.1109/10.841330.

49. Sameni R, Shamsollahi M, Senhadji L. Processing polysomnographic signals, using independent component analysis, 2004.

50. Delorme A, Makeig S. EEGLAB: an open source toolbox for analysis of single-trial EEG dynamics including independent component analysis. *J Neurosci Methods*. 2004;134(1):9-21. doi:10.1016/j.jneumeth .2003.10.009.

51. Mognon A, Jovicich J, Bruzzone L, et al. ADJUST: an automatic EEG artifact detector based on the joint use of spatial and temporal features. *Psychophysiology*. 2011;48(2):229-240. doi:10.1111/j.1469-8986 .2010.01061.x.

52. Nolan H, Whelan R, Reilly RB. FASTER: fully automated statistical thresholding for EEG artifact rejection. *J Neurosci Methods*. 2010;192(1): 152-162. doi:10.1016/j.jneumeth.2010.07.015.

53. Bugli C, Lambert P. Comparison between principal component analysis and independent component analysis in electroencephalograms modelling. *Biometrical J*. 2007;49(2):312-327. doi:10.1002/bimj.200510285.

54. Kendall MG, Stuart A. *The Advanced Theory of Statistics*. 3rd ed. London, UK: Griffin; 1969.

55. Lamothe R, Stroink G. Orthogonal expansions: their applicability to signal extraction in electrophysiological mapping data. *Med Biol Eng Comput*. 1991;29(5):522-528.

56. Lagerlund TD, Sharbrough FW, Busacker NE. Spatial filtering of multichannel electroencephalographic recordings through principal component analysis by singular value decomposition. *J Clin Neurophysiol*. 1997;14(1): 73-82. doi:10.1097/00004691-199701000-0000.

57. Wood CC, McCarthy G. Principal component analysis of event-related potentials: simulation studies demonstrate misallocation of variance across components. *Electroencephalogr Clin Neurophysiol*. 1984;59(3):249-260. doi:10.1016/0168-5597(84)90064-9.

58. Spuler M, Walter A, Rosenstiel W, et al. Spatial filtering based on canonical correlation analysis for classification of evoked or event-related potentials in EEG data. *IEEE Trans Neural Syst Rehabil Eng*. 2014;22(6):1097-1103. doi:10.1109/TNSRE.2013.2290870.

59. Robinson N, Thomas KP, Vinod AP, eds. Canonical correlation analysis of EEG for classification of motor imagery. In: *2017 IEEE International Conference on Systems, Man, and Cybernetics (SMC)*; October 5–8, 2017.

60. Anastasiadou MN, Christodoulakis M, Papathanasiou ES, et al. Unsupervised detection and removal of muscle artifacts from scalp EEG recordings using canonical correlation analysis, wavelets and random forests. *Clin Neurophysiol*. 2017;128(9):1755-1769. doi:10.1016/j.clinph.2017.06.247.

61. Makeig S, Jung TP, Bell AJ, et al. Blind separation of auditory event-related brain responses into independent components. *Proc Natl Acad Sci USA*. 1997;94(20):10979-10984. doi.org/10.1073/pnas.94.20.10979.

62. Debener S, Strobel A, Sorger B, et al. Improved quality of auditory event-related potentials recorded simultaneously with 3-T fMRI: removal of the ballistocardiogram artefact. *Neuroimage*. 2007;34(2):587-597. doi:10.1016/j.neuroimage.2006.09.031.

63. Delorme A, Sejnowski T, Makeig S. Enhanced detection of artifacts in EEG data using higher-order statistics and independent component analysis. *Neuroimage*. 2007;34(4):1443-1449. doi:10.1016/j.neuroimage.2006.11.004.

64. De-xiang Z, Xiao-pei W, Xiao-jing G. The EEG signal preprocessing based on empirical mode decomposition. In: *Proceedings of 2nd International Conference on Bioinformatics and Biomedical* Engineering. 2008: 2131-2134.

65. Yang J-H, Saito Y, Shi Q-W, et al. Empirical mode decomposition method for MEG phantom data analysis. *J Circuit Syst Comp*. 2009;18(8):1467-1480. doi:10.1142/S0218126609005794.

66. Alexei SV, Valentin KV, eds. *Biologically Inspired Cognitive Architectures (BICA) for Young Scientists*. New York, NY: Springer Berlin Heidelberg; 2016.

67. Nik Hisyamudin MN, Turnip A, Pardede J, et al. Artefacts removal of EEG signals with wavelet denoising. *MATEC Web of Conferences*. 2017;135:00058.

68. Ukil A. *Practical Denoising of MEG Data Using Wavelet Transform*. Berlin/Heidelberg: Springer-Verlag; 2006:578-585. doi:10.1007/11893257_65

69. MacCallum M, Almaini AEA. The application of the wavelet transform to polysomnographic signals. In Tang YY, Yuen PC, Li C, Wickerhauser V, eds. *Wavelet Analysis and Its Applications*. New York, NY: Springer Berlin Heidelberg; 2001:284-295.

70. Ellingson ML, Liebenthal E, Spanaki MV, et al. Ballistocardiogram artifact reduction in the simultaneous acquisition of auditory ERPS and fMRI. *Neuroimage*. 2004;22(4):1534-1542. doi:10.1016/j.neuroimage.2004.03.033.

71. Bentley JL. Multidimensional binary search trees used for associative searching. *Commun. ACM*. 1975;18(9):509-517. doi:10.1145/361002.361007.

72. Bono V, Jamal W, Das S, Maharatna K, eds. Artifact reduction in multichannel pervasive EEG using hybrid WPT-ICA and WPT-EMD signal decomposition techniques. In: *2014 IEEE International Conference on Acoustics, Speech and Signal Processing*; May 4–9, 2014; Florence, Italy. doi:10.1109/ICASSP.2014.6854728.

73. Narasimhan SV, Dutt DN. Application of LMS adaptive predictive filtering for muscle artifact (noise) cancellation from EEG signals. *Comput Electr Eng*. 1996;22(1):13-30. doi:10.1016/0045-7906(95)00030-5.

74. Sörnmo L, Laguna P. *Bioelectrical Signal Processing in Cardiac and Neurological Applications*. Amsterdam, the Netherlands and Boston, MA: Elsevier Academic Press; 2005.

75. Sweeney KT, Ward TE, McLoone SF. Artifact removal in physiological signals—practices and possibilities. *IEEE Trans Inf Technol Biomed*. 2012;16(3):488-500. doi:10.1016/j.neucli.2014.11.008.

76. Kaminska A, Cheliout-Heraut F, Eisermann M, et al. EEG in children, in the laboratory or at the patient's bedside. *Neurophysiol Clin*. 2015;45(1):65-74. doi:10.1016/j.neucli.2014.11.008.

77. Andre-Obadia N, Lamblin MD, Sauleau P. French recommendations on electroencephalography. *Neurophysiol Clin*. 2015;45(1):1-17. doi:10.1016/j.neucli.2014.11.002.

78. Wirrell E, Kozlik S, Tellez J, et al. Ambulatory electroencephalography (EEG) in children: diagnostic yield and tolerability. *J Child Neurol*. 2008;23(6): 655-662. doi:10.1177/0883073808314158.

79. American Clinical Neurophysiology. Guideline 2: minimum technical standards for pediatric electoencephalography. *J Clin Neurophysiol*. 2006;23(2):92-96. doi:10.1097/00004691-200604000-00003.

80. Kang PB. Pediatric nerve conduction studies and EMG. In: Blum AS, Rutkove SB, eds. *The Clinical Neurophysiology Primer*. Totowa, NJ: Humana Press Inc; 2007:369-389.

81. Beck SE, Marcus CL. Pediatric polysomnography. *Sleep Med Clin*. 2009;4(3):393-406. doi:10.1016/j.jsmc.2009.04.007.

82. Galloway GM. Intraoperative considerations in the pediatric patient. Chapter 11. *Clinical Neurophysiology in Pediatrics: A Practical Approach to Neurodiagnostic Testing and Management*. New York, NY: Demos Medical Publishing, LLC. 2016:181-186.

83. Schmidt LA, Segalowitz SJ. *Developmental Psychophysiology: Theory, Systems, and Methods*. Cambridge, NY: Cambridge University Press; 2008:xxii, 461.

84. Fujioka T, Mourad N, He C, et al. Comparison of artifact correction methods for infant EEG applied to extraction of event-related potential signals. *Clin Neurophysiol*. 2011;122(1):43-51. doi:10.1016/j.clinph.2010.04.036.

85. Brouillette RT, Lavergne J, Leimanis A, et al. Differences in pulse oximetry technology can affect detection of sleep-disordered breathing in children. *Anesth Analg*. 2002;94(suppl 1):S47-S53.

86. He C, Hotson L, Trainor LJ. Mismatch responses to pitch changes in early infancy. *J Cogn Neurosci*. 2007;19(5):878-892. doi:10.1162/jocn.2007.19.5.878.

87. He C, Hotson L, Trainor LJ. Development of infant mismatch responses to auditory pattern changes between 2 and 4 months old. *Eur J Neurosci*. 2009;29(4):861-867. doi:10.1111/j.1460-9568.2009.06625.x.

88. He C, Hotson L, Trainor LJ. Maturation of cortical mismatch responses to occasional pitch change in early infancy: effects of presentation rate and magnitude of change. *Neuropsychologia*. 2009;47(1):218-229. doi:10.1016/j.neuropsychologia.2008.07.019.

89. He C, Trainor LJ. Finding the pitch of the missing fundamental in infants. *J Neurosci*. 2009;29(24):7718-8822. doi:10.1523/JNEUROSCI.0157-09.2009.

90. Perrin F, Bertrand O, Pernier J. Scalp current density mapping: value and estimation from potential data. *IEEE Trans Biomed Eng*. 1987;34(4):283-288. doi:10.1109/TBME.1987.326089.

91. Perrin F, Pernier J, Bertrand O, et al. Spherical splines for scalp potential and current density mapping. *Electroencephalogr Clin Neurophysiol*. 1989;72(2):184-187. doi:10.1016/0013-4694(89)90180-6.

92. Law SK, Nunez PL, Wijesinghe RS. High-resolution EEG using spline generated surface Laplacians on spherical and ellipsoidal surfaces. *IEEE Trans Biomed Eng*. 1993;40(2):145-153. doi:10.1109/10.212068.

93. Srinivasan R, Nunez PL, Tucker DM, et al. Spatial sampling and filtering of EEG with spline laplacians to estimate cortical potentials. *Brain Topogr*. 1996;8(4):355-366.

94. Chauveau N, Franceries X, Doyon B, et al. Effects of skull thickness, anisotropy, and inhomogeneity on forward EEG/ERP computations using a spherical three-dimensional resistor mesh model. *Hum Brain Mapp*. 2004;21(2):86-97. doi:10.1002/hbm.10152.

Epilogue

The strengths of clinical neurophysiology (CNP) are clear. Measuring signals generated by the nervous system yield objective information on neural function in both a static and dynamic environment. In many cases, patients are able to express their symptoms, though in other cases they may be unable to do so (e.g., anesthetized, asleep, or cognitively impaired). Still, in other situations, the findings are subclinical and measurable only by the CNP procedure itself. The clinical history and neurological examination remain the cornerstone to separate normal from abnormal conditions involving diseases of the nervous system. Anatomic neuroimaging may disclose diagnostic information that represents a crucial element in the neurological evaluation process. However, the electrophysiological integrity of the nervous system is a measureable aspect provided by CNP to address function when neuroimaging is unable to be obtained, is normal, or is unrevealing. CNP is more than EEG and EMG. It involves a host of procedures listed in this book involving both pediatric and adult assessment of central and peripheral neurological function. Artifact exists in all of the procedures and typically impedes interpretation of underlying signals of interest and therefore is considered a "contaminant." However, artifact may also serve as a means of identifying the level of arousal and behavioral state of the patient to add useful information to a CNP procedure (e.g., sleep staging). Extracerebral signals without the appropriate polarity and spatial distribution may appear abnormal when pattern recognition alone is used for interpretation. In the *Atlas*, we cover multiple aspects of CNP. We provide examples and an explanation of common and complex artifacts in the context of their respective procedure to assist busy clinicians by easy access that facilitates visual recognition of challenging waveforms.

It is essential for the interpreter to distinguish a mismatch between electrophysiological potentials produced by the brain and those produced by artifact. Multiple types of artifact may arise from a variety of extracerebral sources leading to pitfalls in interpretation. Some may be difficult to recognize, and challenge the interpreter to separate the physiological signal from abnormality. The reason for the challenging nature of artifact resides in the need to isolate minute waveforms (e.g., evoked potentials [EPs], nerve conduction study [NCS], and EEG) with amplitudes that exist on a scale measured in microvolts. Amplification of CNP signals is therefore necessary to visualize waveforms, and the importance of technology in imparting and reducing artifact cannot be underscored. Low signal-to-noise ratios may be present in some conditions of recording that challenge the distinction of neuronal activity by the interpreter. Furthermore, both physiological artifacts reflecting the behavioral state of the patient and nonphysiological artifacts produced by electrical instruments can occur independently, though often they coexist. Nonphysiological artifact is commonly encountered due to dysfunctional sensors. Although this may be detected readily, it requires "troubleshooting" by an experienced technologist in real time to ensure uninterrupted continuity of the procedure. If the amount of artifact reaches a critical mass, it will eliminate the potential benefit derived from the CNP procedures unless it is corrected. When this is not possible, artifact may produce a pattern of interference that obscures targeted signals, rendering the recording useless. More worrisome is when complex waveforms due to artifact beguile the interpreter into believing that a waveform is abnormal when it is not. The bottom line is, artifact that is misinterpreted as an abnormal physiological signal can impact medical or surgical treatment of a patient.

For most clinicians performing CNP procedures, the significance of artifact is self-evident. For decades, CNP procedures have augmented and extended the reach of the neurological examination. These techniques apply in both children and adults. In many cases, the same CNP procedure has a variety of recording techniques and applications. Therefore, when the usage of the same procedure is modified, different information is obtainable that may lead to the diagnosis that would otherwise not be possible. Such is the case with EEG used in ambulatory monitoring, in-patient video-EEG monitoring, and electrocorticography. In some cases, the information is crucial in management decisions, such as detecting subclinical seizures and nonconvulsive status epilepticus in ICU-EEG monitoring or identifying acute demyelinating polyradiculopathy by EMG and NCS in Guillain–Barré syndrome. Furthermore, some CNP procedures such as MEG are used to influence surgical planning. When artifact is involved, it may falsely impact localization. The impact of artifact in CNP procedures that are performed in the OR may produce erroneous results and influence the surgical approach when EPs and aspects of recording during NIOM are involved. In the sleep laboratory, mixing CNP signals generated by the body and the brain in the usage of polysomnography may combine a variety of artifacts. In the ICU, neuromonitoring involves CNP and non-CNP techniques, requiring multimodal integration. When conclusions are based on artifactual information from misguided CNP results, the information detracts from the clinical neurological evaluation rather than supplementing it.

Although visual inspection continues to be the conventional form of interpreting most CNP examinations, newer software developments seek to eliminate unwanted artifact that prevents interpretation without altering the signal of interest. Newer technologies in digital recording and monitoring techniques employing artifact reduction are currently emerging to improve and optimize CNP recordings. The need to improve our ability to extract, enhance, and validate an underlying signal as one of neural origin when the contour does not make physiological sense is evident. Nevertheless, as we move to the goal of artifact-free CNP procedures, the basis for understanding neurophysiological concepts will remain a key thought process to remember. Irrespective of the type of CNP procedure, realizing that artifact is usually a problem, occasionally helpful, and always important to distinguish from abnormality will serve the interpreter well. In this way, the method of pattern recognition when viewing waveforms will be based upon guidelines and principals to overcome the traps of artifact simply because "it just looks that way."

William O. Tatum, IV, DO

Index